DRUG DISPOSITION DURING DEVELOPMENT

Monographs in Pharmacology and Physiology
Elliot S. Vesell and *Silvio Garattini,* Editors

Volume 1
PHYSIOLOGIC DISPOSITION OF DRUGS OF ABUSE
Louis Lemberger and *Alan Rubin*

Volume 2
DRUG DISPOSITION DURING DEVELOPMENT
Edited by Paolo Lucio Morselli

DRUG DISPOSITION DURING DEVELOPMENT

Edited by

Paolo Lucio Morselli

Department of Clinical Research
L.E.R.S.-Synthelabo
Paris, France

S P Books Division of
SPECTRUM PUBLICATIONS, INC.
New York

Distributed by Halsted Press
A Division of John Wiley & Sons

New York   Toronto   London   Sydney

Copyright © 1977 Spectrum Publications, Inc.

All rights reserved. No part of this book may be reproduced in any form, by photostat, microform, retrieval system, or any other means without prior written permission of the coypright holder or his licensee.

SPECTRUM PUBLICATIONS, INC.
175-20 Wexford Terrace, Jamaica, N.Y. 11432

Library of Congress Cataloging in Publication Data

Main entry under title:

Drug disposition during development.
   (Monographs in pharmacology and physiology ; v. 2)
   Bibliography: p.
   Includes index.
   1. Pediatric pharmacology. I. Morselli, P. L.
II. Series. [DNLM: 1. Drugs--Metabolism. 2. Pharmacology--In infancy and childhood. W1 MO568J v. 2 /
QV38 D791]
RJ560.D78   615'.1   76-47570
ISBN 0-89335-006-0

Distributed solely by the Halsted Press Division of John Wiley & Sons, Inc.
New York, New York
ISBN 0-470-99178-X

Contributors

Bianchetti, Gabrio, Biol.D.
Department of Clinical Research
L.E.R.S.–Synthelabo
58, Rue de la Glacière
75621 Paris Cedex 13, France

Bossi, Laura, M.D.
Laboratory of Clinical Pharmacology
Istituto di Ricerche Farmacologiche "Mario Negri"
Via Eritrea 62
Milano, Italy

Braunlich, Helmut, Dr. Sc.Med.
Institute for Pharmacology and Toxicology
Friedrich Schiller University
Holzmarkt
69 Jena, G.D.R.

De Gaetano, Giovanni, M.D.
Laboratory for Hemostasis and Thrombosis Research
Istituto di Ricerche Farmacologiche "Mario Negri"
Via Eritrea 62
Milano, Italy

Donati, Maria Benedetta, M.D.
Laboratory for Hemostasis and Thrombosis Research
Istituto di Ricerche Farmacologiche "Mario Negri"
Via Eritrea 62,
Milano, Italy

Gomeni, Roberto, Math.D.
Department of Clinical Research
L.E.R.S.–Synthelabo
58, Rue de la Glacière
75621 Paris Cedex 13, France

CONTRIBUTORS

Klinger, Wolfang, D. Sc.Med.
Institute for Pharmacology and Toxicology
Friedrich Schiller University
Holzmarkt
69 Jena, G.D.R.

Latini, Roberto, M.D.
Laboratory of Clinical Pharmacology
Istituto di Ricerche Farmacologiche "Mario Negri"
Via Eritrea 62
Milano, Italy

Mandelli, Marinella, Biol.D.
Laboratory of Clinical Pharmacology
Istituto di Ricerche Farmacologiche "Mario Negri"
Via Eritrea 62
Milano, Italy

Morselli, Paolo Lucio, M.D.
Department of Clinical Research
L.E.R.S.–Synthelabo
58, Rue de la Glacière
75621 Paris Cedex 13, France

Senhouse Rossi, Myriam, M.D.
Laboratory of Tumour Chemotherapy and Immunology
Istituto di Ricerche Farmacologiche "Mario Negri"
Via Eritrea 62
Milano, Italy

Spreafico, Federico, M.D.
Laboratory of Tumour Chemotherapy and Immunology
Istituto di Ricerche Farmacologiche "Mario Negri"
Via Eritrea 62
Milano, Italy

Tognoni, Gianni, M.D.
Drug Information System
Laboratory of Clinical Pharmacology
Istituto di Ricerche Farmacologiche "Mario Negri"
Via Eritrea 62
Milano, Italy

Contents

PREFACE

INTRODUCTION - *by Paolo Lucio Morselli*

1. **Basic Concepts of Pharmacokinetics** 1
   by Roberto Gomeni & Roberto Latini

   Definition of Kinetic Parameters 2
   Absorption Drugs 14
   Solution of the Equations (Mathematical Model) Connected
      with Pharmacokinetic Problems 38
   Conclusions 47
   References 47

2. **Drug Absorption** 51
   by Paolo Lucio Morselli

   Absorption from Elimentary Tract 52
   Absorption from Intramuscular and Subcutaneous
      Injections 53
   Absorption from the Skin 54
   Absorption in Newborns 54
   Absorption in Infants and Children 55
   Conclusions 56
   References 57

3. **Drug Plasma Protein-Binding and Distribution** 61
   by Paolo Lucio Morselli

   Body Compartments 61
   Plasma Protein Binding 62
   Conclusions 65
   References 66

4. **Development of Drug Metabolizing Enzymes** 71
   by Wolfang Klinger

   Significance of the Liver and other Organs 72
   Postnatal Development of the Liver:
      Morphology and Biochemistry 74
   Development of Transport Proteins 75
   Development of Phase I Reactions 75
   Development of Phase II Reactions 80
   Perinatal Inducibility of Biotransformation 81
   Biotransformation and Toxicity During Postnatal
      Development 83
   Conclusions 84
   References 84

5. **Kidney Development: Drug Elimination Mechanisms** 89
   by Helmut Braunlich

   Postnatal Development of Renal Excretion Function
      for Foreign Compounds 90
   Stimulation of Drug Elimination Mechanisms 95
   Development of Renal Drug Excretion 95
   Age Dependent Nephrotoxicity of Drugs 96
   Age Differences in Renal Effectiveness of Drugs 96
   Age Dependent Water and Electrolyte Excretion 97
   References 97

6. **Antineoplastic Agents** **101**
   by Federico Spreafico & Miriam Senhouse Rossi

   Cyclophosphamide 102
   Methotrexate 106
   6-Mercaptopurine 107
   Cytosine-Arabinoside 109
   L-Asparaginase 110
   Vincristine 112

	Actinomycin-d	114
	Adriamycin and Daunomycin	115
	Conclusions	117
	References	118

7. Antibiotics 123
by Gianni Tognoni

    Quality Control of Method Analysis 124
    Assessment of the Clinical Significance of Plasma Levels . . . 124
    Penicillins 126
    Cephalosporins 146
    Aminoglycosides 155
    Tetracyclines 172
    Antitubercolar Agents 177
    Others 183
    Conclusions 191
    References 192

8. Sulfonamides Cotrimoxazole and Urinary Antiseptics 219
by Marinella Mandelli & Gianni Tognoni

    Sulfonamides 219
    Cotrimoxazole 231
    Urinary Antiseptics 236
    References 245

9. Anticoagulants 251
by Giovanni De Gaetano & Maria Benedetta Donati

    Heparin 253
    Oral Anticoagulants 254
    Conclusions 264
    References 265

10. Antipyretic and Nonsteroid Antiinflammatory Drugs 271
by Marinella Mandelli & Paolo Lucio Morselli

    Salicylates 271
    Phenylbutazone 281
    Indomethacin 285
    Pyrazolone Derivatives 288
    Acetanylid, Phenacetin and Acetaminophen 291
    Conclusions 297
    References 297

11. **Antiepileptic Drugs** 311
    by Paolo Lucio Morselli

    Diphenylhydantoin 312
    Phenobarbital 323
    Primidone 331
    Ethosuximide 333
    Carbamazepine 336
    Clonazepam 340
    Di-n-Propylacetate 344
    Conclusions 346
    References 347

12. **Hypnotics** 361
    by Laura Bossi & Paolo Lucio Morselli

    Chloral Hydrate 362
    Glutethimide 365
    Methaqualone 368
    Barbiturates 371
    Benzodiazepines 379
    Conclusions 382
    References 382

13. **Cardiovascular Agents** 393
    by Paolo Lucio Morselli & Gabrio Bianchetti

    Digitalis Glycosides 393
    Antianhytmic Agents 404
    Beta-Adrenergic Receptor Blocking Drugs 409
    Conclusions 418
    References 418

14. **Psychotropic Drugs** 431
    by Paolo Lucio Morselli

    Antipsychotic Drugs 431
    Antidepressant Drugs 439
    Benzodiazepines 449
    Conclusions 459
    References 460

15. **Conclusions** 475
    by Paolo Lucio Morselli

16. **Index** 477

This volume is intended to provide investigators, clinical pharmacologists, pediatricians, general practitioners and medical students with an understanding of the information available up to now on the influence of age on drug disposition and effects from birth to adulthood.

Therapuetic intervention in the newborn, the infant and the child is still in our day based mostly on the trial-and-error principle. It involves conjectural means that are far from the rational approach which in recent years has been developing at the adult level, where careful integration of clinical data with pharmacokinetic knowledge has made possible, in several instances, safer and better therapy.

This monograph is meant to serve as a starting point, an invitation to further, more important work, to everyone who is interested in the field and who feels as I do, that there is a great need to improve our information not only on the kinetics of drugs during development but also on the real efficacy of drugs in the child.

I wish to express my gratitude to Drs. Vesell and Garattini, who offered me such an opportunity, and the colleagues who wrote several of the chapters, to all the friends of the laboratory of Clinical Pharmacology of the Mario Negri Institute, who, with their enthusiastic contribution to many of the studies and observations reported here, made this effort possible; and to the librarians of the Pfeiffer Memorial Library for their careful cooperation in compiling the bibliography, and to Maria Mancini for her great help both in typing and editing.

Milano, January 15, 1976   P.L.M.

Introduction

PAOLO LUCIO MORSELLI

In the last ten years, with the development of clinical pharmacology, of pharmacokinetics and of new analytical techniques, we have gained a better understanding of many of the factors which determine and condition the effects of drugs.

We have learned that the effects of any therapeutic agent are related to the concentration at the site of action, to the time the concentration is maintained and to the speed at which the effective level is reached. We have identified, for many drugs, toxic and therapeutic thresholds, and we are aware that knowledge of physiological variables such as absorption, protein-binding, distribution, metabolism and excretion is essential for achieving optimal therapy. We know that genetic and environmental factors, physiopathological conditions and drug interactions contribute substantially to determining a wide individual variability in drug responses and in drug concentrations at the active sites.

Such a variability in the absence of sufficient pertinent information makes the therapeutic decision a "trial-and-error" experiment.

Among the factors capable of modifying the effects of drugs, age is considered highly significant. However, despite the large body of data from experimental animals, our knowledge of drug disposition in newborns, infants and children and of the toxic effects and therapeutic efficacy in pediatrics is up to now very poor. Systematic studies on drug disposition and effects through the span of the first 15 years of life are totally lacking.

On one hand, we have seen the growth of more and more concern (in both the scientific and non scientific communities) for the real and/or potential toxic effects of drugs in infants and children, and the need for more information has often been stressed. On the other, there have been emotional reactions to a number of accidents, mainly due to lack of knowledge, which have prevented important and effective drugs from being tested or studied in children in controlled situations. This becomes a paradox since disclaimers based on the lack of data perpetuate our ignorance and misuse of drugs in the child. In other words, while we are very well aware of our limited knowledge of drugs in children, while we are fully convinced that we have to know more and that they are "therapeutic orphans," false ethical issues (based on a complete ignorance of the theme of the problem and of its boundaries) have almost completely arrested progress in the field of pediatric clinical pharmacology.

The results of such a paradoxical situation are that therapeutic disasters still occur in children, that their need for safe and effective therapy is not fulfilled and that in our clinical practice we prescribe drugs which have not been tested or recommended for use in children.

In a recent report, Wilson (1975) states that 70% of the drugs listed in the P.D.R. have a form of disclaimer or lack of dosage information for their use in children. Furthermore, the same author points out that about 50% of the drugs released between 1959 and 1971 had disclaimers for their use in children even though they were potentially very useful. As we have said, in contrast with all these disclaimers, based mostly on lack of data, the fact remains that children do require drugs and do receive them.

All responsibility is left to the pediatrician or the general practitioner, and thus, we who do not allow controlled clinical trials in children or routine blood sampling for monitoring of optimal drugs levels, *do* allow uncontrolled clinical trials to be performed every day. We are giving our full and unconditional approval to a situation where not only the needs but also the rights of the patients are not fulfilled.

Again and again we are told that the developing baby is not a miniature adult; however, even today, in our practice, all we do is correct the dose by body weight or surface area and then give the drug blindly.

The newborn, the infant and the young child are developing organisms in which the differences are not only quantitative but also qualitative, and in which the maturation processes do not take place in a gradual and predictable manner. Gastric pH, gastrointestinal motility, arterial blood pressure, regional blood flows and vascular resistances, plasma proteins, bilirubin and FFA concentrations, acid-base equilibrium, body water and fat compartments, metabolic activities, relative size of the liver, brain and other organs, myelin content of the brain, urinary pH and kidney function are all physiological variables which undergo a continuous and substantial change during development and which may remarkably modify the effects of several drugs. Furthermore, infants who require drugs are sick and very seldom are treated with a single drug. Presence of diseases and concomitant therapy may profoundly further modify the drug kinetic profile and hence the therapeutic outcome.

If we consider the situation in an objective manner, we have to realize that, when we start a therapeutic regimen in a child, many are the questions to which we can give either only a partial and incomplete response or no answer at all.

—Are these drugs more or less absorbed in the child?
—How is their distribution changing as a function of the modification of the various body water and fat compartments?
—Do these changes have any impact on the drug's effects?
—What are the metabolic rates at various ages?
—Are the therapeutic and toxic thresholds in the child the same as those observed in adults?
—In the first months, when does a significant modification of the renal excretory capability occur?
—Which or how many of all the factors just mentioned have the most bearing for the drug effects?
—Does the child really require all the compounds we are administering to him?

This monograph has been written not with the aim of answering these questions but as an inducement to improve our information on this very neglected topic, to help begin a new dialogue between the clinical pharmacologist and the pediatrician or the general practitioner. It is an effort to show that some of the information we are looking for is already there in our everyday practice and in the literature, even if diffuse and without any apparent interrelationship, and also to underline the areas where knowledge is extremely scanty or totally absent, the areas where a dedicated effort is most needed.

After a brief introduction to basic pharmacokinetics, the following four chapters will describe the anatomical and physiological events which may contribute to modifying the absorption, protein-binding, metabolism and excretion of various drugs. Subsequently, the kinetic profile of several classes of drugs will be described whenever possible in the newborn, infant and child, keeping the data in adults as a reference point. Unfortunately, for several drugs the information on the child is totally absent.

The lack of systematic studies has made this monograph a difficult task, and we hope it may serve, at least in part, to improve the conscience of our ignorance in this very neglected but extremely important part of our therapeutic activity.

REFERENCES

Binns, T.B. (1974): Better utilisation of medicines. *European Journal of Clinical Pharmacology, 7:* 155-16.
Breckenridge, A. (1971): Pathophysiological factors influencing drug kinetics. *Acta Pharmacologica Toxicologica, 29,* suppl. *3:* 225-232.
Dancis, J. and Hwang, J.C. (eds.) (1974): *Perinatal Pharmacology: Problems and Priorities,* Raven Press, New York.
Davis, J.A. and Dobbing A. (eds.) (1974): *Scientific Foundations of Pediatrics,* Heinemann W. Medical Book, London.
Kretchmer, N. (1975): Perinatal pharmacology: an introduction. In: *Basic and Therapeutic Aspects of Perinatal Pharmacology,* edited by P.L. Morselli, S. Garattini, and F. Sereni, pp. 1-6, Raven Press, New York.
Lasagna, L. (1974): A plea for the "naturalistic" study of medicines. *European Journal Clinical Pharmacology, 7:* 153-154.
Marx, J.L. (1973): Drugs during pregnancy: do they affect the unborn child? *Science, 180,* 174-175.
Mirkin, B.L. (1970): Developmental pharmacology. *Annual Review of Pharmacology, 10:* 255-272.
Morselli, P.L. (1976): Problemas de terapia en la edad pediatrica. In: *Advances en Terapeutica,* edited by J. Laporte and J.A. Salvà. Salvat, Barcelona, 7: 89-99.
Morselli, P.L. (1976a): Pediatric clinical pharmacology routine monitoring or clinical trials? *Intern. Symp. on Clinical Pharmacy and Clinical Pharmacology,* Boston 17-19 Sept. 1975, North Holland, Amsterdam pp. 279-286.
Morselli, P.L. (1976b): Clinical pharmacokinetics in neonates. *Clinical Pharmacokinetics, 1:* 81-98.
Morselli, P.L., Garattini, S. and Cohen, S.N. (eds.) (1974): *Drug Interactions,* Raven Press, New York.
Morselli, P.L., Garattini, S. and Sereni, F. (eds.) (1975): *Basic Therapeutic Aspects of Perinatal Pharmacology,* Raven Press, New York.
Morselli, P.L. and Tognoni, G. (1974): Il servizio di farmacologia clinica in pediatria. *Prospettive Pediatria, 14:* 167-174.
Orzalesi, M. (1975): Problems of drug therapy in the newborn period. In: *Basic and Therapeutic Aspects of Perinatal Pharmacology,* edited by P.L. Morselli, S. Garattini and F. Sereni, pp. 13-20, Raven Press, New York.
Prescott, L.F. (1975): Pathological and physiological factors affecting drug absorption, distribution, elimination and response in man. In: *Handbook of Experimental Pharmacology,* vol. 28, pt. III, pp. 234-257, *Concepts in Biochemical Pharmacology,* edited by J.R. Gillette and J.R. Mitchell, Springer-Verlag, Berlin.
Sereni, F. and Principi, N. (1968): Developmental pharmacology, *Annual Review of Pharmacology, 8:* 453-466.
Shirkey, H. (1968): Therapeutic orphans. *Journal of Pediatrics, 72:* 119-120.
Shirkey, H.C. (1974): Ethical limits of pharmacological research in children. In: *Proceedings, XIV International Congress of Pediatrics,* vol. 3, pp. 206-217, Editorial Medica Panamericana, Buenos Aires.
Special article (1974): Report on the Second European Symposium on Clinical Pharmacology, Evaluation in Drug Control. *European Journal of Clinical Pharmacology, 7:* 145-152.
Stern, L. (1974): Drug experimentation in the perinatal period. In *Proceedings, XIV*

International Congress of Pediatrics, vol. 3, pp. 218-222, Editorial Medica Panamericana, Buenos Aires.

Stern, L. (1975): Drug therapy in the perinatal period. In: *Basic and Therapeutic Aspects of Perinatal Pharmacology,* edited by P.L. Morselli, S. Garattini and F. Sereni, pp. 7-12, Raven Press, New York.

Tognoni, G., Morselli, P.L. and F. Sereni (1975): Ethical and methodological challenges in research in perinatal pharmacology. In: *Basic and Therapeutic Aspects of Perinatal Pharmacology,* edited by P.L. Morselli, S. Garattini and F. Sereni, pp. 423-430, Raven Press, New York.

U.S. Food and Drug Administration (1967): *Proceedings Conference on Pediatric Pharmacology,* G.P.O., Washington.

Weber, W.W. and Cohen, S.N. (1975): Aging effects and drugs in man. In: *Handbook of Experimental Pharmacology,* vol. 28, pt. III, pp. 213-233, *Concepts in Biochemical Pharmacology,* Springer-Verlag, Berlin.

Wilson, J.T. (1972): Pediatric pharmacology: who will test the drugs? *Journal of Pediatrics, 80:* 855-857.

Wilson, J.T. (1975): Pragmatic assessment of medicines available for young children and pregnant or breast feeding women. In: *Basic and Therapeutic Aspects of Perinatal Pharmacology,* edited by P.L. Morselli, S. Garattini, and F. Sereni, pp. 411-421, Raven Press, New York.

Yaffe, S.J. and Juchau, M.R. (1974): Perinatal pharmacology. *Annual Review of Pharmacology, 14:* 219-238.

1

Basic Concepts of Pharmacokinetics

ROBERTO GOMENI
AND
ROBERTO LATINI

Pharmacokinetics is a relatively new scientific discipline which "deals with the mathematical description of biological processes affecting drugs and affected by drugs" (Levy and Gibaldi, 1975). In other words, it is a discipline whose aims are to describe with mathematical expressions the complex fate of a drug in the body, to understand the rules and constants which condition and describe phenomena such as drug absorption, distribution, metabolism and excretion. The objectives of such efforts are a better understanding of drug actions and a better therapeutic use of pharmacological agents (Wagner, 1971; Gibaldi, 1971; Rescigno and Segre, 1972; Rowland, 1972b; Levy and Gibaldi, 1975).

The knowledge of the pharmacokinetic profile of any given drug is today considered an essential element for a rational therapy, and the application of pharmacokinetic knowledge may greatly improve the therapeutic approach. It has, in fact, become evident that intensity and duration of therapeutic and toxic effects of many drugs are closely related to their biological availability and disposition.

The purpose of this chapter is to describe in a simple way the basic pharmacokinetic concepts which may find a useful application at the clinical level and to illustrate briefly how kinetic parameters can be calculated by various methods. A brief section is also dedicated to solution of mathematical models and to curve-fitting using either graphical analysis, or analog or digital computers.

DEFINITION OF KINETIC PARAMETERS

Biological Half-Life (T½)

This term usually defines the time required for any given drug concentration to decrease by one-half. When this parameter is evaluated only by measuring the decay of plasma or serum drug concentrations, it is better defined as the apparent plasma (or serum) half-life. Knowledge of the apparent plasma half-life values for the various drugs today is considered very useful, as it may be helpful to determine optimal dosing intervals during repetitive drug administration. In fact, it is known that average steady-state plasma concentrations are reached, using constant dosing intervals, within a time period equal to 6 half-lives, and that complete drug elimination is achieved within 6 half-lives (Figs. 1a, 1b). The apparent plasma half-life may be calculated from the elimination rate constant Kel (see page 10) since

$$T\frac{1}{2} = \frac{0.693}{Kel} \tag{1}$$

Area $0 \to \infty$ (AUC)

This term defines the area under the plasma concentration curve of the drug (expressed as total drug, free and protein-bound) from the time of administration to an infinite time after a single dose.

Area $0 \to T$ (AUC$_T$)

This term defines the area under the plasma concentration curve during a dosage interval t=(0,T) in the course of repetitive drug administration assuming that equal doses of drug are given at equally spaced time intervals.

Average Steady-State Plasma Concentration

Repetitive drug administration at constant dosing intervals produces a "picket-fence" type curve of drug plasma levels (Fig. 1a) which is reflected in the urinary excretion profile. In other words, when a fixed dose of a drug is administered at regular and constant intervals, the levels of the drug in the plasma (and in the body) reach a state of equilibrium in which the plasma concentration/time curve is the same during any dosing interval. In such a condition, the input of drug into the body is equal to the body output. Theoretically, assuming complete absorption and complete bioavailability, if a drug is administered at dosing

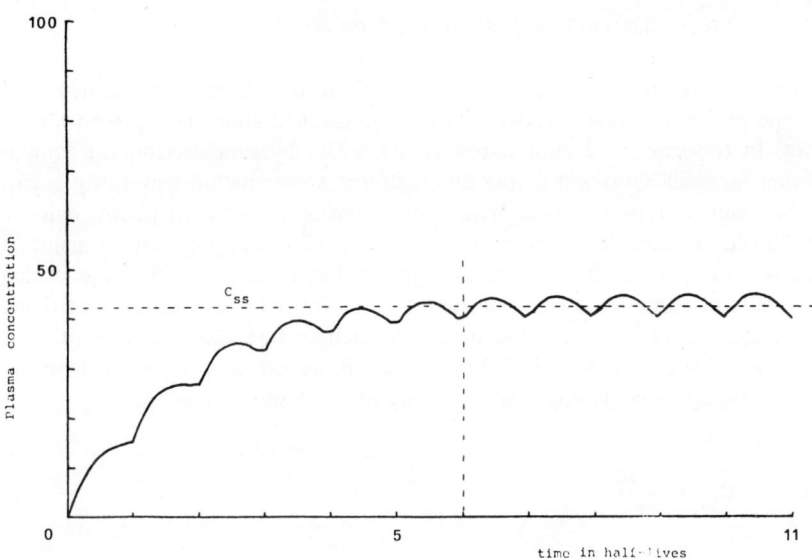

Fig. 1a: The simulated time curve of the plasma concentration of a drug after multiple oral doses, D = 10. The interval between each dose is assumed to be equal to the half-life ($\tau = T\frac{1}{2} = 1$). After 6 oral doses, D, at intervals τ, a plasma concentration is reached which approximates the steady state.

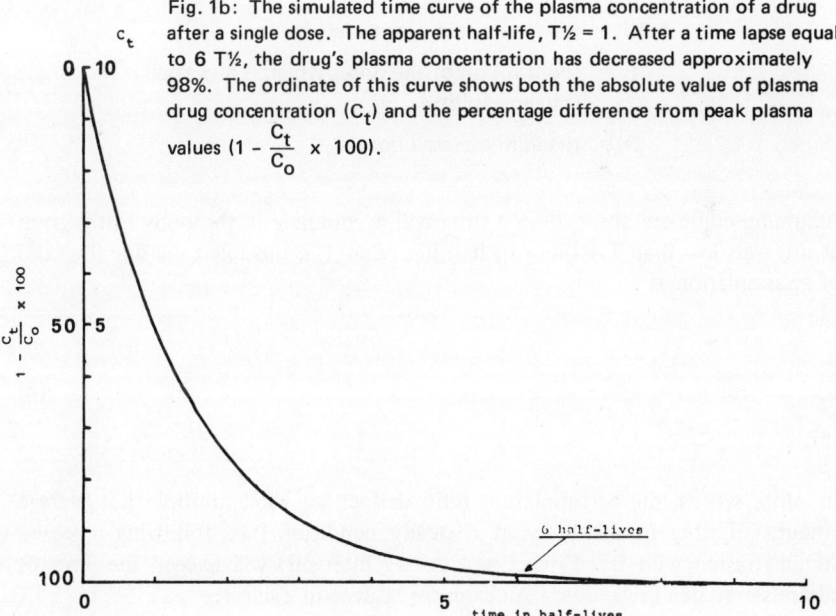

Fig. 1b: The simulated time curve of the plasma concentration of a drug after a single dose. The apparent half-life, $T\frac{1}{2} = 1$. After a time lapse equal to 6 $T\frac{1}{2}$, the drug's plasma concentration has decreased approximately 98%. The ordinate of this curve shows both the absolute value of plasma drug concentration (C_t) and the percentage difference from peak plasma values $(1 - \frac{C_t}{C_o} \times 100)$.

intervals equal to its biological half-life, a steady-state level is approached after a time period equivalent to 4 half-lives and reached after one equal to 6 half-lives. In this case, no accumulation occurs, while, by administering the drug at dosing intervals shorter than the drug half-life, accumulation may easily occur.

In practice, however, even with a drug having an apparent plasma half-life of 100 h, an administration interval of 24 or 12 h is appropriate to maintain steady-state plasma concentrations. This is due to the fact that the dosing interval and elimination rate constant are not the only two factors controlling the plateau level of a drug. Other factors, such as dose and bioavailability, are implicated. Wagner et al. (1965) have proposed the following equations to evaluate the average drug plasma levels after any route of administration:

$$\bar{C}_{ss} = \frac{AUC}{\tau} \tag{2}$$

or

$$\bar{C}_{ss} = \frac{FD}{Kel \, \tau \, Vd} \tag{3}$$

where τ = interval between two doses
AUC = the area under plasma levels
F = the fraction of the doses which is absorbed (bioavailability)
D = the administered dose

Assuming complete absorption, a drug will accumulate in the body if it is given at intervals less than 1.4 times its half-life value. It is possible to define the ratio of accumulation as

$$Ra = \frac{1.4 \, T\frac{1}{2}}{\tau} \tag{4}$$

In other words, the accumulation ratio defines by what multiple the average amount of drug in the body at a steady condition (i.e., following repeated administration with fixed doses and dosing intervals) will exceed the amount administered in a single dose. An example is given in Table 1.

TABLE 1

Accumulation Ratios for Drugs with Different Plasma
Half-Life Values, Administered at Various Dosing Intervals

Plasma Half-life	Dosing Intervals		
	$\tau = 3$ h	$\tau = 6$ h	$\tau = 12$h
3	1.44	0.72	0.36
6	2.89	1.44	0.72
12	5.77	2.89	1.44
24	11.50	5.77	2.89

For a given dose, using equation (2) it is possible to define the value of τ necessary to achieve a desired average asymptotic plasma level since:

$$\tau = \frac{AUC}{C_{ss}} \quad (5)$$

where C_{ss} is the desired plasma level.

The information given by equations (2) and (3) may be very useful in optimizing dose and dosing intervals for those drugs for which estimates of plasma half-life values and AUC are available.

Apparent Volume of Distribution (Vd)

The apparent volume of distribution (Vd) is a proportionality constant in the relationship between the dose administered, or the amount of the drug in the body, and the drug concentration in the plasma. This constant, which is usually expressed in L/kg, has no direct physiological meaning and, in many instances, does not refer to real volume. The apparent volume of distribution may be defined as the volume of body fluids in which the drug appears to be distributed with a concentration equal to that in plasma. With this definition, it is assumed that the body acts as "a single homogeneous compartment with respect to the drug." In a two-compartment open model, the concept applies only to drug concentrations in the postdistributive phase (Rowland, 1972). The concept of volume of distribution assumes that the relative binding of the drug to various tissue components and fluids is independent of the drug concentration, and, in this case, the ratio of the drug concentration in fluids and tissues is constant.

As a consequence, a constant relationship exists between drug concentration in plasma (C) and the amount of drug in the body (A):

$$A = Vd \cdot C \tag{6}$$

The apparent volume of distribution may be calculated either from

$$Vd = \frac{\text{Dose (mg/kg) i.v.}}{C^0 \text{ (mg/l)}} \tag{7}$$

or from

$$Vd = \frac{\text{Dose (mg/kg)}}{\text{AUC Kel}} \tag{8}$$

The method which utilizes the area for the evaluation of Vd has the advantage of being model independent.

The value of this parameter is a characteristic property of any given drug, and usually lipophilic compounds, with high binding to plasma and tissue protein, have a value from 2 or 3 up to 25 L/kg or more. Conversely, water-soluble or very polar compounds have a smaller Vd, which in many instances corresponds to the extracellular water (0.15-0.30 L/kg). When there exists a more or less uniform drug distribution throughout the various body components, the Vd approaches the values of 0.8-1 L/kg. If there is modification of the plasma protein-binding (displacement by other drugs, hypoalbuminemia), or an alteration of physiological attributes such as total body water, adipose tissue fat/lean mass ratio or blood pH, the apparent volume of distribution may vary considerably. For instance, in the case of obesity a very lipophilic drug will have a higher apparent Vd, while the reverse holds true for more polar compounds.

Total Body Clearance (TBCl)

Total body clearance is a very important parameter which may be defined as the portion of the apparent volume of distribution (Vd) cleared from the body per unit time. As a parameter it is much more meaningful than the apparent plasma half-life, since it is derived from the sum of all the clearance or elimination mechanisms. In other words, the total body clearance, written as TBCl, equals metabolic clearance + renal clearance. The upper limit of the total body clearance is given by the flow throughout all the organs of elimination (liver and kidneys) and is approximately 3L/min or 0.042 L/min/kg. To give an example, if we consider a drug which is uniformly distributed in the total body water of a 70 kg man (Vd = 0.6 L/kg), and has a TBCl of 3 L/min, the apparent T½ would be 3.3 min. In the two situations, even with the apparent plasma half-life, of one case 3 times that of the other, the TBCl value is the same; it is the only parameter which really gives a correct approximation of the drug removal rate. Another advantage of this value is that since

$$TBCl = \frac{Dose}{AUC} \tag{9}$$

the parameter is practically model-independent.

Bioavailability or Physiological Availability

This term defines the extent of absorption of a given drug and can be determined by comparison of plasma concentrations of urinary data obtained after both intravenous and oral administration. The comparison is made possible by the assumption that within the same individual Kel and Vd do not change and that, after i.v. administration, the dose is completely available (100%). For the relationship

$$Dose = Kel \cdot Vd \cdot AUC \tag{10}$$

the bioavailability will be

$$Bioavailability = \frac{oral\ Dose}{i.v.\ Dose} \times 100 \tag{11}$$

substituting D,

$$Bioavailability = \frac{oral\ (AUC)}{i.v.\ (AUC)} \times 100 \tag{12}$$

In the case of urinary data.

$$D = \frac{Au\ \infty\ Kel}{Ku} \tag{13}$$

where Ku is the renal excretion rate constant

$$Bioavailability = \frac{oral\ Au\ \infty}{i.v.\ Au\ \infty} \times 100 \tag{14}$$

where Au ∞ is the total amount of drug (drug + metabolites) excreted in the urine.

For the urinary data, the calculation is possible only when no chemical or metabolic conversion of the drug has taken place prior to its entry into the systemic circulation.

First Pass Effect

When a drug is administered by the oral route, in order to reach the systemic circulation it must pass through the liver. Consequently, a considerable fraction of the absorbed drug may be either metabolized or bound by liver tissue proteins during the first pass through the organ, and thus a smaller amount of the drug will reach the systemic circulation than was absorbed. As a result, the area under the plasma concentration curve (AUC) after oral administration will be smaller than that obtained after intravenous administration. In this case, the extent of the unchanged drug reaching the system circulation is referred to as the systemic availability. The magnitude of the first pass effect according to Gibaldi et al. (1971) may be evaluated from

$$R = 1 - \frac{(\text{i.v. dose})}{(\text{i.v. Area}) Q} \tag{15}$$

or

$$R = \frac{Q}{Q + \frac{\text{oral dose}}{\text{oral AUC}}} \tag{16}$$

where R = ratio of $\frac{\text{oral AUC}}{\text{i.v. AUC}}$

and Q = flow rate through the liver (0.7L/min for plasma and 1.5L/min for blood)

Since equation (16) does not require the use of i.v. AUC, it should be applied only in those cases where complete oral absorption has been well documented. It is possible that a drug may have complete bioavailability, documented by urinary data which indicate 100% absorption, but, due to considerable first pass effect, the system availability of the unaltered drug may be very low. Propranolol, alprenolol, lidocaine and desipramine are some common examples of this phenomenon (Shand and Rangno, 1972; Boyes et al. 1971).

Compartment Models

The purpose of pharmacokinetics is to examine the absorption, distribution, metabolism and elimination of various drugs in order to have a better understanding of their pharmacodynamic effects. To reach this objective, mathematical models have been developed which simulate all of the biological processes involved with the kinetic behavior of a drug once it has been introduced into the body. The models most commonly used depict the body as a series of compartments in which the drug (or its metabolites) is uniformly distributed. The term "compartment," in this context, is used to represent a theoretical volume that is identifiable not so much as an anatomical or physiological entity, i.e., an organ or group of organs, but as a body space throughout which the drug is more or less homogeneously distributed. The one- or two-compartment models are those most frequently employed.

In the one-compartment model, the body assumes the characteristics of a homogeneous unit. This model is especially useful in the pharmacokinetic analysis of drug plasma concentrations and of data on urinary excretion after oral or i.m. administration because the distributive phase of the drug is concealed during its absorption. I.v. administration followed by frequent blood sampling limits the one-compartment model since it gives results that are too approximate, and accurate interpretation of the data is impossible. Under these circumstances, it is wiser to use the two-compartment model.

The two-compartment model is based on the assumption that the drug enters the body instantaneously and is uniformly distributed in a so-called central compartment, which is actually similar in volume to the plasma plus that of the highly perfused body tissues, drug distribution in the rest of the body (the peripheral compartment or tissues with lesser blood circulation) occurs at a slower rate. In using this schematic representation, both the elimination process of a drug, whether by renal or biliary route, and its metabolism are assumed to take place in the central compartment. It is important to underline the fact that many other pharmacokinetic models could be developed according to the data available and the specific physiologic considerations in each case. Moreover, the distribution of an individual drug might be studied using different pharmacokinetic models, depending on the information at hand and on the particular objective of the investigation being conducted.

Rate Processes

The movements of drugs across biological membranes, that is, their absorption, diffusion and elimination, are mainly determined by the physicochemical properties both of the drug and the biological milieus with which they interact. The movements can rather easily be described and expressed as mathematical rate processes. The rate processes which are more relevant for human pharmacokinetics are as follows:
—First order rate processes
—Zero order processes
—Capacity-limited processes

First Order Processes

We can speak of first order processes when the transfer rate ($\frac{dC}{dt}$) of drug from side A of a membrane to side B, or from compartment 1 to compartment 2, is directly proportional (K = proportionality constant) to the concentration of the drug (C) on side A of the membrane or in compartment 1. In this case, K is defined as the first order rate constant. Physiological processes which usually follow first order kinetics are drug absorption, drug diffusion, drug metabolism and renal clearance. The disappearance rate from the blood of a given drug which has been administered intravenously may be expressed mathematically according to a first order kinetics as:

$$\frac{dC}{dt} = -K_{el} C \qquad (17)$$

Integrating equation (17), we obtain

$$C = C^o e^{-K_{el}t} \qquad (18)$$

where C^o is the drug concentration at zero time and will depend upon the amount administered.

One property of this equation is that, even when varying the administered dose D, the first order rate constant (Kel) remains unchanged. In many instances it is convenient, in order to simplify its graphical analysis, to transform the equation (18) in a straight line, as

$$lgC = lgC^o - K_{el}t \qquad (19)$$

It is evident (Fig. 2a) that in plotting the equation (19) with a low or a high dose two parallel lines are obtained. It follows that with a first order rate process the apparent half-life value is dose-independent, and the same holds true for parameters such as volume of distribution and body clearance.

Some consequences of first order drug rates:

(1) The biological half-life is dose-independent.
(2) Similarly, the composition of the drug products excreted is independent of the dose administered.
(3) The area-under-the-plotted-curve of blood level vs. time is directly proportional to the dose given, following a single dose, regardless of its size.

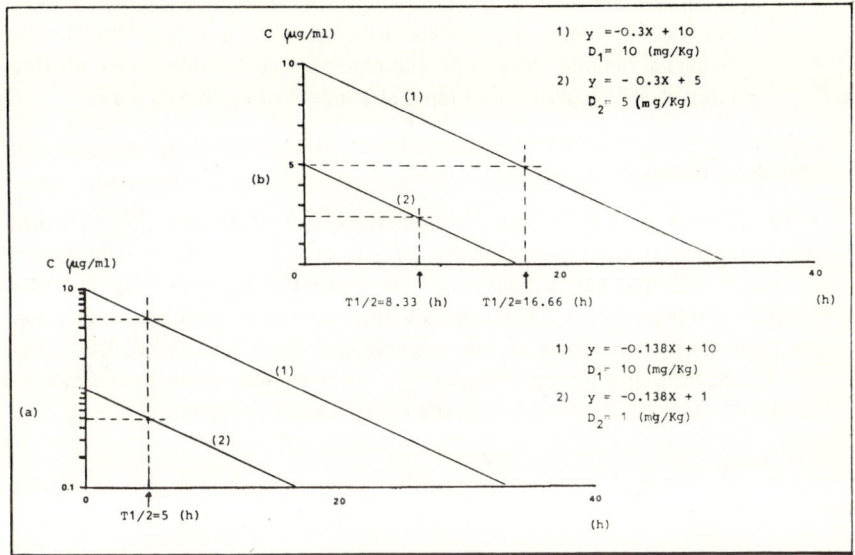

Fig. 2: Plasma drug disappearance curves of the first order rate process (a) and of the zero order rate process (b) are depicted for two different dose levels, D_1 and D_2, where $D_1 > D_2$. It should be noted that with process (a) the apparent half-life is not influenced by changes in dose level, whereas with process (b) the T½ is dose-dependent.

(4) The quantity of drug in the urine is directly proportional to the dose given for all single doses, regardless of their size.
(5) The amount of drug eliminated via the urine in infinite time varies directly with the plasma area, from t=0 to t=∞, after administration of a single dose.
(6) For a wide range of doses, the mean steady-state plasma is directly proportional to the dose that was given.
(7) During a dosage interval, when steady state exists and the intervals are evenly spaced, the amount of unaltered drug recoverable in the urine may vary directly with both the dose and the mean steady-state plasma.
(8) If the same dose is given at regular and equal intervals, the number of drug doses necessary to reach a given percentage of the final steady-state depends upon the relationship of the dosage interval to the drug's half-life and to its concomitant rate of excretion and absorption.
(9) The mean steady-state plasma is directly proportional to the drug's half-life and inversely proportional to body weight, being that the plasma concentration is lower in a great volume of distribution of this is directly proportional to the body weight.

(10) When attained without using a loading dose and with equidistant dosage intervals, the mean steady state is the same as that reached by administering a loading dose plus subsequent maintenance doses at time intervals which allow more rapid attainment of the steady state.

Zero Order Processes

We speak of zero order rate constant when the transfer rate ($\frac{dC}{dt}$) of a drug from compartment 1 to compartment 2 (or in or out of a given compartment) is constant with time and independent from concentration of the drug. A typical example of this process is when a drug is administered by constant i.v. infusion. The mathematical equation of this example (infusion) is described later (page 24). Considering the disappearance of an intravenously given drug from the blood, following zero order kinetics, the mathematical equation is

$$\frac{dC}{dt} = -K_o \qquad (20)$$

and by integration

$$C = C^o - K_o t \qquad (21)$$

It is apparent that (21) is the equation of a straight line. As previously mentioned, if one considers the case of two different C^o, derived from one low and one high drug dose, and plots these two equations, the results are that the half-life increases with the dose (Fig. 2b). In this case, the body clearance is also dose dependent, but the apparent volume of distribution, within a certain range, may be independent from the drug dose.

Capacity-Limited Processes

A rate process is considered capacity-limited, or of the Michaelis-Menten type, when a saturation phenomenon occurs at higher drug concentrations. Under these circumstances, there is usually a zero order process for higher concentrations and a first order process for lower concentrations. Saturation may be present at either of two levels: at that of the enzymes responsible for drug degradation, or at that of the carrier mechanisms involved with active transport of the drug across selected membranes (i.e., tubular secretion and, rarely, intestinal absorption).

Examples of Michaelis-Menten type kinetics have been described for ethanol (Lundqvist and Wolthers, 1958), salicylic acid (Lery et al., 1972) and diphenylhydantoin (Arnold-Gerger, 1970). Where there is a capacity limited process, assuming i.v. administration of a given dose, the rate of drug disappearance can be described as

$$\frac{dC}{dt} = - \frac{Vm\ C}{Km + C} \qquad (22)$$

where Vm is the maximum theoretical rate of the process and Km is the drug concentration at which the rate of the process is equal to one-half of its theoretical maximum rate.

Integrating equation (22), we have

$$tVm = C^o - C + Km\ lg\ \frac{C^o}{C} \qquad (23)$$

In this case, if the drug concentrations (lg C) obtained with two different doses (low and high D) are plotted against time, we obtain the curves reported in Fig. 3.

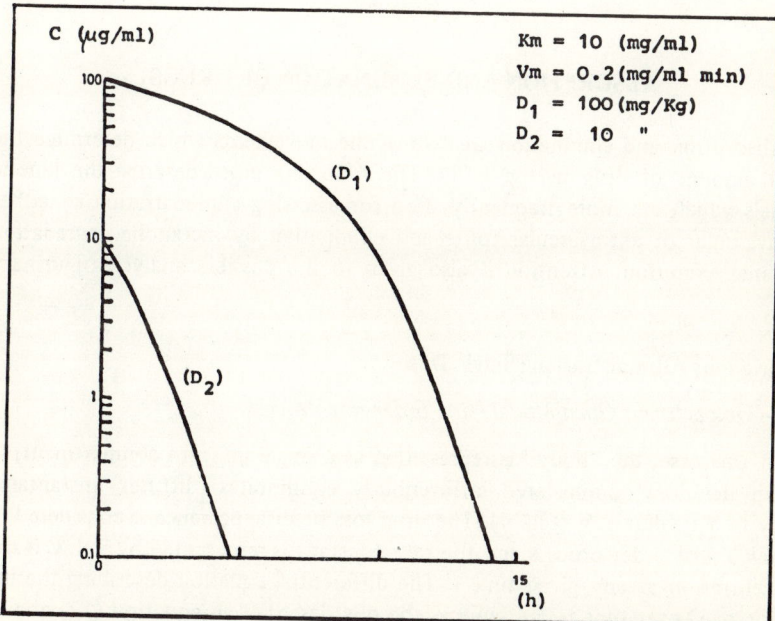

Fig. 3: Plasma drug disappearance curves of the capacity-limited process type for two different dose levels, D_1 and D_2, whre $D_1 > D_2$, are shown in these graphs. It should be noted that the disappearance is linear (first order rate process) only for those plasma concentrations which do not approach the saturation concentration and that the apparent half-life is dose-dependent.

In other words, for concentration below a certain value there is a first order kinetic process, while for higher concentrations a typical capacity-limited process is present.

Some consequences of capacity-limited drug elimination:

(1) The decline of drug levels in the body is not exponential.
(2) The time required to eliminate 50% of a dose increases with increasing doses.
(3) The area-under-the-curve of blood level vs. time is not proportional to the amount of drug absorbed.
(4) The composition of excretion products is affected by dose and dosage form.
(5) It is probable that there is competitive inhibition of the capacity-limited processes by other drugs that are metabolized by the same enzyme or that require the same rate-limiting substance.
(6) In the course of maintenance treatment, severalfold increases in steady-state levels may occur for small increases in the maintenance dose.

ABSORPTION AND ELIMINATION OF DRUGS

Absorption and elimination are two of the movements which determine the total amount of drug in the body. The following pages describe the kinetic models which are more frequently used for assessing administration by either intravascular or extravascular route and elimination by metabolic degradation or renal excretion. Attention is also given to the possible analysis of urinary data.

Intravenous Administration (Single Dose)

One-Compartment Open Model (first order rate process)

In this case, the "body" is represented as a single uniform compartment, in which the dose administered intravenously equilibrates (diffuses) instantaneously in the volume V (Fig. 4). The drug loss or disappearance is considered to follow a first order process and the rate constant is represented by Kel. C is the concentration at any given time t. The differential equation describing the behavior of C over time is the same as the one described in equation (17) above. The slope of the straight line obtained from equation (19) can be computed with the formula

$$\text{Kel} = \frac{\lg C(t_1) - \lg C(t_2)}{(t_2 - t_1)} \tag{24}$$

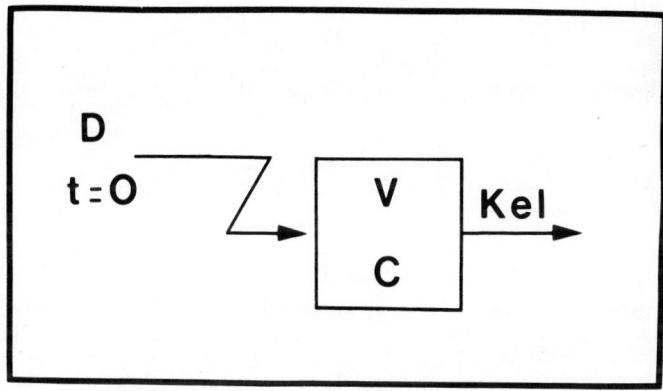

Fig. 4

An example is reported in Fig. 5.

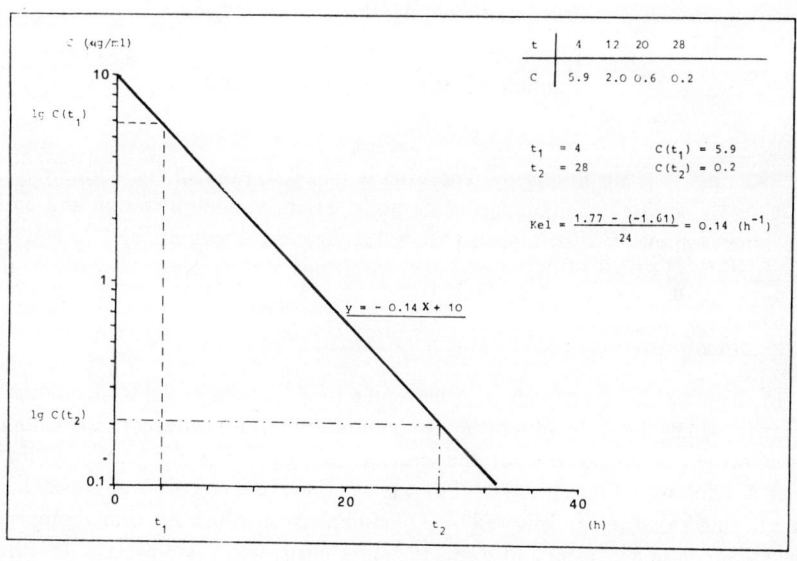

Fig. 5

From these data, the apparent volume of distribution (Vd) and the area under the plasma concentration time (AUC) are easily calculated, so that

$$Vd = \frac{D}{C^o} \qquad (25)$$

and the theoretical area is

$$AUC = \int_0^\infty C\,dt = \int_0^\infty C^o e^{-Kel_{dt}} = \frac{C^o}{Kel} \qquad (26)$$

By using equation (27), it is possible to determine the area under the experimental points and to extrapolate it to infinity by adding a correction factor:

$$AUC^* = \sum_{i=1}^{n} \underbrace{\frac{[C(i+1) + C(i)] \times [t(i+1) - t(i)]}{2}}_{\text{trapezoidal rule}} + \underbrace{\frac{C(n)}{K_{el}}}_{\substack{\text{correction} \\ \text{factor}}} \qquad (27)$$

where   n = number of experimental points

C(n) = last experimental point

Kel = elimination constant (calculated for example between the first and the last experimental point)

An example is given in Fig. 6. The effects of a variation of the administered dose or Kel in an open-compartment model after i.v. administration and with the same volume of distribution (Vd = 1 L/kg) are shown in Figs. 7a and 7b with simulated curves of the plasma concentrations.

One-Compartment Open Model (capacity-limited processes)

In this case, the body may also be represented by a single, uniform compartment in which the drug administered equilibrates instantaneously in the volume V. However, at variance with the previous example, the elimination process does not follow a first order rate, but one can observe a very slow disappearance rate during a first phase followed by a second phase in which the drug disappearance from plasma is faster and seems to follow a first order rate process. In other words, this is a system with a finite capacity. The process can be described by the following equation:

$$-\frac{dC}{dt} = \frac{Vm\,C}{Km + C} \qquad (28)$$

PHARMACOKINETICS

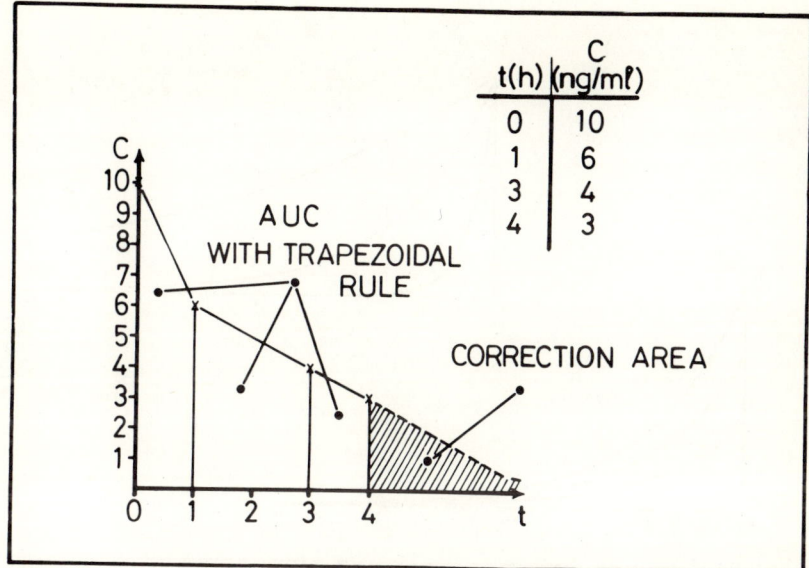

Fig. 6: An example of the calculation of the area under the curve with extrapolation to infinity.

With the equation (24) it is possible to estimate Kel:

$$Kel = \frac{2.3 - 1.09}{4} = 0.3025 \text{ (h}^{-1}\text{)}$$

Area with trapezoidal rule between 0 and 4 $= \frac{(10+6)}{2} + \frac{(6+4)}{2} + \frac{(4+3)}{2} = 21.5$

Correction area $= \frac{C(t=4)}{Kel} = \frac{3}{0.325} = 9.917$

In this example, the AUC* = 21.5 + 9.917 = 31.417 µg/ml h while using definition (26) of area and the estimated value of Kel:

$$AUC = \frac{10}{0.3025} = 33.057 \text{ µg/ml h}$$

From a practical point of view, in order to obtain an initial approximation of the kinetic constant appearing in equation (28), one may express it as

$$-\frac{1}{C}\frac{dC}{dt} = \frac{Vm}{Km + C} \qquad (29)$$

DRUG DISPOSITION DURING DEVELOPMENT

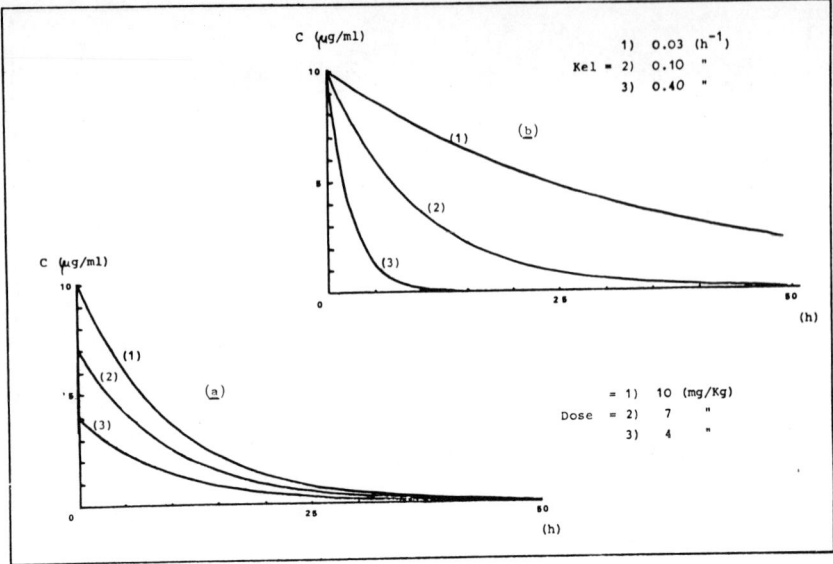

Fig. 7: These graphs represent plasma drug disappearance curves of the one-compartment open-model type in a system defined by the following parameters:

$Kel = 0.1\ (h^{-1})$
$D = 10\ (mg/kg)$
$Vd = 1\ (L/kg)$

Graph (a) demonstrates changes in the curve caused by varying the dose D, while graph (b) shows changes caused by variations in the elimination velocity (Kel).

but

$$-\frac{1}{C}\frac{dC}{dt} = \frac{d\lg C}{dt} \qquad (30)$$

Since

$$\frac{\Delta C}{\Delta t} \simeq \frac{dC}{dt} \quad \text{and} \quad \frac{\Delta \lg C}{\Delta t} \simeq \frac{d\lg C}{dt}$$

$$-\frac{[\lg C(n+1) - \lg C(n)]}{[t(n+1) - t(n)]} \simeq \frac{d\lg C}{dt} = -\frac{1}{C}\frac{dC}{dt} \qquad (31)$$

for values of C between C (n) and C (n + 1) the geometric mean may be used, so that

$$C = \sqrt{C(n) \cdot C(n+1)} \qquad (32)$$

Equation (31) becomes

$$\frac{\lg C(n) - \lg C(n+1)}{t(n+1) - t(n)} = \frac{Vm}{Km + \sqrt{C(n) \cdot C(n+1)}} \qquad (33)$$

that is,

$$\underbrace{\left[\frac{t(n+1) - t(n)}{\lg C(n) - \lg C(n+1)}\right]}_{Y} = \frac{Km}{Vm} + \frac{1}{Vm}\underbrace{\left[\sqrt{C(n) \cdot C(n+1)}\right]}_{X} \qquad (34)$$

Thus if one plots Y vs. X on graph paper according to the relationship

$$Y = \frac{t(n+1) - t(n)}{\lg C(n) - \lg C(n+1)} \quad \text{versus} \quad X = \sqrt{C(n) \cdot C(n+1)} \qquad (35)$$

the result is a linear regression from which it is possible to compute the values

$$\frac{1}{Vm} = \text{the slope of the straight line}$$

$$\frac{Km}{Vm} = \text{the intercept of the straight line at } t = 0$$

A practical example in which a first estimate of Vm and Km is made by simple calculation is reported in Fig. 8.

One must remember that in order to calculate the apparent plasma half-life according to this model, all the considerations made for linear models cannot be applied. However, for instances in which the concentration of the drug is below the Km, the situation corresponds to a first order process. For further considerations see Wagner (1973).

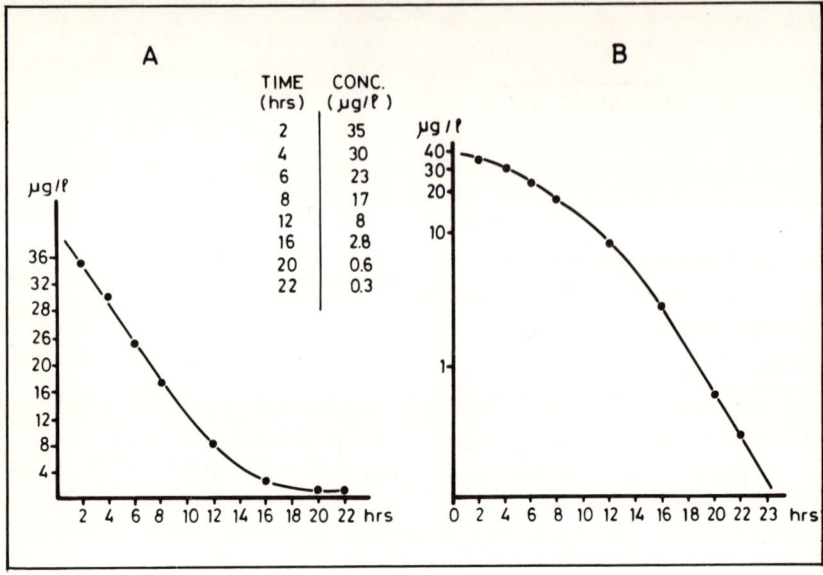

Fig. 8: These graphs simulate plasma drug disappearance curves of the capacity-limited process type, using an arithmetic scale (A) and a semi-logarithmic scale (B). With equation (35) and two different time intervals, 2-4 and 20-22, it is possible to estimate Vm and Kn

$Y_1 = 13.33 \quad\quad Y_2 = 2.90$
$X_1 = 32.40 \quad\quad X_2 = 0.42$

The angular coefficient (K) of the straight line thus projected is calculated from equation (34) using the formula

$$K = \frac{Y_2 - Y_1}{X_2 - X_1} = 0.326$$

moreover, given that

$1/K = Vm = 3.07$ mg/L h

by substituting the value calculated for Vm into equation (34) one obtains the value of Kn:

$Kn = 8.50$ mg/L

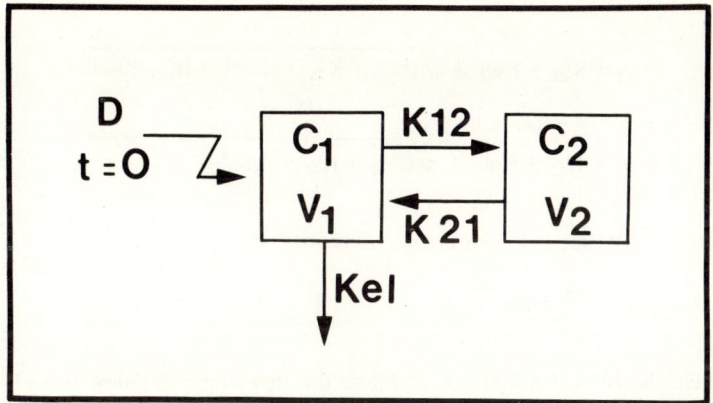

Fig. 9

Two-Compartment Open Model (first order rate process)

Here, the body may be represented as two definite compartments (central and peripheral) with volumes, respectively, V_1 and V_2 (Fig. 9). A similar model is usually used to describe kinetic data when plasma concentrations decline in a biphasic way on a semilogarithmic paper, defining two segments of a straight line. The different rate processes of this model may be described by the following differential equations:

$$\frac{dC_1}{dt} = K_{21} C_2 - (Kel + K_{12}) C_1 \qquad (C_1)_{t=0} = \frac{D}{V_1}$$

$$\frac{dC_2}{dt} = - K_{21} C_2 + K_{12} C_1 \qquad (C_2)_{t=0} = 0$$

(36)

integrating

$$C_1 = \frac{D}{V_1 (\alpha - \beta)} \left[(K_{21} - \beta) e^{-\beta t} - (K_{21} - \alpha) e^{-\alpha t} \right]$$

(37)

$$C_2 = \frac{D K_{12}}{V_1 (\alpha - \beta)} (e^{-\beta t} - e^{-\alpha t})$$

where D = dose

$$\alpha = \frac{1}{2}(K_{12} + K_{21} + Kel) + \sqrt{(K_{12} + K_{21} + Kel)^2 - 4K_{21} Kel} \qquad (38)$$

$$\beta = \frac{1}{2}(K_{12} + K_{21} + Kel) - \sqrt{(K_{12} + K_{21} + Kel)^2 - 4K_{21} Kel} \qquad (39)$$

Mathematically such behavior may be described as

$$C = Ae^{-\alpha t} + Be^{-\beta t} \qquad (40)$$

This behavior indicates that the drug goes through an initial phase (α) in which it diffuses from compartment 1 to compartment 2 and also is simultaneously eliminted from compartment 1. After equilibrium between V_1 and V_2, this phase is followed by the second phase (β), in which drug levels in both compartments decline in parallel due to drug elimination from the central compartment, or compartment 1 (Fig. 10). According to Levy and Gibaldi (1975), this may also be termed the disposition rate constant.

The various kinetic parameters may be expressed as

$$V_1 = \frac{D}{A+B} \quad \text{central compartment volume} \qquad (41)$$

$$V_2 = V_1 \frac{K_{12}}{K_{21}} \quad \text{peripheral compartment volume} \qquad (42)$$

$$K_{21} = \frac{A\beta + B\alpha}{A+B} \quad \text{distribution constant time}^{-1}) \qquad (43)$$

$$K_{12} = \alpha + \beta - K_{21} - Kel \qquad (44)$$

$$Kel = \frac{\alpha\beta}{K_{21}} \quad \text{elimination constant (time}^{-1}) \qquad (45)$$

$$AUC = \frac{A}{\alpha} + \frac{B}{\beta} = \frac{D}{V_1 Kel} \quad \text{area under theoretical curve} \qquad (46)$$

$$TBCl = \frac{D}{AUC} = \frac{D}{\frac{A}{\alpha} + \frac{B}{\beta}} = \frac{D}{\frac{D}{V_1 Kel}} = Kel\, V_1 = \text{Total Body Clearance} \qquad (47)$$

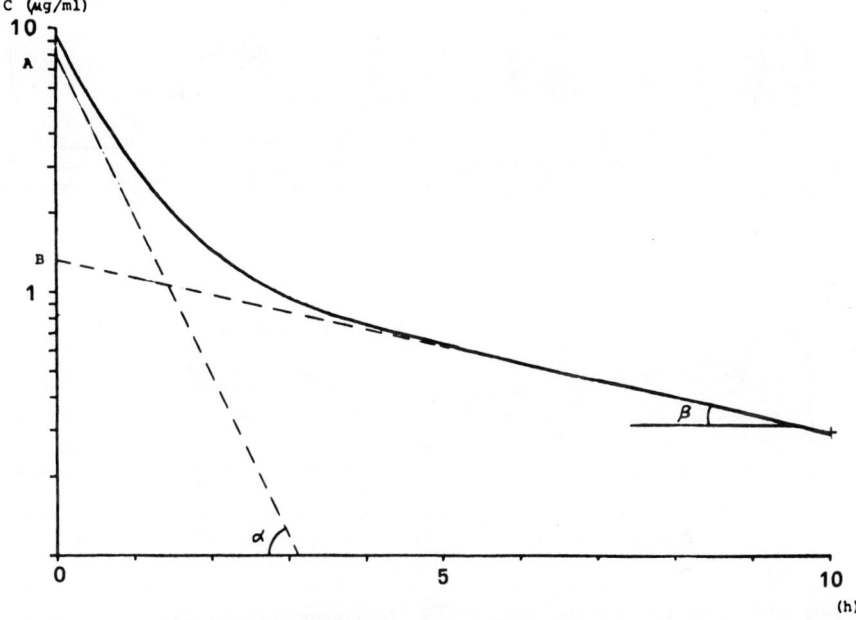

Fig. 10: Plotted semilogarithmically, this figure shows the plasma concentrations in a two-compartment open model after i.v. injections. The curves depicted have been obtained with the "peeling" method, where A and B are the intercepts at time 0 of the two lines with slopes, respectively, α and β.

The total distribution volume may be expressed in several ways:

$$Vd_{ss} = V_1 \frac{(K_{12} + K_{21})}{K_{21}} \quad \text{(Riegelman et al. 1968; Riggs, 1963)} \quad (48)$$

$$Vd\ Area = V_1 \frac{(Kel)}{\beta} \quad \text{(Riegelman et al., 1968; Gibaldi, 1969)} \quad (49)$$

$$V_{dext} = V_1 \frac{(\alpha - \beta)}{(K_{21} - \beta)} \quad \text{(Riegelman et al., 1968)} \quad (50)$$

The effects of a variation of K_{12}, K_{21}, Kel in a two-compartment open model, after i.v. administration, are shown in Fig. 11.

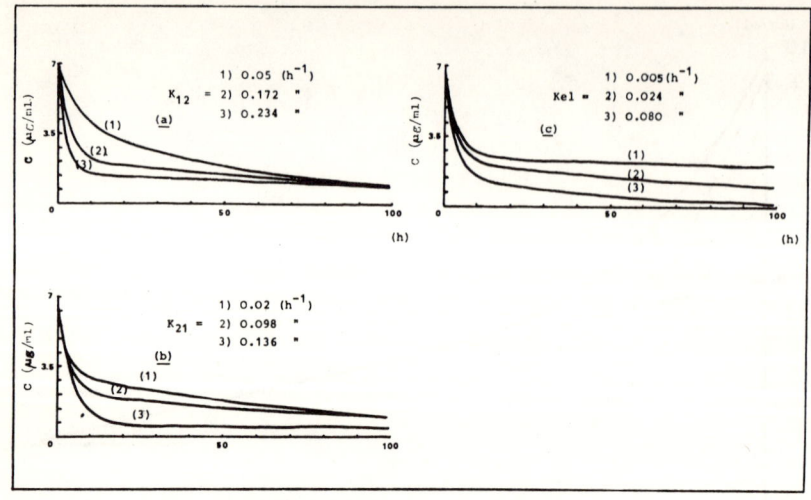

Fig. 11: Plasma drug disappearance curves of the two-compartment open model type are projected in a system defined by the following parameters:

K_{12} = 0.172 (h^{-1})
K_{21} = 0.098 (h^{-1})
Kel = 0.024 (h)
dose = 0.500 (mg/kg)
V_1 = 0.073 (L/kg)

Changes are demonstrated in the curves obtained by varying K_{12} in graph a, K_{21} in graph b and Kel in graph c.

Intravenous Infusion

One-Compartment Open Model (zero order process)

When a drug is administered by intravenous route at a constant rate of infusion, the plasma levels increase according to the equation

$$C = \frac{Ko}{Vd\ Kel}(1 - e^{-Kel\ t}) \qquad (51)$$

where Ko is the infusion rate.

From equation (51) we can immediately deduce that, for approaching $t \to \infty$, C tends asymptotically to the value

$$C_{ss} = \frac{Ko}{Vd\ Kel} \qquad (52)$$

C_{ss} is the drug concentration at the "steady state," or, in other words, in that situation in which as much drug is introduced into as is eliminated from the

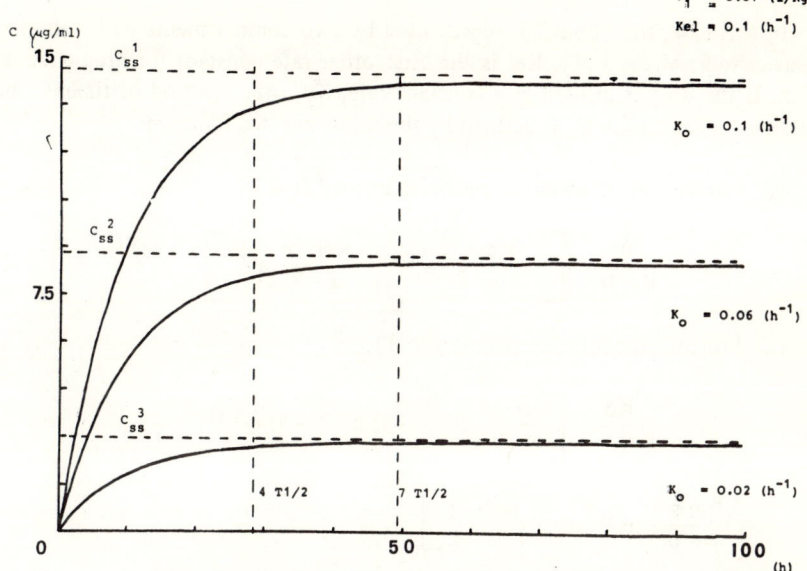

Fig. 12: Simulated curves of the plasma drug levels obtained by the i.v. route at three different rates of infusion (Ko), while the other parameters (Vd and Kel) remain constant. It should be noted that a plasma drug concentration equal to 95% of that at the steady state (C_{ss}) is reached after a time interval equivalent to approximately 4 half-lives (t½ = 6.93 h), and that a plasma level equal to 99% of C_{ss} occurs after approximately 7 half-life equivalents. The steady-state concentration has been calculated according to formula (52).

body time. C is equal to 90-95% when the infusion time reaches a value of about 4 half-lives, but C is equal to 99% of C_{ss} in the infusion time equal to 7 half-lives.

In Fig. 12, the effect of a variation of the infusion rate (Ko) is shown when Vd and Kel are constant. It is apparent that a different Ko leads to a different C_{ss} but that the time interval in which the C_{ss} is attained remains the same.

Stopping the infusion at time t = T, the drug will disappear from plasma according to the equation

$$C = \frac{Ko}{Vd\,Kel} (1 - e^{-Kel\,T}) e^{-Kel(t-T)} \tag{53}$$

Two-Compartment Open Model (zero order process)

In this case, the "body" is represented by two compartments with volumes, respectively; V_1 and V_2; Kel is the first order rate constant for drug elimination. If the drug is infused at a constant rate, Ko, over a period of time T, the plasma concentration C_1 is defined by the following two functions:

(1) For the period when drug is being infused ($t \leq T$)

$$C_1 = \frac{Ko}{Kel\, V_1} \left[1 - \frac{Kel - \beta}{\alpha - \beta} e^{-\alpha t} + \frac{Kel - \alpha}{\alpha - \beta} e^{-\beta t} \right] \quad (54)$$

(2) For the post-infusion period ($t > T$)

$$C_1 = \frac{Ko}{Kel\, V_1} \left[\frac{Kel - \alpha}{\alpha - \beta} (e^{-\beta t} - 1) e^{-\beta T} - 1) e^{-\beta(t-T)} - \frac{Kel - \beta}{\alpha - \beta} (e^{-\alpha T} - 1) e^{-\alpha(t-T)} \right] \quad (55)$$

The plateau value for this model also is

$$C_{ss} = \frac{Ko}{V_1\, Kel} \quad (56)$$

The magnitude of the plateau concentration, C_{ss}, depends upon the rate of infustions (Ko), the elimination rate constant (Kel) and the volume of distribution. The Vd and Kel are fixed values (computed from one- or two-compartment open models after a single i.v. dose) so that the plateau concentration, once more, depends only upon the infusion rate constant (Ko). Conversely, the time required to reach the plateau concentration is independent from the rate (Ko) and is determined solely by the elimination rate constant. Occasionally, the time required to reach the plateau concentration is so long that it may be useful to give a loading dose employing two different constant rates Q_1 over a first period ($0 \leq t < T$), then Q_2 for $t > T$. A method to find the value of Q_1 and Q_2 when the value of T and the desired C_{ss} is known has recently been described by Wagner (1974a).

Extravascular Administration

When a drug is administered by any route of administration other than i.v. injection or infusion, many processes are involved before it reaches the general

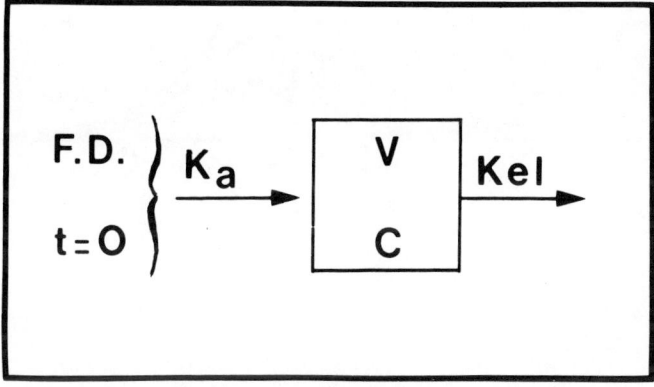

Fig. 13

circulation. Those most frequently implicated are:
- Disintegration of the dosage form
- Dissolution of the active ingredient
- Transport of the active ingredient
- Actual drug absorption

In many instances, the rate of absorption and the total amount absorbed are totally dependent on the relative interplay of these processes. A more detailed description of these factors is given in Chapter 2. The most commonly applied models in routine work following oral or intramuscular administration (the routes of giving drugs most frequently used) are the one-compartment open model and the two-compartment open model.

One-Compartment Open Model (first order rate process)

According to this model, the dose administered is not instantaneously distributed in the compartment which represents the body. Only a fraction (FD), between 0 and 1, reaches the systemic circulation with a peak at time t. The absorption follows a first order kinetic rate (Fig. 13). In this model, drug elimination too is assumed to follow a first order rate process. In other words, during the first phase, plasma levels increase according to a first order rate process, this is followed by a more or less short phase in which the absorption and elimination rates are similar and then by a third phase in which plasma level decay follows a first order rate process. The relative rate of the two processes

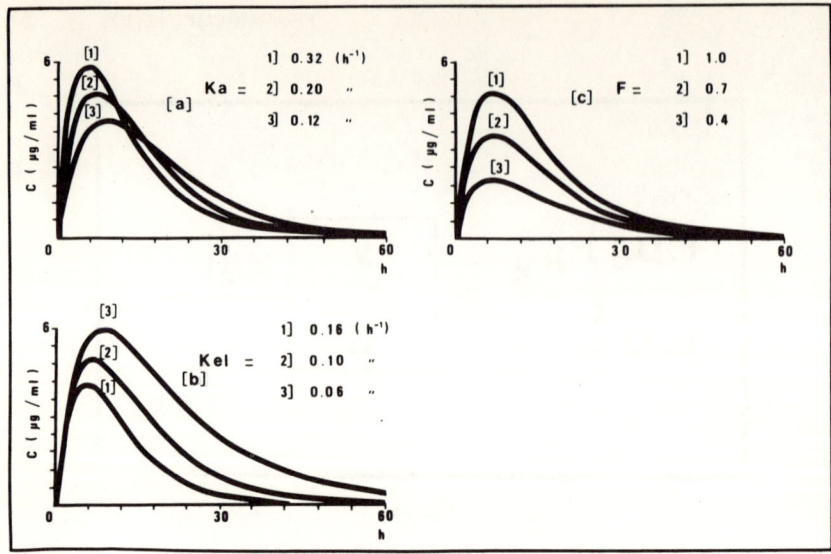

Fig. 14: This graph shows simulated plasma drug disappearance curves of the one-compartment open model type in a system defined by the following parameters:

Ka   = 0.2 (h^{-1})
Kel = 0.1 (h^{-1})
dose = 30 (mg/kg)
F   = 1
vol = 3 (L/kg)

The curves represent results obtained after extravascular drug administration when there are variations in Ka (curve a), Kel (curve b) and F (curve c).

determines the shape of the plasma concentration curve, as illustrated in Fig. 14. This model can be described by the differential equations

$$\frac{dC}{dt} = Ka\, C_1 - Kel\, C \qquad (C)_{t=0} = 0$$

$$\frac{dC_1}{dt} = Ka\, C_1 \qquad (C_1)_{t=0} = \frac{FD}{Vd}$$

(57)

where C   = plasma drug concentration at time t
      C_1 = drug concentration in the compartment from which absorption takes place (for ex. gastrointestinal tract)
      Ka = rate constant of absorption
      Kel = rate constant of elimination
      FD = fraction of dose absorbed
      Vd = apparent volume of distribution

Integrating the second equation, one obtains the formula

$$C_1 = \frac{FD}{Vd} e^{-Kat} \qquad (58)$$

and then, by also integrating the first equation, the following results:

$$C = \frac{FD}{Vd} \frac{Ka}{(Ka - Kel)} (e^{-Kel\, t} - e^{-Kat}) \qquad (59)$$

If the absorption rate is much more rapid than elimination ($Ka \gg Kel$), then the biological half-life of the drug can be computed from the descending part of the curve ($t\frac{1}{2} = \frac{0.693}{Kel}$). The theoretical time after which the plasma concentration reaches its peak value (t max) is given by

$$t_{max} = \frac{1}{Ka - Kel} \lg \frac{Ka}{Kel} \qquad (60)$$

This is dose-independent and depends only upon the constants of absorption and elimination. On the contrary, the value of the maximal peak plasma level depends directly both upon the fraction of the dose which reaches the systemic circulation and upon the absorption and elimination constants according to the equation

$$C_{max} = \frac{FD}{Vd} \left(\frac{Ka}{Kel}\right)^{\frac{Ka}{Ka - Kel}} \qquad (61)$$

It is evident from Fig. 14 that a distributive phase does not seem to exist. In many instances following oral administration, depending on the rate of absorption, a distributive phase may not be apparent; however, this does not mean that a drug has one-compartment characteristics. In the absence of intravenous data, the determination of absorption kinetics on the basis of the oral data alone may give misleading results. A more accurate evaluation may be obtained with the two-compartment open model (see below).

One-Compartment Open Model with Nonlinear Elimination

This model has the same characteristics as the previous model for the absorption phase, but in respect to elimination it follows a capacity-limited kinetics. The differential equation describing the concentration of the drug in the body is

$$\frac{dC}{dt} = \frac{V_m C}{K_m + C} + \frac{FD}{V_d} e^{-K_a t} \tag{62}$$

The kinetic constant relative to the elimination phase is computed as before (Par. 2.1b) and the same holds for the absorption rate constant (Par. 2.4a). In this example, however, it is not possible to use the previous equations for the evaluation of drug bioavailability (page 7) since they presupposed a dose-independent drug clearance. Martis and Levy (1973) have discussed this problem and have developed the equation

$$F = \frac{1}{V_d} \left[\frac{\left[\int_0^\infty \frac{dA_u}{dt} dt\right] \text{oral}}{\left[\int_0^\infty \frac{dC}{dt} dt \quad \text{i.v.}\right]} \right] \tag{63}$$

where A_u is the amount of the drug eliminated at any time after oral administration, and C is the drug concentration after intravenous administration.

Two-Compartment Open Model (first order rate)

This model (Fig. 15) is used to describe pharmacokinetic data when the logarithmic plasma concentration C_1 after the peak concentration in C_2 declines in a biphasic manner according to two segments of a straight line, as shown in Fig. 16. The portion of the curve after the peak is biexponential, consisting of an initial, rapidly declining part which corresponds to the "distribution phase" (α), and a terminal log-linear part which corresponds to the "elimination phase" (β) when an equilibrium exists between the central and "peripheral" compartments. The terms "distributive phase" and "elimination phase" have been placed between quotation marks to indicate that the two processes actually occur not in separate time periods but contemporaneously.

If Ka is the first order rate constant of absorption, K_{12} and K_{21} rate constants for drug distribution between compartments, and Kel the elimination rate constant, the concentration C_1 in the central compartment is given by the equation

$$C_1 = A_1 e^{-\alpha t} + A_2 e^{-\beta t} + A_3 e^{-K_a t} \tag{64}$$

where A_1, A_2 and A_3 are constants defined in equation (68) Ka is the first order rate constant (h^{-1}) ("absorption phase"), α is the fast disposition rate constant (h^{-1}) ("distributive phase") and β is the slow disposition rate constant (h^{-1}) ("elimination phase")

PHARMACOKINETICS   31

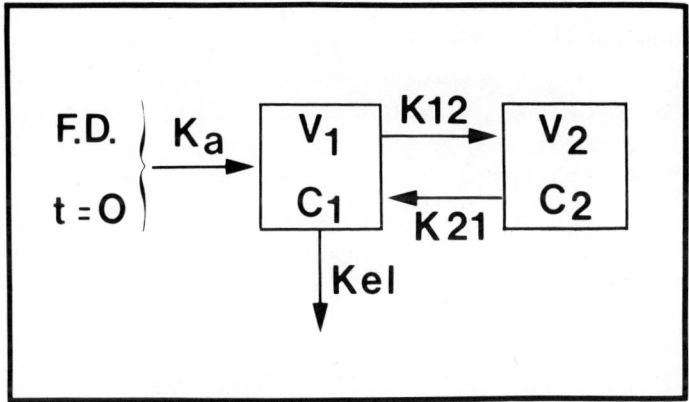

Fig. 15

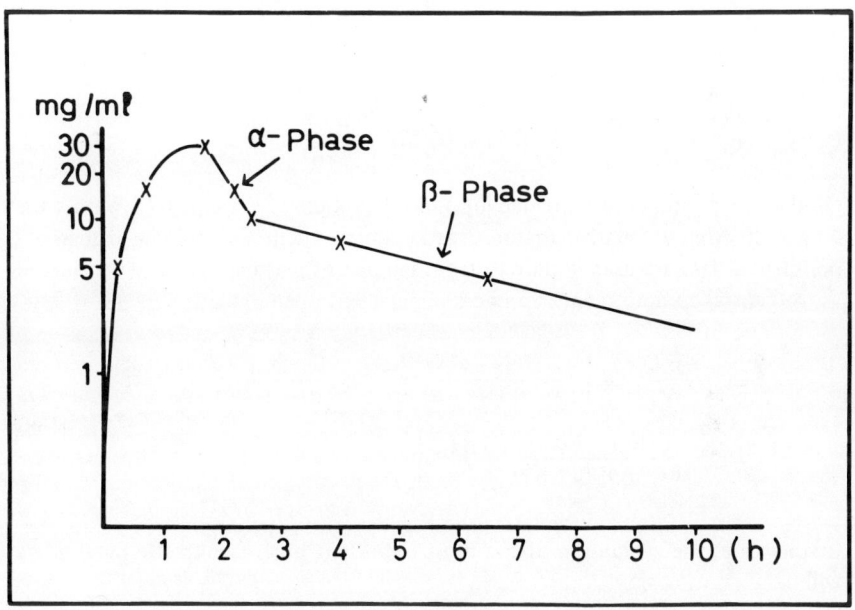

Fig. 16: Simulated curve of the plasma drug concentration obtained after extravascular drug administration, using the two-compartment open model in a system defined by the following parameters:

K_{12} = 0.89740 (h^{-1}) Kel = 0.41668 (h^{-1})
K_{21} = 1.31863 (h^{-1}) D = 1
Ka = 2.43371 (h^{-1}) V_1 = 0.03248 (L/kg)

The α and β are hybrid rate constants and are related to the specific rate constant of this model by the relations

$$\alpha + \beta = K_{12} + K_{21} + Kel \tag{65}$$

$$\alpha\beta = K_{21} \, Kel \tag{66}$$

Describing the rate processes of this model by differential equations, and with C_3 representing the concentration in the site of absorption, the following results:

$$\frac{dC_3}{dt} = Ka\,C_3 \qquad (C_3)_{t=0} = \frac{F\,D}{V_1}$$

$$\frac{dC_1}{dt} = Ka\,C_3 - (Kel + K_{12})C_1 \qquad (C_1)_{t=0} = 0 \tag{67}$$

$$\frac{dC_2}{dt} = K_{12}\,C_1 - K_{21}\,C_2 \qquad (C_2)_{t=0} = 0$$

Of the three equations obtained by the integration of system (67), we discuss here only what is relative to the central compartment C_1. In fact, in man experimental data are usually derived from samples of plasma, generally considered as the central compartment in a two-compartment open model.

$$C_1 = \frac{F\,D}{V_1} Ka \left[\frac{(K_{21} - \alpha)}{(\beta - \alpha)(Ka - \alpha)} e^{\alpha t} + \frac{(K_{21} - \beta)}{(\alpha - \beta)(Ka - \beta)} e^{-\beta t} \right.$$
$$\left. + \frac{(K_{21} - Ka)}{(\alpha - Ka)(\beta - Ka)} e^{-Ka\,t} \right] \tag{68}$$

In this case, the evaluation of the most important pharmacokinetic parameters will be

$$AUC = \frac{A_1}{\alpha} + \frac{A_2}{\beta} + \frac{A_3}{Ka} \tag{69}$$

$$V_2 = \frac{K_{12}}{K_{21}} V_1 \tag{70}$$

$$t\frac{1}{2} = 0.693/\beta \tag{71}$$

$$TBCl = \frac{FD}{AUC} = \frac{FD}{\dfrac{A_1}{\alpha} + \dfrac{A_2}{\beta} + \dfrac{A_3}{Ka}} \tag{72}$$

Urinary Excretion

The rate of elimination from the body for a given drug may also be evaluated by determining its urinary excretion. In a practical sense, this approach is possible only in those cases where the drug is excreted by the kidney in considerable amounts either as such or as metabolites. The excretory process may be described by the differential equation

$$\frac{dAu}{dt} = Kel\, Ab \tag{73}$$

where Au = amount excreted in urine
Ab = amount present in the body

Since the amount in the body is $Ab = Vd\, Cp$, and since in the case of i.v. administration $Cp = C^o\, e^{-Kel\, t}$, we can express equation (73) as

$$\frac{dAu}{dt} = Kel\, Vd\, C^o\, e^{-Kel\, t} \tag{74}$$

A second useful parameter to describe the excretion process is the "renal clearance" of the drug expressed as the proportionality constant between plasma levels and excretion rate:

$$\frac{dAu}{dt} = Cl_r\, Cp \tag{75}$$

where Cl_r = renal clearance and Cp = plasma concentration.

Using equation (74) and substituting, we have

$$\frac{dAu}{dt} = Cl_r\, Co\, e^{-Kel\, t} \tag{76}$$

and then, integrating this differential equation, we have

$$Au = \frac{Cl_r}{Kel} C^o (1 - e^{-Kel\,t}) \qquad (77)$$

If the time is great enough ($t \to \infty$),

$Au = Au\infty$ where

$$Au\infty = \frac{Cl_r}{Kel} C^o$$

Reviewing the data in the literature, one sees that there are two methods generally used to treat the experimental values obtained with urine (Martin, 1967). These are the "sigma minus method" and the "rate method."

The "Sigma Minus Method"

The "sigma minus method" consists of plotting log (Au_∞ - Au) against time, where (Au_∞ - Au) represents the summation (sigma) of the amount of drug excreted, until that time in which the excretion may be considered to be complete (Au_∞), minus the cumulative amount of drug excreted within a time t (Au). In this case, we have

$$\lg (Au\infty - Au) = \lg \frac{Cl_r}{Kel} C^o - Kel\,t \qquad (79)$$

When the drug elimination follows first order kinetics, Kel may be determined from the slope of the terminal (linear section) of the lg "sigma minus" plot. This method necessitates knowledge of Au and, in theory, requires the collection of urine until such time as excretion is complete. Wagner (1963) has suggested that the collection of urine for a period corresponding to 10 half-lives of the drug is usually sufficient for this purpose.

The "Rate Method"

This method was introduced by Swintosky (1957). A log of the rate of drug excretion plotted against time exhibits a terminal linear function of slope equal to -Kel according to the equation

$$\lg \left(\frac{dAu}{dt}\right) = \lg Cl_r\, C^o - Kel\,t \qquad (80)$$

Since it is difficult to obtain the exact rate of excretion of a drug in the urine ($\frac{d\,Au}{dt}$), it is necessary to use the average rate of excretion over a short period of time. From a practical point of view, the log of the amount of drug excreted (Δ Au) in a series of equal intervals (Δ t) is plotted against time, at the middle point of each time interval, and is represented by

$$\lg\left(\frac{\Delta Au}{\Delta t}\right) = \lg Cl_r\, C^o - Kel\, t \tag{81}$$

A practical example with the two methods is reported in Fig. 17, using data on amantadine.

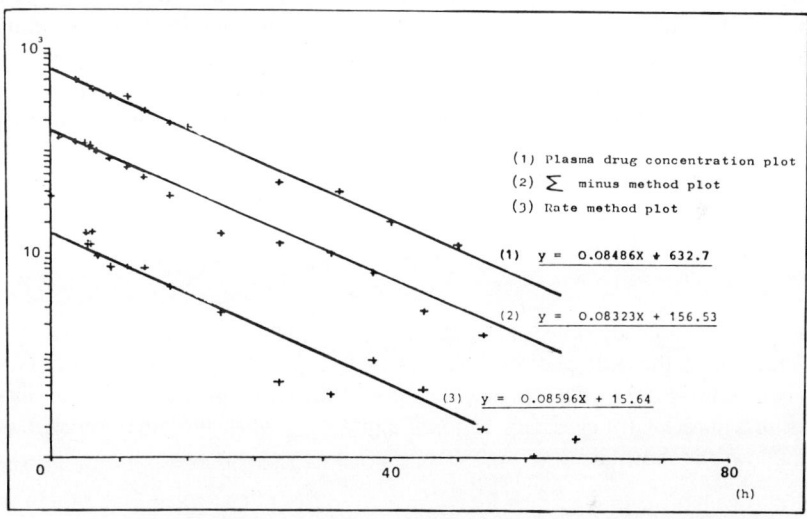

Fig. 17: In man amantadine is excreted by the renal route, completely unchanged; this fact permits the easy processing of urinary data by both the "rate" and the "Σ minus" methods described above. Following are some of the values derived from the respective curves of the graph. It is evident that the elimination rate constant (Kel) obtained from the plasma disappearance data is also well estimated by both "rate" and "Σ minus" methods.

Urine

(1) "Σ minus method"

Kel = 0.08323

$\frac{ClrCo}{Kel}$ = 156.53

r^2 = 0.975; df = 13

(2) "Rate method"

Kel = 0.085961

ClrCo = 15.64

r^2 = 0.954; df = 15

Plasma

Kel = 0.084860

Co = 632.7

r^2 = 0.993; df = 9

Multiple Dosing—Oral and I.V.

In everyday practice, the use of repetitive drug administration is much more frequent than the other kinetic situations described previously. The aim of this method of drug administration, in many instances, is to maintain drug plasma and tissue concentrations above therapeutic thresholds for a prolonged time period. In order to evaluate the correct drug dosages and the appropriate treatment schedule to maintain desired levels, it might be useful to determine the fundamental parameters (Ka_{ss}, Kel, B, FD, Vd) after acute administration by using the various models described in the previous pages. It is, however, possible to derive the same information by utilizing plasma samples or urinary data obtained between two drug administrations. Often the values following the latter method are more reliable and define more exactly the kinetics of a given drug during the course of chronic treatment.

Repetitive drug administration at constant time intervals (τ) which results in the attainment of an average steady-state concentration ($\overline{C}_{ss}$) which may be expressed by the following equation:

$$\overline{C}_{ss} = \frac{FD}{Vd\,Kel\,\tau} \tag{82}$$

As the average steady-state concentration, it is usually assumed to be that value around which the drug plasma concentrations vary in the intervals between two consecutive dosages. Rearranging equation (82), it is possible to determine the dose interval (τ) necessary to reach a given C_{ss} when the other parameters are known, as shown by

$$\tau = \frac{FD}{\overline{C}_{ss}\,Vd\,Kel} \tag{83}$$

The drug accumulation ratio (Ra), which represents the average amount of drug in the body at the steady state ($\overline{A}_{ss}$) and is derived from the amount of drug absorbed following administration of one maintenance dose, is given by the equations

$$Ra = \frac{\overline{A}_{ss}}{FD} \tag{84}$$

$$Ra = \frac{\overline{C}_{ss}\,Vd}{FD} \tag{85}$$

or, by using equation (82), it develops that

$$Ra = \frac{1}{Kel\,\tau} \tag{86}$$

During the course of chronic treatment with regular intervals and fixed doses, the steady-state levels are usually attained in a time equal to 6 plasma half-lives (Fig. 18a). However, in many instances, particularly when there is a very long half-life, it may be desirable to reach steady-state levels in a shorter time. In these cases, it is useful to take advantage of one or two loading doses. The purpose of a loading dose is to reach the desired concentration (C_{ss}) in the body in a short time (Fig. 18b). According to Wagner (1967a, 1974b), the appropriate

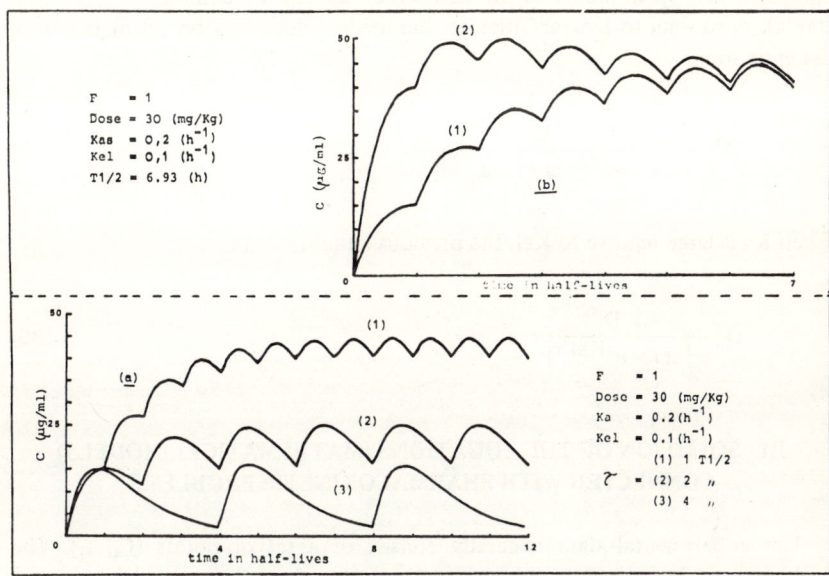

Fig. 18: (a) Three curves are shown which theoretically should result after the repeated administration of the same dose, D = 30, at different time intervals (τ). These intervals have been chosen as being equal to 1, 2 and 4 drug half-lives, respectively. It is apparent that by increasing the time intervals between drug administrations, both the steady-state concentration and the time in which it is reached decrease. (b) The theoretical curve (1) results when the dose, D = 30, is given at intervals, τ = 6.93 (1 half-life); the theoretical curve (2) shows the results after giving an initial loading dose D* = 80 (dose level obtained using formula 88), and successive doses D = 30 at time intervals τ = 6.93, or one half-life.

loading dose D* may be given by

$$D^* = Ra\, D \tag{87}$$

where D is the maintenance dose and
Ra is the drug accumulation ratio

This concept of drug accumulation as the amount of drug built up in the body differs from that of Kruger-Thiemer (1966, 1968) who considered drug accumulation as the build-up of drug concentration. In the case of the one-compartment open model (with first order absorption/elimination rate constants), according to Kruger-Thiemer, the loading dose may be calculated from the equation

$$D^* = \frac{D}{(1 - e^{-Kel\,\tau})(1 - e^{-Kel\,\tau})} \tag{88}$$

When Ka is large relative to Kel, the previous equation reduces to

$$D^* = \frac{D}{(1 - e^{-Kel\,\tau})} \tag{89}$$

III. SOLUTION OF THE EQUATIONS (MATHEMATICAL MODELS) CONNECTED WITH PHARMACOKINETIC PROBLEMS

The experimental data generally consist of a set of points (C_i, t_i). The problem is to fit these data with an equation of the form (linear models).

$$C_i = x_1 e^{-\lambda_1 t_i} + x_2 e^{-\lambda_2 t_i} + \ldots\ldots + x_n e^{-\lambda_n t_i} = \sum_{j=1}^{N} x_j e^{-\lambda_j t_i} \tag{90}$$

and to find the best values of the parameters.

The best method for calculating the parameters involves the minimization of a sum of square function:

$$\text{sum of square} = \sum_{i=1}^{M} (C_i - \sum_{j=i}^{N} x_j e^{-\lambda_j t_i})^2 \qquad (91)$$

where M is the number of compartments.

Daniel and Wood (1971) have demonstrated that equation (91) is statistically valid only when all observations C_i have the same variance. When this is not true, it is necessary to "weight" each point using a modified version of equation (91):

$$\text{sum of square} = \sum_{i=1}^{M} (C_i - \sum_{j=1}^{N} x_j e^{-\lambda_j t_i})^2 W_i \qquad (92)$$

The introduction of the "weight" concept is necessary because different points may have different variances, so that the "weight" of their importance is not equivalent when one is seeking the function that best fits the data. The choice is the mathematical form of the weight Wi depends on whether or not there are replicate observations at each sampling point. If there are multiple observations at each sampling point, the weight may be assumed equal to the inverse of its variance according to Brownlee (1960). When there are single observations at each sampling point, the problem of finding an appropriate weight is difficult to solve, since the experiment itself does not provide any information about the local variance. Ottaway (1973) has discussed this problem comparing more than one method and judging the effect of a particular weight from the goodness-of-fit produced by minimizing the weighting sum of square deviations. The goodness-of-fit may be considered as satisfactory both by using the chi-square test for deciding whether the distribution of data points is uniform on either side of the fitted curve and also by taking into account the proportion of the residual variance associated with points on one or the other side of the fitted curve as an indication of the sensitivity of the residual variance to movement of the curve away from particular data points. On this basis, a "weight" was suggested using the following form:

$$W_i = \frac{1}{(C_i + \hat{C}_i)^2} \qquad (93)$$

C_i is the i-th experimental point and $\hat{C}_i$ is the corresponding computed point.

Precision and Comparison of Parameters

The values of the estimated parameters, especially in equation (91), are usually very sensitive to small changes in the experimental data. This is best measured by comparing the estimated standard deviations of the calculated parameters with the error in the original experimental data. The correlation between the error in the experimental points and the estimated parameters according to Myhill (1967) are reported in Table 2.

TABLE 2

Correlation Between Error in Experimental
Points and Estimated Parameters*

Error in Experimental Points	Error in Estimated Parameters
1%	14%
2%	17%
5%	44%
10%	86%

*Myhill, 1967.

Another important factor which has been investigated is the relationship between the number of experimental points and the standard deviation of the estimated parameters. Glass and De Garreta (1967) have shown that by increasing the number of points from 11 to 21 the standard deviation of the estimated parameters is reduced by about 25-33%. Taking into account these considerations, it would appear that the concept of standard deviation (SD) for the estimated parameters is extremely important.

There are several methods to calculate the SD according to the different methods for the parameter estimation. These include:

—Using graphical analysis
—Calculating during the fitting of regression lines from a variance-covariance matrix
—Using the nonlinear least square regression method

In the latter instance, SD can be calculated as follows:

$$SD = \sqrt{S^2 \, a_{ii}} \qquad (94)$$

where SD = standard deviation of the i-th estimated parameter S^2 = sum of weighted square deviations divided by the degree of freedom (= no. of observations - no. of parameters), a_{ii} = entry for the i-th diagonal element in the matrix A^{-1}, where A is a matrix of the sum of cross-products of the partial derivatives $\frac{\partial C_k}{\partial \theta_j}$, C_k is a function to be fitted and θ_j is the jth unknown parameter of C_k.

Using the second computational method, the computed SD better defined as the "approximate" or "asymptotic" SD is dependent on the selection of correct models with the assumption that the data points are independent and are taken at proper intervals to describe the curve fully. Gennrich (1969) has demonstrated that the asymptotic SD approaches the true SD only as the number of data points approaches infinity. If this hypothesis is true, the value of the asymptotic SD may not always be particularly reliable. The only very reliable method for estimating standard deviation would be to repeat a given experiment several times, calculate a set of parameters for each experiment and compute the mean and standard deviations for each parameter using each of its several estimates.

The asymptotic standard deviation may give some information on the goodness-of-fit of the model. For example, when there is a large SD value relative to the estimated parameter, this indicates that this parameter may not be well determined with the current model or that the fit is not good, possibly because the initial parameter estimates are not close enough to the true values (Westlake, 1971). Sometimes it is desirable to compare values for a given parameter that has been calculated from two different experiments or models. Boxembaum et al. (1974) have discussed an appropriate "t" statistic to compare these values, using the computed asymptotic SD with the relation

$$t = \frac{\theta_{i1} - \theta_{i2}}{\sqrt{(SD_{i1})^2 + (SD_{i2})^2}} \qquad (95)$$

where θ_{i1} and θ_{i2} are, respectively, the estimations of the i-th parameter in the first and second experiment or model and SD_{i1} and SD_{i2} are the relative asymptotic standard deviations.

The degrees of freedom of this comparison are computed with the formula:

df = (number of data points in the first study) +
(number of data points in the second study) −
(number of parameters in the first study) −
(number of parameters in the second study)

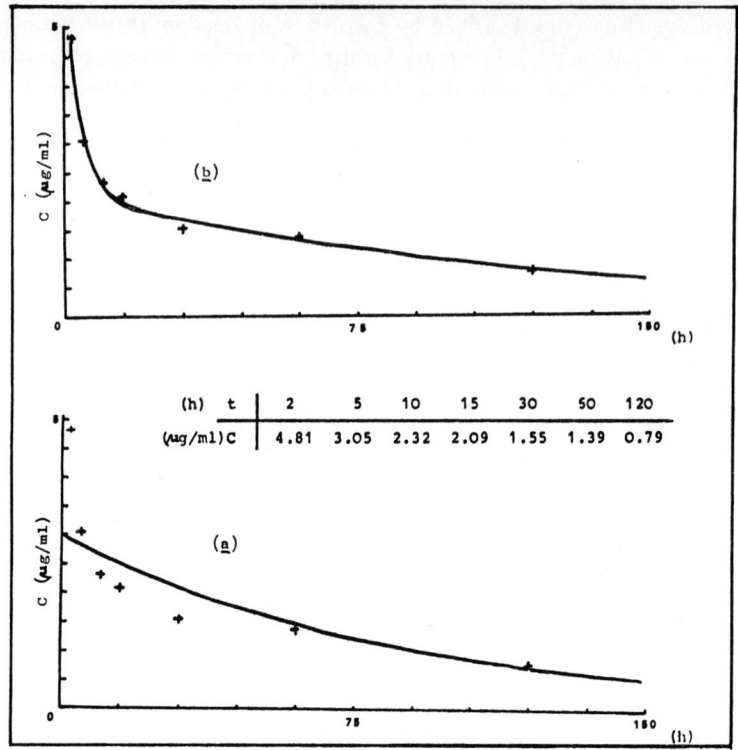

Fig. 19: The fit of experimental data using the one-compartment open model (a) and the two-compartment open model (b).

If one simulates an i.v. administration with the points

$t_{(min)}$	2	5	10	15	30	60	120
$C_{(mg/ml)}$	4.81	3.05	2.32	2.09	1.55	1.39	0.79

they can be studies according to the following models:

(a) the one-compartment open model (Fig. 19a)
(b) the two-compartment open model (Fig. 19b)

Using the NONLIN program to analyze the data, with the first model (2 parameters) the results are

Kel = 0.01168 (l/min)   SD = 0.002889
Co = 2.8926 (mg/ml)   SD = 0.4272

and with the second (4 parameters)

Kel   = 0.02424 (l/min)   SD = 0.004389
K_{12} = 0.1728 (l/min)   SD = 0.05724
K_{21} = 0.09806 (l/min)   SD = 0.02006
Co   = 6.7607 (mg/ml)   SD = 1.0736

If one compares the Kel of the two models,

$$t = \frac{0.02424 - 0.01168}{(0.004389)^2 + (0.002889)^2} = \frac{0.01256}{0.005244} = 2.395$$

df = 7 − 2+7 − 4 = 8

With this df on the t table at 5% significance level there are 2.31, so we can establish that the two Kel are different at 5%.

Curve-Fitting Using Graphical Analysis

This method, also called the "feathering," residual or peeling method, is the most simple and gives appreciable results with one- or two-compartment models but seldom with three- or more compartment models. The usefulness of this method is that it gives preliminary parameter estimates that may be used as starting values for a more refined method, such as nonlinear least square regression, to obtain the "real" value of parameters. This technique depends on the property of equation (90), and considering it in its simplest form

$$C = x_1 e^{-\lambda_1 t} + x_2 e^{-\lambda_2 t} + x_3 e^{-\lambda_3 t}, \qquad (96)$$

at t becomes large, the contributions of the terms

$x_1 e^{-\lambda_1 t} + x_2 e^{-\lambda_2 t}$, in relation to the final term $x_3 e^{-\lambda_3 tx}$, becomes negligible.
Thus

$$C \simeq x_3 e^{-\lambda_3 t} \qquad (97)$$

Taking logarithms we have:

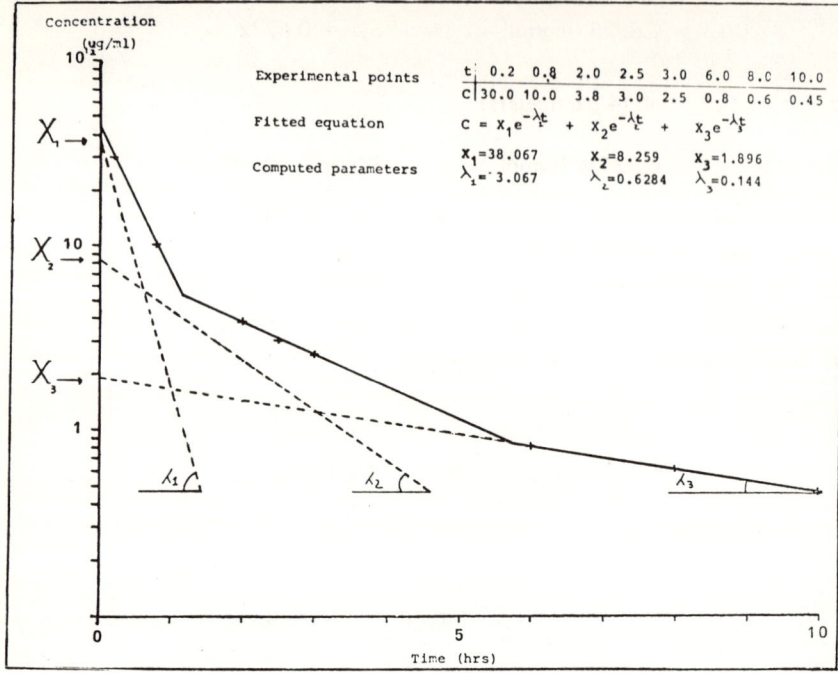

Fig. 20: The graph shows a simulated 3-exponential decline of a drug from plasma. X_1, X_2, X_3 are the intercepts and $\lambda_1, \lambda_2, \lambda_3$ the slopes of the lines of equation, respectively (103), (100) and (97).

$$\lg C = \lg x_3 - \lambda_3 t \tag{98}$$

If the experimental data are plotted in semi-logarithmic graph paper, the straight line given by the equation (98) can be fitted to the last few points (Fig. 20) x_3 can be calculated from the intercept when $t = 0$ and λ_3 from the slope. The next step in the analysis is to subtract the term $x_3 e^{-\lambda_3 t}$ from each of the data points not falling on the above straight line and the resulting curve will be represented by:

$$(C - x_3 e^{-\lambda_3 t}) = x_1 e^{-\lambda_1 t} + x_2 e^{-\lambda_2 t} = C' \tag{99}$$

At this point, the previous considerations must be repeated so that when t becomes large, the contribution of the term $x_1 e^{-\lambda_1 t}$ in relation to the final term $x_2 e^{-\lambda_2 t}$ become negligible and

$$C' \cong x_2 e^{-\lambda_2 t} \tag{100}$$

Taking logarithms we have:

$$\lg C' = \lg x_2 - \lambda_2 t \qquad (101)$$

and with linear regression on a semi-logarithmic scale we can find x_2 and λ_2.

The last step to consider:

$$C' - x_2 e^{-\lambda_2 t} = x_1 e^{-\lambda_1 t} \qquad (102)$$

or

$$C'' = x_1 e^{-\lambda_1 t} \qquad (103)$$

Taking logarithms and considering a regression line, we can find the last value of parameter x_1 and λ_1. The main limitations of this method are that the most accurately determined parameters are those of the last term x_3 and λ_3 and that the accuracy of determination decreases with each successively estimated pair of constants. Another limitation is that the pharmacokinetic parameters computed with this method sometimes overestimate and/or underestimate the corresponding parameters obtained by the least-square solution for this problem, as has been illustrated by Wagner (1967b) and Wagner and Metzler (1967).

Curve-Fitting Using an Analog Computer

This method is very similar to that used in digital computers and consists of a continuous adjustment to the parameters until the oscilloscope tracing matches the experimental curve. The advantage of this method lies principally in its more rapid performance, since analog computers solve differential equations simultaneously whereas in digital computers each operation is carried out sequentially. This fact allows one to have direct information on the sensitivity of each parameter and to test a wide range of values for a particular parameter in a very short time. The disadvantages of this method are that the accuracy of analog computers is on the order of 0.1% to 1%, and these values are related to the number of analog components used. On the other hand, numerical analysis can be carried out with an accuracy greater than 10^{-6}. In addition, with analog technique it is not even possible to calculate approximate values for the standard deviations of the parameter estimates. Because of these limitations, this method of calculation is seldom used, but it is possible to find some examples of this approach in the literature. Robertson and Cohn (1963) used it to investigate a four-compartment model for calcium metabolism and it was utilized by Cerasi and Anderson (1971) for the study of interrelationships between blood glucose and plasma insulin concentrations during glucose infusion. Kirschner et al. (1973) employed the analog computer for simulation of the blood and urine levels after multiple doses, independently varying the magnitude of doses and the time period between doses.

Curve-Fitting Using a Digital Computer

This method uses a digital computer program to carry out the necessary mathematical steps in minimizing the sum of square function (91) or (92). All procedures require initial estimates of x_i and λ_i for the values of the parameters, and, with an iterative method, these values can be modified until the sum of square (91) or (92) becomes minimal; the resulting final values of the parameters are thus the best estimates. The most important problem with this iterative method is that the initial estimates must be close to the final values if the calculation is to converge on a set of final parameters for which the sum of square function has a true minimum. The most suitable for obtaining the initial estimates is the preliminary use of graphical analysis. A number of digital computer programs are available for funding pharmacokinetic parameters and for simulating pharmacokinetic data. Among these are SAAM (Berman and Weiss, 1974), NONLIN (Metzler, 1969) and BMDX 85 (Dixon, 1973).

Comparison of Pharmacokinetic Models

In pharmacokinetic analysis, equations with different number of exponentials are sometimes used to fit the same experimental data. For this reason, it is important to define a method for comparing the different data or, even better, to find which equation provides a good interpretation of the experiment. To test whether or not the goodness-of-fit is improved with additional parameters Maudel (1964) has discussed the use of the F ratio test:

$$F = \frac{WSS_1 - WSS_2}{WSS_2} \times \frac{df_2}{df_1 - df_2} \quad (df_1 > df_2) \tag{104}$$

WSS_1 and WSS_2 are, respectively, the weighted sum of squared deviations obtained from the first and second models, df is the degree of freedom = number of the experimental data points minus the number of parameters.

The F ratio obtained may be compared to the critical value derived from a table where the numerator has $(df_1 - df_2)$ degrees of freedom and the denominator has df_2 degrees of freedom. In comparing the fit obtained from the two examples, with the NONLIN program it is evident that the weighted sum of squared deviations of the one-compartment model is $WSS_1 = 0.00402$, with $df_1 = 5$, and for the second model, $WSS_2 = 0.00447$, with $df_2 = 3$. It is important to remember that in these calculations the points have been weighted according to the formula (93). Using the formula (104),

$$F = \frac{0.00402 - 0.000447}{0.000447} \times \frac{3}{5 - 3} = 11.9899$$

and the F table for the corresponding degrees of freedom, we have F = 9.55 at 5%. Therefore, we can conclude that in this case the two-compartment model is better suited for our data, moreover, this is the obvious conclusion from simply comparing the fit of the two different graphs (Fig. 19).

CONCLUSIONS

The aim of this chapter was to illustrate in a relatively simple way some basic concepts of applied pharmacokinetics, which could be useful for interpreting and utilizing clinical data in a more rational way. This practical approach, which appears to be validated by the following chapters, needs to be extended. Only from a wider use of kinetic concepts at a clinical level will it be possible to derive constructive criticism, eventual validation of theoretical concepts and a more precise definition of its real meaning and impact for a more rational and safer therapy.

REFERENCES

Arnold, K. and Gerber, N. (1970): The rate of decline of diphenylhydantoin in human plasma. *Clinical Pharmacology and Therapeutics, 11:* 121-134.

Berman, M. and Weiss, M.F. (1974): *User's manual for SAAM,* Public Health Service, National Institute of Health, Bethesda.

Boxenbaum, H.G., Riegelman, S. and Elashoff, R.M. (1974): Statistical estimations in pharmacokinetics. *Journal of Pharmacokinetics and Biopharmaceutics, 2:* 123-148.

Boyes, R. N., Scott, D.B., Jebson, P.J., Godman, M.J. and Julian, D.G. (1971): Pharmacokinetics of lidocaine in man. *Clinical Pharmacology and Therapeutics, 12:* 105-116.

Brownlee, K.A. (1960): *Statistical Theory and Methodology in Science and Engineering,* pp. 306-307, Wiley, New York.

Cerasi, E. and Anderson, B. (1971): An analogue computer model for the insulin response to glucose infusion. *Simulation,* June, 243-255.

Daniel, C. and Wood, F.S. (1974): *Fitting Equations to Data,* Wiley-Interscience, New York.

Dixon, W.J. (173): *BMD Biomedical Computer Programs,* pp. 387-396, University of California Press.

Gennrich, R. (1969): Asymptotic procedures in nonlinear least square estimation. *Annals of Statistics, 40:* 633-643.

Gibaldi, M. (1969): Effect of mode of administration on drug distribution in a two-compartment open system. *Journal of Pharmaceutical Sciences, 58:* 327-331.

Gibaldi, M. (1971): Pharmacokinetic aspects of drug metabolism, *Annals of the New York Academy of Sciences, 179:* 19-31.
Gibaldi, M. Boyes, R.N. and Feldman, S. (1971): Influence of first-pass effect on availability of drugs on oral administration. *Journal of Pharmaceutical Sciences, 60:* 1338-1340.
Glass, H.I. and De Garreta, A.C. (1967): Quantitative analysis of exponential curve fitting for biological applications. *Physics Medical Biology, 12:* 379-388.
Kirschner, L., Simon, T.H. and Rasmussen, C.E. (1973): Analog computer program for simulating variable dosing regimens. *Journal of Pharmaceutical Sciences, 62:* 117-121.
Krüger-Thiemer, E. (1966): Formal theory of drug dosage regimens. I. *Journal of Theoretical Biology, 13:* 212.
Krüger-Thiemer, E. and Pelikan, E.W. (1968): Qualitative and quantitative definitions of drug accumulation. *Pharmacologist, 10:* 166.
Levy, G. and Gibaldi, M. (1975): Pharmacokinetics. In: *Handbook of Experimental Pharmacology*, V. 28, pt. 3, *Concepts in Biochemical Pharmacology*, edited by J.R. Gillette and J.R. Mitchell, pp. 1-34, Springer-Verlag, Berlin.
Levy, G., Tsuchiya, T. and Amsel, L.P. (1972): Limited capacity for salicyl phenolic glucuronide formation and its effect on the kinetics of salicylate elimination in man. *Clinical Pharmacology and Therapeutics, 13:* 258-268.
Lundquist, F. and Wolthers, H. (1958): The kinetics of alcohol elimination in man. *Acta Pharmacologica et Toxicologica, 14:* 265-289.
Martin, B.K. (1967): Drug urinary excretion data—some aspects concerning the interpretation. *British Journal of Pharmacology and Chemotherapy, 29:* 181-193.
Martis, L. and Levy, R.H. (1973): Bioavailability calculations for drugs showing simultaneous first-order and capacity-limited elimination kinetics. *Journal of Pharmacokinetics and Biopharmaceutics, 1:* 283-294.
Maudel, J. (1964): *The Statistical Analysis of Experimental Data*, Wiley-Interscience, New York.
Metzler, C.M. (1969): *A User's Manual for NONLIN Technical Report 7292/69/7292/005*, November 25, Upjohn Co., Kalamazoo, Michigan.
Myhill, J. (1967): Investigation of the effect of data error in the analysis of biological tracer data. *Biophysical Journal, 7:* 903.
Ottaway, J.H. (1973): Normalization in the fitting of data by iterative methods. *Biochemical Journal, 134:* 729-736.
Rescigno, A. and Segre, G. (1966): *Drug and Tracer Kinetics*, Blaisdell, Waltham.
Riegelman, S., Loo, J. and Rowland, M. (1968): Concept of a volume of distribution and possible errors in evaluation of this parameter. *Journal of Pharmaceutical Sciences, 57:* 128-133.
Riggs, D.S. (1963): *Mathematical Approach to Physiological Problems*, p. 209, Williams & Wilkins, Baltimore.
Robertson, J.S. and Cohn, S.H. (1963): Use of an analog computer in studies of strontium and calcium metabolism in man. *Annals of the New York Academy of Sciences, 108:* 122-127.
Rowland, M. (172a): Influence of route of administration on drug availability. *Journal of Pharmaceutical Sciences, 61:* 70-74.
Rowland, M. (1972b): Drug administration and regimens. In: *Clinical Pharmacology*, edited by K.L. Melmon and H.F. Morrelli, pp. 21-60, McMillan, New York.
Shand, D.G. and Rangno, R.E. (1972): The disposition of propranolol. I. Elimination during oral absorption in man. *Pharmacology* (Basel), *7:* 159-168.
Swintosky, J.V. (1957): Excretion equations for interpretation for digitoxin. *Nature* (London), *179:* 98-99.

Wagner, J.G. (1963): Some possible errors in the plotting and interpretation of semilogarithmic plots of blood level and urinary excretion data. *Journal of Pharmaceutical Sciences, 52:* 1097-1101.
Wagner, J.G. (1967a): Drug accumulation. *Journal of Clinical Pharmacology, 7:* 84-88.
Wagner, J.G. (1967b): Use of computers in pharmacokinetics. *Clinical Pharamacology and Therapuetics, 8:* 201-218.
Wagner, J.G. (1971): *Biopharmaceutics and Relevant Pharmacokinetics*, Drug Intelligence, Hamilton Hill.
Wagner, J.G. (1973): Properties of the Michaelis-Menten equation and its integrated form which are useful in pharmacokinetics. *Journal of Pharmacokinetics and Biopharmaceutics, 1:* 103-121.
Wagner, J.G. (1974a): A safe method for rapidly achieving plasma concentration plataus. *Clinical Pharmacology and Therapeutics, 16:* 691-700.
Wagner, J.G. (1974b): Loading and maintenance doses of digoxin in patients with normal renal function and those with severely impaired renal function. *Journal of Clinical Pharmacology, 15:* 329-338.
Wagner, J.G. and Metzler, C.M. (1967): Estimation of rate constants for absorption and elimination from blood concentration data. *Journal of Pharmaceutical Sciences, 56:* 658-659.
Wagner, J.G., Northam, J.I., Alway, C.D. and Carpenter, O.S. (1965): Blood levels of drug at the equilibrium state after multiple dosing. *Nature* (London), *207:* 1301-1302.
Westlake, W.J. (1971): Problems associated with analysis of pharmacokinetic models. *Journal of Pharmaceutical Sciences, 60:* 882-885.

2

Drug Absorption

PAOLO LUCIO MORSELLI

Absorption is a fundamental process by which drugs are delivered from their sites of administration into the bloodstream. In every instance (given by oral route, by rectal suppositories, intramuscularly, subcutaneously or topically), in order to reach the circulation, drugs have to cross barriers such as the cell lipoidal membranes and/or the endothelial walls. Such a crossing generally takes place by passive diffusion, according to a nonsaturable process in which the transfer is directly proportional to the concentration gradient and to the lipid/water partition coefficient of the drug. Even if structurally related, drugs are generally transferred independently, and at the level of passive diffusion they do not interfere with each other. Other mechanisms such as active transport, filtration through pores and pynocitosis play a very little role for most of the thereapeutic agents, with the exception of vitamines.

A detailed description of the various factors regulating and modifying drug absorption is not among the aims of this chapter (the reader may refer to the excellent reviews of Wagner, 1968; Levine, 1970; Schanker, 1971; Binns, 1971; Katz and Pulsen, 1971; Prescott, 1974). After a brief summary of the actual knowledge of the process, we will focus on the known and/or possible causes and conditions which may signficantly modify absorption of several drugs in the course of development. Examples taken from the literature and from our own experience will be brought to bear. The topic of drug absorption during development has never been studied or reviewed systematically, and most of the reports available refer to the first month of life. For infants and children, the data are very scarce when compared with those for adults, however, they do suggest that some important differences may be present at these ages.

ABSORPTION FROM THE ALIMENTARY TRACT

In order to be absorbed, a drug must be present in aqueous solution, at the surface of the cell membrane, preferably in a non-ionized form. This implies that physicochemical factors linked to the drug itself and to the pharmaceutical formulation, as well as anatomical and physiological variables such as status of the intestinal mucosa, gastric pH and gastric emptying time, and the presence of other agents or food material, play a very important role (Wagner, 1968; Levine, 1970; Schanker, 1971; Prescott, 1974). Acidic drugs are mostly ionized at pH over 5-6; the reverse holds true for basic compounds and vice versa. Since ionized drugs do not cross the biological membranes to any appreciable extent, it is understandable that the gastrointestinal pH conditioning the degree of ionization may considerably affect the rate of transfer (Schanker, 1971). However, although this general rule may be taken as a useful theoretical guideline *in vivo* in man, pH does not seem to be the most important determinant for the absorption rate. Dissolution rate of the administered form and gastric motility appear to be at least as important, as shown by several recent reports by Prescott (Prescott and Nimmo, 1971; Heading et al., 1973; Prescott, 1973, 1974, 1975).

Presence or absence of bile salts and modifications of gastrointestinal blood flow may also modify drug absorption of several compounds, interfering with gastric emptying, intestinal transit time and drug removal rate (Nightingale et al., 1971; Jusko et al., 1971; Diamond et al., 1970; Lundgren 1974; Crouthamel et al., 1975; Wilkinson, 1975).

The morphology and functions of the alimentary tract are not constant, varying almost continuously from birth till senescence (Smith, 1951; Bender, 1965; Yaffe and Yuchau, 1974; Miller and Holzel, 1974; Weber and Cohen, 1975). Such an ongoing modification may considerably affect the rate of absorption of several compounds. The most striking changes occur during the first month of life. After that time, there occurs a slow maturation toward the adult pattern, followed by a steady-state condition for about 20-25 years with a subsequent progressive reduction of secretions, motility and blood flow (Spencer, 1964; Bender, 1965; Weber and Cohen, 1975).

As said before, for simplicity we can assume that the two major factors regulating the gastrointestinal absorption of drugs are *pH-dependent diffusion* and *gastric emptying time*. In the neonate, these two physiological variables undergo continuous changes due to maturation and are remarkably different from those present in grown-up children and adults.

The gastric pH at birth is usually between 6 and 8 but within a few hours drops to values of 3 to 1. Subsequently, till the 8th-10th day of life, the acid secretion is greatly reduced or practically absent, with a condition of more or less relative achloridia. The acid secretion is closely related to the development of the gastric mucosa, and consequently, in premature newborns, the secretion of gastric acids is less than in full-term newborns. Adult values for gastric acidity are usually reached only after 3 years of age (Smith, 1951; Yaffe and Yuchau, 1974; Weber and Cohen, 1975).

The gastric emptying time in a neonate is considerably prolonged (up to 6-8 h) and approaches adult values only after 6-8 months. The peristalsis is very irregular, completely unpredictable and only practically dependent on the feeding habit (Smith, 1951).

Other factors which could play a role are the progressive bacterial growth, the gradual maturation of biliary function and the readjustment of the splanchnic circulation. It has, in fact, been shown that the intestinal microorganism may play a part in the metabolism of several compounds (Scheline, 1968), even if the extent to which they may act upon several compounds before absorption is not yet established. Diet and age have in any case a considerable influence on the nature of the gastrointestinal flora (Scheline, 1968, Weber and Cohen, 1975). The biliary function, although present, is not yet fully developed (Watkins et al., 1973; Murphy and Signer, 1974), and this may have some influence on the absorption as well as on the disposition pattern of drugs which undergo enterohepatic cycle after conjugation with glucuronic acid. In this respect, it may be worthwhile to remember that the β-glucoronidase activity in the newborn may be 7-fold the adult value (Kandall et al., 1973; Yaffe and Yuchau, 1974). Malabsorption syndromes are often associated with an increased deconjugation of bile acids in the small intestine, probably because of a small bowel contamination, and the steatorrhea encountered in premature and full-term newborns may also be related to the inadequate solubilization of fat in the duodenum due to the low bile acid secretion (Murphy and Signer, 1974).

ABSORPTION FROM INTRAMUSCULAR AND SUBCUTANEOUS INJECTIONS

The three main factors conditioning the rate of absorption of a drug administered in aqueous solution either subcutaneously or intramuscularly are: the ease of penetration through the endothelial capillary walls, the surface area over which the solution has spread, and the rate of blood flow through the area. As recently shown by several authors, the absorption rate and the amount absorbed may significantly change by using different muscles for injections (Meyer and Zelechowski, 1971; Reeves et al., 1974; Schwartz et al., 1974; Vukovich et al., 1975). The observed differences are clearly correlated with regional blood flow, which differs considerably among various muscles both at rest and during exercise (Evans et al., 1975; Wilkinson, 1975). As shown by Nora et al. (1964) for insulin and by Schwartz et al. (1974) for lidocaine, the different rates of absorption are not without significance as to the effectiveness of the drug.

In the neonate, the intramuscular absorption rate may change remarkably during the first days of life in relation to the maturational adaptation and changes in the relative blood flows of the various muscles. Additional variables may be the presence of hypoxic conditions and vasocostriction reactions to exposure to an unduly cold environment (Orzalesi, 1975). Furthermore, the skeletal muscle mass and the subcutaneous fat tissue are considerably reduced (about 25% of body weight) with a higher percentage of water (Widdowson, 1974). Finally, muscular contractions capable of increasing the dispension of the injected solutions are relatively inefficient. During further development, the relative proportion of subcutaneous fat to skeletal muscles undergoes marked changes. Up to the age of 7 years there is a tendency to put on fat, but subsequently the rate of increase of subcutaneous tissue slows down, while the muscular growth greatly increases in boys but not in girls (Widdowson, 1974; Marshall and Tanner, 1974). Sex differences in the intramuscular absorption probably related to different blood flows and absorptive surface have recently been described by Vukovich et al. (1975).

ABSORPTION FROM THE SKIN

Skin, unlike intestine, is designed to prevent absorption (Binns, 1971). The status of the skin, the vehicle in which the drug is dissolved and the drug itself are important variables. Hydration of the skin and rise in temperature usually greatly improve permeability. There are several indications that cutaneous absorption occurs more rapidly and to a greater extent in newborns and infants, probably because of the thinner stratum corneum and the higher degree of hydration (Widdowson, 1974). The permeability of the skin tends to reduce as age increases (Kopelman, 1973). The rate and extent of dermal absorption are without doubt causative factors in the toxicity of hexachlorophene and salicylic acid ointments in newborns and infants (Curle et al., 1971; Lockart, 1972; Kopelman, 1973; Stern, 1975; Wechselberg, 1968).

ABSORPTION IN NEWBORNS

On the basis of the previous considerations, a different bioavailability for drugs given either orally or intramuscularly is not surprising in the neonate. The possible differences are, however, not always in the same direction, and, depending on the physicochemical properties of the compounds and on the route of administration, there may be either an increased or a reduced absorption.

The relative achloridric condition of the first 6-8 days of life gives cause to the higher bioavailability of penicillin G, ampicillin and nafcillin observed in the neonate (Huang and High, 1953; O'Connor et al., 1965; Silverio and Pole, 1973).

On the contrary, Wallin et al. (1974) and Boreus et al. (1975) report that oral absorption of phenobarbital is not only delayed but also reduced in newborns up to 15 days, while the drug is efficiently and more rapidly absorbed if administered by intramuscular route (see Chapter 12). A delayed oral absorption in the newborn has been observed for nalidixic acid (Rohwedder et al., 1970), gentamicin (McCracken and Jones, 1970), diphenylhydantoin (Jalling et al, 1970), cephalexin (Boothman et al., 1973) and acetaminophen (Levy et al., 1975). A difference in the absorption rate of rifampicin between the 1st and 3rd day of life has been reported by Acocella et al. (1969). On the other hand, an oral absorption comparable to that observed in older children has been reported for various sulfonamides, phenylbutazone and cotrimoxazole (Fichter and Curtis, 1956; Gladtke, 1968; Krauer et al., 1968; Sereni et al, 1968, Dost and Gladtke, 1969; Brumfitt et al., 1973). An efficient absorption after oral administration has also been found for digoxin, while the compound is absorbed very slowly and in an unpredictable manner if it is administered by intramuscular route (Assael et al, 1974; Morselli, 1976). Reasons for the delayed and reduced absorption could be, in addition to the low relative blood flow often present in cardiopathic newborns, the tissue necrosis which may frequently be associated with digoxin intramuscular administration, as recently demonstrated by Steiness et al. (1974). A reduced absorption following intramuscular administration has also been described for colymycin in newborns on the 1st but not on the 3rd day of life (Muratore et al., 1967).

Diazepam is readily and efficiently absorbed after both oral and intramuscular administration (Morselli et al., 1973; Morselli, 1977) (see Chapter 14), provided that no extemporary dilutions with aqueous medium are performed. In such a case, a precipitation may occur, both within the syringe and at the injection site, and the following absorption may be very slow indeed (peak up to 6-8 h).

ABSORPTION IN INFANTS AND CHILDREN

The available data on drug disposition in infants and children, although considerably less numerous than those pertaining to newborns, suggest that in normal conditions absorption (following oral, rectal or intramuscular administration) is either comparable to or faster than that of adults.

A reduced absorption may be observed in some particular cases or conditions, as those reported for diphenylhydantoin by Jalling et al. (1970) in infants and by Borofsky et al. (1973) in one child. The compound, however, is generally efficiently absorbed in children if administered by oral route (see Chapter 12). Other examples of reduced absorption are those described by Marget (1971) in two infants with celiac disease, and by Elliot et al. (1964), who found an impaired absorption of ampicillin in children with diarrhea. At variance with these findings, the oral absorption of cotrimoxazole is not altered by gastroenteritis

(Lewin et al., 1973; Fowle et al., 1975; Marks, 1975), and Mehta et al. (1974) also reported normal absorption of chloramphenicol in P.C.M. syndromes. Two distinct patterns of absorption (prompt and delayed) for both nalidixic acid and ampicillin were found by Nelson et al. (1972) in infants and children suffering from acute shigellosis. The differences in absorption rate did not, however, seem to have any effect on the clinical response.

For many other drugs no differences were noticed in infants and children as compared with adults. Among these we may keep in mind salicylate and phenylbutazone (see Chapter 10), digoxin (see Chapter 13) and various sulfonamides and antibiotics (Gladtke, 1974; also Chapters 7 and 8). A clear trend toward faster absorption may be observed in infants and in children up to 10-13 years of age with several anticonvulsant drugs, such as ethosuximide, dipropylacetate, clonazepam and phenobarbital, following oral intake (see Chapter 11). Similarly, faster absorption may be observed in infants and children with diazepam administered by oral, intramuscular or rectal route (Marcucci et al., 1970; Garattini et al., 1973; Agurell et al., 1975; also Chapter 14).

In children Winsberg et al. (1974) invariable observed a very rapid absorption of imipramine, with peak levels reached within 2-4 hr. The rapidity of absorption, the greater proportion of the lean body mass and the reduced plasma protein-binding (observed for imipramine in children by the same authors) may favor higher drug concentration in the CNS, and partially account for the relatively early clinical response in children (Winsberg et al., 1974). For the same reason, and considering also the potential toxic cardiac effects of this class of drugs, the use of a single dose at bedtime should be discouraged.

CONCLUSIONS

Most of the reported studies were not designed or performed with the specific aim of evaluating absorption; the information which can be derived is in most cases indirect and must perforce be taken with a certain degree of caution. Despite these drawbacks, however, it does appear that, at least for some classes of compounds, absorption (especially gastrointestinal) may undergo significant modification with age. Whether these alterations are critical in regard to the therapeutic effect cannot be determined on the basis of the actual data.

The increased gastrointestinal absorption rate observed in children in the case of highly lipophilic compounds may be of some interest both for the reason described above and because it may very often be associated with a faster disappearance rate of the drug. These conditions would suggest that, at least in children, several divided doses during the day might be more rational than only one or two daily drug administrations.

On the basis of the information available it emerges that despite the large number of data on bioavailability and absorption in adults, our knowledge relative to infants and children, in various pathological conditions, is quite limited. Such a lack of knowledge stresses the importance of more observation and studies on the effect of age and its possible influences on therapuetic outcome.

REFERENCES

Acocella, G., Buniva, G., Flauto, U. and Nicolis, F.B. (1969): Absorption and elimination of the antibiotic rifampicin in newborns and children. In: *Progress in Antimicrobial and Anticancer Chemotherapy*, pp. 755-760, University of Tokyo.

Agurell, S., Berlin, A., Ferngren, H. and Hellström, B. (1975): Plasma levels of diazepam after parenteral and rectal administration in children. *Epilespia, 16:* 277-283.

Assael, B.M., Mandelli, M., Visconti, U., Marini, A., Sereni, F. and Morselli, P.F. (1974): Farmacocinetica della Digossina nel neonato e nel lattante. In: *Atti del Convergno di Studio sulla Digitale*, pp. 83-93, Boheringer, Milano.

Bender, A.D. (1965): The effect of increasing age on the distribution of peripheral blood flow in man. *Journal of the American Geriatric Society, 13:* 192-198.

Binns, T.B. (1971): The absorption of drugs from the alimentary tract, lungs and skin. *British Journal of Hospital Medicine, 6:* 133-142.

Boothman, R., Kerr, M.M., Marshall, M.J. and Burland, W.L. (1973): Absorption and excretion of cephalexin by the newborn infant. *Archives of Disease in Childhood, 48:* 147-150.

Boréus, L.O., Jalling, B. and Kallberg, N. (1975): Clinical pharmacology of phenobarbital in the neonatal period. In: *Basic and Therapeutic Aspects of the Perinatal Pharmacology*, edited by P.L. Morselli, S. Garattini and F. Sereni, pp. 331-340, Raven Press, New York.

Borofsky, L.G., Louis, S. and Kutt, H. (1973): Diphenylhydantoin in children (pharmacology and efficacy). *Neurology, 23:* 967-972.

Brumfitt, W., Hamilton-Miller, J.M.T. and Kosmidis, J. (1973); Trimethoprim-suflamethoxazole: the present position. *Journal of Infectious Diseases, 128*, suppl.: S778-S791.

Crouthamel, W.G., Diamond, L. Dittert, L.W. and Doluisio, J.T. (1975): Drug absorption, VII: Influence of mesenteric blood flow on intestinal drug absorption in dogs. *Journal of Pharmaceutical Sciences, 64:* 664-671.

Curley, A., Hawk, R.E., Kimbrough, R.D., Natheson, G. and Finberg, L. (1971): Dermal absorption of hexachlorophene in infants. *Lancet, 2:* 296-297.

Diamond, L., Doluisio, J.T. and Crouthamel, W.G. (1970): Physiological factors affecting intestinal drug absorption. *European Journal of Pharmacology, 11:* 109-114.

Dost, F.H. and Gladtke, E. (1969): Pharmakokinetik des 2-Sulfanilamido-3-methoxypyrazin beim kind (Elimination, entereale Absorption, Verteilung and Dosierung). *Arzneimittel-Forschung, 19:* 1304-1307.

Elliott, R.B., Stokes, E.J. and Maxwell, G.M. (1964): Ampicillin in paediatrics. *Archives of Disease in Childhood, 39:* 101-105.

Evans, E.F., Proctor, J.D., Fratkin, M.J., Velandia, J. and Wasserman, A.J. (1975): Blood flow in muscle groups and drug absorption. *Clinical Pharmacology and Therapeutics, 17:* 44-47.

Fichter, E.G. and Curtis, J.A. (1956): Sulfonamide administration in newborn and premature infants. *Pediatrics, 18:* 50-58.

Fowle, A.S.E., Bye, A., Hariri, F., Middlemiss, D. and Naficy, K. (1975): The dosage of Co-trimoxazole in childhood. *European Journal of Clinical Pharmacology, 8:* 217-222.

Garattini, S., Marcucci, F., Morselli, P.L. and Mussini, E. (1973): The significance of measuring blood levels of benzodiazepines. In: *Biological Effects of Drugs in Relation to Their*

Plasma Concentrations, edited by D.S. Davies and B.N.C. Prichard, pp. 211-255, MacMillan, London.

Gladtke, E. (1968): Pharmacokinetic studies of phenylbutazone in children. *Il Farmaco* (ed. sci.), *23:* 897-906.

Gladtke, E. (1974): Enteral absorption and renal excretion of drugs in relation to age. In: *Proceedings, XIV International Congress of Pediatrics*, Vol. 3, pp. 195-199, Editorial Medica Panamericana, Buenos Aires.

Heading, R.C., Nimmo, J., Prescott, L.F. and Tothill, P. (1973): The dependence of paracetamol absorption on the rate of gastric emptying. *British Journal of Pharmacology, 47:* 415-421.

Huang, N.N. and High, R.H. (1953): Comparison of serum levels following the administration of oral and parenteral preparations of penicillin to infants and children of various age groups. *Journal of Pediatrics, 42:* 657-668.

Jalling, B., Boréus, L.O., Rane, A. and Sjöqvist, F. (1970): Plasma concentrations of diphenylhydantoin in young infants. *Pharmacologia Clinica, 2:* 200-202.

Jusko, W.J., Levy, G., Yaffe, S.J. and Allen, J.E. (1971): Riboflavin absorption in children with biliary obstruction. *American Journal of Diseases of Children, 121:* 48-52.

Kandall, S.R., Thaler, M.M. and Erickson, R.P. (1973): Intestinal development of lysosomal and microsomal β-glucuronicase and bilirubin uridine diphosphoglucuronyl transferase in normal and jaundiced rats. *Journal of Pediatrics, 82:* 1013-1019.

Katz, M. and Poulsen, B.J. (1971): Absorption of drugs through the skin. In: *Handbook of Experimental Therapeutics*, V. 28, pt. 1, *Concepts in Biochemical Pharmacology*, edited by B.B. Brodie, J.R. Gillette and H.S. Ackerman, pp. 103-174, Springer-Verlag, Berlin.

Kopelman, A.E. (1973): Cutaneous absorption of hexachlorophene in low-birth-weight infants. *Journal of Pediatrics, 82:* 972-975.

Krauer, B., Spring, P. and Dettli, L. (1968): Zur pharmakokinetik der Sulfonamide im ersten Lebensjahr. *Pharmacologia Clinica, 1:* 47-53.

Levine, R.R. (1970): Factors affecting gastrointestinal absorption of drugs. *American Journal of Digestive Diseases, 15:* 171-188.

Levy, G., Kahanna, N.N., Soda, D.M., Tsuzuki, O. and Stern, L. (1975): Pharmacokinetics of acetaminophen in the human neonate: formation of acetaminophen glucuronide and sulfate in relation to plasma bilirubin concentration and D-glucaric acid excretion. *Pediatrics, 55:* 818-825.

Lewin, E.B., Klein, J.O. and Finland, M. (1973): Trimethoprim-sulfamethoxazole: absorption, excretion, and toxicity in six children. *Journal of Infectious Diseases, 128*, suppl.: 618-621.

Lockhart, J.D. (1972); How toxic is hexachlorophene? *Pediatrics, 50:* 229-235.

Lundgren, G. (1974): The circulation of the small bowel mucosa. *Gut, 15:* 1005-1013.

Marcucci, F., Mussini, E., Morselli, P.L., Garattini, S., Libretti, A. and Zaccala, M. (1970): Osservazioni sul metabolismo delle benzodiazepine nell 'uomo. In: *Atti II Riunione Nazionale della Società Italana di Neuropsicofarmacologia*, pp. 63-70, Arti Grafiche Pacini Mariotti, Pisa.

Marget, W. (1971): Special aspects of cephalosporin therapy in infants and children. *Postgraduate Medical Journal, 47*, suppl.: 54-57.

Marks, M.I. (1975): Pharmacokinetics and efficacy of trimethoprim-sulfamethoxazole in the treatment of gastroenteritis in children. *Canadian Medical Association Journal, 112:* 33S-34S.

Marshall, W.A. and Tanner, J.M. (1974): Puberty. In: *Scientific Foundations of Paediatrics*, edited by J.A. Davis and J. Dobbing, pp. 124-151, Heinemann W. Medical Book, London.

McCracken, G.H. and Jones, L.G. (1970): Gentamicin in the neonatal period. *American Journal of Diseases of Children, 120:* 524-533.

Mehta, S., Kalsi, H.K., Raman, J. and Mathur, V.S. (1974): Chloramphenicol metabolism in children with P.C.M. In: *Proceedings, XIV International Congress of Pediatrics*, Vol. 3, pp. 203-204. Editorial Medica Panamericana, Buenos Aires.
Meyer, M.B. and Zelechowski, K. (1971): Intramuscular lidocaine in normal subjects. In: *Lidocaine in the Treatment of Ventricular Arrhythmias*, edited by D.B. Scott and D.G. Julian, pp. 161-168, Livingstone, Edinburgh.
Miller, V. and Holzel, A. (1974): Growth and development of endodermal structures. In: *Scientific Foundations of Pediatrics*, edited by J.A. Davis and J. Dobbing, pp. 281-296, Heinemann W. Medical Book, London.
Morselli, P.L. (1977): Problemas de terapia en la edad pediatrica. In: *Avances en Terapeutica*, edited by J. Laporte and J.A. Salvà, Salvat, Barcelona, in press.
Morselli, P.L. (1976): Pediatric clinical pharmacology–routine monitoring for clinical trials? In: *Clinical Pharmacy and Clinical Pharmacology*, edited by Gouvera, Tognoni, and Van der Kleijn, North Holland Biomedial Publisher, pp. 279-284.
Morselli, P.D., Garattini, S. and Cohen, S. (eds.) (1974): *Drug Interactions*, Raven Press, New York.
Morselli, P.L., Principi, N., Tognoni, G., Reali, E., Belvedere, G., Standen, S.M. and Sereni, F. (1974³): Diazepam elimination in premature and full term infants and children. *Journal of Perinatal Medicine, 1:* 133-141.
Muratore, A., Colarizi, P. and Orzalesi, M. (1967): Assorbimento livelli ematici e modalità di eliminazione della colimicina nel neonato. *Minerva Nipiologica, 18:* 141-146.
Murphy, G.M. and Signer, E. (1974): Bile acid metabolism in infants and children. *Gut, 15:* 151-163.
Nelson, J.D., Shelton, S., Kusmiesz, H.T. and Haltalin, K.C. (1972): Absorption of ampicillin, and nalidixic acid by infants and children with acute shigellosis. *Clinical Pharmacology and Therapeutics, 13:* 879-886.
Nightingale, C.H., Axelson, J.E. and Gibaldi, M. (1971): Physiologic surface-active agents and drug absorption. VII. Effect of bile flow on sulfadiazine absorption in the rat. *Journal of Pharmaceutical Sciences, 60:* 145-147.
Nora, J.J., Smith, D.W. and Cameron, J.R. (1964): The route of insulin administration in the management of diabetes mellitus. *Journal of Pediatrics, 64:* 547-551.
O'Connor, W.J., Warren, G.H., Edrada, L.S., Mandala, P.S. and Rosenman, S.B. (1965): Serum concentrations of sodium nafcillin in infants during the perinatal period. *Antimicrobial Agents and Chemotherapy, 5:* 220-222.
Orzalesi, M. (1975): Problems of drug therapy in the newborn period. In: *Basic and Therapeutic Aspects of Perinatal Pharmacology*, edited by P.L. Morselli, S. Garattini and F. Sereni, pp. 13-20, Raven Press, New York.
Prescott, L.F. (1973): Variation in drug response due to disease. In: *International Aspects of Drug Evaluation and Usage*, edited by A.J. Jonhan and M.F. Grayson, Chruchill Livingstone, London.
Prescott, L.F. (1974): Drug absorption interactions–gastric emptying. In: *Drug Interactions*, edited by P.L. Morselli, S. Garattini and S.N. Cohen, pp. 11-20, Raven Press, New York.
Prescott, L.F. (1975): Pathological and physiological factors affecting drug absorption, distribution, elimination and response in man. In: *Handbook of Experimental Pharmacology*, V. 28, pt. III, *Concepts in Biochemical Pharmacology*, edited by J.R. Gillette and J.R. Mitchell, pp. 234-257, Springer-Verlag, Berlin.
Prescott, L.F. and Nimmo, J. (1971): Generic inequivalence–clinical observations. *Acta Pharmacologica Toxicologica, 29*, suppl. 3: 288-303.
Reeves, D.S., Bywater, M.J., Wise, R. and Whitmarsh, V.B. (1974): Availability of three antibiotics after intramuscular injection into thigh and buttock. *Lancet, 2:* 1421-1422.
Rohwedder, H.-J., Simon, C. Kübler, W. and Hohfnauer, M. (1974): Untersuchungen

über die Pharmakokinetik von Jalidixinsäure bei Kindern Verschiedenen Alters. *Zeitschrift für Kinderheikunde, 109:* 124-134.
Schanker, L.S. (1971): Drug absorption. In: *Fundamentals of Drug Metabolism and Drug Disposition,* edited by B.N. La Du, H.G. Mendel and E.L. Way, pp. 22-40, Williams & Wilkins, Baltimore.
Scheline, R.R. (1968): Drug metabolism of intestinal microorganisms. *Journal of Pharmaceutical Sciences, 57:* 2021-2037.
Schwartz, M.L., Meyer, M.B., Covino, B.G., Narang, R.M., Sethi, V., Schwartz, A.J. and Kamp, P. (1974): Antiarrhythmic effectiveness of intramuscular Lidocaine: influence of different injection sites. *Journal of Clinical Pharmacology, 14:* 77-83.
Sereni, F., Perletti, L., Marubini, E. and Mars, G. (1968): Pharmacokinetic studies with a long-acting sulfonamide in subjects of different ages. *Pediatrics Research, 2:* 29-37.
Silverio, J. and Poole, J.W. (1973): Serum concentrations of ampicillin in newborn infants after oral administration. *Pediatrics, 57:* 578-580.
Smith, C.A. (1951): *The Physiology of the Newborn Infant.* 2nd ed., pp. 180-198, C.C. Thomas, Springfield.
Spencer, R.P. (1964): Variation of intestinal activity with age: a review. *Yale Journal of Biology and Medicine, 37:* 105-129.
Steiness, E., Svendsen, D. and Rasmussen, F. (1974): Plasma digoxin after parenteral administration local reaction after intramuscular injection. *Clinical Pharmacology and Therapeutics, 16:* 430-434.
Stern, L. (1975): Drug therapy in the perinatal period. In: *Basic and Therapeutic Aspects of Perinatal Pharmacology,* edited by P.L. Morselli, S. Garattini and F. Sereni, pp. 7-12, Raven Press, New York.
Vukovich, R.A., Brannick, L.J., Sugerman, A.A. and Neiss, E.S. (1975): Sex differences in the intramuscular absorption and bioavailability of cephradine. *Clinical Pharmacology and Therapeutics 18:* 215-220.
Wagner, J. (1968): Biopharmaceutics influence of formulation on therapeutic activity. 1. Definition, scope and relationship to gastrointestinal physiology. *Drug Intelligence, 2:* 30-34.
Wallin, A., Jalling, B. and Boréus, L.O. (1974): Plasma concentrations of phenobarbital in the neonate during prophylaxis for neonatal hyperbilirubinemia. *Journal of Pediatrics, 85:* 392-397.
Watkins, J.B., Ingall, D., Szczepanik, P., Klein, P.D. and Lester, R. (1973): Bile-salt metabolism in the newborn. Measurement of pool size and synthesis by stable isotope technique. *New England Journal of Medicine, 288:* 431-434.
Weber, W.W. and Cohen, S.N. (1975): Aging effects and drugs in man. In: *Handbook of Experimental Pharmacology,* V. 28, pt. 3, *Concepts in Biochemical Pharmacology,* edited by J.R. Gillette and J.R. Mitchell, pp. 213-233, Springer-Verlag, Berlin.
Wechselberg, K. (1968): Salizylsäure-Vergiftung durch perkutane resorption 1% iger Salizylvaseline. *Pädiatrische Praxis, 7:* 431-433.
Widdowson, E.M. (1974): Changes in body proportions and composition during growth. In: *Scientific Foundations of Pediatrics,* edited by J.A. Davis and J. Dobbing, pp. 153-163, Heinemann W. Medical Book, London.
Wilkinson, G.R. (1975): Pharmacokinetics of drug disposition. Hemodynamic considerations. *Annual Review of Pharmacology, 15:* 11-27.
Yaffe, S.J. and Juchau, M.R. (1974): Perinatal pharmacology. *Annual Review of Pharmacology, 14:* 219-238.

3

Drug Plasma Protein – Binding and Distribution

PAOLO LUCIO MORSELLI

The time of onset, the intensity and the duration of the effects of any drug depend not only on its absorption and elimination, but also on its distribution kinetics in the various tissues and body compartments (Goldstein et al., 1968; Butler, 1971; Keen, 1971). The size of body water compartments and adipose tissue depots, the cardiac output, the regional blood flow, the organ perfusion pressure, the permeability of cell membranes, the acid-base balance and the degree of binding to plasma and tissue proteins are all physical variables whose modification can significantly alter the distribution of many drugs in the body and hence their effects. Each of these factors may vary substantially during development and may condition changes in drug distribution.

Despite the importance of these factors for the drug effect, the information relative to drug distribution and drug protein-binding in course of development is rather scarce. Most of the data refer, in fact, to the perinatal period, whereas for infants and children reports are very few indeed. On the basis of the available data, we will consider two main aspects: variation of body compartments and plasma protein-binding.

BODY COMPARTMENTS

The newborn is characterized by a very high content in total body water and a low fat content. The amount of total body water ranges from 70% to 78% of body weight in the full-term newborn, and it may be as high as 85% in the premature. After birth there is a progressive decrease, with a concomitant increase in fat, adult values (60-58%) being reached at about 12 months. Extracellular water is also very high at birth (45-47%), then drops to 27-25% after 12-14 months and reaches adult values (17%) at the 10th-15th year. On the contrary, the intracellular water, low at birth (32-34%), rises gradually to 43% at 3 months, drops again between 1 and 2 years and stabilizes around a value of 40-41% after 3-5 years (Edelman et al., 1952; Früs-Hansen, 1956, 1961; Yaffe and Yuchau, 1974; Widdowson, 1974; Weber and Cohen, 1975). The percentage of fat is about 16% of body weight at birth, rises to 22-24% within the first 3-12 months, falls to 8-12% over the next 4 years, then rises to 18% at 10-11 years in boys, and further in girls (Widdowson, 1974).

It is understandable that since drugs are distributed between extracellular water and depot fat according to their lipid/water partition coefficient, the relative variations of these two body compartments may influence a different drug distribution according to the physicochemical properties of each single drug. Additional factors may be the relative acidosis present in newborns, and the progressive changes in hemodynamics with a regular constant increase of organ perfusion pressures and changes in regional blood flows (Payne, 1974; Shinebourne, 1974; Houston and Oetliker, 1974).

PLASMA PROTEIN-BINDING

Drug-binding to plasma proteins is a reversible interaction between a small molecule (the drug) and a macromolecule (the protein) where the degree and the extent of the interaction depends on several factors such as the type and the amount of binding protein, the type and amount of drug, the affinity constant of the drug for the protein and the eventual presence of other substances and/or physiopathological conditions capable of modifying the drug/protein interaction (Meyer and Gutman, 1968; Goldstein et al., 1968; Keen, 1971; Settle et al., 1971; Solomon, 1971; Davison, 1972; Reidenberg and Affrime, 1973; Anton, 1973).

In the newborn, a decreased plasma protein-binding has been well documented for several drugs. Such a reduced binding is due to the concurrent presence of several causes capable of modifying the drug/protein interaction. Although plasma albumin is present at concentrations equivalent to those found in adults, it is different qualitatively and the total protein content is markedly lower (5-6 g/100 ml than in grown-up children and adults, mainly for the low gamma globulin levels, which further drops in the first 2 months and reach adult values only between 7 and 12 years of age (Gitlin and Boesman, 1966; Miyoshi et al., 1966; Allansmith et al., 1968; Hyvarinen et al., 1973; Weber and Cohen, 1975). Total plasma proteins reach values equivalent to those in adults at about

10-12 months (Ecobichon and Stephens, 1973; Windorfer et al., 1974). In addition to the lower protein content, other factors capable of altering the binding in the neonate are the presence of fetal ablumin (which shows a lower affinity for drugs), high concentration of bilirubin and free fatty acids, other endogenous competing substances and a lower blood pH (Miyoshi et al., 1966; Odel, 1973; Spector et al., 1973; Krasner et al., 1973; Gugler et al., 1974; Windorfer et al., 1974; Kapitulnick et al., 1975, Levy, 1975). Still another factor which may play a significant role in drug distribution and disposition in the newborn is the relative or absolute absence at birth, in the neonatal liver, of the Y protein (Levi et al., 1970; Litwack et al., 1971; Weber and Cohen, 1975). There are today evidences that Y protein is the major anion-binding protein (see Chapter 4), and according to Kunin et al. (1973) several antibiotics bind to such a protein.

Plasma Protein-Binding and Apparent Volume of Distribution in the Newborn

As said before, while the plasma protein-binding is in most instances reduced, the apparent volume of distribution may be either increased or decreased, depending on the relative lipid solubility of the molecule and the relative ratio between extracellular water and adipose tissue. Several authors have reported a reduce salicylate plasma protein-binding in the newborn (Berhman and Battaglia, 1967; Ganshorn and Kurz, 1968; Palmisano and Cassady, 1969; Krasner et al., 1973; Windorfer et al., 1974). In premature newborns, the binding is even lower than in full-term infants, and in both, as in children and adults, the free fraction increases by increasing the plasma concentration (Krasner et al., 1973; Windorfer et al., 1974; Levy and Yaffe, 1974). Krasner and Yaffe, (1975) have observed in newborns a reduced association constant (1.7 x 10^5 M^{-1} against 4 x 10^5 M^{-1}) and have hypothesized that this may be due to the presence of dialyzable factors capable of diminishing the proteins' affinity for salicylate. A different binding affinity has also been hypothesized by Windorfer et al. (1974). This is in agreement with the fact that salicylate levels over 2-3 mg/100 ml may reduce the mean reserve albumin-binding capacity (Palmisano and Cassady. 1969) and concentration over 10 mg/100 ml may double the free fraction of bilirubin in newborns' plasma (Øie and Levy, 1975). Because of the elevated association constant of bilirubin (10^7 M^{-1}), the phenomenon can only be explained assuming the presence of other mechanisms capable of modifying the affinity of albumin for bilirubin. In this respect, it has to be remembered that an elevated concentration of FFA is capable of modifying the salicylate effect on bilirubin (Odell, 1973). Because of the reduced binding and the higher extracellular fluid volume, the apparent volume of distribution of salicylate in the neonate is higher than that observed for similar concentrations in grown-up children and adults (EArle, 1961; Levy and Garrettson, 1974; Garrettson et al., 1975) (see Chapter 10). Furthermore, the relative hypoxemia and the lower blood pH may contribute to increasing salicylate tissue levels and hence the toxic risk. At variance with what is currently thought, and in agreement with a previous report of Crawford and Hooi (1968), Levy et al. (1975) have recently observed that salicylate binding in neonatal plasma is appreciably higher than in maternal plasma. Reasons for such a finding are very probably the reduced albumin plasma concentration in the last month of pregnancy together with an elevated total lipid plasma level (Reboud et al., 1963, Bobok et al., 1974). These observations, however, are not applicable to all drugs, since bupivacaine (Tucker et al., 1970) and diazepam (Kanto et al., 1974) are less bound to umbilical cord plasma than to the corresponding maternal plasma.

An increased volume of distribution in the neonate clearly related to decreased binding to plasma proteins has been described for phenylbutazone (Gladtke, 1968) and phenobarbital (Boreus et al., 1975). The free fraction of phenobarbital, already high (60-64%) in normobilirubinemic newborns, may be as high as 72% in hyperbilirubinemia (Ganshorn and Kurz, 1968; Ernhebo et al., 1971). Similarly, the free fraction of diphenylhydantoin seems to be strictly related to the total bilirubin concentration and to the FFA levels (Ernhebo et al., 1971; Rane et al., 1971; Fredholm et al., 1975). In good agreement with these observations, an increased volume of distribution of diphenylhydantoin in the neonate has been reported by Rane (1974), while an increased red blood cell/plasma ratio in the newborn (0.84 vs. 0.78 in adults) has been described by Borondy et al. (1973).

An increased digoxin red blood cell/plasma ratio associated with a lower binding to cord serum has been found by Gorodischer et al. (1974), and digoxin myocardial and skeletal muscle concentrations higher than those found in children and adults have been described in 5 newborns by Kim et al. (1974). Recently, we could observe in 3 prematures and 2 full-term newborns an apparent volume of distribution similar to that found in adults but lower than that computed in infants and children (Morselli et al., 1977).

Other drugs for which a decreased plasma protein-binding has been described in newborns are sulphaphenazol (Chignell et al., 1971), sulfamethoxine and sulfamethoxydiazine (Ganshorn and Kurz, 1968), sulfamethoxypyrazine (Sereni et al., 1968), benzylpenicillin and ampicillin (Ernhebo et al., 1971), nafcillin (Krasner et al., 1973), imipramine (Pruitt and Dayton, 1971), desmethylimipramine (Rane et al., 1971) and pentobarbital (Short et al., 1975).

At variance with what has been observed for salicylate, Krasner and Yaffe (1975) could not ascertain any difference between cord serum and adult serum in the diazepam binding properties. In agreement with this, the reduced adipose tissue in the newborn and the drug's very high lipid solubility would account for the tendency of the apparent volume of distribution of diazepam in neonates, both premature and full-term, to be rather lower than that computed in adults (Morselli, 1977).

Plasma Protein-Binding and Apparent Volume of Distribution in Infants and Children

Few data are available on these two physiological variables in infants and children. As a general rule, it may be said that there is a progressive tendency toward a decreased volume of distribution with increasing age. This happens for most of the drugs cited in the previous paragraphs. A different behavior with an increased apparent volume of distribution in infants and children up to 5 years has been observed for digoxin (Morselli et al., 1975) and diazepam (Morselli, 1977). Although specific studies are lacking, it seems from recent reports that drug plasma protein-binding reaches adult values at about 12-14 months of age (Ecobichon and Stephens, 1973, Windorfer et al., 1974). However, Winsberg et al. (1974) described attainment of adult values for imipramine plasma protein-binding at only 10-13 years. A decreased binding of salicylic acid in children with Down's syndrome has been reported by Ebady and Kugel (1970).

CONCLUSIONS

Important changes in apparent volume of distribution and plasma protein-binding may occur for several drugs in the perinatal period. Such differences seem to be fewer in infants and children. Even without specific data, it is understood that, as in adults (Prescott, 1973, 1975), pathological situations such as kidney and liver diseases, as well as cardiac failure and malabsorption syndromes, can condition reduced binding and/or altered volume of distribution.

From a practical point of view, the reduced plasma protein-binding and the consequent increase in the apparent volume of distribution observed with several drugs in newborns, along with the possible interactions which may occur between drugs and endogenous substrates, may have very important reflections and consequences relative to the therapeutic and/or toxic effects. It has also to be remembered that because of expanded volume of distribution, a given plasma level in the newborn may reflect a plasma/tissue ratio higher than that in adults, with a greater amount of drug in the body tissues than the same plasma concentration would indicate in older children and adults.

Finally, it is worthwhile to remember, once again, that highly bound drugs such as sulfonamide, salicylate and diphenylhydantoin are capable of displacing bilirubin from plasma albumin, leading to toxic bilirubin concentrations in brain of susceptible infants (Silverman et al., 1956; Odel, 1959; Schiff et al., 1971; Stern, 1972; Anton, 1973). On the contrary, the *in vitro* displacing effect of injectable formulas of caffeine and diazepam, has been shown to be due not to the two drugs but to the sodium benzoate contained in the preparation (Krasner, 1973; Adoni et al., 1973), and its occurrence *in vivo* appears very unlikely.

REFERENCES

Adoni, A., Kaptulnik, J., Kaufmann, N.A., Ron, M. and Bondheim, S.H. (1973): Effect of maternal administration of diazepam on the bilirubin-binding capacity of cord blood serum. *American Journal of Obstetrics and Gynecology, 115:* 577-579.

Allansmith, M., McClellan, B.H., Butterworth, M. and Maloney, J.R. (1968): The development of immunoglobin levels in man. *Journal of Pediatrics, 72:* 276-290.

Anton, A.H. (1973): Increasing activity of sulfonamides with displacing agents: a review. *Annals of the New York Academy of Sciences, 226:* 273-292.

Behrman, R.E. and Battaglia, F.C. (1967): Protein binding of human fetal and maternal plasmas to salicylate. *Journal of Applied Physiology, 22:* 125-130.

Bobok, I., Czákó, G., Csernyánsky, H. and Ludmany, K. (1974): Lipoids in maternal cord and newborn cord serum. *Acta Paediatrica Academiae Scientiarum Hungaricae, 15:* 95-100.

Boréus, L.O., Jalling, B. and Kallberg, N. (1975): Clinical pharmacology of phenobarbital in the neonatal period. In: *Basic and Therapeutic Aspects of Perinatal Pharmacology,* edited by P.L. Morselli, S. Garattini and F. Sereni, pp. 331-340, Raven Press, New York.

Borondy, P., Dill, W.A., Chang, T., Buchanan, R.A. and Glazko, A.J. (1973): Effect of protein binding on the distribution of 5,5-diphenyldantoin between plasma and red cells. *Annals of the New York Academy of Sciences, 226:* 82-87.

Butler, T.C. (1971): The distribution of drugs. In: *Fundamentals of Drug Metabolism and Drug Disposition,* edited by B.N. La Du, H.G. Mandel and E.L. Way, pp. 44-62, Williams & Wilkins, Baltimore.

Chignell, C.F., Vesell, E.S., Starkweather, D.K. and Berlin, C.M. (1971): The binding of sulfaphenazole to fetal-neonatal and adult human plasma albumin. *Clinical Pharmacology and Therapeutics, 12:* 897-901.

Crawford, J.S. and Hooi, H.W.Y. (1968): Binding of salicyclic acid and sulphanilamide in serum from pregnant patients, cord blood and subjects taking oral contraceptives. *British Journal of Anaesthesiology, 40:* 825-833.

Davison, C. (1971): Protein binding. In: *Fundamentals of Drug Metabolism and Drug Disposition,* edited by B.N. La Du, H.G. Mandell and E.L. Way, pp. 63-75, Williams & Wilkins, Baltimore.

Earle, R., Jr. (1961): Congenital salicylate intoxication. Report of a case. *Medical Intelligence, 265:* 1003-1004.

Ebadi, M.S. and Kugel, R.B. (1970): Alteration in metabolism of acetylsalicylic acid in children with Down's syndrome. Decreased plasma binding and formation of salicyluric acid. *Pediatrics Research, 4:* 187-193.

Ecobichon, D.J. and Stephens, D.S. (1973): Perinatal development of human blood esterases. *Clinical Pharmacology and Therapeutics, 14:* 11-17.

Edelman, I.S., Haley, H.B., Schloerb, P.R., Sheldon, D.B., Früs-Hansen, B.J., Stoll, G. and Moore, F.D. (1952): Further observations on total body water. I. *Surgery, Gynecology and Obstetrics, 95:* 1-12.

Ehrnebo, M., Agurell, S., Jalling, B. and Boréus, L.O. (1971): Age differences in drug binding by plasma proteins: studies on human foetuses, neonates and adults. *European Journal of Clinical Pharmacology, 3:* 189-193.

Fredholm, B.B., Rane, A. and Persson, B. (1975): Diphenylhydantoin binding to proteins in plasma and its dependence on free fatty acid and bilirubin concentration in dogs and newborn infants. *Pediatrics Research 9:* 96-130.

Früs-Hansen, B. (1956): Changes in body water compartments during growth. *Acta Paediatrica, 110,* supl. 46.

Früs-Hansen, B. (1961): Body water compartments in children: changes during growth and related changes in body composition. *Pediatrics, 28:* 169-181.
Ganshorn, A. and Kurz, H. (1968): Unterschiede zwischen der Proteinbindung Neugeborener and Erwachsener und ihre Bedeutung für die pharmakologische Wirkung. *Naunyn-Schmiedebergs Archiv für Pharmakologie und Experimentelle Pathologie, 260:* 117-118.
Garrettson, L.K., Procknal, J.A. and Levy, G. (1975): Fetal acquisition and neonatal elimination of a large amount of salicylate. *Clinical Pharmacology and Therapeutics, 17:* 98-103.
Gitlin, D. and Boesman, M. (1966): Serum α-fetoprotein, ablumin and λ-globulin in the human concepts. *Journal of Clinical Investigation 45:* 1826-1838.
Gladtke, E. (1968): Pharmacokinetic studies on phenylbutazone in children. *Il Farmaco* (ed. sci), *23:* 897-906.
Goldstein, A., Aronow, L. and Kalman, S.M. (1968): *Principles of Drug Action: The Basis of Pharmacology*, J. Wiley & Sons, New York.
Gorodischer, R., Krasner, J. and Jaffe, S.J. (1974): Serum protein binding of digoxin in newborn infants. *Research Communications in Chemical Pathology and Pharmacology, 9:* 387-390.
Gugler, R., Shoeman, D.W. and Azarnoff, D.L. (1974): Effect of in vivo elevation of free fatty acids on protein binding of drugs. *Pharmacology, 12:* 160-165.
Houston, I.B. and Oetliker, O. (1974): The growth and the development of the kidneys. In: *Scientific Foundations of Pediatrics*, Ch. 7, pp. 297, edited by J.A. Davis and J. Dobbing, Heinemann W. Medical Book, London.
Hyvarinen, M., Zeltzer, P., Oh, W. and Stiehm, E.R. (1973): Influence of gestational age on serum levels of α-1-fetoprotein, IgG globulin and albumin in newborn infants. *Journal of Pediatrics, 82:* 430-437.
Kanto, J., Erkkola, R. and Sellman, R. (1974): Perinatal metabolism of diazepam. *British Medical Journal, 1:* 641-642.
Kapitulnik, J., Horner-Mibashan, R., Blondheim, S.H., Kaufmann, N.A. and Russel, A. (1975): Increase in bilirubin-binding affinity of serum with age of infant. *Journal of Pediatrics, 86:* 442-445.
Keen, P. (1971): Effect of binding to plasma proteins on the distribution, activity and elimination of drugs. In: *Handbook of Experimental Pharmacology*, V. 28, pt. 1, *Concepts in Biochemical Pharmacology*, edited by B. B. Brodie, H.S. Gillette and H.S. Ackerman, pp. 213-233, Springer-Verlag, Berlin.
Kim, P.W., Yanagi, R., Jrasula, R.W., Soyka, L.F., Levitsky, S. and Hastreiter, A.R. (1974): Post-mortem digoxin concentration in infants. In: *Proceedings, 47th Scientific Session*, American Heart Association, Nov. 18-21, Dallas, Texas.
Krasner, J. (1973): Fluorescent properties of bovine serum ablumin-bilirubin complex, *Biochemical Medicine, 7:* 135-144.
Krasner, J. and Yaffe, S.J. (1975): Drug-protein binding in the neonate. In: *Basic and Therapeutic Aspects of Perinatal Pharmacology*, edited by P.L. Morselli, S. Garattini and F. Sereni, pp. 357-366, Raven Press, New York.
Krasner, J., Giacoia, G.P. and Yaffe, S.J. (1973): Drug-protein binding in the newborn infant. *Annals of the New York Academy of Sciences, 226:* 101-114.
Kunin, C.M., Craig, W.A., Kornguth, M. and Monson, R. (1973): Influence of binding on the pharmacologic activity of antibiotics. *Annals of the New York Academy of Sciences, 226:* 214-224.
Levi, A.J., Gatmaitan, Z. and Arias, I.M. (1970): Deficiency of hepatic organic anion binding protein, impaired organic anion uptake by liver and physiologic jaundice in newborn monkeys. *New England Journal of Medicine, 283:* 1136-1139.

Levy, G. (1975): Salicylate pharmacokinetics in the human neonate. In: *Basic and Therapeutic Aspects of Perinatal Pharmacology*, edited by P.L. Morselli, S. Garattini and F. Sereni, pp. 319-330, Raven Press, New York.
Levy, G. and Garrettson, L.K. (1974): Kinetics of salicylate elimination by newborn infants of mothers who ingested aspirin before delivery. *Pediatrics, 53:* 201-210.
Levy, G., Procknal, J.A. and Garretson, L.K. (1975): Distribution of salicylate between neonatal and maternal serum at diffusion equilibrium. *Clinical Pharmacology and Therapeutics, 18:* 210-214.
Levy, G. and Yaffe, S.J. (1974): Relationship between dose and apparent volume of distribution of salicylate in children. *Pediatrics, 54:* 713-717.
Litwack, G., Ketterer, B. and Arias, I.M. (1971): Ligandin: a hepatic protein which binds steroids bilirubin, carcinogens and a number of exogenous organic anions. *Nature, 234:* 466-467.
Meyer, M.C. and Guttman, D.E. (1968): The binding of drugs by plasma proteins. *Journal of Pharmaceutical Sciences, 57:* 895-918.
Miyoshi, K., Saijo, K., Kotani, Y., Kashiwagi, T. and Kawai, H. (1966): Characteristic properties of fetal human albumin (Alb. F) in isomerization equilibrium. *Tokushima Journal of Experimental Medicine, 13:* 121-132.
Morselli, P.O. (1977): Problemas de terapia en la edad pediatrica. In: *Avances en Terapetuica*, edited by J. Laporte and J.A. Salvà, Slavat, Barcelona, in press.
Morselli, P.L., Assael, B.M., Gomeni, R., Mandelli, M., Marini, A. Reali, E., Visconti, U. and Sereni, F. (1975): Digoxin pharmacokinetics during human development. In *Basic and Therapeutic Aspects of the Perinatal Pharmacology*, edited by P.L. Morselli, S. Garattini and F. Sereni, pp. 377-392, Raven Press, New York.
Odell, G.B. (1959): Studies in kernicterus. I. The protein binding of bilirubin. *Journal of Clinical Investigation, 38:* 823.
Odell, G.B. (1973): Influence of binding on the toxicity of bilirubin. *Annals of the New York Academy of Sciences, 226:* 225-237.
Øie, S. and Levy, G. (1975): Effect of certain drugs and drug metabolites on bilirubin binding in albumin solution and in plasma of newborns and adults, in press.
Palmisano, P.A. and Cassady, G. (1969): Salicylate exposure in the perinate. *Journal of the American Medical Association, 209:* 556-558.
Payne, W.W. (1974): Biochemical adaptations at birth. In: *Scientific Foundations of Pediatrics*, edited by J.A. Davis and J. Dobbing, Ch. 8, pp. 86-94, Heinemann W. Medical Book, London.
Prescott, L.F. (1973): Variation in drug response due to disease. In: *International Aspects of Drug Evaluation and Usage*, edited by A.J. Jonhan and M.F. Grayson, Churchill Livingstone, London.
Prescott, L.F. (1975): Pathological and physiological factors affecting drug absorption, distribution, elimination and response in man. In: *Handbook of Experimental Pharmacology*, V. 28, pt. III, *Concepts in Biochemical Pharmacology*, edited by J.R. Gillette and J.R. Mitchell, pp. 234-257, Springer-Verlag, Berlin.
Pruitt, A.W. and Dayton, P.G. (1971): A comparison of the binding of drugs to adult and cord plasma. *European Journal of Clinical Pharmacology, 4:* 59-62.
Rane, A. (1974): Urinary excretion of diphenylhydantoin metabolites in newborn infants. *Journal of Pediatrics, 85:* 543-545.
Rane, A., Lunde, P.K.M., Jalling, B., Yaffe, S.J. and Sjöqvist, F. (1971): Plasma protein binding of diphenylhydantoin in normal and hyperbilirubinemic infants. *Journal of Pediatrics, 78:* 877-882.
Reboud, P., Groulade, J., Groslambert, P. and Colomb, M. (1963): The influence of normal pregnancy and the post partum state on plasma proteins and lipids. *American Journal of Obstetrics and Gynecology, 86:* 820-828.

Reidenberg, M.M. and Affrime, M. (1973): Influence of disease on binding of drugs to plasma proteins. *Annals of the New York Academy of Science, 226:* 115-126.
Schiff, D. Chan, G. and Stern, L. (1971): Fixed drug combinations and the displacement of bilirubin from albumin. *Pediatrics, 48:* 139-141.
Sereni, F., Perletti, L., Marubini, E. and Mars, G. (1968): Pharmacokinetic studies with a long-acting sulfonamide in subjects of different ages. *Pediatric Research, 2:* 29-37.
Settle, W., Hegeman, S. and Featherstone, R.M. (1971): The nature of drug-protein interaction. In: *Handbook of Experimental Pharmacology*, V. 28, pt. I, *Concepts in Biochemical Pharmacology*, edited by B. B. Brodie, J.R. Gillette and H.S. Ackerman, pp. 175-186, Springer-Verlag, Berlin.
Shinebourne, E.A. (1974): Growth and development of the cardiovascular system. Functional development. In: *Scientific Foundations of Pediatrics*, Ch. 13b, pp. 198-213, edited by J.A. Davis and J. Dobbing, Heinemann W. Medical Book, London.
Short, C.R., Sexton, R.L. and McFarland, I. (1975): Binding of ^{14}C-salicylic acid and ^{14}O-pentobarbital to plasma proteins of several species during the perinatal period *Biology of the Neonate, 26:* 58-66.
Silverman, W.A., Anderson, D.H., Blanc, W.A. and Crozier, D.N. (1956): A difference in mortality rate and incidence of kernicterus among premature infants allotted to two prophylactic antibacterial regimens. *Pediatrics, 18:* 614-621.
Solomon, H.M. (1971): Competition between drugs and normal substrates for plasma and tissue binding sites. In: *Handbook of Experimental Pharmacology*, V. 28, pt. I, *Concepts in Biochemical Pharmacology*, edited by B.B. Brodie, J.R. Gillette, and H.S. Ackerman, pp. 234-239, Springer-Verlag, Berlin.
Spector, A.A., Santos, E.C., Ashbrook, J.D. and Fletcher, J.E. (1973): Influence of free fatty acid concentration on drug binding to plasma albumin. *Annals of the New York Academy of Sciences, 226:* 247-258.
Stern, L. (1972): Drug interaction. II. Drugs, the newborn infants and the binding of bilirubin to albumin. *Pediatrics, 49:* 916-918.
Tucker, G.T., Boyes, R.N. and Bridenbaugh, P.O. (1970): Binding of anilide-type local anesthetics in human plasma. II. Implications in vivo, with special reference to transplacental distribution. *Anesthesiology, 33:* 304-314.
Weber, W.W. and Cohen, S.N. (1975): Aging effects and drugs in man. In: *Handbook of Experimental Pharmacology*, V. 28, pt. 3, *Concepts in Biochemical Pharmacology*, edited by J.R. Gillette and J.R. Mitchell, pp. 213-233, Springer-Verlag, Berlin.
Widdowson, E.M. (1974): Changes in body proportions and composition during growth. In: *Scientific Foundations of Pediatrics*, Ch. 12, p. 153, edited by J.A. Davis and J. Dobbing, Heinemann W. Medical Book, London.
Windorfer, A., Jr., Kuenzer, W. and Urbanek, R. (1974): The influence of age on the activity of acetylsalicylic acid-enterase and protein salicylate binding. *European Journal of Clinical Pharmacology, 7:* 227-231.
Winsberg, B.G., Perel, J.M. Hurwic, M.J. and Klutch, A. (1974): Imipramine protein binding and pharmacokinetics in children. In: *The Phenothiazines and Structurally Related Drugs*, edited by I.S. Forrest, C.J. Carr and E. Usdin, pp. 425-431, Raven Press, New York.
Yaffe, S.J. and Juchau, M.R. (1974): Perinatal pharmacology. *Annual Review of Pharmacology, 14:* 219-238.

4

Development of Drug Metabolizing Enzymes

WOLFGANG KLINGER

Nearly all drugs are highly lipid-soluble. This lipid-solubility is necessary for the permeation of membranes during absorption, for the drug's distribution and for its availability at the receptor sites. On the other hand, this property is the reason for the reabsorption of the drug after biliary or glomerular excretion. Drugs and foreign substances, which are not metabolized by the highly specific enaymes of carbohydrate, lipid or protein metabolism for the production of energy, would stay in the organism for weeks and months, recycled by continuous reabsorption in the gut and the kidneys, if they were not biotransformed to the more hydrophilic metabolites which are more suitable for excretion. These more polar substances are, with few exceptions, less effective and less toxic (Remmer, 1966).

Drugs and foreign compounds are characterized by an extremely high structural variability; therefore, the enzymes responsible for their biotransformation are of low substrate specificity. There are at least two typical biotransformation reactions which frequently occur in parallel or stepwise. Generally, three major processes occur during the biotransformation of a compound:

(1) Uptake into the cell, with the participation of cytoplasmic organic anion-binding acceptor or transport proteins, called "y" and "z." Excretion out of the cell might also result from similar mechanisms.
(2) Phase I reactions, e.g., hydroxylation, reduction and hydrolysis at the main reaction types.
(3) Phase II reactions, e.g., conjugations.

Abbreviations

ADH	Alcohol dehydrogenase
BSP	Bromsulfthaleine
cyt	Cytochrome
ER	Endoplasmic reticulum
GA	Glucuronic acid
GT	Glucuronyltransferase
mfO	Mixed-function oxidase
NAD	Nicotinamide-adenine-dinucleotide
$NADH_2$	Nicotinamide-adenine-dinucleotide, red.
NADP	Nicotinamide-adenine-dinucleotide-phosphate
$NADPH_2$	Nicotinamide-adenine-dinucleotide-phosphate, red.
RER	Rough endoplasmic reticulum
RNA	Ribonucleic acid
SER	Smooth endoplasmic reticulum
UDPG	Uridine-diphosphate-glucose
UDPGA	Uridine-diphosphate-glucuronic acid
UDPG-DH	Uridine-diphosphate-glucose-dehydrogenase

The data compiled here refer primarily to man. Unfortunately, but understandably in ethical terms, the development of biotransformation in man has not been investigated to the extent that it has been in different laboratory animals. Animal data are included in our discussion when the available data in man, especially those derived from pharmacokinetic studies, support the assumption that the findings in animals can be extrapolated to man.

SIGNIFICANCE OF THE LIVER AND OTHER ORGANS

The liver is considered the main organ of drug metabolism: most of the enzymes catalyzing phase I and phase II reactions are located in the endoplasmic reticulum, which, upon homogenization of the liver, is recovered as microsomes. The microsomes are of two kinds, rough (RER) and smooth (SER), depending on whether or not the microsomal vesicles are derived from reticulum studded with ribosomes. In the normal adult liver, about 10-15% of the whole protein belongs to the ER (Remmer and Merker, 1965), and, within this fraction, about 20% belongs to the final oxidase of a so-called "electron transport" chain, cyt P-450 (Estabrock, 1971). This hemoproteid binds CO and has a characteristic

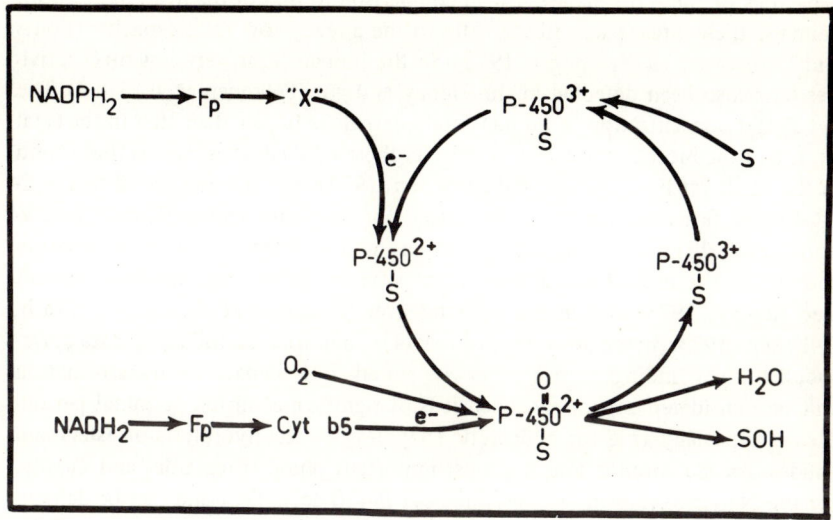

Fig. 1: S = substrate; Fp = flavorprotein (Estabrook, 1971).

absorption peak at 450 mμ in its reduced form with CO as a ligand. The entire system is made up of different components (Fig. 1): $NADPH_2$ acts as an electron donor to a flavoprotein, often designated the so-called "$NADPH_2$-cyt c-reductase," which acts as the cyt P-450-reductase. Between this and the cyt P-450, there is an unknown structure termed "X," whose existence in the liver cell has not yet been verified. The enzyme cyt P-450, as the final oxidase, is the oxygen-activating component which binds the drug in its oxidized form; the drug is then reduced by the above-mentioned $NADPH_2$-cyt P-450-reductase, and, thereafter, it binds molecular oxygen and accepts a second electron, very probaby via reduced cyt b_5 from $NADH_2$ (Estabrook, 1971). One oxygen atom is incorporated into the drug, and water is formed through a simultaneous reduction of the other oxygen atom. Finally, the hydroxylated compound and water are split off, and the cycle starts again. By this system, commonly called "mixed-function oxidase" (mfO); aromatic and aliphatic compounds are hydroxylated, and the N- and O-dealkylations, S-oxydation and nitro- and azo-reduction of suitable compounds occur. Moreover, physiological compounds such as steroids and fatty acids are also hydroxlated by the same system (Conney and Kuntzman, 1971).

In animals, cyt P-450 and other constituents of the microsomal electron transport chain as well as mfO reactions can be detected in kidney and lung tissue (see Klinger, 1973; Fouts and Devereaux, 1973), but the biotransformation capacities of these organs are low in comparison to that of the liver, in newborn animals, these organs contribute little to the already low total capacity (Fouts and Devereaux, 1973; Klinger, 1973). In the human fetus, very low mfO activities have also been detected in the kidney and gut (Pelkonen et al., 1969). The cyt P-450 concentration in human fetal adrenals is higher than that in the fetal liver, and the biotransformation activity in these adrenals is as high as that found in the adult rat liver (Juchau and Perdersen, 1973). The significance of this finding for the fetus and neonate is not clear, for the pharmacokinetic data in newborns (Morselli et al., 1974) correspond very well with the low biotransformation activity of the liver that has been demonstrated in fetal and newborn animals (see Klinger, 1973) and in human fetal liver (Pelkonen et al., 1969, 1971a,b; Pelkonen, 1973a,b; see Morselli et al., 1974). Therefore, all following data correspond to liver findings, if not otherwise stated. Extrahepatic biotransformation will be considered separately when it is of significance in the perinatal period. This is especially true for hydrolytic enzymes, for the hydrolysis of esters and amides, for glucuronidation, the most important phase II reaction, and, finally, for the N-hydroxylation, which is not cyt P-450-dependent and can be demonstrated to have high activity in the lung (Uehleke, 1973). An overview of the phase I and II reactions considered here is given in the tables below.

POSTNATAL DEVELOPMENT OF THE LIVER: MORPHOLOGY AND BIOCHEMISTRY

The substructural picture of the rat liver cell shows an adult pattern at the 5th-7th day of life (Franke and Klinger, 1967). On the other hand, in the human fetus, around the 3rd month of gestation, the hepatic cells have already attained essentially complete differentiation (Zamboni, 1965). Immediately after birth, the blood supply of the liver changes (Martius et al., 1957), and this could contribute to restrictions in the functional state. In the rat, during the postnatal period, there are changing patterns in the microsomal phospholipids (Dallman et al., 1969), and the phospholipid protein-quotient increases (Dallner et al., 1966). The age-dependent concentrations of NAPD and NAD (Raiha, 1961) do not limit the microsomal electron transport chain in the perinatal period. The gluc-6-P-dehydrogenase, which is important for the reduction of NAD and NADP, has practically the same activity in the human fetal liver as in that of the adult (Messina et al., 1973; Pelkonen et al., 1971). The cyt P-450 concentration and the activity of the other constituents of the microsomal electron transport chain show a species-dependent development, which has been demonstrated for the rat (Muller et al., 1971; McLeod et al., 1972; see Uehleke, 1973), the pig (Short et al., 1972), the rabbit (Fouts and Devereaux, 1973) and the guinea pig (Kuenzig et al., 1974). For man, similar investigations can be quoted, having been carried out with liver microsomal preparations from early human fetuses obtained at legal abortion (Yaffe et al., 1970; Ackermann and Rane, 1972; Rane and Sjöquist, 1972; Pelkonen et al., 1969, 1971a,b; Pelkonen, 1973a), from two newborn infants at post-mortem (Soyka, 1970) and from human adult liver after surgical biopsy (Ackermann, 1970, 1972; Ackermann and Heinrich, 1970). While one group found cyt P-450 concentration to be as high in the fetal as in the adult human liver (see Rane and Sjöquist, 1972), the other group detected, respectively, no and very low concentrations of the enzyme (Pelkonen et al., 1971a,b; Pelkonen, 1973a). Drug metabolizing activities have also been determined in needle biopsies of human liver (Schoene et al., 1972). Since it is not known at present which step of the microsomal electron transport chain is rate-limiting (McLeod et al., 1972; Short et al., 1972; Klinger et al., 1974), as it is not clear whether it is the same step in all species and at all ages, and as the developmental pattern of different cyt p-450-dependent biotransformation reactions varies considerably (see Klinger, 1973), the development of the overall enzymic acitivity for the different biotransformation reactions will be considered in the following chapters.

DEVELOPMENT OF TRANSPORT PROTEINS

The capacity, i.e., the concentration of the cytoplasmic acceptor or transport proteins y and z found in the liver cell, and in other organs at distinctly lower concentrations, develops postnatally not only in rats and guinea pigs but also in primates. It has been suggested that in man the postnatal development of BSP clearance, as well as the excretion of conjugated bilirubin, is limited by the capacity of these acceptor proteins (Levi et al., 1970).

DEVELOPMENT OF PHASE I REACTIONS

Dehydrogenation: Ethanol Oxidation

ADH activity develops in both animals and man mainly during the postnatal period. In the human fetal liver, it is detectable in the 2nd month of gestation, but adult values are reached only at the age of 5 years (Räihä and Pikkarainen, 1971). In the fetal liver, there is one isoenzyme detectable; in the newborn, two; and in the adult, four (Pikkarainen and Räihä, 1969).

Cyt P-450 Dependent Mixed-function Oxidation

Investigations of the development of drug biotransformation reactions in different animal species show, in essence, that the capacity of animal fetuses in this regard is very low or negligible (see Klinger, 1973). With human fetal liver preparations, the metabolism of various substrates was about one-third of that found with preparations of the adult liver (Rane and Ackermann, 1972; Pelkonen, 1973; Pelkonen and Kärki, 1973; Pelkonen et al., 1973). Worth mentioning is the very high variability in the prenatal specimens, to the extent that, in some cases, the activity in fetal liver may be higher than in adult liver; these unexpected results have been obtained using early fetal liver. Pharmacokinetic investigations in newborns, however, demonstrate, that after birth the capacity for the oxidative biotransformation of drugs must be very low. For example, the newborn metabolizes diazepam at a much lower rate than does the adult (Kanto et al., 1974; Morselli et al., 1974), and both amidopyrine (Reinicke et al., 1970) and amobarbital (Krauer et al., 1973) have longer-lasting blood levels than in the adult.

It must be concluded from the preceding studies that the early human fetus may have a rather high capacity to oxidize drugs, but in the perinatal period the effectiveness of this system is rather low. This is possibly due to the competition of endogeneous substrates, e.g., steroids (Kardish and Feuer, 1972) and fatty acids, with the drugs at the binding site of cyt P-450. Well-proven is the high capacity of human fetal liver, but also of other fetal organs, to hydroxylate steroids. It has been suggested that these hydroxylations are effected through a mechanism other than the usual process involved in hydroxylation of foreign compounds (Waddell, 1972).

N-hydroxylation: The Flavin-mediated N-Oxidation of Secondary and Tertiary Amines

The developmental pattern of these oxidations varies in rats and rabbits. In rats, a first peak at 2-3 days and a second higher one at 27 days after birth have been demonstrated, however, in rabbits, a continuous increase with a maximum at an age of about 40 days was detected (Uehleke, 1973). For the developmental course in man, no data are available.

Reduction

The process of nitro-reduction is only partly cyt P-450-dependent; activity can be demonstrated with microsomes, as well as with cyt P-450-free cytosol. With the cytoplasmic fraction, no definite postnatal development of activity has been observed (Klinger, et al., 1974), but this reaction has (at least partly) been recognized as being not yet fully developed in immature babies because of certain clinical events. The low activity of nitro-reduction in immature babies was the partial cause of death in several premature infants. These babies had been treated with chloramphenicol on a dose schedule developed for adults (see Done, 1964), because, at that time, the "immaturity" of biotransformation reaction in newborns was not known. Chloramphenicol is first reduced on the nitro group and then conjugated (see Done, 1964).

TABLE 1
Phase I Reactions

Reaction Type	Subcellular Location	Cofactors	Examples
I. Dehydrogenation	Liver cytosol	Alcohol and aldehyde dehydrogenase	Ethanol Acetaldehyde
II. Cyt P-450-dependent mixed-function oxidation	Liver microsomes	$NADPH_2$ $NADH_2$ O_2	
1. Hydroxilation of aromates			Acetanilide Chlorpromazine
2. Hydroxilation of aliphates			Hexobarbital Pentobarbital
–N-dealkylation	(Hydroxylation of the N-alkyl group and splitting of aldehyde)		Amidopyrine
–O-dealkylation	(Hydroxylation of the O-alkyl group and splitting of aldehyde)		Codeine

TABLE 1 continued

Phase I Reactions

Reaction Type	Subcellular Location	Cofactors	Examples
3. Oxidation of heteroatoms			
–N-oxidation of primary arylamines			Phenacetine
–S-oxidation			Chlorpromazine Phenothiazines
4. Oxidative deamination			Amphetamine Methamphetamine
III. N-hydroxylation of tertiary amines	Liver and lung microsomes	NADPH$_2$ O$_2$	
IV. Reduction			
1. Nitro-reduction	Liver microsomes and liver cytosol	NADPH$_2$ NADH$_2$	Chloramphenicol

2. Azo-reduction	Liver microsomes and liver cytosol	NADPH$_2$ NADH$_2$	Prontosil Azo dyes
V. Hydrolysis			
1. Hydrolysis of esters	Liver cytosol and liver microsomes Blood plasma – all organs		Procaine Acetylsalicylic acid Atropine
2. Hydrolysis of amides			Procainamide
VI. Oxidative desulfuration	Liver microsomes and liver cytosol	NADPH$_2$ NADH$_2$ O$_2$	
1. Conversion of P = S → P = O			Parathione
2. Conversion of C = S → C = O			Thiobarbiturates

Hydrolysis

Hydrolysis is not the most important biotransformation reaction for drugs such as procaine, pethidine, meprobamate, paroxone, acetylsalicylic acid. In all animals, and in all organs, hydrolytic activity develops postnatally (see Klinger, 1973). The same is true for man, and the blood esterases especially have been found to possess very low activity at birth, reaching adult values only after a few weeks of extrauterine life (Jones and McCance, 194; Ecobichon and Stephens, 1973; Windorfer et al., 1974).

Oxidative Desulfuration

In animals, the ability to convert thiobarbiturates to oxobarbiturates, and thioalkylphosphates to oxoalkylphosphates, develops primarily postnatally (see Klinger, 1973), direct or indirect data for man are not available.

DEVELOPMENT OF PHASE II REACTIONS

Glucuronidation

In general, in various animal species the glucuronidation of different substrates (the ether or ester-linkage of OH or carboxylic groups to C-1 of glucuronic acid) has different developmental patterns. There are not only species differences, but also differences in the postnatal development of the glucuronidation of various substrates within one species (see Klinger, 1973). It is, therefore, impossible to extrapolate animal data to man. In man, most investigations of glucuronidation are connected with bilirubin glucuronidation and postnatal hyperbilirubinemia. The human fetal liver is capable of glucuronidation of bilirubin (Bakken, 1970) or steroids (Diczfalusy, 1959; Kaufmann, 1960), but the capacity for glucuronidation is not fully developed at birth. The increase in this capacity is different for different substrates (bilirubin, azetanilid, o-aminophenol, p-nitrophenol, 4-methylumbelliferon; see Klinger, 1973). At a gestational age of 4 months, in the human fetal liver GT activity is detectable (Hartiala, 1971), at the same age, the glucuronidation capacity is fully developed (Vest, 1959).

Conjugation with Sulfate

Even in early gestation, sulfation activity is detectable. The liver develops especially high activity in the human fetus, but sulfation also occurs in other organs (kidney, lung, etc.). Relatively high activities have been established for the sulfation of steroids and particularly, for estrogens (Diczfalusy et al., 1961; Pulkkinen, 1966). In all organs, the activity with different substrates develops fully only in the postnatal period (Pulkkinen, 1966).

Conjugation with Glutathione (Mercapturic Acid Conjugation)

The only example of this process that has been widely investigated is the conjugation of BSP. BSP has been used in pediatrics for many decades, it is well-known that the elimination velocity is low in prematures, as well as in mature newborns, and that adult values are reached at an age of 6 months (see Klinger, 1973). Since BSP elimination is dependent on transport mechanisms, the postnatal development of BSP elimination may be a function of the organic anion-binding proteins as well. Animal studies have shown that conjugation activity is low is fetuses and in newborns, and that it develops postnatally.

Acetylation

Fichter and Curtis (1955) found a low acetylation of sulfonamides in prematures and mature newborns. The pharmacokinetics of these drugs in children are summarized by Gladtke (1971). As with many of the other reactions, hepatic acetylation ability develops postnatally.

Conjugation with Glycine

The simplest example of this process is the conversion of benzoic acid to hippuric acid. The conjugation of p-aminobenzoic acid is also used as a liver function test in pediatrics. Full activity, up to the adult level, is reached in normal children at the age of 8 weeks (Vest and Salzberg, 1965). The glycine conjugation capacity can be enhanced by the administration of glycine (Vest, 1965).

PERINATAL INDUCIBILITY OF BIOTRANSFORMATION

An increased de novo synthesis of the proteins and enzymes involved in the biotransformation of foreign compounds begins some hours after the administration of an inducer. First, higher activities of the mfO-reactions are measurable; thereafter, an elevation of microsomal protein is detectable (Remmer and Merker, 1965) and an increase of the SER can be seen electromicroscopically. With continued administration of an inducer, the liver parenchymal cell increases, resulting in hypertrophy and, in young animals, hyperplasia. Not only are some constituents of the microsomal membranes synthesized at a higher rate, but there is also slower breakdown, especially of lipids (see Klinger, 1973). In all species, induction is possible in the newborn. A great number of drugs have been

TABLE 2
Phase II Reactions

Reaction Type	Subcellular Location	Cofactors	Examples
I. Glucuronidation	Liver microsomes and liver cytosol Gut, kidney	UDPG UDPGA NAD	Morphine
II. Conjugation with sulfate	Liver cytosol liver microsomes Many organs and tissues	PAPS	Phenols Steroids
III. Conjugation with glutathione (mercapturic acid conjugation)	Liver cytosol		BSP Chemotherapeutical agents
IV. Acetylation	Liver cytosol	CoA-acetate	Sulfonamides INH
V. Conjugation with glycine	Liver mitochondria	CoA-benzoic acid	Benzoic acid p-Aminobenzoic acid

tested in animals as inducers, among them are phenobarbital, barbital, diphenylhydantoin, phenylbutazone, diazepam and nicethamide (see Klinger, 1973). As the inducers are able to increase the activity not only of mfO-reactions but also of glucuronidations, their use has been proposed for the teatment of hyperbilirubinemia in newborns (Fouts, 1965; Klinger, 1965; Yaffe, 1966).

Since 1968, there have been numerous reports on the effect of phenobarbital, nicethamide, diazepam and phenylbutazone (see Gmyrek et al., 1971). The best results were obtained when the inducers had already been administered to the mother in the last days pre-partum. Many of these investigations were conducted in an attempt to solve the problem of whether or not prenatal induction was possible (see Klinger, 1973). While Bakken (1970) believed bilirubin to be the physiological inducer for its own glucuronidation and the conjugate to be the trigger for the excretion (Bakken, 1970a), Winsnes and Bratlid (1973) could not confirm these plausible statements in experiments with rats. This question has been investigated carefully in several different species. It is well documented now that prenatal induction is possible in the mouse (Richards, 1973), the rabbit (Windorfer, 1972) and, last but not least, in man (Pelkonen et al., 1971; Sereni et al., 1973; Morselli et al., 1974). The perinatal enhancement of biotransformation reactions not only accelerates the glucuronidation and excretion of bilirubin and the biotransformation of drugs, but also increases their variability (Sereni, 1973). As the influence on the biotransformation of steroids in the newborn has not been clear until now, the general treatment of newborns, or at least of prematures, does not seem to be justified (Windorfer, 1974b).

The increase of bilirubin elimination by treatment with orotic acid is believed to be due to an increased formation of UDPGA; in this way, it is acting rather specifically on the glucuronidation processes only (Gmyrek et al., 1971; Hinkel et al., 1973). This induction of bilirubin elimination by potent inducers, such as phenobarbital, is also possible in genetically defective children. The congenital familial non-hemolytic jaundice of Crigler-Najjar, a hereditary GT-deficiency, can be treated with phenobarbital and other inducers (see Klinger, 1973), and hyperbilirubinemia in gluc-6-dehydrogenase-deficient newborn infants can be prevented by phenobarbital administration (Meloni et al., 1973).

BIOTRANSFORMATION AND TOXICITY DURING POSTNATAL DEVELOPMENT

The chloramphenicol tragedy 15 years ago (see Done, 1964) showed that unexpected toxic reactions in premature infants were the result of pharmacokinetic peculiarities in the perinatal period. After administration, of one single dose, toxic reactions, or even death, can occur within minutes. In these cases, it is unlikely that biotransformation is an important factor. Biotransformation is a limiting factor when toxic reactions or death are delayed or occur after administration of several doses of a drug. With chloramphenicol, no significant differences between the concentration in blood and the distribution volume are found after a single dose in neonates or adults, but there are major differences in the rate of elimination. Repeated daily administration of the same dose to neonates and adults will result in higher blood levels in the neonates and in ashen-gray cyanosis and death in premature and mature newborn babies (Done, 1964). This example indicates that the comparison of the acute LD 50 of a drug in newborn animals with that in the adult cannot provide reliable information on biotransformation, the slow rate of which may be responsible for toxicity after repeated administrations. It must be recommended, therefore, that not only the LD 50 (see Goldenthal, 1971) but also the main biotransformation routes and the biological activity of the metabolites should be determined in newborn and infant animals if a drug is proposed for use in neonates or infants.

CONCLUSIONS

Biotransformation activity—i.e., transport of the drug or foreign compound into the cell, phase I and phase II reactions and transport of the metabolites out of the cell—is low during the perinatal period. The only exceptions are the hydroxylation and sulfation of steroids in the fetus. The main organ for biotransformation in the perinatal period is the liver, the same as in adults. Relatively high activities have been found in the lung for N-oxidation of secondary and tertiary amines, in the gut for glucuronidation, and in kidney and lung for sulfation. The low biotransformation activity in the perinatal period is not due to insufficient cofactor availability. Biotransformation activity in the neonate may be enhanced by induction, which is possible even during late gestation. At present the mechanisms which regulate biotransformation activity and its development are not known.

REFERENCES

Ackermann, E. (1970): Die Demethylierung von Aminophenazon und Codein in der Leber des Menschen. Eine Untersuchung über den mikrosomalen Elektronentransport. *Biochem. Pharmacol., 19:* 1955.

Ackermann, E. (1972): Entalkylierung von Äthylmorphin und p-C-Hydroxylierung von Anilin in Lebermikrosomen von Menschen und von männlichen und weiblichen Rattan. *Biochem. Pharmacol., 19:* 2169.

Ackermann, E. and Heinrich, I. (1970): Die Aktivität der N- und O-Demethylase in der Leber des Menschen. *Biochem. Pharmacol. 19:* 327.

Ackermann, E. and Rane, A. (1972): The liver microsomal monooxygenase system in the human fetus: distribution in different centrifugal fractions. *Clin. Pharmacol. Ther. 13:* 652.

Bakken, A.F. (1970a): Bilirubin excretion in newborn human infants. I. Unconjugated bilirubin conjugation. *Acta Paediat. Scand., 59:* 148.

Bakken, A.F. (1970b): Bilirubin excretion in newborn infants. II. Conjugated bilirubin as a possible trigger for bilirubin excretion. *Acta Paediat. Scand. 59:* 153.

Conney, A.H. and Kuntzman, R. (1971): Metabolism of normal body constituents by drug-metabolizing enzymes in liver microsomes. In: *Handbook of Experimental Pharmacology,* V. XXVIII, pt. 2, *Concepts in Biochemical Pharmacology,* p. 401, edited by J.R. Gillette and J.R. Mitchell, Springer-Verlag, Berlin.

Dallman, P.R., Dallner, G., Bergstrand, A. and Ernster, L. (1969): Heterogeneous distribution of enzymes in submicrosomal membrane fragments. *J. Cell Biol., 41:* 357.

Dallner, G., Siekevitz, P. and Palade, G.E. (1966): Biogenesis of endoplasmic reticulum membranes. I. Structural and chemical differentiation in developing rat hepatocyte. *J. Cell Biol., 30:* 73.

Diczfalusy, E. (1959): Metabolism des oestrogènes chez le foetus et le nouveau-né. *Bull. Soc. Belge Gynéc. Obstét. 28:* 459.

Diczfalusy, E., Cassmer, O., Alonso, C. and DeMiquel, M. (1961): Oestrogen metabolism in the human foetus. III. Nature of conjugated oestrogen formed by the foetus. *Acta Endocr.* (Copenhagen) *38:* 31.

Done, A.K. (1964): Developmental pharmacology, *Clin. Pharmacol. Ther. 5:* 432.

Ecobichon, D.J., and Stephens, D.S. (1973): Perinatal development of human blood esterases. *Clin. Pharmacol. Ther., 14:* 41.

Estabrook, R.W. (1971): Cytochrome P-450–its function in the oxidative metabolism of drugs. In: *Handbook of Experimental Pharmacology,* V. XXVIII, pt. 2, *Concepts in Biochemical Pharmacology,* edited by J.R. Gillette and B.B. Brodie, p. 264, Springer-Verlag, Berlin.

Fichter, E.G. and Curtis, J.A. (1955): Sulfonamide administration in newborn and premature infants. *Amer. J. Dis. Child., 90:* 596.

Fouts, J.R. and Devereaux, Th. (1973): Developmental aspects of hepatic and extrahepatic drug-metabolizing enzyme systems: microsomal enzymes and components in rabbit liver and lung during the first month of life. *J. Pharmacol. Exper. Ther., 183:* 458.

Franke, H. and Klinger, W. (167): Untersuchungen zum Mechanismus der Enzyminduktion. X. Die Wirkung von Barbital auf die Substruktur der Leberzellen von Ratten verschiedener Alters. *Acta Biol. Med. Germ. 18:* 99.

Gladtke, E. (1971): Pharmakokinetik von Chemotherapeutika in Abhängigkeit vom Lebensalter. *Mschr. Kinderheilk., 119:* 105.

Gmyrek, D., Pietsch, I., Kalz, Wiegans, U. und Schmehl, U. (1971): Zur medikamentösen Prophylaxe der Neugeborenenhyperbilirubinämie. 1. Einfluß von Phenylbutazon auf Bilirubinspiegel und Extrazellularraum. *Dtsch. Ges. Wesen, 26:* 681.

Goldenthal, E.I. (1971): A compilation of LD 50 values in newborn and adult animals. *Tox. Appl. Pharmacol., 18:* 185.

Hartiala, K. (1971): The glucuronidation pathway. *Chem. Biol. Interactions, 3:* 274.

Hinkel, G.K., Schwarze, R. and Kintzel, H.W. (1973): Optimale Orotsäuredosierung zur Verhütung der toxischen Hyperbilirubinämie Frühgeborener. *Acta Paediatr. Acad. Sci. Hung., 13:* 367.

Jones, P.E.H. and McCance, R.A. (1949): Enzyme activities in the blood of infants and adults. *Biochem. J., 45:* 464.

Juchau, M.R. and Pedersen, M.G. (1973): Drug biotransformation reactions in the human fetal adrenal gland. *Life Sci. II, 12:* 193.

Kanto, J., Errkola, R. and Sellman, R. (1974): Perinatal metabolism of diazepam. *Brit. Med. J.,* 641.

Kardish, R. and Feuer, G. (1972): Relationship between maternal progesterones and the delayed drug metabolism in the neonate. *Biol. Neonate, 20:* 58.

Kaufmann, H.J. (1960): Die Gefährdung Frühgeborener und Neugeborener durch Arzneimittel. *Dtsch. Med. Wschr., 85:* 1090.

Klinger, W. (1965): Untersuchungen zum Mechanismus der Enzyminduktion bei Ratten und Mäusen. *Habilitationsschrift Jena.*

Klinger, W. (1973a): Biotransformation in der Leber und extrahepatische Biotransformation. In: *Entwicklungspharmakologie,* edited by H. Ankermann, P. 51, VEB Verlag Volk und Gesundheit, Berlin.

Klinger, W. (1973b): Amidopyrine-N-demethylation by lung 9000 x g supernatant of newborn and adult rats. *Acta Biol. Med. Germ., 31:* 467.

Klinger, W., Muller, D., Reichenbach, F., Kleeberg, U., Lubbe, H. and Rein, H. (1974): Developmental aspects of the microsomal electron transport chain in the rat. *Internat. Symp. Perinatal Pharmacology,* Milan, 17-19 June.

Krauer, B., Draffan, G.H., Williams, F.M., Clare, R.A., Dollery, C.T. and Hawkins, D.F. (1973): Elimination kinetics of amobarbital in mothers and their newborn infants. *Clin. Pharmacol. Ther., 14:* 442.

Kuenzig, W. and Kamm, J.J. (1972): Perinatal development of the hepatic mixed function oxidase system in the guinea pig. *Fed. Proc.,* Abstr., *31:* 595.

Kuenzig, W., Kamm, J.J. Boublik, M., Jenkins, F. and Burns, J.J. (1974): Perinatal drug metabolism and morphological changes in the hepatocytes of normal and phenobarbital-treated guinea pigs. *J. Pharmacol. Exp. Ther., 191:* 32.

Levi, A.M., Gatmaitan, Z. Arias, I.M. (1970): Deficiency of hepatic organic anion-binding protein, impaired organic anion uptake by liver and "physiologic" jaundice in newborn monkeys. *New England J. Med., 283:* 1136.

McLeod, S.M., Renton, K.W. and Eade, N.R. (1972): Development of hepatic microsomal drug-oxidizing enzymes in immature male and female rats. *J. Pharmacol. Exper. Ther., 183:* 489.

Martius, G., Zimmer, F. and Fackler, F. (1957): Untersuchungen über die Leistungsfähigkeit der Leber in den ersten Lebenstagen. *Arch Gynäk., 188:* 539.

Meloni, T., Cagnazzo, G., Dore, A. and Cutillo, St. (1973): Phenobarbital for prevention of hyperbilirubinemia in glucose-6-phosphate dehydrogenase-deficient newborn infants. *J. Pediatr. 82:* 1048.

Messina, A.M., Chacko, C.M. and Nadler, H.L. (1972): Gluc-6-PDH in the developing human liver. *Proc. Soc. Exper. Biol. Med., 139:* 778.

Morselli, P.L., Mandelli, M., Tognoni, G., Principi, N., Pardi, G. and Sereni, F. (1974): Drug interactions in the human fetus and in the newborn infant. In: *Drug Interactions,* edited by P.L. Morselli, S. Garattini and S.N. Cohen, S. 239, Raven Press, New York.

Müller, D., Förster, D., Dietze, H., Langenberg, R. and Klinger, W. (1973): The influence of age and barbital treatment on the content of cytochromes P-450 and b_5 and on the activity of glucose-6-phosphatase in microsomes of rat liver and kidney. *Biochem. Pharmacol., 22:* 905.

Pelkonen, O. (1973a): Drug metabolism and drug-induced spectral interactions in human fetal liver microsomes. *Biochem. Pharmacol., 22:* 2357.

Pelkonen, O. (1973b): Drug metabolism in the human fetal liver—relationship to fetal age. *Arch. Int. Pharmacodyn., 202:* 281.

Pelkonen, O., Arvela, P. and Kärki, N.T. (1971a): 3,4-Benzpyrene and N-methylaniline metabolizing enzymes in the immature human foetus and placenta. *Acta Pharmacol. Toxicol., 30:* 385.

Pelkonen, O., Kaltiala, E.H., Larmi, T.K.I. and Kärki, N.T. (1973): Comparison of activities of drug-metabolizing enzymes in human fetal and adult livers. *Clin. Pharmacol. Therap., 14:* 840.

Pelkonen, O. and Kärki, N.T. (1971): Demonstration of cyt P-450 in human foetal liver microsomes in early pregnancy. *Acta Pharmacol. Toxicol., 30:* 158.

Pelkonen, O. and Kärki, N.T. (1973): 3,4-Benzpyrene and aniline are hydroxylated by human fetal liver but not by placenta at 6-7 weeks of fetal age. *Biochem. Pharmacol., 22:* 1538.

Pelkonen, O., Vorne, M., Jouppila, P. and Kärki, N.T. (1971b): Metabolism of chlorpromazine and p-nitrobenzoic acid in the liver, intestine and kidney of the human foetus. *Acta Pharmacol. Toxicol. 29:* 284.

Pelkonen, O., Vorne, M. and Kärki, N.T. (1969): Drug-metabolizing activity in the liver, intestine and kidney of human foetus. *Acta Phys. Scand., 77,* Suppl. 330: 69.

Pikkarainen, P. and Räihä, N.C.R. (1969): Change in alcohol dehydrogenase isoenzyme pattern during development of human liver. *Nature, 222:* 563.

Pulkkinen, M. (1966): Sulphate conjugation during development, in human, rat, and guinea pig. *Acta Physiol., Scand., 66:* 115.

Räihä, N.C.R. (1961): Variations in pyridine nucleotides in liver of fetal, newborn and adult guinea pigs. *Amer. J. Physol., 201:* 961.

Räihä, N.C.R. and Pikkarainen, P.H. (1971): The development of alcohol dehydrogenase and its isoenzymes. In: *Metabolic Changes Induced by Alcohol,* edited by G.A. Martini and Ch. Bode, S. 1, Springer-Verlag, Berlin.

Rane, A. and Ackermann, E. (1972): Metabolism of ethylmorphine and aniline in human fetal liver. *Clin. Pharmacol. Ther., 13:* 663.

Rane, A., and Sjöqvist, F. (1972): Drug metabolism in the human fetus and newborn infant. *Pediat. Clin.* (North Amer.), *19:* 37.

Reinicke, C., Rogner, G., Frenzel, J., Maak, B. and Klinger, W. (1970): Die Wirkung von Phenylbutazon und Phenobarbital auf die Amidopyrin-Elimination, die Bilirubin-Gesamtkonzentration im Serum und einige Blutgerinnungsfaktoren bei neugeborenen Kindern. *Pharmacologia Clinica, 2:* 167.

Remmer, H. (1966): Die Elimination von Arzneimitteln durch enzymatischen Abbau in der Leber. *Der Internist, 7:* 413.

Remmer, H. and Merker, H.J. (1965): Effect of drugs on the formation of smooth endoplasmic reticulum and drug metabolizing enzymes. *Ann. N.Y. Acad. Sci., 123:* 79.

Richards, Th. C. (1973): Histochemical changes in developing mouse liver after administration of phenobarbital. *Amer. J. Anatom., 138:* 449.

Schoene, B., Fleischmann, R.A. and Remmer, H. (1972): Determination of drug metabolizing enzymes in needle biopsies of human liver. *Europ. J. Clin. Pharmacol., 4:* 65.

Sereni, F., Mandelli, M., Principi, N., Tognoni, G., Pardi, G. and Morselli, P.L. (1973): Induction of drug metabolizing enzyme activities in the human fetus and in the newborn. *Enzyme, 15:* 318.

Short, C.R., Maines, M.D. and Westfall, B.A. (1972): Postnatal development of drug-metabolizing enzyme activity in liver and extrahepatic tissues of swine. *Biol. Neonate, 21:* 54.

Soyka, L.F. (1970): Isolation and characterisation of reduced nicotinamide adenine dinucleotide phosphate: ferri cyt c oxidoreductase and identification by cyt b_5 in the liver of human infants. *Biochem. Pharmacol., 19:* 945.

Uehleke, H. (1973): The role of cyt P-450 in the N-oxidation of individual amines. *Drug Metab. and Disp., 1:* 299.

Vest, M. (1959): Studien zur Entwicklung des Glukuronid-Bildungsvermögens der Leber bei Neugeborenen. Das Verhalten des Aminophenol-Glukuronids in Blut nach Verabreichung von Acetanilid. *Schweiz. Med. Wschr., 89:* 102.

Vest, M.F. (1965): The development of conjugation mechanisms and drug toxicity in the newborn. *Biol. Neonat.* (Basel), *8:* 258.

Vest, M.F. and Salzberg, R. (1965): Conjugation reactions in the newborn infant: the metabolism of paraaminobenzoic acid. *Arch. Dis. Child., 40:* 97.

Waddell, W.J. (1972): Localisation and drug metabolism in the fetus. *Fed. Proc., 31:* 52.
Windorfer, A. (1972): Steigerung der Glukoronidierungsrate in der Neugeborneenperiode durch therapeutische Phenobarbitaldosen. *Zschr. Kinderheilk., 113:* 33.
Windorfer, A. (1974): Wiegefahrlos sind die modermen Methoden zur Behandlung des physiologischen Neugeborenenikterus? *Klin Pädiat., 186:* 92.
Windorfer, A., Kuenzer, W. and Urbanek, R. (1974): The influence of age on the activity of acetylsalicylic acid-esterase and protein-salicylate binding. *Europ. J. Clin. Pharmacol., 7:* 227.
Winsnes, A. and Bratlid, D. (1973): Effects of bilirubin loading of pregnant rats on hepatic UDP-glucuronyltransferase activity in the offspring. *Biol. Neonat., 22:* 367.
Yaffe, S.J., Rane, A., Sjöqvist, F., Boréus, S.-O. and Orrenius, S. (1970): The presence of a monooxygenase system in human fetal liver microsomes. *Life Sci., 9:* II, 1189.
Zamboni, L. (1965): Electron microscopic studies of blood embryogenesis in humans. I. The ultrastructure of the fetal liver. *J. Ultrastructure Res., 12:* 509.

5

Kidney Development: Drug Elimination Mechanisms

HELMUT BRAUNLICH

The most important organ for drug excretion is the kidney. At the time of birth, the development and maturation of renal excretion mechanisms for drugs is not completed, the different renal functions develop at various rates (Barnett and Vesterdal, 1955; Braunlich, 1973; McCance, 1950; Rohwedder, 1968; Schreiter, 1966). Generally, the basic age differences in the renal excretion mechanisms of drugs can be predicted. Nevertheless, experimental data are necessary for each drug on its particular route of renal excretion since many drugs are excreted by different mechanisms. Therefore, it is impossible to predict the age-related differences in renal excretion of a given drug, and it becomes necessary to investigate the age differences in renal excretion for each single class of compounds. Knowledge of the renal excretion mechanisms and their age-dependence is of great practical importance. The age differences in renal excretion of drugs are greater for substances with predominant or selective renal excretion without preceding biotransformation, but many metabolites also are excreted predominantly by the kidney (Klinger, 1973).

A great number of renal functions are characterized by having a diurnal rhythm, in the dark period, renal functions are generally diminished. This diurnal rhythm in kidney function is not fully developed during the neonatal period (Mills, 1966; Stanbury and Thomson, 1951; Krauer, 1975). The age differences in renal excretion are, therefore, smaller if 24 hr periods are compared than if only shorter periods of the day are considered.

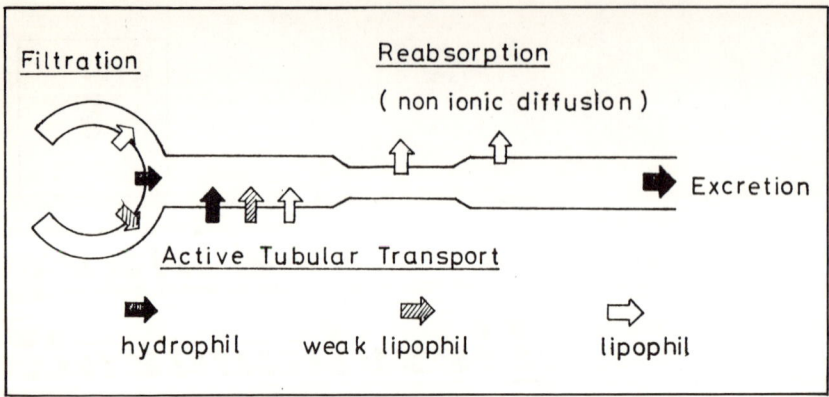

Fig. 1: Drug movement in the kidney (Scheler, 1969).

POSTNATAL DEVELOPMENT OF RENAL EXCRETION FUNCTION FOR FOREIGN COMPOUNDS

In the kidney, three patterns of drug movement have been demonstrated (Fig. 1):

— glomerular filtration
— tubular secretion by active transport mechanisms
— reabsorption (nonionic diffusion), which acts contrarily to glomerular filtration and active tubular transport

Drugs are excreted into the urine either by glomerular filtration and tubular secretion, or by glomerular filtration alone. During the early postnatal period, the three patterns of movement of drugs are characterized by development and maturation (see Weiner, 1971).

Thus far, in the early postnatal period active tubular transport of drugs from the lumen of the renal tubules into tubular cells has not been demonstrated. The renal reabsorption of amino acids, uric acid and glucose is mediated by an active tubular transport; these transport mechanisms, therefore, are not fully developed in the postnatal period of life (Kretchmer et al., 1963; Weiner, 1971).

Glomerular Filtration

Characteristics. Most drugs are excreted by glomerular filtration. The binding of drugs to serum proteins diminishes the renal excretion by this route. The

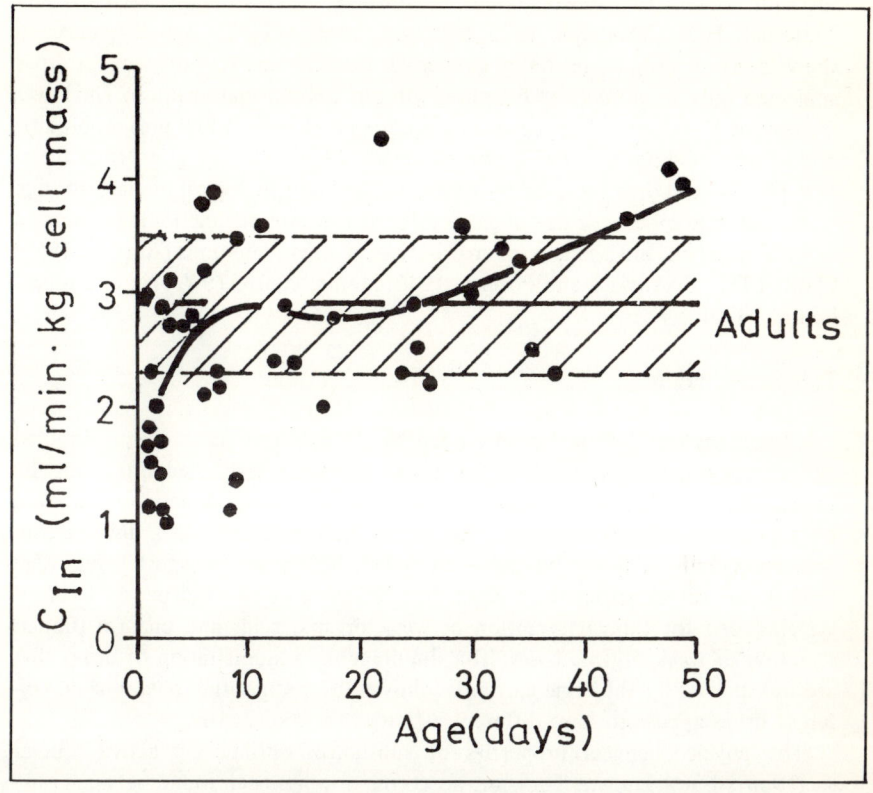

Fig. 2: Postnatal development of glomerular filtration rate (inulin clearance) (Schreiter, 1966).

velocity of renal drug excretion by glomerular filtration is not influenced by physicochemical properties. Since there are a great number of pores in the glomerular membranes, not only lipophilic but also hydrophilic, drugs are excreted by filtration. The glomerular filtration rate can be estimated by drugs which are selectively filtered without biotransformation (Inulin). At most, glomerular filtration amounts to about 20% of the whole drug excretion capacity of the kidney under conditions of maximum load (Balint, 1965; Berman and Mishra, 1972; Weiner, 1971; Zufarov, 1974).

Postnatal development (Fig. 2). It has been proven that the kidneys produce urine during the fetal period (Ehrnebo et al., 1971; Kobyletzki, 1971), but quantitative determinations are not available. During the postnatal period, the glomerular filtration rate is small and the renal excretion of drugs by glomerular filtration occurs to a lesser extent in newborns than in adults (Barnett and Vesterdal, 1955; Braunlich, 1973; Schreiter, 1966) (Fig. 2). Age differences in the velocity of drug excretion by glomerular filtration are very distinct for drugs subjected only to glomerular filtration without tubular reabsorption. The lower glomerular filtration rate in newborns is compensated by a low protein-binding rate of drugs (Braunlich, 1973; Ehrnebo et al., 1971). The low glomerular filtration rate in newborns is caused by functional and morphological immaturity due to the small number and size of glomeruli, the low rate of functioning glomeruli to total number, and the lack of maturation of single nephrons (Arataki, 1953; Clark, 1957; Gruenwald and Popper, 1940; McIntosh, 1957; Webber and Blackbourn, 1970).

Tubular Secretion

Characteristics. Tubular secretion can be characterized as an active, directed and energy-requiring transport. The active transport is carried out from the lumen into the cell, and the movement of drugs in the other direction is achieved by a passive penetration process. The carrier transport begins if a distinct concentration limit in blood plasma is exceeded. Maximum transport values (Tm values) can be estimated for a given drug. There exist two independent carrier systems, one for tubular secretion of weak organic acids and one for tubular secretion of weak organic bases. The simultaneous administration of drugs that are transported by the same carrier is followed by competition phenomena. Different drugs appear to have different affinities for the carriers.

The physicochemical properties of substances optimal for active tubular secretion are not known. Thus far, no correlation has been found between physicochemical properties and velocity of active tubular secretion. Drugs that are excreted by tubular secretion competitively inhibit the renal tubular excretion of endogenous products of metabolism, e.g., bilirubin. At present, it must be determined experimentally whether or not a given drug is excreted by tubular secretion. Active tubular transport of a drug is evidently proven if its accumulation by renal cortical slices can be demonstrated. An active tubular transport pattern is also implied by the existence of a higher renal excretion than corresponding glomerular filtration rate. A passive enrichment of drugs in renal cortical slices, renal tubular reabsorption, or an extrarenal elimination process must be excluded as a causative factor. The excretion capacity of tubular secretion is very high but limited (Tm values). A full saturation of renal excretion capacity may be easily reached for drugs that are 80% tubular-secreted (Balint, 1965; Braunlich, 1973; Calcagno and Rubin, 1963; Deetjen, 1965; Hirsch, 1972; Hock et al., 1970; Rennick, 1972; Schreiter, 1966; Weiner, 1971).

Postnatal development (Fig. 3). The Tm values for tubular secretion are smaller in newborns than in adults. Consequently, the drug accumulation ability in renal cortical slices from newborn rats is lower than that in adult specimens

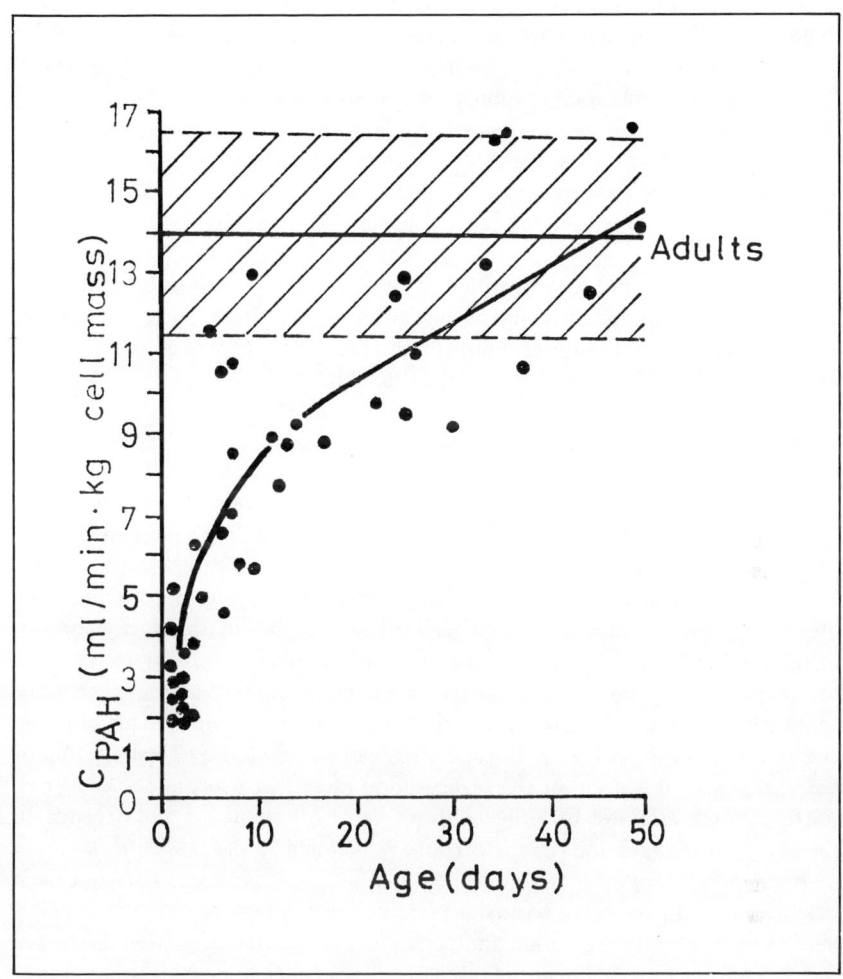

Fig. 3: Postnatal development of tubular secretion function (PAH clearance) (Schreiter, 1966).

(Barnett et al., 1948; Bertram et al., 1970; Braunlich, 1973; Dicker and Shirley, 1971; Hook et al., 1970; Schreiter, 1966; Whittam, 1960). The tubular secretion rate for many drugs is lower in newborns than in adults (Fig. 3). Age differences in excretion velocity can be demonstrated, especially after the administration of drugs in high doses with consequent saturation of the carriers (antibiotics, sulfonamides). However, this is not the ideal example to cite in showing age differences in renal drug excretion by tubular secretion.

The reasons for the small carrier capacity in the newborn is yet to be determind. The following factors are considered to be the limiting ones:

- The mass of functioning tubular cells is smaller.
- The length of the tubuli is not fully developed.
- The blood flow in the peritubular area is not sufficient.
- The energy supply processes are immature.
- The velocity of carrier transport is lower than in adults.

Unfortunately, it is not known which of these is really the limiting factor in the active tubular secretion of drugs in newborns (Clark, 1957; Ecker and Hook, 1974; Gruenwald and Popper, 1940; Hirsch et al., 1971; Kim et al., 1972; Kleinman and Lubbe, 1972; Kretchmer et al., 1963; McIntosh, 1957).

Tubular Reabsorption (Nonionic Diffusion)

Characteristics. Tubular reabsorption is a passive process in which drugs are moved from the tubular lumen into the tubular cell. The drug's physicochemical properties are very important factors in determining the reabsorption rate. Lipophilic drugs are reabsorbed to a large extent, but the hydrophilic metabolites of lipophilic drugs cannot be reabsorbed. Because of this fact, biotransformation limits the reabsorption rate of lipophilic drugs. For reabsorption from the tubular lumen into the tubular cell, the nonionic form of a drug is necessary (nonionic diffusion); therefore, the reabsorption rate varies with the pH of urine, and the reabsorption of weak organic acids can be reduced by alkalinization of the urine. A modification of the reabsorption rate of weak organic acids by pH-shifting is very effective for drugs with pK values of about 7.4 and depends on the extent of pH variation (Dootjen, 1965; Weiner and Mudge, 1964).

Postnatal development. Age differences in nonionic processes have not been demonstrated. In the early postnatal period, a smaller reabsorption rate is plausible, the concentration of urine and consequently, the concentration difference for drugs from tubular lumen to tubular cell is smaller in newborns because of the smaller length of renal tubuli. The penetration of drugs through the tubular membrane is also slower in the newborn (Berlin-Heimendahl, 1964; Kerpel-Fronius, 1972; Kretchmer et al., 1963). Since there is a less degree of biotransformation, the reabsorption rate of these unchanged drugs is often higher in newborns (Klinger, 1973). This age difference in renal excretion is caused by the age-dependence of the extrarenally located elimination mechanisms.

Age differences in the pH value of urine are well known. The production and renal excretion of basic compounds is not fully developed in newborns; therefore, in this age group the urine pH is lower than in adults (Berlin-Heimendahl, 1964; Clark, 1957; Kerpel-Fronius, 1972; McCance and Finck, 1947; Zufarov, 1974). Because of the acid urine of newborns, a high reabsorption rate for weak organic acids is to be expected, and yet the reabsorption rate for weak organic bases is low (Deetjen, 1965; Weiner and Mudge, 1964).

STIMULATION OF DRUG ELIMINATION MECHANISMS

An increase in biotransformation of drugs can be produced by induction of microsomal enzymes. In this way, the low biotransformation capacity of newborns can be raised to adult values (see Klinger, 1973). The renal excretion capacity for drugs that are tubularly secreted can be stimulated by repeated administration of drugs, thus loading the carrier capacity for an extended period of time. This stimulation of tubular transport is probably due to a more intensive synthesis of carrier protein (Berkhin and Galyuteva, 1974; Rennick, 1972). In renal cortical slices of rats pre-treated with p-amino hippuric acid or penicillin, the accumulation rate for p-amino hippuric acid was specifically stimulated (Berkhin and Galyuteva, 1974; Hirsch, 1972; Hirsch and Hook, 1970). The accumulation rate in renal cortical slices from newborn rats and dogs was thereby raised to adult values (Ecker and Hook, 1974; Hirsch and Hook, 1970; Kim et al., 1972). The renal excretion of tubularly secreted substances can also be stimulated by the repeated administration of foreign substances (Bernhardt et al., 1973), and clinical observations regarding this phenomenon have been published (Rind and Gladtke, 1965; Traeger et al., 1974). The stimulation of renal drug excretion in newborns at no time exceeds the normal values for adults.

It is of practical importance that the repeated administration of drugs might influence the pharmacokinetics and stimulate their renal excretion. In fact, the diminution of effectiveness sometimes seen after prolonged administration of a drug may be a result of this process. Repeated administration of a drug by influencing the glomerular filtration or the tubular reabsorption rate might also stimulate the renal excretion.

DEVELOPMENT OF RENAL DRUG EXCRETION

Age-dependent differences of the renal excretion of drugs can be established for a great number of compounds. In most cases, the renal excretion is lower in newborns than in adults. Because of the different physicochemical properties and the contribution of the three patterns of renal drug movement, a prediction in renal excretion velocity according to age differences is difficult. For a great number of drugs, the renal excretion pattern has already been studied (Braunlich, 1973; Done, 1965; Dost and Gladtke, 1969; Kellner, 1971; Kobyletzki and Althammer, 1967; Krauer et al., 1968; Natochin, 1974; Neussel and Olbing, 1972; Rohwedder and Goll, 1970; Sereni and Principi, 1968; Weingartner, 1973; Yaffe and Juchau, 1974; Yaffe and Rane, 1971). The slow renal excretion of drugs in newborns must always be considered during therapy, usually, the dosage should be reduced. Dosage calculation considering only the factor of the smaller body weight is not the correct method of modification. Even drugs with low toxicity should be given to newborns at prolonged intervals between administration since there is a decrease in renal excretion velocity.

AGE-DEPENDENT NEPHROTOXICITY OF DRUGS

Many drugs are nephrotoxic agents, and their nephrotoxic effect is not caused by a sensitivity of the kidney to drugs. As a result of the different forms of renal drug movement and the concentrating mechanisms for urine, a high drug concentration in urine can be attained. The active tubular secretion, as well as tubular reabsorption, of the drugs produces a high drug concentration in the tubular cells, subsequently, the concentration of the urine causes a higher drug concentration in urine than in plasma. Thus the nephrotoxicity of these substances is caused by the kidney's excretion functions for drugs.

The drug excretion mechanisms which are responsible for the enrichment of these substances in the kidney are not fully developed in newborns. The age differences in the development of kidney function are the reason for the low nephrotoxicity of drugs excreted by the kidney in the newborn. The age-dependence of drug toxicity has been studied for some foreign substances excreted by the kidney, and these experiments prove the low nephrotoxicity of drugs that are excreted by tubular secretion in the neonatal period (Terracini and Palestro, 1966; Wachstein and Robinson, 1965; Yeary et al., 1966). Reports of higher nephrotoxicity of drugs in newborns are explained, in most cases, by the use of high dosages not correctly modified for age. There are no indications that any drugs have a distinct kidney-damaging effect in the neonatal period when the correct dosage is used (Kaufmann, 1965; Nyhan, 1961).

AGE DIFFERENCES IN RENAL EFFECTIVENESS OF DRUGS

The almost selective renal effect of diuretics is caused by the accumulation of these drugs in the tubular cells as a consequence of their active transport. Thus diuretics reach their highest concentration in the body at the same site where they are acting. Since the tubular secretion function for drugs is not fully developed in neonates, the maximal diuretic effect in newborns can be obtained only by administration of a higher dosage than in adults. This is evident for thiazide diuretics and organic mercurial compounds (Braunlich and Kersten, 1971; Frenzel et al., 1974).

AGE-DEPENDENT RENAL WATER AND ELECTROLYTE EXCRETION

When considering the therapeutic use of infusion solutions in the newborn, it is necessary to understand that renal excretion functions for water and electrolytes are not fully developed and that there is an immaturity of hormonally regulated electrolyte exchange in the tubuli. In newborns, the renal excretion of sodium is very slow during saline infusion. Excretion in newborns is influenced by an intensive exchange for this ion for hydrogen ions and potassium; as a result, the pH values of the urine are low and potassium is lost (Ames, 1953; Braunlich, 1973; Calcagno, 1954; Frenzel et al., 1974; Jahrig et al., 1972; McCance and Young, 1941; Ziegler and Fomon, 1971; Zweymuller, 1971). Disturbances in acid-base balance are more easily provoked in this age group than in adults since the production of basic substances is not fully developed in the neonate (Berlin-Hei-Mendahl, 1964; Kerpel-Fronius, 1972; McCance and Finck, 1947). Finally, the repeated daily administration of sodium chloride is followed by an accelerated maturation of renal sodium excretion ability. In experimental studies in rats, the same value as that for adults was attained on the 19th day of life (Braunlich and Puschmann, 1972).

REFERENCES

Ames, R.G. (1953): Urinary water excretion and neurohypophysical function in full-term and premature infants shortly after birth. *Pediatrics, 12:* 272.
Andersen, J.B., Rosdahl, N. and Vejlsgaard, R. (1972): Aspects of pharmacology of gentamicin in newborn infants. *Acta Paed. Scand., 61*: 343.
Arataki, M. (1926): The postnatal growth of the kidney, with special reference to the number and size of the glomeruli. *Amer. J. Anat., 36:* 399.
Axline, St. G., Yaffe, S.J. and Simon, H.J. (1967): Clinical pharmacology of antimicrobials in premature infants. II. Ampicillin, methicillin, oxacillin, neomycin and colistin. *Pediatrics, 39:* 97.
Balint, P. (1965); Nierenclearance. Technik, Bewertung, Ergebnisse. *Fischer Verlag Jena.*
Bauer, B. (1971): Elektrolytclearance bei Fruhgeborenen in der ersten Lebenswoche. *Mschr. Kinderheilk., 119:* 302.
Barnett, H.L. (1940): Renal physiology in infants and children: method for estimation of glomerular filtration rate. *Proc. Soc. Exp. Biol. Med., 44:* 654.
Barnett, H.L., Hare, McNamara, H. and Hare, R.S. (1948): Influence of postnatal age on kidney function of premature infants. *Proc. Soc. Exp. Biol. Med., 69:* 55.
Barnett, H.L. and Vesterdal, J. (1955): The physiological and clinical significance of immaturity of kidney function in young infants. *J. Pediat., 42:* 99.
Berkhin, E.B. and Galyuteva, G.I. (1974): Significance of genetic induction in the action of thyroidin and trijodthyronine on the tubular secretion of the kidneys. *Farmakologia i Toksikologia* (Moskau), *37:* 513.
Berlin-Heimendahl, S.V. (1964): Besonderheiten des Wasser-, Mineral- und Saurebasenstoff-

wechsels in den ersten Lebenstagen. *Dtsch. Med. Wschr., 89:* 2425.
Berman, L.B. and Misra, R.P. (1972): Molecular nephrology. *Amer. J. Med., 53:* 701.
Bernhardt, G., Braunlich, H., Dietze, C., Lungershausen, W. and Schade, R. (1973): Beschleunigung der renalen Ausscheidung von p-Aminohippursaure bei Ratten verschiedenen Alters durch wiederholte Zufuhr von Fremdstoffen. *Acta Biol. Med. Germ., 31:* 423.
Bertram, D., Rind, H. and Gladtke, E. (1970): Die Elimination von para-Aminohippursaure beim Kind. *Zschr. Kinderheilk., 108:* 208.
Braunlich, H. (1973): In: *Entwicklungspharmakologie* (edited by H. Ankermannn), S. 127, Verlag Volk und Gesundheit, Berlin.
Braunlich, H. and Kersten, L. (1971): Der Einfluß von Diuretika auf die renale Ausscheidung von Wasser und Ionen bei Ratten verschiedenen Alters. *Acta Biol. Med. Germ., 27:* 149.
Braunlich, H. and Puschmann, R. (1972): Die Entwicklung der renalen Ausscheidung von Natrium und Kalium in der postnatalen Periode bei der Ratte. *Acta Biol. Med. Germ., 28:* 89.
Calcagno, Ph. L. and Rubin, M.J. (1963): Renal extraction of para-aminohippurate in infants and children. *J. Clin. Invest., 42:* 1632.
Calcagno, Ph. L., Rubin, M.J. and Weintraub, D.H. (1954): Studies on the renal concentrating and diluting mechanisms in the premature infant. *J. Clin. Invest., 33:* 91.
Clark, S.L. (1957): Cellular differentiation in the kidneys of newborn mice studied with the electron microscope. *J. Biochem. Biophys. Cytol., 3:* 349.
Deetjen, P. (1965): Tubularer Transport schwacher organischer Sauren und Basen. In: *Normale und pathologische Funktion des Nierentubulus* edited by K.J. Ulrich and K. Hierholzer, S. 19, Verlag Hans Huber, Bern and Stuttgart.
Dicker, S.E. and Shirley, D.G. (1971): Rates of oxygen consumption and of anaerobic glykolysis in renal cortex and medulla of adult and newborn rats and guinea pigs. *J. Physiol.* (Lond.), *212:* 235.
Done, A.K. (1965): Developmental pharmacology. *Clin. Pharmacol. Ther., 5:* 432.
Dost, F.H. and Gladtke, (1969): Pharmakokinetik des 2-Sulfanilamido-3-methoxy-pyrazin beim Kind (Elimination, enterale Absorption, Verteilung und Dosierung). *Arzneimittelforsch., 19:* 1304.
Ecker, J.L. and Hook, J.B. (1974): Accumulation of p-aminohippuric acid by separated renal tubules from newborn and adult rabbits. *J. Pharmacol. Exp. Therap., 190:* 352.
Ehrnebo, M., Agurell, S., Jalling, B. and Boreus, L.O. (1971): Age differences in drug binding by plasma proteins: studies on human foetuses, neonates and adults. *Europ. J. Clin. Pharmacol., 3:* 189.
Frenzel, J., Braunlich, H., Schramm, D. and Kersten, L. (1947): Renale Wirkungen von cyclopenthiazid in der Neugeborenenperiode. *Acta Paed. Hung., 15:* 157.
Gruenwald, P. and Popper, H. (1940): The histogenesis and physiology of the renal glomerulus in early postnatal life: histological examinations. *J. Urol.* (Baltimore), *43:* 452.
Guthamm, H. and May, W. (1930): Gibt es eine intrauterine Nierensekretion? *Arch. Gynak., 141:* 450.
Hirsch, G.H. (1972): Stimulation of renal organic base transport by uranyl nitrate. *Canad. J. Physiol. Pharmacol., 50:* 533.
Hirsch, G.H., Cowan, D.F. and Hook, J.B. (1971): Histological changes in normal and drug induced development of renal PAH transport. *Proc. Soc. Exp. Biol. Med., 137:* 116.
Hirsch, G.H. and Hook, J.B. (1970): Maturation of renal organic acid transport: substrate stimulation by penicillin and p-aminohippurate (PAH). *J. Pharmacol. Exp. Therap.,* 103.
Hook, J.B., Williamson, H.E. and Hirsch, H. (1970): Functional maturation of renal PAH-transport in the dog. *Canad. J. Physiol., 48:* 169.

Jahrig, K., Zollner, H. and Margies, D. (1972): Osmolar clearance and clearance of total electrolytes in newborn infants. *Biol. Neonate, 20:* 93.

Kaufmann, H.J. (1965): Die Gefahrdung der Neugeborenen durch Medikamente. *Padiat. Prax., 4:* 1.

Kellner, R. (1971): THAM-Ausscheidung bei Fruhgeborenen. *Dtsch. Ges. wesen, 26:* 361.

Kerpel-Fronius, E. (1972): Das Azidoseproblem in der Neonatologie. *Padiat. Padol., 7:* 109.

Kim, J.K., Hirsch, G.H. and Hook, J.B. (1972): In vitro analysis of organic ion transport in renal cortex of the newborn rat. *Pediat. Res., 6:* 600.

Kleinman, L. and Lubbe, R.J. (1972): Factors affecting the maturation of renal PAH extraction in the new-born dog. *J. Physiol., 223:* 411.

Klinger, W. (1973): In: *Entwicklungspharmakologie,* edited by H. Ankermann, S. 51, Verlag Volk und Gesundheit, Berlin.

Kobyletzki, D.V. (1971): Pharmakokinetik und Pharmakologie. In: *Fortschritte der perinatalen Medizin* edited by E. Saling and K.A. Huter, S. 110, Georg Thieme, Stuttgart.

Kobyletzki, D.V. and Althammer, H. (1967): Experimentelle Untersuchungen zur perinatalen Pharmakokinetik von Nitrofurantoin. *Int. J. Clin. Pharm., 1:* 120.

Krauer, B., Dettli, P. and Spring, L. (1968): Zur Pharmakokinetik der Sulfonamide im 1. Lebensjahr. *Pharmacol. Clin., 1:* 47.

Kretchmer, N., Greenberg, R.E. and Sereni, F. (1963): Biochemical basis of immaturity. *Ann. Rev. Med., 14:* 407.

McCance, R.A. (1950): Renal physiology in infancy. *Amer. J. Med., 9:* 229.

McCance, R.A. and Finck, M.A. v. (1947): Urinmenge in Abhangigkeit vom Lebensalter. *Arch. Dis. Child., 22:* 200.

McCance, R.A. and Young, W.F. (1941): The secretion of urine by newborn infants. *J. Physiol., 99:* 265.

McIntosh, R. (1957): On growth and development. *Arch. Dis. Child., 32:* 261.

Mills, J.N. (1966): Human circadian rhythms. *Physiol. Rev., 46:* 128.

Natochin, Y.V. (1974): Renal pharmacology: comparative, developmental and cellular aspects. *Ann. Rev. Pharmacol., 14:* 75.

Neussel, H. and Olbing, H. (1972): Zur Pharmakokinetik von Carbenicillin bei Kindern nach intramuskularer In jektion. *Int. J. Clin. Pharmacol., 5:* 444.

Nyhan, W.L. (1961): Toxicity of drugs in the neonatal period. *J. Pediat.* (St. Louis), *59:* 1.

Rennick, C. (1972): Renal excretion of drugs: tubular transport and metabolism. *Ann. Rev. Pharmacol., 12:* 141.

Rind, H. and Gladtke, E. (1965): Die Aktivierung der Sulfonamidelimination bei reifen und unreifen Neugeborenen durch Complamin. *Klin. Wschr., 43:* 904.

Rohwedder, H. J. (1968): In: *Fortschritte der Padologie,* Bd. II, edited by F. Linneweh, S. 218, Springer-Verlag, Berlin.

Rohwedder, H.-J. and Goll, U. (1970): Untersuchungen uber die Pharmakokinetik von Gentamycin bei Kindern. *Dtsch. Med. Schr., 95:* 1171.

Scheler, W. (1969): Grundlagen der Allgemeinen Pharmakologie. *Fischer Jena,* S. 274.

Schreiter, G. (1966): Neuere physiologische und klinische Aspekte der Nierenfunktion. *Dtsch. Ges. wesen, 21:* 433.

Sereni, F. and Principi, N. (1968): Developmental pharmacology. *Ann. Rev. Pharmacol., 8:* 453.

Stanbury, S.W. and Thomson, A.E. (1951): Diurnal variation in electrolyte excretion. *Clin. Sci., 10:* 268.

Terracini, B. and Palestro, G. (1966): Effect of two nephrotoxic agents on newborn rats. *Experientia* (Basel), *22:* 297.

Traeger, A., Stein, G., Fritze, Ch., Braunlich, I. and Braunlich, H. (1974): Untersuchungen zur Beschleunigung der renalen Ausscheidung von p-Aminohippursaure nach wiederholter Zufuhr bei verschieden alten Menschen. *Dtsch. Ges.wesen, 29:* 1129.

Wachstein, M. and Robinson, M. (1965): Neonatal resistance to nephrotoxic renal tubular necrosis in the rat. *Fed. Proc., 24:* 619.

Webber, W.A. and Blackbourn, J. (1970): The permeability of the glomerulus to large molecules. *Lab. Invest., 23:* 1.

Weiner, I.M. (1971): Excretion of drugs by the kidney. In: *Handbook of Experimental Pharmacology,* Vol. XXVIII, p. 328.

Weiner, I.M. (1967): Mechanisms of drug absorption and excretion. The renal excretion of drugs and related compounds. *Ann. Rev. Pharmacol., 7:* 39.

Weiner, I.M. and Mudge, G.H. (1964): Renal tubular mechanisms for excretion of organic bases and acids. *Amer. J. Med.* (N.Y.), *36:* 743.

Weingartner, L. (1973): Zur Urinausscheidung von Klostrimazol in verschiedenen Altersabschnitten beim Kind. *Int. J. Clin. Pharmacol., 8:* 131.

Whittam, R. (1960): Sodium and potassium movements in kidney cortex slices from newborn animals. *J. Physiol.* (Lond.), *153:* 358.

Yaffe, S.J. and Juchau, M.R. (1974): Perinatal pharmacology. *Ann. Rev. Pharmacol., 14:* 219.

Yaffe, S.J. and Rane, A. (1971): Developmental aspects of pharmakokinetics. *Acta Pharmacol. Toxicol.* (Kopenh.), *29,* Suppl. 3: *240.*

Yeary, R.A., Benish, R.A. and Finkelstein, M. (1966): Acute toxicity of drugs in newborn animals. *J. Pediat.* (St. Louis), *69:* 663.

Ziegler, E.E. and Fomon, S.J. (1971): Fluid intake, renal solute, and water balance in infancy. *J. Pediat.* (St. Louis), *78:* 561.

Zufarov, K.A. (1974): Structural bases of filtration, absorption and secretion. "Medicine" Publishing House, Uzbek, SSR, Taschkent.

Sweymuller, E. (1971): Storungen des Elektrolythaushaltes aus der Sicht des Padiaters. *Wien. Klin. Wschr., 83:* 541.

6

Antineoplastic Agents

FEDERICO SPREAFICO
and
MIRIAM SENHOUSE ROSSI

As is true for any other drug, the major determinants of the therapeutic activity of antineoplastic agents are represented by the interrelationship of several factors, including the physicochemical nature of the compound, its manner and route of administration, the characteristics of its absorption, binding, distribution and metabolism, and the interaction of the drug with its cellular target. Already substantiated in many areas of pharmacology, consideration of the quantitative and qualitative aspects of the physiological disposition of antitumoral agents is of utmost importance in the development of rationalized cancer chemotherapeutic designs. Indeed, it can be argued that knowledge of the pharmacokinetic parameters of the drugs employed is more important in cancer chemotherapy than in many other fields of therapeutics. Not only does a narrow margin between ineffectiveness and excessive toxicity often exist for these agents, but a further complication to sound treatment is represented by the fact that the mode of action of the agent may limit its effectiveness to only one phase of the cell cycle. For example: in the case of a phase-specific drug, beyond a certain concentration no further cytotoxic activity will be gained, thus the scheduling of drug administration to achieve and maintain this effective concentration will be critical and, obviously, dependent on the distribution and elimination of the compound.

Scheduling must also take into account the damage inflicted on normal cell populations, and for both categories of agents—but especially for non-phase-specific agents—the timing of doses is heavily influenced by this type of consideration (Skipper et al., 1970).

Unfortunately, the possibility of coherently integrating the biochemical, pharmacokinetic and cell population kinetic factors is currently restricted to a few well-characterized experimental systems; not only is current knowledge of the cellular kinetics of human neoplasms still severely limited but this ignorance also extends to many basic aspects of the pharmacology of available antineoplastic compounds. For many of these drugs, the pharmacokinetics has thus far been investigated only in animals or in a small number of patients who were, moreover, frequently affected by different types of neoplasms. For other cytotoxic agents, their metabolism is still a matter of discussion or the analytical methods for their measurement simply are not available.

A number of antitumoral compounds have brief half-lives in the circulation and are administered in low doses. They have a rapid metabolism and/or a spontaneous degradation, and one finds chemically related compounds in the tissues, especially in the case of the antimetabolites. All of these factors compound the difficulty of pharmacokinetic investigation; however, the acquisition of such basic information, which is necessary in order to materially advance anti-cancer treatment, is currently the object of active investigation at multiple levels. One cannot consider this an easy task for a number of reasons. Tumors of the same type, for instance, frequently display different sensitivity to a given drug, a fact which hampers the possibility of comparing variations in scheduling based on pharmacokinetics. The last few years have seen definite improvements in cancer treatment through the use of combination chemotherapy; however, the influence that one antitumoral has on the metabolism and disposition of other members of the combination, or the effects that one cycle of treatment exerts on the pharmacokinetics of following cycles, has not yet been given systematic attention, even at the experimental level. On the other hand, the ethical restraints in conducting this type of investigation in cancer patients need not be emphasized.

Given the fact that the clinical pharmacology of antineoplastic agents is still at its inception, the problem of possible age-related differences in the metabolism of these drugs—e.g., differences between adults and children, and differences within the pediatric age group—has been studied very little, although the possible consequences of such discrepancies are important in designing the safest and most effective treatment schedules. Accordingly, this chapter will be devoted to an examination of the existing knowledge on several antitumorals chosen for their paradigmatic characteristics or for their frequent use in pediatric oncology. The discussion will explore some of the implications of pediatric physiology on the pharmacodynamics of these drugs.

CYCLOPHOSPHAMIDE

Cyclophosphamide (Cy) is one of the more frequently employed alkylating agents and, as such, has been the object of extensive investigation. This non-

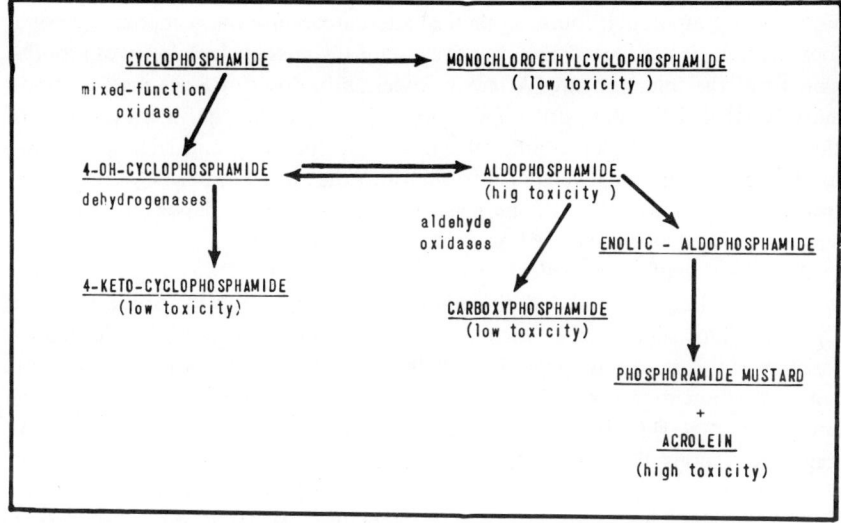

Fig. 1: Proposed metabolic pathways of cyclophosphamide (modified from Connors et al., 1974).

ionized, lipid-soluble compound was originally synthesized in 1958 and is metabolically inactive without *in vivo* biotransformation. The necessary activation occurs primarily in the liver where Cy is converted by microsomal mixed-function oxidases into active alkylating derivatives. In spite of a long series of studies, the biotransformation pathway has still not been completely clarified, and a hypothetical scheme is presented in Fig. 1 from the work done by Hill et al. (1972). The activated metabolites reach the periphery via the blood circulation, and there is rapid uptake by all body tissues, including the brain, since these agents easily penetrate the blood-brain barrier. Although the Cy derivatives are more active against rapidly reproducing cells, the metabolites actually have a non-phase specific mode of action, and the concentration of the active products at the target sites greatly influences the extent of cell-killing in sensitive tissues. It is evident, therefore, that hepatic microsomal activity, the relative production and stability of metabolites (active or inactive) and the degree of elimination by the patient are the most important clinical factors controlling the effectiveness of Cy.

In the clinical situation, the route of administration is another important variable because it determines the rate of absorption of the parent compound. When given orally, Cy is only partially absorbed, with 17-30% of the administered drug eliminated unchanged in the stools (Bagley et al., 1973). The oral route, with increments in the dosage to account for fecal loss, is used primarily in maintenance treatment, whereas Cy is commonly given intravenously for induction of remission. The intramuscular route, a practical alternative since the compound is not a local irritant, is used less frequently because of the possible variability of absorption from the injection site. After i.v. injection in doses of 6–80 mg/kg, radioactively labeled Cy was very rapidly distributed into the equivalent of 64% of the body weight (Bagley et al., 1973). Its lipid solubility and lack of protein-binding permit an equally rapid diffusion into the tissues, where Cy concentration equilibrates with that of the plasma. Cy is then either deposited in the tissues, eliminated by renal excretion or activated in the liver.

The plasma half-life in patients previously unexposed to Cy averages 6.5 h, but with five consecutive daily administrations Bagley et al. (1973) found that the Cy T½ became successively shorter. Given the nonionizing, lipid-soluble characteristics of Cy, it would appear less likely that either increased tissue uptake or renal excretion were accountable for the increasing rate of Cy plasma disappearance; rather, it would suggest that a change in the rate of hepatic activation might be responsible. In fact, Mouridsen et al. (1974) reported that in their patients the rate of Cy plasma disappearance seemed to be determined predominantly by the rate of hepatic biotransformation. In addition, prior patient treatment with allopurinol, a drug often used concomitantly with the antineoplastic agents to prevent urate nephropathy, resulted in the prolongation of the Cy T½ (Bagley et al., 1973). The mechanism of this drug interaction is currently unknown.

Cy is excreted almost exclusively by the kidney, but extensive tubular reabsorption occurs, and only a small amount of the unaltered drug is found in the urine. Bagley et al. (1973) reported that less than 20% of the Cy dose was recovered in the urine over a wide range of o.v. doses. The mean renal clearance of Cy in adults is only 10.7 ml/min (Cohen et al., 1971), a value not only consistent with the nonionized nature of the drug, but also indicative of extensive tubular reabsorption. This process of renal recycling ensures that most of the administered drug, an average of 88% according to Cohen et al. (1971), will undergo biotransformation by being circulated to the liver. Renal excretion, in contrast, is the major route of elimination for the more polar, less lipid-soluble Cy metabolites, this then being the basis for the cystitis which frequently results with Cy treatment.

Hepatic activation of the parent compound is a rapid process, and the metabolites pass swiftly into the bloodstream; this decrease in liver concentration of the biotransformation products is compensated for by the efflux of tissue-stored Cy, which, in turn, is circulated to the liver and activated. The alkylating metabolites in the plasma appear to be at least 50% protein-bound, and the average alkylating activity of the unbound metabolites is maintained in the plasma for a minimum of 24 h in most patients (Bagley et al., 1973). The requirement for microsomal enzyme activation exposes Cy to the possibility of increased activation by induction of the hepatic enzymes, thus affecting, as previously mentioned, the plasma T½ and the peak levels of alkylating activity. Although this effect has been clinically investigated in only a relatively small number of patients, pre-treatment with phenobarbital (Jao et al., 1972) or with prednisone for several days (Faber et al., 1974) has resulted in an increased rate of Cy activation, however, the overall influence of induction on the therapeutic effect of the drug has not, thus far, been entirely explained.

With the clarification of the biotransformation pathway and the identification of cytotoxic metabolites (Connors et al., 1974; Colvin et al., 1973), it has become apparent that the pharmacokinetics of both the parent compound and the alkylating agents, plus the interaction of the latter, are the pertinent factors in Cy therapeutics (Chabner et al., 1975b). In principle, the therapeutic efficacy of a non-phase-specific agent such as Cy should not be modified by altering its rate of transformation, as the concentration-by-time product of the active metabolites would remain essentially constant. However, since under the influence of an inducer or an inhibitor the relative rates and/or ratios of various pathways leading to cytotoxically active or inactive metabolites could be affected, the possibility that modification in biological activity could result cannot be overlooked. In fact, Spreafico et al. (1974) have observed changes in Cy anti-leukemic activity in animals pre-treated with phenobarbital. Moreover, as various antitumors, and Cy in particular (Spreafico et al., 1974), have been shown to alter the level of microsomal enzymes in animals, undoubtedly the pharmacokinetics (Mouridsen et al., 1974) and, possibly, the *in vivo* performance of this cytotoxic agent could be different when used in single doses, in repeated daily doses or in combination with other antineoplastic agents. Clinically, this point, as well as the existence of age-related differences in Cy activation, have not been investigated to any significant extent.

The dosage requirements for Cy, using apparently optimal antitumoral activity and minimal toxicity for a certain therapeutic goal as guidelines, are best calculated, as is the case with all antitumorals, on the basis of body surface area rather than weight (Mellet, 1974). Dosage modifications according to age have been reported by few investigators (Finkelstein et al., 1969) and usually on a per weight basis, not per body surface area, thus precluding accurate comparisons between dosage levels in adults and children. In practice, the amounts used in both pediatric and adult age groups have been the same, without notable differences in toxic manifestations when the doses are calculated by surface area. Theoretically, limitations in hepatic biotransformation due to functional insufficiency should be seen only in neonates, where hepatic immaturity is reflected in a decreased mixed-function oxidase activity that then reaches adult levels by early infancy (see Chapter 9); keeping this fact in mind, it would be necessary to modify dosage levels of Cy for reasons of hepatic function only in the exceptional case where the drug was being used in the newborn or young infant or where liver function studies were abnormal. Adequate renal function is certainly of great clinical importance in determining the need to alter the dosage for an individual patient. Bagley et al. (1973) reported prolonged retention of alkylating metabolites in the presence of moderate renal insufficiency in their patients. This finding is significant when considering the dosage requirements in children under 2 years of age, since in this age group normal kidney function demonstrates decreased glomerular filtration, and an even greater reduction in tubular reabsorption, than found in adult norms.

Another important consideration in utilizing Cy in the pediatric patient is the effect of this antitumoral on the gonadal tissue. Several cases of amenorrhea and testicular atrophy during and after treatment with Cy have been reported (Fairley et al., 1972), and this finding is especially relevant in the pediatric use of the drug. Further studies of this particularly distressing side effect are necessary in order to better define its relationship with the age of the patient, pre- or postpubertal, and with dosage schedules.

METHOTREXATE

Methotrexate (MTX) was originally introduced clinically for the treatment of childhood leukemia (Farber et al., 1948) but has since found wide use in oncological chemotherapy due both to its significant activity against a wide range of neoplasms (Chabner et al., 1975a) and to the availability of a specific antidote, i.e., folinic acid. The major mechanism of action of MTX is through a reversible, competitive binding to the intracellular enzyme, dihydrofolate reductase, thus causing tetrahydrofolate depletion and the consequent blockage of DNA synthesis (Werkheiser, 1963; Johns et al., 1964). Folinic acid, being on the other side of the metabolic block, when given within an appropriate interval of MTX administration is able to partially mitigate the effect of the cytotoxic agent on normal cells. In addition to its inhibition of DNA synthesis, MTX can also depress RNA and protein synthesis; consequently, the drug is classified as a cell cycle phase-specific agent "with limitation," a mode of action which renders MTX quite schedule-dependent for its effectiveness. Under experimental conditions, phase-specific agents are generally most efficient in killing tumor cells when given either at frequent intervals or by prolonged infusion. Non-phase-specific cytotoxic agents, on the contrary, are more active therapeutically with intermittent high-dosage schedules. For an in-depth discussion of these important aspects of pharmacodynamics in cancer chemotherapy, the reader is referred to the several excellent reviews available, among them Skipper et al. (1970) and Jusko (1971).

In man, the degree of MTX absorption from the g.i. tract appears to be a saturable process, since small amounts, e.g., 0.1 mg/kg, are rapidly and completely absorbed, whereas doses on the order of 10 mg/kg are slowly and incompletely taken up. Accordingly, MTX is often used parenterally in order to obtain more controlled plasma levels. In the plasma, MTX binds up to 70% to proteins, primarily albumins, a process which can be influenced by the co-administration of organic acids such as salicylic acid or sulfisoxazole (Henderson et al., 1965). As a class, the antifolates have probably been the most investigated of all the antineoplastic agents, particularly as regards their disposition, and an elaborate pharmacokinetic model has been proposed (Bischoff et al., 1971). In both man and animals, the plasma disappearance curve is triphasic, with T½ values, in man, after i.v. doses of 30 mg/sq. meter, being 0.75, 3.5 and 26.9 h, respectively; since the therapeutic effect and drug toxicity depend much more on the duration of an effective plasma drug level than on the height of the level, the last phase is clinically the most important (Huffman et al., 1973). The drug does have an enterohepatic recirculation, but fecal excretion is of minor importance. The major elimination route is urinary, and 50–90% of the drug is thus excreted over a 48 h period, most of this being in the first 8 h after administration. As in the case of other lipid-insoluble drugs, MTX is primarily excreted unaltered, and, because it is a weak organic acid, this drug is not only filtered by the glomeruli but also actively secreted by the tubules. Not unexpectedly, the concomitant administration of other weak inorganic acids (salicylates, etc.) can influence the drug's renal clearance.

After this initial elimination, only small amounts of MTX are found in the urine, largely as metabolites, and residual amounts of the agent can be recovered from the kidney, liver and spleen even several weeks following its administration. It is apparent that impaired renal function would markedly influence the dynamics of this antineoplastic agent. Freemen-Narrod et al. (1974) observed two different patterns in the elimination of MTX in man. In their study, some of the adults and all children showed a relatively rapid plasma clearance, with an apparent T½ of 90 min, after i.v. dosing; under the same conditions, the other adults displayed plasma half-lives of 6–8 h. Although renal function indices were normal in all of the individuals, the differences in creatinine clearance (above or below 80 ml/min) correlated with the fast or slow elimination of MTX from the plasma. The limited number of patients in this study does not allow one to draw definitive conclusions without further investigation of this pharmacokinetic finding, yet the fact that all of the children were "rapid" MTX eliminators suggests that the pediatric age group may handle the drug in a manner different from most adults. Certainly, a more thorough examination of this phenomenon is merited in order to determine its full clinical significance, i.e., its pertinence to the drug's therapeutic efficacy and toxic side effects.

6-MERCAPTOPURINE

First synthesized in 1953, 6-mercaptopurine (6-MP) is, chemically, a sulfur analog of hypoxanthine (6-hydroxypurine) and of adenine (6-aminopurine), and was the first member of the large thiopurine series to demonstrate significant antineoplastic potential. The drug is still in use as one of the components in combination therapy for acute leukemia in childhood and as immunosuppressive agent. The exact biochemical mode of action of 6-MP, mediated through its conversion to ribonucleoside monophosphate, continues to elude investigators in some of its aspects because of its complexity; the major sites of activity appear to be represented by inhibition of de novo purine biosynthesis and at the purine nucleotide interconversion steps (Calabresi and Parks, 1970; Henderson and Paterson, 1973). Thus the formation of DNA and RNA could be blocked, as well as that of coenzymes, along with the additional possibility of thiopurine incorporation into nucleic acids. This drug demonstrates its greatest effect during the S-phase of the cell cycle, but, because of its complex interference with the cell synthetic machinery, it possesses an element of self-limitation (Skipper et al., 1970).

6-MP is only partially absorbed by the gastrointestinal tract, and, on the average, 50% of an oral dose is recoverable in the feces (Loo et al., 1968). The compound, when taken orally, reaches lower peak plasma levels and is excreted more slowly than when given parenterally (Elion, 1967). After intravenous injection, approximately 19% of the 6-MP is bound to plasma proteins (Loo et al., 1968). The plasma T½ of an i.v. dose, according to the most recent studies, is different in children and in adults. In the pediatric patient, the average T½ is 21 min, but in the adult the apparent T½ averages 47 min (Loo et al., 1968). These findings certainly would suggest an age-related difference in the drug's pharmacokinetics.

6-MP and its metabolites have a wider volume of distribution than that of total body water, as is true for other drugs that undergo extensive degradation in the body. Despite this fact, the CSF/plasma ratio of this agent is never more than 1/5, even after i.v. dosing, indicating that 6-MP passes the blood-brain barrier with difficulty. Cell uptake of the antitumoral agent from the extracellular fluid is rapid, but a large percentage of the intracellular compound is inactivated by xanthine oxidase to form 6-thiouric acid, which is then catabolized to uric acid. The concomitant administration of allopurinol was, therefore, proposed by Elion et al. (1963) as a means of increasing antineoplastic activity by augmenting the fraction of the drug dose available for anabolism to the nucleotide forms. Experimentally, this combination has been described as being more active in man. On a practical basis, there is little to be gained clinically beyond the sparing of the drug; moreover, data on the pharmacokinetic changes of 6-MP, observed using concomitant treatment with allopurinol, are contradictory. Elion et al. (1963) originally described a reduction in the amount of the drug excreted as thiouric acid; however, more recently Coffey et al. (1972) did not find any significant changes in the pharmacokinetics of 6-MP in patients also treated with the xanthine oxidase inhibitor. These latter results have indicated that an alternate catabolic pathway probably exists for the cytotoxic agent, so that when the xanthine oxidase pathway is blocked, the thiopurine is rapidly degraded by this secondary route. This alternative pathway is assumed to involve the formation of methylthiopurine, which is subsequently metabolized via a different enzyme system.

This antitumoral agent is excreted exclusively by the kidneys; approximately 20% of an i.v. 6-MP dose is recoverable in the urine within 6 h in all age groups (Loo et al., 1968). A larger percentage of the sulfate derivatives of the drug are also found in the urine in the same time period. As mentioned previously, with oral administration of the drug the rate of elimination is somewhat slower. Because the kidneys play such an important role in the excretion of this agent, the existence of renal insufficiency in a patient would necessitate modification of the dosage in order to obtain therapeutic, not toxic, 6-MP plasma levels. For the same reason, the reduced glomerular filtration rate that is physiological in children under 2 years of age would require usage of lower doses, per body surface area, than those needed to obtain equivalent plasma levels in older children and adults. The findings of Loo et al. (1968), however, which suggest an accelerated rate of 6-MP biotransformation in children, add to the renal function another factor to be considered that would have a contrasting effect on the pharmacodynamics of this antineoplastic drug in very young children. Clearly, more thorough investigation of the age-related differences in 6-MP metabolism is necessary in order to obtain maximum therapeutic efficacy of this drug in the pediatric patient.

CYTOSINE ARABINOSIDE

Cytosine arabinoside (Ara-C) differs from naturally occurring cytidine and deoxycytidine by having arabinose, rather than ribose or deoxyribose, as its sugar moiety. The cytostatic action of Ara-C is apparently due to an inhibitory action on DNA polymerase by Ara-C triphosphate in competition with deoxycytidine triphosphate. RNA synthesis and cell maturation are not primarily affected, although, in principle, sufficient cellular damage may be caused by inhibiting DNA synthesis to incur metabolic death of the cell even after removal of the metabolic block. Ara-C is considered a cell cycle phase-specific antineoplastic agent and would seem to exert its cytostatic action principally in the latter part of the S-phase of the cellular growth cycle (Skipper et al., 1970). This mode of action has therapeutic significance because it implies that the rate of cell kill is independent of the Ara-C concentration, above a minimal threshold level, and that by prolonging the duration of the agent in the body an increasing number of cells would reach the appropriate cell phase to be inhibited.

Given this specific fact of Ara-C cytotoxicity, the drug is usually given intravenously, sometimes intrathecally, and seldom by other routes because of its poor or variable absorption (Finkelstein et al., 1970; Ho and Frei, 1971). The prolonged infusion method is most commonly used in order to obtain and maintain therapeutically adequate levels. The most recent pharmacokinetic studies show that Ara-C has a biphasic plasma disappearance curve with the average apparent T½ of the short phase being 11 to 12 min and that of the long phase 111 to 157 min (Ho and Frei, 1971; Wan et al., 1974). These results were obtained in a small number of adults using doses ranging from 47 mg to 3,000 mg/sq. meter of body surface area that were given in a single rapid i.v. injection or by infusion. Previous pharmacokinetic studies had reported monophasic plasma disappearance curves with half-lives varying from 30 to 60 min in adults (Creasey et al., 1966) and averaging 30 min in children (Finkelstein et al., 1970).

Although widely distributed in the body, Ara-C has demonstrated only limited penetration of the blood-brain barrier, with a CSF/plasma ratio of 0.4 resulting in studies by Ho and Frei (1971). The drug appears to follow one of two metabolic pathways: part of the dose is deaminated, mainly by the liver and kidney, to form the therapeutically inert uracil analog Ara-U, while the other part is activated by kinases to Ara-C triphosphate, the actual antineoplastic agent. Besides some indications that the deamination route is a rate-limited process, thus dose-dependent (Ho and Frei, 1971), it is not yet known which factors favor the conversion of the inactive parent compound into the cytotoxic agent.

Ara-C is excreted exclusively by the kidney, and the rate or renal clearance in the adult has been reported as being 90 ml/min (Dedrick et al., 1973). Within 24 h after administration of the radioactive compound, investigators found about 8% of the dose recoverable in the urine as unaltered Ara-C and approximately 70% as the labeled uracil analog (Ho and Frei, 1971). Working with children, Finkelstein et al. (1970) reported about 90% recovery of total radioactivity in the urine, consisting of less than 10% Ara-C and the rest Ara-U, within 24 h after i.v. administration of the labeled compound.

Clinical evidence would support the fact that Ara-C is metabolized and excreted in a similar manner by children and adults alike, but specific pharmacokinetic information to substantiate this hypothesis is currently lacking. Considering that Ara-C is partly deactivated and partly activated by the liver, and that it is eliminated only via the kidney, in those patients with hepatic and/or renal function indices less than adult norms, dosage modifications might be needed to prevent undue toxicity from the drug. This should probably be taken into account when using Ara-C in the neonate and infant up to 2 years old, where physiological liver and/or kidney limitations would influence the metabolism and excretion of this agent. Toxic manifestations, including gastrointestinal symptoms and bone marrow depression, are the same in both adults and children (Lampkin et al., 1972).

L-ASPARAGINASE

L-asparaginase (L-Asnase), an enzyme derived from bacteria, is used primarily as an antineoplastic agent in acute leukemia. Although at least two sources of the enzyme are known, from *E. coli* and from *Erwinia carotovora*, only the former, and specifically that fraction designated as EC_2, has found practical use thus far (Whitecar et al., 1970; Schwartz, 1970). The mode of action of L-Asnase is unique in cancer chemotherapy since it is based on the fact that some tumor cells, lacking the normal complement of the enzyme L-asparagine synthetase, are unable to synthesize the amino acid L-asparagine. Outside of the cell, L-Asnase catalyzes the hydrolysis of L-asparagine to aspartic acid and ammonia, thus depriving the dependent tumor cells of their extracellular source of vital nutrient (Whitecar et al., 1970). It is possible, however, that other mechanisms, perhaps involving the cell membrane, could also play a role. Curiously enough, not all tumor cells in the same pathological classification display equal susceptibility to the cytotoxic action of this agent.

This cytotoxic enzyme cannot be administered orally because of its destruction by intestinal juices. In order to obtain more reliable blood levels, it is normally given intravenously, but i.m. injection and intrathecal administration have also resulted in significant plasma levels of the enzyme (Ho et al., 1971). As a macromolecular protein, L-Asnase has physicochemical properties which affect its distribution in the body, for example, after i.v. administration there is limited drug penetration of the blood-brain barrier, and the enzyme even enters the extravascular space poorly (Ho et al., 1970). Being a protein of bacterial origin, the enzyme can induce a strong antibody response in patients which then significantly influences its plasma disappearance curve (Schwartz, 1970). It is not surprising, therefore, that the pharmacokinetics of L-Asnase demonstrate considerable variation from patient to patient, and that these differences do not appear to be related to the usual factors, such as age, sex, diagnosis or extent of disease (Ho et al., 1970). The effect of this immunological response has been noted both in children and in adults (Schwartz, 1970).

After a single rapid i.v. injection, the initial L-Asnase plasma level appears to be dose-related. The subsequent plasma disappearance curves may be monophasic or biphasic, and are not influenced by either the dose or the source of the enzyme. Ho et al. (1970) reported finding an exponential curve in L-Asnase plasma levels, with half-lives that ranged from 8 to 30 h. Interestingly enough, in those patients receiving daily doses of the enzyme there was a cumulative increase in the plasma levels but no change in the individual patient's T½. Haskell et al. (1972), using crystallized enzyme, obtained biphasic plasma half-lives in their patients, with the average apparent T½ of the short phase being 4 to 9 h and the long T½ being 1.4 to 1.8 days. These authors also found that there seemed to be rapid binding of L-Asnase at sites that were in, or close to, the intravascular space after a single i.v. injection. In addition, they reported that the amino acid L-asparagine was undetectable in the blood as long as there were L-Asnase plasma levels.

In keeping with its physicochemical and antigenic properties, L-Asnase is not excreted in any appreciable quantities in either the urine or bile (Ho et al., 1971). It is believed that sequestration by the reticuloendothelial system serves as the major route of elimination in man. This method of excretion proceeds slowly, with enzyme activity detectable in the blood 13 to 22 days after a single i.v. injection in patients who have shown a minimal immunological response to the drug (Ohnuma et al., 1970).

Considering its mechanism of action, it is not surprising that the toxic side effects of L-Asnase are numerous and quite different from those of the other cytotoxic agents. Symptoms of biochemical abnormalities due to depletion of L-asparagine and L-glutamine, such as neurological deficits (Weiss et al., 1974), symptoms of drug sensitivity, including anaphylaxis (Capizzi et al., 1971), evidence of coagulation disorders, and insulin-responsive, nonketonic hyperglycemia (Whitecar et al., 1970) are some of the manifestations of L-Asnase toxicity. The diabetic effect seems to be dose-related since it usually occurs only at daily dosage levels greater than 25,000 i.u. per sq. meter of body surface area. In children, the side effects are generally the same as in adult patients, the dosage levels per body surface area being similar in both age groups. Dosage levels range from less than 1,000 to more than 400,000 units L-Asnase/sq. meter daily, the smaller amounts being used in those patients who have a negligible immunologic response. The therapeutic efficacy of the enzyme is thus not strictly dose-dependent, and prompt results are obtained in the responsive patient without prolonged treatment (Lampkin et al., 1972). In the absence of specific data to the contrary, and given the duration of L-Asnase plasma levels in adults, Pratt et al. (q970) assume that the pharmacokinetic patterns of the enzyme are similar in children, and they suggest weekly, rather than daily, administration of the drug as a means of decreasing its toxic manifestations. They further report, from clinical observation, that the extension of treatment beyond a 2-week period does not enhance the therapeutic effect of the drug.

VINCRISTINE

In any discussion of pediatric oncology, vincristine (VCR) must be included because of its presence, in combination with a steroid and other agents, in most of the current therapeutic procotols for leukemia. To cite an example, one of the classical protocols for acute lymphoblastic leukemia consists of vincristine and prednisone to induce remission and then maintenance the methotrexate and 6-mercaptopurine. VCR and its analog, vinblastine, are the clinically important agents of the vinca alkaloid group, both having a complex, and only partially elucidated, mode of action. Although these agents are generally regarded as metaphase-arresting drugs, since they disrupt the mitotic spindle by interfering with microtubular proteins, other mechanisms are probably also operative in causing cell death with VCR (Madoc-Jones and Mauro, 1974).

The lack of information of a precise mode of action extends into the areas of the pharmacology and pharmacokinetics of this cytotoxic agent. For instance, the other vinca alkaloids seem to be erratically absorbed from the g.i. tract, but specific information concerning VCR is not available. This drug is administered only the the i.v. route, with precautions taken to prevent local irritation due to extravasation. Although comparable data on VCR have not been published, the study recently reported (Owellen and Hartke, 1975) on the pharmacokinetics of vinblastine in humans merits consideration in this discussion. Radioactive vinblastine (0.20 to 0.25 mg/kg) was administered to two adults via a 1 min i.v. infusion, both patients had normal renal and liver function studies. The antineoplastic agent showed a biphasic plasma clearance pattern, with the T½ for the alpha, or short, phase being 4.25 and 4.78 min, respectively, and the T½ for the beta, or prolonged, phase being 185 and 195 min in the respective cases. The volume of distribution (V_d) for the central compartment was 29.7 L and 39.4 L, while the total V_d was 86.4 L and 111.4 L, respectively. The vinblastine was bound extensively to blood components in the following order: plasma→platelets→RBC→WBC; this latter finding supports previous experimental evidence that the vinca alkaloids bind to serum proteins (Donigan and Owellen, 1973). Therefore, VCR should have, if it follows the pattern of vinblastine, a biphasic T½ wide body distribution and, according to Johnson et al. (1963), preferential uptake by enoplastic tissue. Morasca et al. (1969), in a study on 14 children, showed that there was measurable VCR activity in the serum of some of the patients for up to 4 h after a dose of 0.1 mg/kg VCR was given by 1 h i.v. infusion. All of the children had a definite level of VCR serum activity for at least 2 h after the infusion was stopped that tapered off at varying rates. Because of differences in the age of the subjects, in the dosage levels, in the means of administration and in the means of measuring VCR activity, the two studies cannot actually be compared, yet there is a strong suggestion that VCR pharmacokinetics follows the same open, two-compartment system described above in the vinblastine study.

VCR does not appear to pass the blood-brain barrier, and intrathecal administration in animals has consistently produced overwhelming paralysis (Adamson et al., 1965) Very little is known about the actual metabolism of the vinca alkaloids, including VCR, except that the liver is involved. VCR elimination is thought to be largely via the bile, although, in their study with vinblastine, Owellen and Hartke (1975) found appreciable mounts of unaltered drug and metabolites in the urine over a 72 h period after this VCR analogue had been given.

The possibility of age-dependent differences in VCR pharmacokinetics has not been explored to any extent. A similar dose of the drug, 1 to 2 mg/sq. meter, is used in both adult and pediatric therapy. Greenwald (1973), however, mentions that clinically children seem to tolerate dose levels that would cause more serious toxicity in adults; this fact might be indicative of a difference in pharmacokinetics and/or metabolism between the two age groups. Mention has already been made of VCR's use in combination with other agents; as discussed previously, the reciprocal influences that the combined cytotoxic agents may have on their individual absorption, distribution and metabolism patterns are still "terra incognita." In view of its wide use in pediatric oncology, the almost total lack of pharmacokinetic data on VCR in humans, and especially in children, would seem a significant gap in chemotherapeutic knowledge.

ACTINOMYCIN-D

Actinomycin-D (Act-D) deserve mention in this chapter on antineoplastic agents in pediatrics since this antibiotic, derived from a species of *Streptomyces*, has been found useful in the treatment of Wilm's tumor, a neoplastic condition most frequently occurring in childhood (Goldberg, 1965; Greenwald, 1973). Its cytotoxicity is due to its binding to double-stranded DNA, thus preventing the action of the RNA polymerases, and subsequent ribonucleotide synthesis (Schwartz et al., 1968). DNA synthesis can also be blocked, but apparently only at higher concentrations (Schwartz, 1974).

Oral administration of Act-D proved much less effective than by parenteral routes, indicating poor g.i. absorption. The only method of administration of any clinical significance is i.v. because of the antibiotic's local inflammatory action (Philips et al., 1960; Goodman and Gilman, 1965). In the past, dosage schedules have been determined by general assessment of the drug's therapeutic efficacy, but there is no pharmacological basis of treatment to correlate with the clinical response, and hence little pharmacokinetic data (Frei, 1974a).

There is very rapid clearance of i.v. Act-D from the blood, little antibiotic activity being detectable within 2 min of injection because of the drug's wide tissue distribution. In animals, however, preferential uptake of Act-D by the liver, kidney and submaxillary glands, due to unknown mechanisms, have been observed (Schwartz et al., 1968) so that concentrations can be reached in these organs far exceeding levels necessary to inhibit RNA synthesis. A selective tissue toxicity has been hypothesized from these experimental studies, but similar data pertaining to humans are not available. Also lacking is specific information relating to Act-D passage across the blood-brain barrier and the brain tissue levels that are attained with the common dosages. Act-D is very limitedly metabolized and is excreted mostly via the liver. Fifty percent of the total dose was found unchanged in the bile, while only 10% was recoverable in the urine in animal experiments (Goodman and Gilman, 1965).

As with many of the antineoplastic agents, treatment schedules have developed along empirical lines. Currently, the same dose per sq. meter is generally used in both children and adults, with the particulars of the treatment course varying somewhat in individual cases. The commonly used daily dosage level is 450 mg./sq. meter given for 5-7 days (Frei, 1974b). In view of its effectiveness against Wilm's tumor, this agent is sometimes utilized in infants under one year of age and, indeed, even in the newborn. Considering the role played by the liver in the disposition of the drug, and the immaturity of certain hepatic functions in early infancy, undoubtedly the pharmacodynamics of Act-D are different in this age group, and dosage modifications would be necessary. Fortunately, in recent years it has been recognized that the great majority of nephroblastomas presenting during the first year of life, e.g., congenital Wilm's tumor, are significantly less aggressive and pathologically more benign, and necessitate only nephrectomy (Bolande, 1974). Chemotherapy with Act-D, then, is generally used only in children one year of age and older, however, up to 2 years of age physiological limitations in kidney function, although the renal route would not appear the major pathway for Act-D elimination, might be sufficient to alter the pharmacokinetics of the drug.

The adverse side effects of Act-D mostly involve rapidly proliferating tissue and appear to be cumulative (Goldin and Johnson, 1974). Myelosuppression or g.i. symptoms might become severe enough to limit treatment (Henry and Marlow, 1943). Since this drug has radiomimetic properties, special precautions regarding dosage levels and treatment schedules must be considered, regardless of age, in any patient receiving previous radiotherapy.

ADRIAMYCIN AND DAUNOMYCIN

The last place in this necessarily brief examination of cytoxic agents must be given to 2 of the new antineoplastic compounds, Adriamycin (AM) and Daunomycin (DM). AM is the object of much current interest because of its remarkably high therapeutic activity on a wide spectrum of clinical neoplasma (Editorial, 1974). While AM is under active investigation in a range of combinations, DM is used almost exclusively in the treatment of acute leukemia (Greene et al., 1972). The two antibiotics differ only in that a hydrogen ion in the acetyl moiety of DM has been replaced by a hydroxyl group in AM, yet this small structural variation apparently is the cause of a number of pharmacological differences that are only partially explainable at this time. The two drugs are thought to have the same biochemical mode of action in binding to DNA, possibly by intercalation between base pairs, thereby inhibiting the nucleic acid polymerases.

In experimental systems, and also clinically, AM exhibits a higher therapeutic index than does DM, despite the fact that *in vitro* DM appears to be the more active against many types of cells. Differences in drug uptake by cells have been observed, yet they do not appear to explain the different activity of the two analogues in a given system. The metabolism of DM seems somewhat more extensive and less rapid than that of AM, but the available analytical methods are not entirely satisfactory, and the possible cytotoxic activity of the metabolites has not been fully clarified. Both AM and DM are degraded mainly in the liver and excreted via the biliary system without enterohepatic circulation. At the present time, 2 mechanisms do appear to play a role in giving AM greater clinical effectiveness: the operationally lower immunodepressive activity of this analogue and its tendency to accumulate more readily than DM in peripheral tissues (Spreafico et al., 1975).

Routinely, both drugs are given intravenously and have a biphasic plasma disappearance curve, the first phase of which is interpreted as redistribution. After a single bolus i.v. dose averaging 60 mg/sq. meter, the mean short plasma T½ of AM is 1.1 h and the mean long T½, 16.7 h (Benjamin et al., 1974). For DM at 180 mg/sq. meter by rapid i.v. bolus, the short plasma half-life is 0.75 H and the long T½, 55 h (Alberts et al., 1971), although Huffman et al. (1972), with improved analytical methods, shortened this last T½ to 46 h. With both AM and DM, high levels of metabolites appear in the blood soon after administration of the parent compounds and undergo a distribution phase in which a biphasic plasma T½ is also evident. The decelerated, but parallel, pharmacokinetic pattern of DM is demonstrated by the less rapid formation and excretion of metabolites; there is even some indication of metabolism of DM by the circulating erythrocytes (Alberts et al., 1971). In contrast to the wide general tissue distribution of AM and DM, with high levels of the latter found in kidney, pancreas, spleen, liver and lung (Alberts et al., 1971; Juffman et al., 1972), the brain tissue levels of DM have been shown to be minimal, and the low CSF levels obtained after AM administration indicate that it, too, passes the blood-brain barrier with difficulty (Benjamin, 1974). This is not an unexpected finding given the low lipid solubility of both antibiotics.

Urine excretion of the two agents and of their metabolites play only a minor role in the drugs' elimination from the body. In urine collected for 5 days after a single bolus i.v. injection of AM, less than 6% of the dose was recoverable, three-fifths of this as the unaltered antibiotic and the rest as the metabolites (Benjamin et al., 1974), while in urine collected for the same period after DM injection, 23% of the dose was recoverable (Huffman et al., 1972) as both antibiotic and metabolites. The kidney is, therefore, only marginally involved in the elimination of AM and has somewhat more involvement in the excretion of DM. On the other hand, the catabolism of AM and DM by the liver, their subsequent excretion via the biliary tract, without intestinal reabsorption, accounts for the major route of drug and metabolite elimination (Arena et al., 1971).

A single, high-dosage, intermittent treatment schedule has been recommended in using AM (Benjamin et al., 1974). This suggestion, based both on the pharmacokinetic nature of the drug and on its mode of cytotoxic action, might also be applied to DM treatment schedules. Being essentially cell cycle non-phase-specific in their action, both AM and DM are concentration-dependent in respect to the rate of their cell kill. The demonstration of their presence in tissues for a protracted period after rapid i.v. injection (Yesair et al., 1972), and the prolonged plasma T½ of both drugs, indicate that a therapeutically effective and clinically convenient treatment schedule can be obtained using widely spaced injections of relatively high doses.

The importance of hepatic functional integrity in the metabolism of AM was first shown by Benjamin et al. (1974) when they reported that patients with compromised hepatic function had altered pharmacokinetic patterns with quadrupling of drug plasma levels per dose over normal values. Because of the likelihood of accentuated toxicity under these circumstances (Pratt and Shanks, 1974), AM, and probably also DM, should be given in reduced doses whenever a patient has signs of hepatic insufficiency. The total antineoplastic activity of the antibiotic is not changed, however, when the drug dose is reduced, because of a decrease in the rate of drug metabolism. Under these conditions, the interrelationship between drug concentration and the duration of drug in the body is altered in such a way that the therapeutically important C x T values remain practically the same. Obviously, the maintenance of equivalent antineoplastic activity does not hold true in those instances where drug metabolism is normal, but the dosage must be reduced due to hypersensitivity to the drugs' side effects, e.g., in post-radiotherapy patients with increased tendencies toward bone marrow suppression.

Using the above criteria, the hepatic immaturity of early infancy would necessitate dosage modification on the rare occasion when AM or DM would be used in this age group. Benjamin et al. (1974) reported that mild hyperbilirubinemia appeared to be a reliable indication of decreased ability to metabolize AM. No other age-related reasons for dosage alteration of either drug would seem to exist, although specific pharmacokinetic data in children are not available.

The most common dose-limiting factors with AM and DM are serious toxic complication—myelosuppression, mucositis and cardiomyopathy. This last complication, apparently characteristic of these antibiotics, is particularly insidious because of its post-treatment appearance and its tendency to cause severe cardiac failure. There is clinical evidence that this irreversible cardiac damage is dose-related (Lefrak et al., 1973), and consequently total AM dosage of 550 mg/sq. meter is considered the upper limit to be used in adults without danger of permanent cardiac sequelae. Ample evidence exists, however, that children, particularly those with no history of prior radiotherapy, can tolerate higher doses of DM (Tan et al., 1967) and AM (Gilladoga et al., 1974) without serious side effects. Unfortunately, the reasons behind this discrepancy in drug tolerance, seemingly related to age and possibly related to pharmacokinetics, have not as yet been investigated.

CONCLUSIONS

From the brief discussion presented above, which encompasses representative examples of the most common antineoplastic agents currently employed in pediatric oncology, one can draw two general conclusions. The first has been emphasized frequently throughout the chapter, i.e., the limited knowledge presently available on the pharmacological characteristics of the individual drugs in children. Such data as do exist are restricted to only a handful of agents and are limited in breadth, having been obtained on small numbers of patients, often under nonstandardized conditions. This unexplored area is all the more unfortunate since direct evidence has been obtained which indicates that age-related differences might exist in the handling of these compounds, in addition to the reasonably predictable idiosyncrasies based on the peculiarities of pediatric physiology. In principle, these differences involve characteristics which could have important consequences on the responses and side effects in cancer chemotherapeutics. One aspect on which the interest of clinicians and researchers should be focused is the reciprocal pharmacokinetic effects exerted by antineoplastic agents when more than one is used at the same time in one patient. This is an important feature, as combination cancer chemotherapy is, at present, the most common clinical practice, having demonstrated significant therapeutic advantages when compared with using the agents singly. A second area which bears investigation, actually a logical extension of the previous aspect, is the influence that previous treatment with these agents, singly or in combination, might have on the successive use of the same of different antitumoral compounds. This is an area which is virtually unexplored, even experimentally, and which, with the new trends toward more complex treatment of neoplastic disease, might reveal unsuspected methods for improving therapeutic results.

The second conclusion to be gathered from the material discussed in this chapter is that we need to fill in the missing pharmacological information in order to more efficiently utilize the cytotoxicity of these compounds. Recent developments in the field of pediatric pharmacology would indicate a growing awareness of the importance of pharmacokinetics (Jusko, 1972; Morselli et al., 1975), although with the antineoplastic agents clinical considerations serve as a limiting factor against their thorough pharmacokinetic investigation in children. Certainly, with more careful planning, and with greater cooperation between pediatric oncologists and pharmacologists, many of the gaps in our knowledge can be filled without losing sight of the primary therapeutic objectives.

REFERENCES

Adamson, R.H., Dixon, R.L., Ben, M., Crews, L., Shohet, S.B. and Rall, D.P. (1965): Some pharmacologic properties of vincristine. *Archives Internationales de Pharmacodynamie et de Therapie, 157:* 299-311.
Alberts, D.S., Bachur, N.R. and Holtzman, J.L. (1971): The pharmacokinetics of daunomycin in man. *Clinical Pharmacology and Therapeutics, 12:* 96-104.
Arena, E., d'Alessandro, N., Dusonchet, L., Gebbia, N., Gerbasi, F., Pallazo, A.M., Raineri,

A., Rausa, L. and Tubaro, E. (1971): Analysis of the pharmacokinetic characteristics, pharmacological and chemotherapeutic activity of 14-hydroxydaunomycin (Adriamycin) a new drug endowed with an antitumor activity. *Arzneimittel-Forschung, 21:* 1258-1263.
Bagley, C.M. Jr., Bostick, F.W. and De Vita, V.T., Jr. (1973): Clinical pharmacology of cyclophosphamide. *Cancer Research, 33:* 226-233.
Benjamin, R.S. (1974): Pharmacokinetics of adriamycin (NSC-123127) in patients with sarcomas. *Cancer Chemotherapy Reports, 58:* 271-273.
Benjamin, R.S., Wiernik, P.H. and Bachur, N.R. (1974): Adriamycin chemotherapy — efficacy, safety and pharmacologic basis of an intermittent single high-dosage schedule. *Cancer, 33:* 19-27.
Bischoff, K.B., Dedrick, R.L., Zaharko, D.S. and Longstreth, J.A. (1971): Methotrexate pharmacokinetics. *Journal of Pharmaceutical Sciences, 60:* 1128-1133.
Bolande, R.P. (1974): Congenital and infantile neoplasia of the kidney. *Lancet, 2:* 1497-1499.
Calabresi, P. and Parks, R. (1970): In: *The Pharmacological Basis of Therapeutics,* edited by L.S. Goodman and A. Gilman, pp. 1372, 4th ed., Macmillan, New York.
Capizzi, R.L., Bertino, J.R., Skeel, R.T., Creasey, W.A., Zanes, R., Olayon, C., Peterson, R.G. and Handschumacher, R.E. (1971): L-Asparaginase: clinical, biochemical, pharmacological and immunological studies. *Annals of Internal Medicine, 74:* 893-901.
Chabner, B.A., Myers, C.E., Coleman, C.N. and Johns, D.G. (1975a): The clinical pharmacology of antineoplastic agents. I. *New England Journal of Medicine, 292:* 1107-1113.
Chabner, B.A., Myers, C.E., Coleman, C.N. and Johns, D.G. (1975b): The clinical pharmacology of antineoplastic agents. II. *New England Journal of Medicine, 292:* 1159-1168.
Coffey, J.J., White, C.A., Lesk, A.B., Rogers, W.I. and Serpick, A.A. (1972): Effect of allopurinol on the pharmacokinetics of 6-mercaptopurine (NSC 755) in cancer patients. *Cancer Research, 32:* 1283-1289.
Cohen, J.L., Jao, J.Y. and Jusko, W.J. (1971): Pharmacokinetics of cyclophosphamide in man. *British Journal of Pharmacology, 43:* 667-680.
Colvin, M. Padgett, C.A. and Fenselau, G. (1973): A biologically active metabolite of cyclophosphamide. *Cancer Research, 33:* 915-918.
Connors, T.A., Cox, P.J., Farmer, P.B., Foster, A.B. and Jarman, M. (1974): Some studies of the active intermediates formed in the microsomal metabolism of cyclophosphamide and isophosphamide. *Biochemical Pharmacology, 23:* 115-129.
Creasey, W.A., Papac, R.J., Markiw, M.E., Calabresi, P. and Welch, A.D. (1966): Biochemical and pharmacological studies with 1-β-D arabinofuranosylcytosine in man. *Biochemical Pharmacology, 15:* 1417-1428.
Dedrick, R.L., Forrester, D.D., Cannon, J.N., ElDareer, S.M. and Mellett, L.B. (1973): Pharmacokinetics of 1-β-D-Arabinofuranosylcytosine (ARA-C) deamination in several species. *Biochemical Pharmacology, 22:* 2405-2417.
Donigian, D.W. and Owellen, R.J. (1973): Interaction of vinblastine, vincristine and colchicine with serum proteins. *Biochemical Pharmacology, 22:* 2113-2119.
Editorial (1974): Adriamycin and the heart. *Lancet, 1:* 1325.
Elion, G.B., Callahan, S., Nathan, H., Bieber, S., Rundles, R.W. and Hitghings, G.H. (1963): Potentiation by inhibition of drug degradation: 6-substituted purines and xanthine oxidase. *Biochemical Pharmacology, 12:* 85-93.
Elion, G.B. (1967): Biochemistry and pharmacology of purine analogues. *Federation Proceedings, 26:* 898-904.
Faber, O.K., Mouridsen, H.T. and Skovsted, L. (1974): The biotransformation of

cyclophosphamide in man. *Acta Pharmacologia et Toxicologica, 35:* 195-200.
Fairley, K.F., Barrie, J.U. and Johnson, W. (1972): Sterility and testicular atrophy related to cyclophosphamide therapy. *Lancet, 1:* 568-569.
Farber, S., Diamond, L.K., Mercer, R.D., Sylvester, R.F. and Wolff, V.A. (1948): Temporary remissions in acute leukemia in children produced by folic antagonist 4-amethopteroylglutamic acid (Aminopterin). *New England Journal of Medicine, 238:* 787-793.
Finkelstein, J.Z., Hittle, R.E. and Hammond, G.D. (1969): Evaluation of a high dose cyclophosphamide regimen in childhood tumors. *Cancer Research, 23:* 1239-1242.
Finkelstein, J.Z., Scher, J. and Karen, M. (1970): Pharmacologic studies of titrated cytosine arabinoside (NSC 63878) in children. *Cancer Chemotherapy Reports, 54:* 35-39.
Freeman-Narrod, M., Gerstley, B.J., Treat, C., Engstrom, P.F. and Bornstein, R. (1974): Variations in the half-life of methotrexate in man. *Proceedings of the American Association for Cancer Research, 15:* 49.
Frei, E., III (1974a): S.A. Waksman conference on actinomycins: closing remarks. *Cancer Chemotherapy Reports, 58:* 121.
Frei, E., III. (1974b): The clinical use of actinomycin. *Cancer Chemotherapy Reports, 58:* 49-54.
Gilladoga, A.C., Tan, C.T., Phillips, F.S., Sternberg, S.S., Tang, C.K., Wollner, N. and Murphy, M.L. (1974): Cardiac status of forty children receiving adriamycin (Adr) over 495 mgs/m^2 and animal studies. *Proceedings of the American Association for Cancer Research, 15:* 107.
Goldberg, I.H. (1965): Mode of action of antibiotics. II. Drugs affecting nucleic acid and protein synthesis. *American Journal of Medicine, 39:* 722-752.
Goldin, A. and Johnson, R.K. (1974): Evaluation of actinomycins in experimental systems. *Cancer Chemotherapy Reports, 58:* 63-77.
Goodman, L.S. and Gilman, A. (eds.) (1965): *The Pharmacological Basis of Therapeutics*, 3rd. ed., pp. 1354-1393, Macmillan, New York.
Greene, W., Huffman, D., Wiernick, P.H., Schimeff, S., Benjamin, R. and Bacur, N.R. (1972): High dose daunorubicin therapy for acute non-lymphocytic leukemia — correlation of response and toxicity with pharmacokinetics and intracellular daunorubicin reductase activity. *Cancer, 30:* 1413-1427.
Greenwald, E.S. (1973): *Cancer Chemotherapy*, 2nd. ed., Medical Examination Publ. Co., New York.
Haskell, C.M., Canellos, G.P., Cooney, D.A. and Hardesty, C.T. (1972): Pharmacologic studies in man with crystallized L-asparaginase (NSC-109229). *Cancer Chemotherapy Reports, 56:* 611-614.
Henderson, E.S., Adamson, R.H. and Oliverio, V.T. (1965): The metabolic fate or tritiated methotrexate. II. Absorption and excretion in man. *Cancer Research, 25:* 1018-1024.
Henderson, J.F. and Paterson, A.R.P. (1973): In: *Nucleotide Metabolism: An Introduction*, p. 148, Academic Press, New York.
Henry, M.C. and Marlow, M. (1973): Preclinical toxicologic study of actinomycin D (NSC-3053). *Cancer Chemotherapy Reports, 4,* pt. 3, no. 1: 77-84.
Hill, D.L., Laster, W.R., Jr. and Struck, R.F. (1972): Enzymatic metabolism of cyclophosphamide and nicotine and production of a toxic cyclophosphamide metabolite. *Cancer Research, 32:* 658-665.
Ho, D.H., Carter, C.J., Thetford, B. and Frei, E., III (1971): Distribution and mechanism of clearance of L-asparaginase (NSC-109229). *Cancer Chemotherapy Reports, 55:* 539-545.
Ho, D.H.W. and Frei, E., III (1971): Clinical pharmacology of 1-β-D-arabinofuranosyl cytosine. *Clinical Pharmacology and Therapeutics, 12:* 944-954.
Ho, D.H.W., Thetford, B., Carter, C.J.K. and Frei, E., III (1970): Clinical pharmacologic

studies of L-asparaginase. *Clinical Pharmacology and Therapeutics, 11:* 408-417.
Huffman, D.H., Benjamin, R.S. and Bachur, N.R. (1972): Daunorubicin metabolism in acute nonlymphatic leukemia. *Clinical Pharmacology and Therapeutics, 13:* 895-905.
Huffman, D.H., Wan, S.H., Azarnoff, D.L. and Hoogstraten, B. (1973): Pharmacokinetics of methotrexate. *Clinical Pharmacology and Therapeutics, 14:* 572-579.
Jao, J.Y., Jusko, W.J. and Cohen, J.L. (1972): Phenobarbital effects on cyclophosphamide pharmacokinetics in man. *Cancer Research, 32:* 2761-2764.
Johns, D.G., Hollingsworth, J.W., Cashmore, A.R., Plenderleith, I.H. and Bertino, J.R. (1964): Methotrexate displacement in man. *Journal of Clinical Investigation, 43:* 621-629.
Johnson, I.S., Armstrong, J.G., Gorman, M. and Burnett, J.P., Jr. (1963): The vinca alkaloids: a new class of oncolytic agents. *Cancer Research, 23:* 1390-1427.
Jusko, W.J. (1971): Pharmacodynamics of chemotherapeutic effects: dose-time-response relationship for phase non-specific agents. *Journal of Pharmaceutical Sciences, 60:* 892-895.
Jusko, W.J. (1972): Pharmacokinetic principles in pediatric pharmacology. *Pediatric Clinics of North America, 19:* 81-100.
Lampkin, B.C., McWilliams, N.B. and Mauer, A.M. (1972): Treatment of acute leukemia. *Pediatric Clinics of North America, 19:* 1123-1140.
Lefrak, E.A., Pitha, J., Rosenhein, S. and Gottlieb, J.A. (1973): A clinicopathologic analysis of adriamycin cardiotoxicity. *Cancer, 32:* 302-314.
Loo, T.L., Luce, J.K., Sullivan, M.P. and Frei, E., III (1968): Clinical pharmacologic observations on 6-mercaptopurine and 6-methyl thiopurine ribonucleoside. *Clinical Pharmacology and Therapeutics, 9:* 180-194.
Madoc-Jones, H. and Mauro, F. (1974): Site of action of cytotoxic agents in the cell life cycle. In: *Handbook of Experimental Pharmacology,* V. 38, pt. I, edited by A.C. Sartorelli and D.G. Jones, pp. 205-219, Springer-Verlag, Berlin.
Mellett, L.B. (1974): Pharmacodynamics and pharmacokinetic measurements of antitumor agents. *Clinical Pharmacology and Therapeutics, 16:* 231-242.
Morasca, L., Rainisio, C. and Masera, G. (1969): Duration of cytotoxic activity of vincristine in the blood of leukemic children. *European Journal of Cancer, 5:* 79-80.
Morselli, P.L., Garattini, S. and Sereni, F. (eds.) (1975): *Basic and Therapeutic Aspects of Perinatal Pharmacology.* Raven Press, New York.
Mouridsen, H.T., Faber, O. and Skvosted, L. (1974): The biotransformation of cyclophosphamide in man: analysis of the variation in normal subjects. *Acta Pharmacologica et Toxicologica, 35:* 98-106.
Ohnuma, T., Holland, J.F., Freeman, A. and Sinks, L.F. (1970): Biochemical and pharmacological studies with L-asparaginase in man. *Cancer Research, 30:* 2297-2305.
Owellen, R.J. and Hartke, C.A. (1975): The pharmacokinetics of 4-acetyl tritium vinblastine in two patients. *Cancer Research, 35:* 975-980.
Philips, F.S., Schwartz, H.S., Sternberg, S.S. and Tan, C.T.C. (1960): The toxicity of actinomycin D. *Annals of the New York Academy of Sciences, 89:* 348-360.
Pratt, C.B. and Shanks, E.C. (1974): Doxorubicin in treatment of malignant solid tumors in children. *American Journal of Diseases in Children, 127:* 534-536.
Pratt, C.B., Simone, J.V., Zee, P., Aur, R.J.A. and Johnson, W.W. (1970): Comparison of daily versus weekly L-asparaginase for the treatment of childhood acute leukemia. *Journal of Pediatrics, 77:* 474-483.
Schwartz, H.S. (1974): Some determinants of the therapeutic efficacy of actinomycin D (NSC 3053), adriamycin (NSC 123127) and daunorubicin (NSC 83142). *Cancer Chemotherapy Reports, 58:* 55-62.
Schwartz, H.S., Sodergren, J.E. and Ambaye, R.Y. (1968): Actinomycin D: drug

concentrations and actions in mouse, tissues, and tumors. *Cancer Research, 28:* 192-197.
Schwartz, M.K. (1970): The distribution and clearance of L-Asparaginase. In: *Recent Results in Cancer Research,* V. 33, edited by E. Grundmann and H.F. Oettgen, pp. 58-63, Springer-Verlag, New York.
Skipper, H., Schabel, F.M., Jr., Mellett, L.B., Montgomery, J.A. Wikoff, L.J., Lloyd, H.H. and Brockman, R.W. (1970): Implications of biochemical, cytokinetic, pharmacologic and toxicologic relationships in the design of optimal therapeutic schedules. *Cancer Chemotherapy Reports, 54:* 431-450.
Spreafico, F., Donelli, M.G., Vecchi, A., Bossi, A. and Garattini, S. (1974): Factors modifying the activity and toxicity of anticancer agents. In: *Recent Results in Cancer Research,* V. 49, edited by G. Mathe and R.K. Oldham, pp. 88-94, Springer-Verlag, Berlin.
Spreafico, F., Mantorani, A., Vecchi, A. and Tagliabue, A. (1975): Comparative pharmacological aspects of adriamycin and daunomycin in experimental animals. *Cancer Research,* in press.
Tan, C., Taasaka, H., Yu, K.P., Murphy, L. and Karnofsky, D. (1967): Daunomycin antitumor antibiotic in the treatment of neoplastic disease: clinical evaluation with special reference to childhood leukemia. *Cancer, 20:* 333-353.
Wan, S.H., Huffman, D.H., Azarnoff, D.L., Hoogstraten, B. and Larsen, W.E. (1974): Pharmacokinetics of 1-β-D arabinofuranosyl cytosine in humans. *Cancer Research, 34:* 392-397.
Weiss, H.D., Walker, M.D. and Wiernik, P.H. (1974): Neurotoxicity of commonly used antieoplastic agents. I. *New England Journal of Medicine, 291:* 75-81.
Werkheiser, W.C. (1963): The biochemical, cellular and pharmacological action and effects of the folic acid antagonists. *Cancer Research, 23:* 1277-1285.
Whitecar, J.P., Jr., Bodey, G.P., Harris, J.E. and Freireich, E.J. (1970): L-Asparaginase. *New England Journal of Medicine, 282:* 732-734.
Yesair, D.W., Schwartzbach, E., Schuck, D., Denine, E.P. and Asbell, M.A. (1972): Comparative pharmacokinetics of daunomycin and adriamycin in several animal species. *Cancer Research 32:* 1177-1183.

7

Antibiotics

GIANNI TOGNONI

The wide use of antinfectious agents in perinatal and pediatric practice has led to the creation of a large body of literature, recently carefully reviewed and discussed (Gardner, 1974; Harrod and Stevens, 1974; McCracken and Eichenwald, 1974a,b; McCracken, 1974). However, it is with some difficulty that a comprehensive picture on antibiotic disposition and metabolism can be extracted from these excellent papers because of the heterogeneity in their content and their diversity of approach. Few studies exist that are specifically concerned with the pharmacological aspects of antimicrobial therapy as it applies to pediatrics. This fact represents the consequence of two conditions which acted concurrently until a short time ago. One of these factors was the relatively limited development of a pediatric-oriented clinical pharmacology (Sereni and Principi, 1968; Yaffe and Juchau, 1974; Kretchmer, 1975); secondly, the main orientation of the majority of the papers dealing with antimicrobial agents was toward giving practical directions for therapy. Antibiotic therapy from its inception has suffered from being thought of mostly as a clinical and bacteriological problem. In addition, pharmacologists have been only limitedly interested in this field.

There is no doubt that the main problems in antimicrobial therapy concern when and how to use these drugs (Smith, 1973; O'Grady and Lambert, 1973; Editorial, 1974a; Tager and Speizer, 1975; Kunin, 1975); certainly, substantial improvement in their use can be provided by careful consideration of antibiotic choice and availability in hospital practice (Macaraeg et al., 1971; Lorian and

Topf, 1972; Maki et al., 1973a,b; Noone and Safi, 1973; Zemen et al., 1974; May et al., 1974; McGowan and Finland, 1974; Shoji et al., 1974; Simmons and Stolley, 1974), by controlling the emergence of resistant and dangerous strains (Finland, 1973; Maki et al., 1973b, Rolinson, 1973b, Bartlett and Finegold, 1974; Driessen, 1975) and by a better understanding of the manner in which microorganisms act and interact with host defenses (Alexander, 1974a; Bodey, 1974; Wolff, 1974; Smith, 1975). All of these points are also applicable in pediatric practice, where, if anything, the problems of organization, sampling procedures, and assessment of outcome are even more precarious (Stewart and Moghadam, 1972; Kazemi et al., 1973; Sprunt et al., 1973; Diamant and Diamant, 1974; Garcia de Olarte et al., 1974; Ironside, 1974; Stevenson, 1974; Knittle et al., 1975). At the same time, it has become evident that the availability of good pharmacokinetic data can help to clarify similarities and differences between products with long clinical use and the newly marketed molecules. The following points have provoked our attention in the more recent publications, and seem to be providing new data at a very fast rate.

QUALITY CONTROL OF METHODS ANALYSIS

In addition to the fact that clinicians and bacteriologists have long considered their own approach quite adequate, the methods of antibiotic analysis in body fluids and the parameters for estimation of their activity are very often not sufficiently standardized to allow a comparison of the pharmacological data obtained by different groups. This fact represents an extra variable, besides those derived from differences in strain sensitivity, hospital environment and clinical conditions (Garrod and Waterworth, 1971; Stokes and Whitby, 1971; Jalling et al., 1972; Ericsson and Malmborg, 1973; Andrews et al., 1974; Gavan, 1974).

ASSESSMENT OF THE CLINICAL SIGNIFICANCE OF PLASMA LEVELS

The practice of measuring antibiotic activity in biological fluids is not new. However, not enough data have been accumulated, nor is there as yet sufficiently comprehensive knowledge to allow the use of the available information in actual clinical situations (Rolinson, 1973a; Kunin, 1974, Wagner, 1974). The application of a pharmacokinetic approach to antimicrobial therapy represents a challenge to clinical pharmacologists. Their investigative models must take into consideration the duration and extension of diffusion processes into various tissues and tissue compartments where the same antibiotic is supposed to act against different microorganisms. The relationship between serum levels and actual drug concentration within infected tissue is far from being clear, despite the fact that for every product we can rely on data describing its presence in the various districts of the body (Weinstein, 1970a; Nelson, 1971; Kunin et al., 1973; Klastersky et al., 1974a; Romankiewicz, 1974; Babb, 1975; Prescott, 1975).

The models which have been developed (tissue cages, skin windows, fibrin clots) offer very useful, if not entirely analogous, approximations to the real situation (Chisholm et al., 1973; Dawes, 1973; Barza et al., 1974a,b; Barza and Weinstein, 1974a). The results obtained with these experimental models allow a better definition of clinically useful information, such as:

(1) the value of continuous infusion vs. intermittent injections in achieving effective tissue levels.
(2) the half-life of various compounds within the tissues, a factor which could be critical for the growth-inhibiting effect on different bacteria.
(3) the relative influence of protein-binding and/or of the physicochemical properties of the molecule on the diffusion capacity.

Very little, if any, data are yet available on the pharmacokinetics of antibiotics given in combinations. Clinically, this type of antimicrobial therapy is used more extensively than most authoritative reviews would suggest (Klein, 1974; Jawetz, 1975). Combination chemotherapy appears useful principally in those seriously ill patients where the distribution and penetration of antibiotics in different tissues and compartments have changed, together with host defense mechanisms. Of course, information regarding all these parameters would be most helpful in conjunction with clinico-bacteriological indices (MacGregor and Beaty, 1972; Editorial, 1974a; Mulholland et al., 1973; Geddes and Williams, 1973; Cattell, 1974; Lykkegaard Nielsen et al., 1974; Pesnel et al., 1973; Weitzman and Berger, 1974).

Naturally, the problems of antibiotic chemotherapy are even more complex during the perinatal period, when organs and compartments are constantly developing and marked variability in kinetic parameters is bound to exist (see preceding chapters). Investigations specifically designed to gather pharmacokinetic information are currently in progress at several centers, and their results will contribute to defining more accurately the validity of new and old therapeutic schemes (McCracken and Kaplan, 1974). With increased study of the mode of disposition and metabolism of antibiotics, new points of reference should be established that would help to clarify the existing problems. Hopefully, the rapid accumulation of data will ensure the obsolescence of the present review and reveal the advantages of enlarging the multicenter and multidisciplinary approach (Orzalesi, 1975; Tognoni et al., 1975). Only recently, in fact, has some effort been made among various investigators to share their data and results, and as a consequence of this interaction the necessary cross-citations between pediatric and pharmacological literature, indicating interdisciplinary cooperation, will hopefully become the norm (Garfield, 1974).

Based on these premises, the following paragraphs will try to interpret and present the existing data, derived from sources with variable reliability and with some inconsistencies. As will be seen, a gap in the available information exists between that of the perinatal age group and the adult. This lack of continuity in the pharmacological data reflects the previously mentioned prevailing clinical approach in pediatric chemotherapy: however, one can surmise that this picture will change when new and carefully controlled data are developed, as has happened with other classes of drugs. The criteria for choice of the antibiotics discussed in the following chapter, in addition to considering the availability of data, have been dictated by the relative importance of different agents in general and pediatric practice (Garrod et al., 1973; Symposium, 1974). Data refer to humans if not otherwise specified.

PENICILLINS

The number of compounds which belong to this class has been constantly increasing over the years. Efforts have been directed toward developing molecules able to cover different clinical needs more completely and more satisfactorily. Many penicillins now on the market differ both in their spectrum of antimicrobial activity and in their pharmacokinetic properties. The characteristics of the new penicillins, their advantages and their relative therapeutic value have been reviewed and extensively discussed very recently (Rolinson and Sutherland, 1973; Thrupp, 1974; Neu, 1975). An effort has been made in the present discussion to select from the literature those recent developments that seemed pertinent to the purpose of this publication.

The compounds have been classified in three groups according to some of their pharmacological properties. Each group is accompanied by a table in which a synopsis of the interesting pharmacokinetic data is presented. The compounds of Table 1 have been chosen as the main representatives of subgroups whose members share similar pharmacological and antimicrobial properties, the most significant molecules belonging to each subgroup are then described in more detail in Tables 2 and 3. Attention has been given to some general patterns of distribution, and to the discussion of those penicillins which have found wider application in pediatric practice and for which specific information is available for comparison with adult data.

Data on drug distribution and half-life most frequently have been obtained using volunteers, who, unfortunately, do not represent an accurate model for disease states, where very high dosages often are employed (Bergan and Øydvin, 1974). Classification criteria have been taken from a well-known textbook (Garrod et al., 1973) and from an extensive review (Rolinson and Sutherland, 1973). A very detailed presentation of the spectra of activity and of relative MIC values can be found in these publications. Some points deserve specific comment, as they are more thoroughly documented in the literature and are useful in the evaluation of the schematic data reported in Tables 1, 2, and 3.

Table 1. Pharmacokinetic Parameters Relative to Different Groups of Penicillins

Compound	Preferred Route of Administration	Serum Protein-Binding (%)	Clearance (ml/min/1.73m^2) Total	Clearance (ml/min/1.73m^2) Renal	App. Vd (L)	App. Serum T½ (min)	Urinary Excretion (% of dose)
Penicillin G (benzylpenicillin)	Parenteral	46-58 59-65	550	340-1,050	37-47	25-56	60-85
Ampicillin	Oral Parenteral	15-29	260-420	130-270	29-48 18.8*	35-95	19-44 55-95
Dicloxacillin	Oral Parenteral	96-98	156	88 113	20	42	36-73
Methicillin	Parenteral	15-60	560	350	22	30	
Carbenicillin	Parenteral	47-70	93-189		10-21	45-80	
Indanyl-carbenicillin	Oral				11-22	34-51	

*Volume of distribution at steady state.

Data presented in this table are taken from the following sources (markedly different data reflect the state of the information in this field): Bulger et al., 1964; Levy, 1967; Kunin, 1967; Gibaldi and Schwartz, 1968; Rosenblatt et al., 1968; Plaut et al., 1969; Dittert et al., 1970; Hoffman et al., 1970; Kampmann et al., 1972, 1973; Jusko and Lewis, 1973; Rolinson and Sutherland, 1973; Bergan and Øydvin, 1974; Loo et al., 1974; Hoffler et al., 1974; Lund et al., 1974; Brogden et al., 1875a; Hansen et al., 1975; Simon et al., 1975.

Table 2. Penicillinase Stable and Acid Stable Penicillins

Compound	Preferred Route of Administration	Protein-Binding (%)	Clearance (ml/min/1.73m^2) Total	Clearance (ml/min/1.73m^2) Renal	App. Vd (L)	App. Serum T½ (min)	Urinary Excretion (% of active compound)
Nafcillin	Parenteral	87-90	410	160	44-57	33	36-38
Oxacillin	Parenteral	92-94	380-500	190-226	29	24	25-55
Cloxacillin	Oral	94-96	122-180	101-162	24	25-39	28-68
	Parenteral				7.13 ± 1.47		
Dicloxacillin	Oral	96-98	157	80-113	20	42	27-73
	Parenteral						
Flucloxacillin	Oral	95	110-140	68-108	8.16 ± 1.30	46	42-75*
	Parenteral					53 ± 2	21-59†

*After i.m. administration.
†After oral administration.
Papers from which data have been taken are the following: Kunin, 1967; Gibaldi and Schwartz, 1968; Rosenblatt et al., 1968; Dittert et al., 1970; Doluisio et al., 1970; Kind et al., 1970; Bodey et al., 1972; Rolinson and Sutherland, 1973; Barza and Weinstein, 1974b; Bergan and Øydvin, 1974; Hellstroöm et al., 1974a,b.

Table 3. Pharmacokinetic Data on Ampicillin-Like Penicillins

Compound	Perferred Route of Administration	Serum Protein-Binding (%)	Clearance (ml/min/1.73m^2) Total	Clearance (ml/min/1.73m^2) Renal	App. Serum T½ (min)	Urinary Excretion (% of active compound)
Ampicillin	Parenteral Oral–50% absorption in fasting state	15-29	260-420	130-270	35-95	55-95
Pivampicillin	77-82% Oral absorption	See ampicillin	See ampicillin		48-69	62-74
Amoxicillin	88.7 ± 4.5% Oral absorption	17	240-290		40-90	60-80

Sources: see Table 1.

A good deal of effort has gone into the development of molecules which consistently are totally absorbed in their active, unchanged form. Among the isoxazolyl penicillins, increased bioavailability by the oral route has been obtained starting with oxacillin, proceeding to cloxacillin then to dicloxacillin (Gravenkemper et al., 1965; Hellström, et al., 1974a,b) and flucloxacillin. The absorption of the last two molecules has been found to range between 55 and 80% of the administered dose, it can be considered equivalent to that observed after i.m. injection. Interestingly enough, a more rapid absorption has been measured following the oral, rather than the i.m., route with no differences between antibiotic given in capsule or oral-suspension from (Naumann, 1966; Doluisio et al., 1969, Nauta and Mattie, 1975). Food, however, can delay and significantly decrease the process of absorption.

The sodium indanyl-ester of carbenicillin, which is rapidly hydrolized *in vivo* to give carbenicillin, is 40% absorbed when given by the oral route. Therapeutic levels cannot be measured in serum and tissues; only the urinary concentrations are effective acting against Pseudomonas and indole-positive Proteus species and *Escherichia coli.* The use of this compound, therefore, has been advocated for urinary tract infections, even though the frequency of reinfections of superinfection casts doubts on the validity of this indication (Holloway and Taylor, 1974; Cox, 1973; Naumann and Rosin, 1973; Hodges and Perkins, 1973; Knirsch et al., 1973). The problem of increasing resistance to carbenicillin should also be considered. Some authors deny this fact, when sufficiently high doses are employed (Fiedelman, 1974). New compounds related to carbenicillin have been proposed very recently. Carfecillin, like indanyl-carbenicillin has some indication in specific urinary tract infections due to Pseudomonas strains (Wilkinson et al., 1975). Sulbenicillin has the same kinetic behavior as carbenicillin (Hansen et al., 1975). Tircacillin shows a slightly higher *in vitro* activity, with very similar pharmacokinetic properties (Libke et al., 1975). The low and erratic absorption of oral ampicillin has led to the preparation of some pharmacologically inactive esters, hetacillin, metampicillin, pivampicillin. These compounds hydrolize very rapidly (T½ of hetacillin 11 ± 2 min), to give ampicillin (Jusko et al., 1973; Kirby and Kind, 1967). Because it is representative of the others in this group, only pivampicillin (Sinkula and Yalkowsky, 1975) has been cited in the accompanying tables. The absorption is dose-dependent (92%, 85%, 77%, respectively, after 250, 500, 1,000 mg) (Loo et al., 1974). Relatively low absorption (45-50%) has been shown for hetacillin (Jusko and Lewis, 1973). Amoxicillin absorption, on the other hand, can be considered to be complete within 2 h and does not seem to be influenced by the presence of food (Lund et al., 1974; Zarowny et al., 1974). No difference in absorption of ampicillin in respect to its different formulations (anhydrous vs. trihydrate form) can be demonstrated. The variability that is observed can be attributed to individual patterns of absorption (Lode et al., 1974, Mayersohn and Endreny, 1973;

Dugal et al. 1974). Of all the compounds in this class, amoxycillin represents the best alternative when the oral route is preferred because its observed pattern of absorption is very close to that seen after i.m. administration (Kosmidis et al., 1973; Neu, 1974; Pearson, 1974; Brogden et al., 1975a).

As is evident from the reported data, the penicillins include compounds which are both very strongly and very weakly protein-bound. At present, agreement is incomplete about the clinical significance of this parameter. The discussion on protein-binding has been centered mainly on its influence on the antibiotics' penetration of the tissues and on the modificiations of antimicrobial activity (Kunin, 1967; Kunin et al., 1973). Data obtained *in vitro* (Barza and Weinstein, 1974a), in experimental models *in vivo* (Chisholm et al., 1973, Barza et al., 1974a,b) and in actual clinical situations with pediatric patients (Nelson, 1971; Baciocco and Iles, 1971; Howell et al., 1972) have allowed some conclusions to be drawn. These assumptions hold true at least for the types of tissues that have been investigated (joint effusions, clots, abscesses).

Penetration is directly related to the concentration of free, rather than total, antibiotic in the serum, and peak levels, rather than the AUC, seem to be important in determining the extent of tissue penetration after a single parenteral administration. Repeated intermittent bolus administration appears to produce higher serum levels than continuous infusion (Barza and Weinstein, 1974b). The importance of high peak serum levels is possibly demonstrated by the data showing better penetration into purulent respiratory secretions and interstitial fluid by amoxicillin compared to ampicillin (May and Ingold, 1974; Tan et al., 1974). High individual variability is observed in serum-tissue ratios, and values ranging from 0.01 (continuous infusions of penicillin given at 75 mg/kg/day over 9 days) to 36 have been reported for children from 21 months to 12 years old (Nelson, 1971). Different conditions of inflammation and vascularization of the infected area, changes in pH and the location of an abscess are some of the major factors to be considered (Kunin, 1974). Moreover, correlation between the thickness of a clot and the speed of its penetration by antibiotic has been shown so that with equivalent serum levels a range of intervals from 26 to 200 min was necessary to have measurable amounts of penicillin in clots of varying thickness (O'Connell and Plaut, 1969).

Penicillins are rapidly excreted; therefore, when given in small doses they would seldom achieve therapeutically adequate levels in the tissues fluids (Chisholm et al., 1973). The diffusion of penicillins from the bloodstream into the CSF is poor, when the meninges are not inflamed. In addition, a mechanism of active transport from CSF to blood in dogs has been demonstrated for benzyl penicillin (Dixon et al., 1969). This action, which proceeds against a concentration gradient, could play a role in determining the low pencillin concentrations frequently observed in the CSF of patients. Ampicillin penetration into the CSF seems proportional to the existing degree of meningeal inflammation, although a high rate of variability has been observed. Concentrations ranging from 0.03 to 38 µg/ml have been reported, with CSF-serum ratios varying from 0 to 100% (Thrupp et al., 1966).

The possible therapeutic importance of high, sustained antibiotic concentrations at the tissue level is supported by recent data on the killing activity of penicillin inside human phagocytes containing gonococci. In this study, there was direct proportionality between the concentration of penicillin in the culture medium and its ability to prevent growth of intracellular bacteria (Veale et al., 1975) (for possible clinical implications on the choice of penicillins see Wilcox, 1974; May and Ingold, 1974). Significantly, the state of hydration has been shown to influence antibiotic uptake in renal tissue, with dehydration decreasing the penetration of carbenicillin in the severely diseased human kidney (Whelton et al., 1973; Romankiewicz, 1974). For a more comprehensive discussion of the various factors which might play a role in determining the penicillins' distribution from vascular to extravascular compartments in disease states, the reader is referred to the articles by Levy (1967), Giusti (1973) and Prescott (1975).

The degree of protein-binding is particularly significant when comparing various isoxazolyl penicillins. Whereas oxacillin, cloxacillin, dicloxacillin and flucloxacillin total levels are in a relationship of 1:2:4:4 free levels reflecting probable drug activity show a ratio of 1:2:2:4 (Bodey et al., 1972; Kunin et al. 1973). At present, few data are available about binding to specific tissue proteins and its influence on drug distribution (see Kunin et al., 1973, for oxacillin; Johnson et al., 1974, for ampicillin in dogs [both refer to liver]).

Little quantitative information has been reported on the type and extent of metabolic degradation processes of the penicillins. A recent report gives data about the breakdown in man of a range of penicillins by two routes, β-lactam hydrolysis and side-chain removal (Cole et al., 1973), and Table 4 summarizes the results. According to this report, no differences were observed for drugs given by oral vs. i.m. routes. These data confirm the hypothesis that, besides differences in absorption, the extent of metabolic inactivation, which probably occurs in the liver, influences the blood level differences of isoxazolyl penicillins (Rosenblatt et al., 1968; Kind et al., 1970). An increase of metabolic degradation by the liver was seen in cases with decreased renal function (Kunin and Finland, 1959; Bulger et al., 1964). This effect was seen primarily during chronic treatment. An acute infusion in the presence of markedly diminished GFR or anuria only resulted in curves of penicillin serum levels, which suggested no extrarenal elimination of the drug (Plaut et al., 1969). On the other hand, severe liver function impairment alone, as found in cirrhotic patients, does not seem to require dosage modification for ampicillin. In this latter condition, a higher than normal apparent Vd has been noted, accompanied by lower plasma levels, prolonged retention in the body and a tripling of the normal metabolic biliary clearance (30% of the administered dose vs. 10% in normal subjects)

Table 4. Urinary Recovery of Various Penicillins and
Their Metabolites (0-12 h)

	Route	Penicillin (% of dose)	Penicilloic Acid (% of dose)	6-Aminopenicillanic Acid (% of dose)
Benzyl penicillin	Oral	66.4 ± 26.5	15.6 ± 12.7	0
	i.m.			
Phenoxymethyl penicillin	Oral	25.9 ± 12.3	34.4 ± 19.7	≲1%
Oxacillin	Oral	16.9 ± 13.2	16.1 ± 13.3	0
Cloxacillin	Oral	38.1 ± 17.9	11.1 ± 12.9	0
Dicloxacillin	Oral	32.9 ± 20.0	3.8 ± 7.6	/
Flucloxacillin	Oral	40.6 ± 30.1	3.7 ± 5.1	/
Ampicillin	Oral	25.8 ± 17.1*	6.7 ± 5.9	Traces
		43.3 ± 18.2**	10.8 ± 6.4	
	i.m.	72.5 ± 21.0	10.0 ± 4.1	
Amoxicillin	Oral	49.1 ± 13.4*	24.7 ± 10.7	/
		63.4 ± 18.8**	20.2 ± 11.4	
Methicillin	i.m.	75.0 ± 13.3	10.0 ± 4.1	/
Carbenicillin	i.m.	81.5 ± 8.6	1.8 ± 4.0	/

* and ** Respectively, after 500 and 250 mg.
Adapted from Cole et al., 1973.

(Jusko and Lewis, 1975; see, however, Simon et al., 1975, who reported 30% of the dose being metabolized).

No agreement exists about the degree of correlation of creatinine clearance with the serum half-life, even if higher and significantly prolonged levels are observed in subjects with impaired renal function. This is not surprising due to the relatively minor role of glomerular filtration compared to that of tubular excretion (Nauta and Mattie, 1975). An inverse relationship between penicillin half-life and endogenous creatinine clearance has been shown by other authors, and the same effect can be seen in relationship to increasing age (Kampmann et al., 1972; Simon et al., 1975). The rate of variability of this finding, however, is so high as to make the development of precise calculations difficult. There have been no instances of direct renal toxicity ascribed to the pencillins, however, when using very high dosages of parenteral penicillin G in patients with impaired renal function, an assessment of serum levels has been recommended, to avoid seizures (Plaut et al., 1969; Fossieck and Parker, 1974). The interstitial nephritis caused by methicillin therapy (Aerenlund Jensen et al., 1971) has been recently associated with the presence of antitubular basement-membrane antibodies. It has been suggested, therefore, that the high amount of methicillin secreted by the proximal renal tubules could possibly result in the formation of an immunogenic complex (Border et al., 1974; Flax, 1974).

Specific attention has been given to the effect of probenecid administration on the kinetic behavior of penicillins. At present, there is general agreement on the fact that probenecid causes an artificial impairment of renal function and induces a more generalized reduction of the tissue compartment, leading to a decreased Vd and higher levels of circulating penicillins. A larger fraction of the drugs then becomes available for metabolism for a longer period (Gibaldi and Perrier, 1972). With probenecid, a decrease in the urinary excretion of unchanged ampicillin from 73.5% to 56% has been observed (Gibaldi and Schwartz, 1968). In the same study, the decreased biliary excretion due to the effect of probenecid was found to be compensated for by higher blood levels, which, in turn, provoked higher bile levels, possibly due to passive diffusion from the blood (Lund et al., 1974). The longer half-life in blood (from the previous 35-95 min to 75-260 min with probenecid) corresponded to a longer half-life in bile (from 70 to 120 min), with a consequent prolonged duration of therapeutic levels (Kampmann et al., 1973). Amoxicillin, under these circumstances, behaved like ampicillin (Karney et al., 1974). These data have also been confirmed for nafcillin, which is largely removed by the liver and whose hepatic clearance was shown to be diminished after probenecid administration (Barza and Weinstein, 1974b). These same authors suggest that investigations should be conducted to verify the possibility that the high serum levels seen with renal impairment could be misleading with respect to the actual amount of drug available at tissue level. Other drugs secreted by the same proximal tubulur transport mechanism, such as phenylbutazone and sulfinpyrazone, have been shown to significantly increase penicillin half-life. This increase is additive to that induced by renal pathology and age-induced impairment of tubular secretion (Kampmann et al., 1972).

Disposition of penicillins during development. The discussion of the disposition of various types of penicillins in the pediatric age group has been organized around single compounds or drug subgroups according to the availability of data and the specificity of the problems involved. Interestingly, more specific information is available for the early postnatal period. Maturation of renal function (Barnett et al., 1949; Broberger, 1973), variation of gastric acidity and, to a minor degree, differences in protein-binding (Ganshorn and Kurz, 1968; Ehrnebo et al., 1971) have been shown to be common factors which influence the disposition of this class of compounds.

Penicillin G, Procaine Penicillin and Benzathine Penicillin

Two main sets of data have been produced over the thirty years in which these compounds have been used; one set was compiled soon after the introduction of antibiotics on the market (Barnett et al., 1949; Huang and High, 1953), and the second, gathered recently, documents the picture more completely (McCracken et al., 1973; Klein et al., 1973; Kaplan and McCracken, 1973). Results of the first group of investigations are summarized in Table 5. Some conclusions are easily drawn from the data thus presented. The oral route is no longer used for the administration of acid-sensitive penicillins, but it is evident how the presence of lower acidity can affect the disposition of the antibiotic in neonates. Values similar to those found in adults are reached only at about 3 years of age. In this series of patients, a clear-cut distinction is found not only between infants and children, but also between infants younger or older than 6 months of age.

The degree of development of renal function is the other major factor to be considered. Sodium and procaine penicillin clearances of 90 ml/min/1.73 m^2 and 596.2 ml/min/1.73 m^2, respectively, have been measured in prematures and in children. This means that 17% the amount of renal function existed in premature infants as compared to children, when values were corrected for surface area, and 34% when corrected for body weight (Barnett et al., 1949). Daily determinations of serum penicillin levels in a premature infant over a 10-day period showed equivalent peak serum levels at 0.5 h (after the second day) but a steady decrease from a high of 9.6 µg/ml to 0.6 µg/ml was present on subsequent days at 6 h, possibly indicating progressive renal maturation (Huang and High, 1953). An increase in renal clearance for all penicillins after 5 days of life has been shown to be present in prematures and has also been suggested in full-term infants for the benzathine penicillins (Klein et al., 1973). Decreased protein-binding of benzyl penicillin (from about 60% to about 49%) has been documented in the serum of neonates at birth and in that of hyperbilirubinemic newborns (Ehrnebo et al., 1971). No specific data are available to allow an evaluation of the clinical significance of this finding.

Recent series of data for penicillin G are shown in Table 6 and for procaine and benzathine penicillin in Table 7. Slightly lower serum levels of penicillin have been observed in premature infants less than 2,000 g than in those weighing 2,000-3,500 g (14-15 µg/ml and 18-20 µg/ml). Apparent serum half-life seemed, however, independent of birth weight and inversely correlated with age and creatinine clearance. This suggests a role of minor importance for the secretory tubular route in the early neonatal period, whereas only 10% of the dose is thought to be excreted by glomerular filtration in adults (McCracken et al., 1973). To the contrary, penicillin clearance greater than that of inulin has been reported in premature infants (Barnett et al., 1949). Older infants and children (2.75-11.6 yrs) are considered to have renal function like adults (Barnett et al., 1949), and a serum half-life of 49 min measured using a group in this age range. Furthermore, a similar half-life was also measured in the tonsils of these patients (Kaplan et al., 1974b).

The disposition of benzathine penicillin G has been recently discussed with particular emphasis on its significance in controlling nursery outbreaks of

Table 5. Serum Levels Following Oral and Intramuscular Administration of K Penicillin and Procaine Penicillin (22,000 units/kg)

Group	Route	Age	Peak Time (h)		Peak Level (U/ml)		6 h Level (U/ml)	
			K Pen.	Proc. Pen.	Range K. Pen.	Proc. Pen.	K Pen.	Proc. Pen.
Premature newborns	Oral	24 h - 35 d	2.0	2.0	0.25-4.0 (2.18)	0.5-16 (3.25)	<0.03-4.0 (1.05)	0.125-2.0 (0.95)
Full-term newborns	Oral	24 h - 12 d	0.5	2.0	0.5-8.0 (3.50)	1.0-4.0 (2.50)	0.06-1.00 (0.30)	0.5-2.0 (1.06)
Infants	Oral	2 w - 2 yr	0.5	0.5	0.12-4.0 (1.57)	0.12-2.0 (0.82)	<0.015-0.06 (<0.037)	<0.015-0.06 (0.01)
Children	Oral	2 yr - 13 yr	0.5	0.5	0.25-4.0 (1.32)	0.25-1.0 (0.46)	(<0.015)	(0.003)
Premature newborns	i.m.	24 h - 35 d	0.5-6 (<24 h) 0.5 (7-35 d)	2.0	8.0-64.0 (23.0)	1.0-16.0 (8.7)	0.5-32.0 (7.0)*	0.5-12 (3.5)
Full-term newborns	i.m.	24 h - 12 d	0.5	2.0	16.0-64.0 (36.0)	3.0-16.0 (7.9)	0.5-16.0 (5.45)**	1.0-8.0 (3.8)
Infants	i.m.	2 w - 2 yr	0.5	0.5	12.0-48.0 (18.8)	0.5-12.0 (3.6)	<0.015-0.03 (0.01)	0.25-2.0 (0.85)
Children	i.m.	2 yr - 13 yr	0.5	2.0	8.0-24.0 (13.8)	1.0-8.0 (4.3)	<0.015-0.06 (0.005)	<0.015-1.0 (0.47)

* <24 h = mean: 24.0 (U/ml); 7-35 d = 1.3 U/ml.
** <24 h = mean: 12.0 (U/ml); 4-12 d = 1.1 U/ml.
( ): Mean value - h = hours, d = days, w = weeks, y = years.

Table 6. Penicillin G Disposition In Newborns

	Peak Time (h)	Peak Level** (μg/ml)	Serum Half-Life Range and Mean (h)	Urinary Excretion* (%)
0-6 Days (mean: 3.2) 25.000°	1	7.8-35.1 (22.0 ± 2.1)	1.4-9.7 (3.3)	32.4
0-6 Days (mean: 3.7) 16.650°	1	17.1-36.0 (24.8 ± 1.3)	2.0-7.0 (3.2)	30.6
0-6 Days (mean: 2.5) 50.000°	1	35.8	–	–
> 7 Days (mean: 8.0) 25.000°	0.5	7.5-41.1 (22.3 ± 3.5)	1.9-3.9 (2.3)	36.8
7-13 Days (mean: 9.5) 16.650°	0.5-1	5.3-25.5 (15.9 ± 1.7)	1.2-2.2 (1.7)	27.4
> 14 Days (mean: 18.5) 16.650°	0.5	5.7-29.1 (14.0 ± 3.2)	0.9-1.9 (1.3)	26.4
> 7 Days (mean: 15.7) 50.000°	1	33.8	–	–

°Dosages are given as units/Kg/dose.
*For those receiving 16.650 U/Kg, values are of a 0-8 h period; for other groups, 0-12 h.
**Mean values ± S.E. in brackets.
Adapted from McCracken et al., 1973.

streptococcal infection and on its use for the therapy of minor streptococcal disease on the neonate and of congenital syphilis. Available data seem to suggest that a single intramuscular dose is effective in curing minor infections (Klein et al., 1973) and in treating those luetic infants without neurosyphilis. Long, sustained activity of 1-3 weeks was found in tonsils (Breese and Disney, 1958) and in urine (Klein et al., 1973) with benzathine penicillin usage, but no antibacterial activity was found in the CSF in three of the four cases studied. Aqueous penicillin G and procaine penicillin are thus the drugs of choice to treat

Table 7. Procaine and Benzathine Penicillin Disposition in Newborns

	Peak Time (h)	Mean Peak Level (µg/ml)	Detectable Activity in Serum	Urinary Excretion (%)
Benzathine penicillin 50.000 U/Kg/dose				
Klein et al., 1973	13	1.23	5-7 days	–
Kaplan and McCracken, 1973	24	1.05 (range: 0.38-2.1)	12 days*	
Procaine penicillin 50.000 U/Kg/dose McCracken et al., 1973				
0-6 days (mean: 3.6)	2-12	7.4-8.8	24 h (1.5 µg/ml)	29.8 (0-12 h)
7 days (mean: 9.1)	4 h	5-6	24 h (0.5 µg/ml)	16.8 (0-12 h)

*In four out of five newborns.

CNS involvement as they allow therapeutic concentrations to be reached in the CSF (McCracken and Kaplan, 1974). No differences seemed to exist in the renal clearance of procaine penicillin and of aqueous penicillin, even if it is not clear why a lower percentage of excretion was reported for the older group of newborns shown in Table 7 (McCracken et al., 1973).

Ampicillin, Amoxicillin and Isoazoxazyl Penicillins

The parenteral route is the means of administration most widely used for ampicillin, and, in the future, will be even more so since the introduction of amoxicillin, a drug which seems to fit the need for a therapeutically equivalent oral treatment. Data about ampicillin disposition after i.m. and i.v. administration are presented separately. Tables 8 and 9 summarize the available information for premature and full-term newborns, respectively.

As in the case with penicillin, the stage of renal maturation probably plays the major role in determining changes in apparent serum half-life of ampicillin; the wide dispersion of data suggests a continuous, but not uniform, maturation. Apparently, this process is more regular after 1-2 days in term rather than in premature infants (Axline et al., 1967; Boe et al., 1967); moreover, a significant difference was observed in those values obtained before and after 2 weeks of age. The percentage of urinary excretion of ampicillin appeared to be independent

Table 8. Ampicillin Disposition in Premature Newborns

	Peak Time (h)	Peak Level Range (µg/ml)	T½ (h)	Trough Level at 12 h (µg/ml)	Urinary Excretion (0-12 h) (%)
Axline et al., 1967					
10 mg/Kg/dose					
2-7 days	1	13-19	4.0	1	22%
8-14 days			2.8		
15-30 days			1.7	n.d.	32%
31-68 days			1.6		
Kaplan et al., 1974a					
1-2 days					
50 mg/Kg/dose (i.m.)	0.5-1	80-134		7-75	
75 mg/Kg/dose (i.m.)	0.5-2	98-206	6.2*	20-42	40***
100 mg/Kg/dose (i.m.)	1-2	126-298	4.7*	51-65	
7-8 days (after repeated doses)					
50 mg/Kg/dose	0.5-1	82-188		5-88	
75 mg/Kg/dose	0.5-1	124-165	2.0*	29-38	67***
100 mg/Kg/dose	1-2	168-278	3.5**	33-81	

* and ** Range of values for the age group, independent of dosage: 3.1-9.7 and 1.4-5.3, respectively.
***Mean values for respective age groups: range of cumulative data, 19-79.

Table 9. Ampicillin Disposition in Full-Term Newborns

	Peak Time (h)	Peak Level Range (μg/ml)	T½ (h)	Trough Level at 12 h (μg/ml)
Boe et al., 1967				
25 mg/Kg dose				
1 day	1	57.3 ± 2.2	3.4	6.1 ± 1.0
4-5 days	1	47.3 ± 5.2	2.2	1.4 ± 0.5
Kaplan et al., 1974a				
1-2 days				
(after 1-2 doses)				
50 mg/Kg/dose	1-2	36-99	4.7*	4-55
75 mg/Kg/dose	1-2	78-172		13-55
100 mg/Kg/dose	1-2	128-232	3.1*	9-30
7-8 days				
(after 11-15 doses)				
50 mg/Kg/dose	0.5-1	78-86	2.3	5-11
75 mg/Kg/dose	1	102-176		8-14
100 mg/Kg/dose	1	120-257	1.8	5-45

*Range for this age group: 1.7-10.0.

of the baby's age and the dosage, and seemed to correlate with creatinine clearance. Repeated dosing did not seem to influence the kinetics of the drug. The lower serum levels observed at the end of therapy in the series of Kaplan et al. (1974a) would seem to be attributed to the increasing age of the infants.

Protein-binding has never been determined in *in vivo* studies. *In vitro* experiments under physiological conditions of temperature and pH showed a binding capability in the neonate that was 50% of that seen in adults with a range of 7.6-12.1% and 19.3-24.3%, respectively, for less-than-24-hour neonates and for adult volunteers (Ehrnebo et al., 1971). No data have been found regarding possible differences in liver metabolism and biliary excretion in the pediatric age group. Penetration of ampicillin into the CSF is good when the meninges are inflamed and tends to decline as the pathological changes subside, however, it does not seem possible to correlate quantitatively the degree of inflammation, as measured by WBC, protein and sugar content of CSF, and the degree of penetration. Curiously enough, in meningitis due to *H. influenzae* and *D. penumoniae* there seems to be better CSF penetration than in cases of meningococcal meningitis (Taber et al., 1967; Wilson and Haltalin, 1975). Both the intravenous and the intramuscular route give good results, allowing therapeutic levels to be achieved and maintained. Higher and more prolonged serum levels have been observed after i.m. than after i.v. administration, with CSF levels closely following the same pattern, and a much higher concentration has been measured in the subdural fluid than in CSF (Wilson and Haltalin, 975). Furthermore, there is suggestive evidence that CSF penetration is quicker in infants than in children, although no specific data are available to substantiate this claim (McCracken, 1974).

No differences have been demonstrated in the apparent half-life in children and in adults. This also holds true for patients (3 mos-2.5 yrs old) with congenital heart defects, where a normal total clearance, 329-448 ml/min, has been measured after continuous infusion. Half-life values of 0.9-1.1 h that were obtained in these patients were independent of age. A lower clearance (97-122 ml/min), doubled serum levels, and identical values of half-life have been observed in children with great vessel transposition compared with those with other heart defects and with normal adults (Vietor et al., 1974).

Absorption after oral ampicillin administration is said to be good in fasting subjects (McCracken, 1974). It should be noted, however, that low erratic absorption was seen in infants 1 to 11 months, and in newborns 15-30 days old. In these babies, levels as low as one-tenth of those reached after i.m. administration were observed (Marget and Wagner, 1967). The same low values plus a fairly high incidence of gastrointestinal disturbances have also been reported in more recent studies (Bass et al., 1974). Better absorption resulted when the drug was given in drops as compared with capsules. Interestingly enough, a threefold increase of the AUC with respect to that in adults was measured in newborns 24-48 h old. The anhydrous form resulted in better serum levels than the trihydrate, giving an AUC ratio of 1.33. Alterations in the general conditions of pH and hydration did not seem to influence the absorption pattern, according to Silverio and Poole (1973). The investigations of Sabra et al. (1973), while open to criticism ethically, did agree with these findings. Individual differences between patients of the same age, i.e., good and poor absorbers, have also been described (Nelson et al., 1972).

Amoxicillin is an antibiotic, similar to ampicillin, that has been introduced quite recently. The important characteristics of better, more regular absorption and of lower incidence of gastrointestinal side effects that have been observed in adults also seem to hold true in pediatric patients (McCracken, 1974; Brogden et al., 1975a). Equivalent doses of the two antibiotics give serum levels of amoxicillin which are more than double those observed with ampicillin. Different results have been reported in severely ill pre-term newborns who started being treated within the first 48 hours of life. Amoxicillin did not appear to be better absorbed than ampicillin. On the contrary 3 h serum levels after repeated treatment show more sustained levels for ampicillin. Absorption is not modified in pathological situations, such as acute shigellosis, but in this specific case, unfortunately, the pharmacological advantage does not compensate for the limited amoxicillin activity against shigella infection. The course of illness in those shigellosis patients treated with amoxicillin did not differ significantly from that observed with the use of a placebo (Nelson and Haltalin, 1974).

Peak absorption of amoxicillin has been documented at 3 h after the dose was given (2-3 wks), and the serum half-life was reported to be 3 times longer than in adults. On the other hand, infants of 1-2 years of age showed an absorption peak at 2 h, with a plasma half-life comparable to that seen in adults (0.8-1.9 h) (Simon and Toeller, 1974). Amoxicillin in granulated form gives an earlier peak serum level (0.5 h), but at 1-4 h after a dose no differences in serum level is seen compared with the capsulated form (Nishimura et al., 1973). In children, higher urinary excretion has been described for amoxicillin than for ampicillin, and greater metabolic degradation has been documented. As yet, there is no evidence to support the clinical advantages of the high levels of amoxicillin that are reached in sputum and bronchial secretions (Brogden et al., 1975a).

As yet, very few data have been published that deal with the clinical pharmacology of isoazoxazyl penicillins, antibiotics that can be administered either orally or parenterally (Grossman and Ticknor, 1966; O'Connor et al., 1966; Marget and Wagner, 1967, Axline et al., 1967). Highly variable serum levels are seen following oral administration. A better and faster absorption is documented for dicloxacillin. In a recent study, flucloxacillin has been shown to be well absorbed in premature newborns less than 1 week of age. When ampicillin and flucloxacillin are given together, the absorption of ampicillin is delayed and decreased (Cohen et al., 1975).

Methicillin

No comprehensive studies on methicillin have been made after those of Boe et al. (1967) and Axline et al. (1967), in premature and full-term newborns. Pertinent data are presented in Table 10. The only more recent information on this antibiotic since those studies is a measurement of the protein-binding, which was shown to be lower in the newborn than in adults (35.3 ± 0.95% of free drug vs. 25.8 ± 0.73%) (Ganshorn and Kurz, 1968).

Carbenicillin

The specific activity of this drug against some indole-positive proteus species and *Pseudomonas aeruginosa* is the main reason why carbenicillin is sometimes preferred to the other penicillins in treating neonatal infections. Acknowledgment of the clinical usefulness of the antibiotic, however, resulted in a thorough documentation of its pharmacological properties (Nelson, 1970; Ross et al., 1970, with the accompanying discussion). To our knowledge, three papers have been published dealing to some extent with the disposition patterns in the

Table 10. Methicillin Disposition in Neonatal Age

	Age (days)	Peak Time (h)	Serum Peak Level (μg/ml)	Serum T½ (h)	Vd (% BW)	Urinary Excretion (%)
Premature newborns Axline et al., 1967 20 mg/Kg (i.m.)	4-7	1	36.2-41.6	2.4	25-35	31 (0-6 h)
	11-14			1.8		
	17-33			1.4		42 (0-6 h)
Boe et al, 1967 25 mg/Kg (i.m.)	4-5	1	47.6 ± 2.7	3.3	—	—
	13-15		52.2 ± 2.9	1.0	—	—
	26-30		37.8 ± 2.2	1.4	—	—
Full-term newborns Boe et al., 1967 25 mg/Kg (i.m.)	24 h	1	60.1 ± 2.3	3.3	—	—
	4-5		47.1 ± 2.0	1.3	—	—
	8-9		41.1 ± 2.0		—	—
	13-15		35.1 ± 1.7	0.9	—	—
	16-30		27.7 ± 0.9	0.8	—	—

Table 11. Serum Half-Life (h) of Carbenicillin According to
Birth Weight and Postnatal Age

Birth Weight	Age (days)				
	1-3	4-7	8-14	15-21	22-45
Nelson and McCracken, 1973					
< 2,000 g					
75 mg/Kg	5.5	5.9	4.3	2.9	
100 mg/Kg		5.6	3.6		
> 2,000 g					
75 mg/Kg	5.7	2.9	2.4		
100 mg/Kg	5.4	2.9	2.1		
< 2,000 g	6.5^a	6.6^b	4.4^c	2.9*	–
2,000-3,000 g	6.7^a	2.9^b	2.2^c	–	1.5^d
> 3,000 g	4.7^a	2.9^b	2.2^c	1.5*	1.6^d
Morehead et al., 1972	1-7 days				
< 2,500 g					
50 mg/Kg	3.3				
100 mg/Kg	3.5				
> 2,500 g					
50 mg/Kg	4.0				
100 mg/Kg	2.7				

*Single case.
a,b,c,d: Ranges of values for the whole group: 3-13.6; 1.8-11.6; 1.8-5.8; 1.3-1.6 respectively.

pediatric age group (Simon et al., 1971; Morehead et al., 1972; Nelson and McCracken 1973). Relevant data from these investigations have been collected in Table 11. A dividing line between infants <2,000 g and >2,000 g was suggested as an indication for dosing intervals of every 8 h and every 6 h, respectively; a further division within these groups was proposed according to the gestational age. Supposedly, no changes in disposition occur in premature infants until 7 days after birth. On the contrary, in full-term newborns 3 days are enough to induce a clear-cut modification in the handling of carbenicillin (Nelson and McCracken, 1973). The variability of reported data is very high. A limit of 7 days of age was proposed for both premature and full-term infants by Simon et al. (1971). who assigned practically the same values of apparent serum half-life to both groups. However, the extreme variability of these results deserves mention, this being particularly true during the first week of life in which ranges of trough serum levels of 8.5-80 µg/ml and 5.9-95 µg/ml have been measured (Morehead et al., 1972).

General patterns have emerged which suggest that carbenicillin disposition depends mainly on maturation of renal function. A rough correlation has been proposed between the percentage of urinary excretion of carbenicillin within 12 h after dosing and the creatinine clearance, between the carbenicillin serum half-life and the creatinine clearance, and between the serum half-life and age of the patient (Nelson and McCracken, 1973). Both intravenous and intramuscular administration gave essentially the same patterns, with higher levels after i.v. administration for the first 90 min, and an overlapping curve thereafter (Morehead et al., 1972), in which they referred to single i.v. injections of high doses of carbenicillin; the proposed apparent volume of distribution was 50% of body weight for premature infants and 59% for the full-term newborn. A peak level at 1 h after i.m. injection has also been documented by Panero and Orzalesi (personal communication), whose serum levels were lower than those seen by Morehead et al. (1972), and in agreement with those of Neussel and Olbing (1972). The same authors give half-life values for full-term, normal-weight newborns which are in agreement with Nelson and McCracken (1973); there was a progressive decrease from 4.5 h on day 1, to 3.8 on days 3-4, to 3.5 on days 7-11, to 2.5 h on days 13-26. Therefore, following i.m. administration a lower, delayed peak was seen in newborns compared with that in infants and in children (peak level at 1-2 h and 1 h, respectively). Higher variability was also observed in the younger group than in the older infants (peak levels: 89 μg/ml ± 46 and 143 μg/ml ± 37) (Neussel and Olbing, 1972). With 12 h after it was given, 36% of the carbenicillin dose was excreted in the low-birth-weight infant, and 61% in normal-birth-weight newborns, both groups under 7 days of age (Morehead et al., 1972). Other investigators found that 40-45% of the dose was excreted in full-term newborns during the first 4 h after i.v. administration (Simon et al., 1971).

Data have been obtained for infants and children following single i.v. injections of 100 and 200 mg/kg of carbenicillin (Simon et al., 1971). Serum levels were dose-related, and a slightly longer half-life was seen following the higher dosage (110 min vs. 100 min). No difference in the mean serum half-life of carbenicillin were observed between infants 3-12 months and children 2-6 years old, being 110 min in both groups. The apparent volume of distribution in the two groups was 67% and 50% of body weight, respectively. Moreover, a further decrease in this parameter was seen in schoolchildren (7-12 years), whose values are identical with adult values (app. Vd: 26% B.W., with apparent serum half-life of 90 min). In those pathological situations with some degree of impaired renal function, such as cardiac insufficiency and myxedema, there are higher serum half-life values. Not unexpectedly, clinical improvement following therapeutic treatment in these cases is accompanied by a return to normal values. A 66% increase in serum half-life is seen with concomitant administration of probenecid (from 60 to 100 min in 5 healthy adult volunteers). From 60 to

80% of the administered dose of carbenicillin is excreted in urine within 6 h in pediatric patients after the neonatal period.

CEPHALOSPORINS

The clinical significance of this class of antibiotics and their place in the therapy of infectious diseases have been extensively reviewed by Saslaw (1970). Thrupp (1974) and Owens et al. (1975). These reviews have even gone so far as to ask "whither the cephalosporins" (Hamilton-Miller and Brumfitt, 1974). Growing importance has been given to the fact that these antibiotics should not be used too often, both because of the frequent emergence of bacterial resistance and because of their relative high cost. Consequently, there is an increasing concensus that they should be used only as a second choice after the penicillins. Complete agreement does not exist regarding the clinical significance of the cross reactivity between these two classes of drugs, and allergic reactions similar to those occurring with penicillins have been observed following treatment with cephalosporins. The relative resistance to enzymatic degradation of both penicillins and cephalosporins is discussed very cleary in recent works (Kuwahara et al., 1970; Jackson et al., 1973; Hewitt, 1973a; Owens et al., 1975).

The introduction on the market of many new cephalosporin derivatives (Fig. 1) has not resulted in any substantial improvement in the efficacy of this antibiotic family. Despite differences in their pharmacokinetic properties and their spectra of activity, the products available at present can actually be considered comparable in their therapeutic effectiveness (Garrod, 1974). New derivatives, such as the cephamycins, which are closely related to cephalosporins, have been developed and are presently being investigated but, as yet, the data are too scanty to allow any meaningful evaluation (Editorial, 1973; Williams and Andrews, 1974; Owens et al., 1975). The research for a cephalosporin with an ideal profile thus far has not been successful (Wise, 1974).

For the purpose of this review, data have been summarized in a general scheme in order to give a synoptic profile of the individual drugs (Table 12). Agreement exists regarding some of the general properties such as route of administration, relative degree of protein-binding and metabolic degradation. A wide range of variation, however, is evident when data relative to single parameters are compared in different papers. A choice has been made in favor of those papers, which deal more specifically with pharmacokinetics (see references quoted in Table 12). Authors will be mentioned in the following discussion only when their data suggest a distinct comment, or differ significantly from other sources.

Analytical techniques for cephalosporins allow monitoring of drug levels within a reasonable time interval (Noone, 1973). More specific methods are being developed which permit a more quantitative and specific assessment of

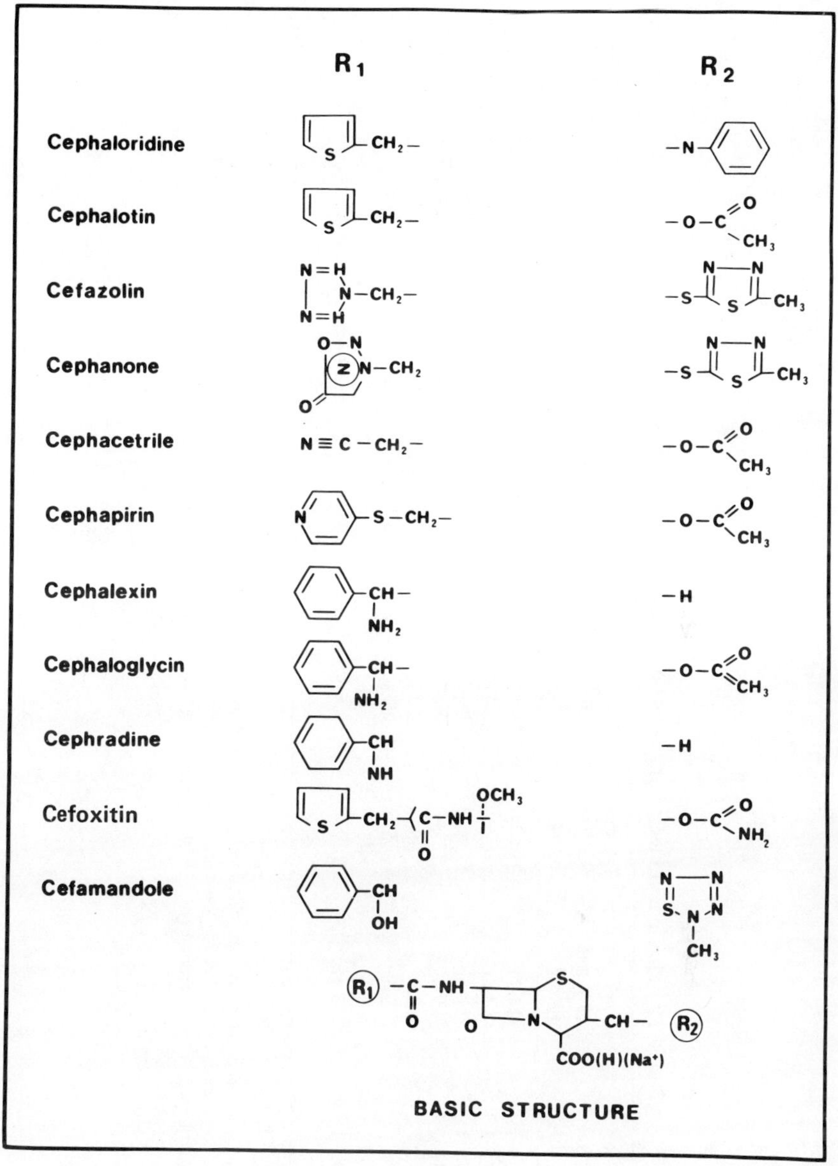

	R_1	R_2
Cephaloridine		
Cephalotin		
Cefazolin		
Cephanone		
Cephacetrile		
Cephapirin		
Cephalexin		
Cephaloglycin		
Cephradine		
Cefoxitin		
Cefamandole		

BASIC STRUCTURE

Fig. 1

small amounts of the drug itself (Cooper et al., 1973). Only two of the compounds are better absorbed when given by the oral route. These are cephalexin (CX) and the more recent cephradine (CD), both of which are considered absolutely equivalent from the point of view of their clinical usefulness (Williams and Beddes, 1973; Garrod, 1974). A peak serum level is observed approximately

Table 12. Pharmacokinetic Parameters of Some Cephalosporin Antibiotics

Drug	Peak* Time (h)	Peak Level* μg/ml	Protein-Binding (%)	Half-Life (h)	App. Vd L/1.73 m²	Clearance ml/min/1.73 m² Serum	Clearance ml/min/1.73 m² Renal	Urinary Excretion (%-24 h)
Cephaloridine	1	16-21	20-24	1.1-1.5	13-20	145-190	105-150	64-85
Cephalotin	0.5-1	7.6	56-69	0.4-0.7	18-25	410-530	210-320	37-62
Cefazolin	0.5-1	18,48	63-85	1.6-2.6	10-15	56-110	47-77	60-97
Cefacetrile	0.5-0.7	19,47	22,34	0.8-2.0	12-20	180-440	180-390	88-100
Cephanone	1	36	88	2.3-2.6	10-13	54-58	43-51	95
Cefalexin	1	10-18	15 / 41	0.9-1.1	13-18	376	240-265	96
Cephradine	0.5-1	12-16	12 / 6	0.5-1.0	19-29	511-641	290-470	55-94

*After 0.5 g either i.m. or p.o. (see text).

Papers from which data have been taken are the following: Nissenson et al., 1972; Bergeron et al., 1973; Craig et al., 1973; Kirby and Regamey, 1973; Levison et al., 1973; Simon et al., 1973a; Westenfelder et al., 1973; Barza and Weinstein, 1974b; Hodson and Holloway, 1974; Cohn et al., 1974; Naumann and Reintjens, 1974; Regamey et al., 1974; Zaki et al., 1974; Welling et al., 1974; Lode et al., 1975.

1 h after administration, and it increases proportionally with doses as high as 1 g. With CD, even earlier absorption has been observed when the equivalent dose was given in the form of a suspension compared with that of capsules, but no differences in comparative AUC were measured (Zaki et al., 1974). Oral absorption is said to be almost complete and only delayed and prolonged by concomitant eating, which causes great variability in peak times and serum levels (O'Callaghan et al., 1971; Griffith and Black, 1970). Despite the altered absorption when food is present, no change in the percentage excreted in urine has been observed in studies conducted with CX (Gower and Sash, 1969).

The parenteral administration of CX does not seem to offer any definite advantages; besides its painfulness, the i.m. administration gives lower blood levels than the oral route and a dyspnoic reaction has been observed after intravenous injection (Solberg et al., 1973). Pain at the site of injection is a property shared by many of the cephalosporins. Cefalotin (CT) is the most painful, while cefaloridine (CR) seems to be the least. The addition of 1% lidocaine to the injectable solution to overcome this drawback did not seem to influence the degree of absorption in studies with cefacetrile (CTR), even if an earlier peak at 30 min was observed compared with the usual peak at 45-60 min (Wise and Reeves, 1974). In addition, CT has been reported to cause phlebitis after i.v. administration independently from modifications of the pH of the solution (Carrizosa et al., 1974). The site of injection with i.m. administration appears to be one of the factors that influence the pharmacokinetics of the various cephalosporins. With CTR, higher peak levels are obtained when it is injected into the thigh, while buttock injection gives more prolonged levels (Wise and Reeves, 1974). In another study, the deltoid appeared to assure better absorption than injection into the gluteus and vastus lateralis (Vukovich et al., 1975), although it is noteworthy that the use of the same site for repeated injections caused lower absorption of cefazolin (CZ) (Welling et al., 1974). After i.m. administration of CD, a striking difference in absorption rate has been observed between males and females (K_1, M: s.70 ± 0.34/h; F: 1.16 ± 0.17) and was more evident when the gluteus was used, moreover, the AUC was also significantly different (Vukovich et al., 1975).

CZ has been the object of many comparative studies because of the therapeutic advantages claimed due to its high serum concentrations and its longer serum half-life. Peak CZ plasma levels can usually be measured about 1 h after i.m. administration and 15 min after a single i.v. injection. Extensive protein-binding, however, limits the amount of drug available for antibacterial activity. When the free fractions of the two drugs are compared, CR gives peaks 3 to 4 times higher than CZ; about 4 h after their administration, this difference no longer exists. Mean serum bactericidal activity follows the same pattern as the levels of free serum fractions (Bergeron et al., 1973). Nevertheless, when corrected for protein-binding, serum levels of CZ are still 3 times higher than those of CT (Craig et al., 1973). An inhibitory index of the free antibiotic has been calculated for different cephalosporins against various bacterial strains, according to this test, CR and cefamandole seem to be favored but this *in vitro* measure does not correspond with the clinical efficacy rating (Griffith, 1974).

The extent of protein-binding also seems to correlate with the apparent volume of distribution, thus it is very low for CZ. Decreased binding, as seen in azotemic patients, leads to a significant increase in the volume of distribution (23.0 ± 43 1/1.73 m^2) (Craig et al., 1973). Cephanone shares the same properties as CZ, including the same degree of protein-binding and a prolonged half-life due to low serum and renal clearances (Kirby and Regamey, 1973). Interestingly, a significant decrease in the serum half-life, the volume of distribution and the renal (but not total) clearance have been observed for CZ after repeated dosages over a period of 4 days (Welling et al., 1974), while, in contrast, in studies with CX no change in T½ has been reported after 5 administrations (Gower and Dash, 1969).

In the absence of renal impairment, there is no accumulation of any of the cephalosporins. Of this entire group of compounds, CT has the shortest half-life and the highest clearances. Particularly noteworthy are those results reported after the use of chemical instead of microbiological analytical techniques. CT, as an example, is shown to have a half-life of 11 ± 1 min (Cooper et al., 1973; Anders et al., 1975). As is also evident from the urinary data, this cephalosporin is not excreted entirely via the kidney. It undergoes an extensive metabolic degradation to give rise to deacetylated derivative, which has markedly reduced antibacterial activity and a half-life of 17.6 ± 3.2 min (Griffith and Black, 1971). A minor route of extrarenal elimination is also hypothesized for CR to account for that portion of the dose not found in urine (Kirby and Regamey, 1973).

Cephalosporins are excreted by both glomerular filtration and tubular secretion. This latter process is thought to be low for CR but high for CT (Regamey et al., 1974). Probenecid delays renal excretion, giving higher and prolonged serum levels of the antibiotics (Kirby and Regamey, 1973, for clarification on the possible mechanisms of action of probenecid, see discussion under penicillins). A half-life increased from 50 to 107.1. min has been measured when probenecid was given to patients taking oral CX (Gower and Dash, 1969). Likewise, an increase in T½ from 60 to 90 min was reported for CTR when probenecid was given; alkalinzation did not seem to modify urinary excretion of CTR (Wise and Reeves, 1974). Diuretics did not alter the pattern of urinary excretion of CT (Tice et al., 1975).

There has been much attention given to the changes in pharmacokinetic parameters in patients with renal impairment. In general, under these circumstances the cephalosporins demonstrate a prolonged half-life and the affected patients should be considered at risk if high doses of antibiotic are employed. CR has been more frequently implicated as one of the compounds of this class that should be considered nephrotoxic. There is no clear explanation for this kidney-damaging effect. Experimental data show, however, that other drugs acting at the tubular level, such as probenecid, protect from nephrotoxicity (Hewitt, 1973a). Reports of renal failure have also been associated with CT (Burton et al., 1974) and often occur when a combination of gentamicin and one of the cephalosporins has been given (Bobrow et al., 1972, Klastersky et al., 1974c, see also under gentamicin section). Unlike the other cephalosporins, CT, because of its metabolism by the liver, is usually not considered to need dosage modification in patients with renal insufficiency, but, in general, factors such as age, creatinine clearance of less than 20-30 ml/min, concomitant use of other drugs, dehydration and combination with diuretics seem to be the major risk components that require dosage adjustments (Bechtol, 1972; Giusti, 1973). Both CT and cephapirin have been shown to be responsible for the occurrence of a serum sickness-like illness in 100% of adult volunteers receiving high i.v. doses for a prolonged period (Sanders et al., 1974).

Tissue permeability and the rate of diffusion are not easily compared among the different cephalosporins. The available information on this aspect is scanty and, furthermore, has been obtained in different pathological situations. Lacking a comprehensive evaluation of tissue distribution of this class of antibiotics, a few of the clinically pertinent findings are briefly mentioned here (for a comprehensive review of single compounds, see Owens et al., 1975; Orsolini, 1970; Griffith and Black, 1971; Cimmino and Garaci, 1973). Biliary tract levels appear, generally, to parallel serum levels, but a highly variable ratio between the serum and gall bladder or common duct levels can be observed. CZ reaches higher levels than CR and CT in the gall bladder and common duct. Clinically useful levels are also obtained with CX, whereas no therapeutic concentrations have been observed with CTR (Brogard et al., 1970, 1973; Shibata and Fujii, 1970; Ratzan et al., 1974). In studies with CX the mean ratio of gall bladder bile concentration to serum concentration was 22 in normal patients, while in patients with gall bladder disease the ratio was 17 (Ram and Watanatittan, 1974). The same authors also give higher values for common duct concentrations and underline that great differences are to be expected according to the degree of hepatic dysfunction and the timing of the samplings. It is important to remember that any obstruction to bile flow markedly reduces the appearance of antibiotics in the bile (Acocella et al., 1968; Babb et al., 1974; Ratzan et al., 1974).

Cephalosporin penetration seems to be low into sinus secretions, and no correlation has been shown between the local antibiotic concentration and its clinical efficacy (for CD, see Axelsson and Brorson, 1974). Higher penetration in sputum during the acute phase of bronchitis has been shown for CX. A lower ratio sputum/serum is found with increasing inflammation (Halprin and McMahon, 1973). In osseous tissue, a bacterially active concentration is reached in both normal and chronically inflamed tissue, with bone sampling, one-tenth to one-fourth of the serum levels of CT and CTR have been measured (Hierholzer et al., 194). An antibiotic concentration sufficient to reach MIC for staphylococcus aureus is measurable in the skin after an i.m. administration of a single dose of CX. CZ and CD are found in experimentally produced skin blisters in amounts which reflect their protein-binding (34% and 71%, respectively, of total serum levels) (Simon et al., 1973a). The experimental model of an implanted subcutaneous fibrin clot has been applied to CR and CT. Antibiotic accumulation occurs within the clot after repeated administrations and after the third dose a concentration of 50% of that in serum is reached (Barza et al., 1974a). With these same cephalosporins, CR and CT, penetration in inflammatory exudates and in infected lymph nodes takes place within 2 h after systemic administration (Reller et al., 1973; Pickering et al., 1973).

The passage of cephalosporins into the CSF is increased when there are inflamed meninges, but the concentration reaches levels that are therapeutic only for staphylococcal infections (Taber et al., 1967; Vianna and Kaye, 1967; Pickering et al., 1974; Crosson, 1975). CSF concentrations as high at 15 μg/ml are reported to occur after repeated i.v. administration of high doses of CTR (3 g every 6 h) (Maurice et al., 1973). A range of concentrations of 0.15-46.5 μg/ml has been measured with CT, however, and an unacceptably high rate of failure was present even at higher levels (Brown et al., 1970). Experimental data show that probenecid could possibly increase CSF concentrations of CRT and CZ (Dacey and Sande, 1974). Brain tissue/blood concentrations ranging from 1/70 to 1/6 for CT and from 1/40 to 1/6 for CR have been found (Griffith and Black, 1971).

Cephalosporin disposition during development. Data for this age group are particularly scanty and do not allow a systematic presentation to be made. Available information is given for each compound.

Cephalothin

Using a specific analytical method, Anders et al. (1975) found half-life values (14.9 ± 1.9 min) not significantly different from those obtained in adults in a group of patients ranging in age from 2 months to 17 years. In a similar group (3 months to 13 years of age), lower serum levels and scarce penetration in infected tissue have been reported for CT when compared with CZ, with an insignificant difference in clinical efficacy (Pickering et al., 1974).

Cephaloridine

Few data on drug disposition in newborns, infants and children have been published (Walker and Maisog, 1969). Following i.m. administration in newborns, the peak serum level is observed in 3-4 h; in infants and children (4 weeks-2 years and 2 years old, respectively), the peak serum level is reached between 2 and 3 h. This level remains fairly constant as long as 6 h in newborns, whereas it declines in the other groups. The apparent serum half-life is about 3 h in infants, and about 2.2 h in children. In newborns, great variability in serum levels (20-40 µg/ml after 15 mg/kg) is seen. This wide variation was also reported by Keay et al. (1967), who, in addition, did not observe differences between normal and low-weight newborns. A single daily dose of 30 mg/kg was considered sufficient for therapeutic coverage. Similar levels, with less variability, are reached in infants and children following a 25 mg/kg i.m. dose (Walker and Maisog, 1969).

Cefazolin

The only information available about this antibiotic in the neonatal age group has been found in a short report containing limited data on peak levels and urinary excretion in premature and full-term newborn babies (Nakazawa et al., 1972). The peak serum level occurred 1 h after i.m. administration; urinary recovery of 61.5% of the administered dose over 7 h was obtained in premature infants, while 41.4% was recovered from full-term newborns over the same period. Kinetic patterns similar to those seen in adults are documented for groups of patients ranging from 1 month to 15 years of age (Kobayashy et al., 1970; Gold et al., 1973; Khan, 1973). In purulent tissues particularly, good penetration has been measured, which would seem to parallel serum concentration (Pickering et al., 1974).

Cefalexin

Certainly, more and comparatively better data have been published about this orally absorbed cephalosporin (Donnisen and Davison, 1970). Table 13 summarizes the findings of different authors. The absorption rate is significantly lower in premature (1-4 weeks of age) than in full-term babies (1-2 weeks old), and slighter, but constant, increase is evident from 1-2 weeks to 3 weeks-12 months, to 2-6 years, to 7-12 years (Simon et al., 1970). In newborns, absorption has been calculated to be about 60% of that seen in adults (Boothman et al., 1973); moreover, slower absorption has been noted after higher dosages (Simon et al., 1970; von Harnack, 1971). This latter finding, however, was not confirmed by Boothman et al. (1973), who reported an earlier and proportionally higher peak following a higher dosage (50 mg/kg vs. 15 mg/kg), with a second peak seen 8 h after the administration. Additional studies have shown that a single oral dose gives higher serum levels in babies under 3 months than in older infants (Walker and Gonzalez, 1971); higher, more regular levels have also been measured in 6-month-old infants than in those 9-12 months old (Marget and Daschner, 1969). Serum levels in excess of 8 µg/ml, and sustained for as long as 12 h, have been reported following a single oral dose of 15 mg/kg in a large series of newborn infants (MacMillan, 1971); no precise definition of the age limits is given in this particular report. Unfortunately, the great dispersion and paucity of the reported cases make it difficult to draw definite conclusions. The differences

Table 13. Cephalexin Disposition in Pediatric Age

	Age Group	Dose (mg/kg)	Peak Time (h)	Peak Level (μg/ml) Range	Peak Level (μg/ml) Mean	Trough Level (h)	App. Serum T½ (h)	Urinary Excretion (%) (0-14 h)
Marget and Daschner, 1969	9-22 d	50	3	15-40	22	—	5	73-100 (0-12 h)
	< 6 mo	25	2	12-22	17	—	4	
	9-12 mo	25	1	5-25	10	—	2.5-3	
Simon et al., 1970	premature (1-4 wk)	25	4-5		15.6	6	3.7 ± 0.4	—
	full-term (1-2 wk)	25	2.5		12.4	4.5	3.4 ± 0.2	—
	infants (3 wk-12 mo)	25	1.5-2		15.2	4.5	1.5 ± 0.2	—
	children (2-6 yr)	25	2		26.2	—	1.3 ± 0.1	—
	(7-12 yr)		1.5-2		26.2	—	1.1 ± 0.1	—
Cockburn et al., 1972	premature (0-8 d)	15	4-5	2.5-13	7.5	12-14	—	60
Boothman et al., 1973	full-term (0-3 d)	15	4	5-15	—	—	—	17-59
		50	2-3	20-30	—	—	—	18-64
Helwig et al., 1972	< 1 yr	27.4	2	1-180	9.82	—	—	—
	> 1 yr	17.4	1		25.15	—	—	—

in serum half-life are the result of changing rates of absorption and elimination, both of which increase progressively with age (Simon et al., 1970). A lower and delayed peak has been observed in children with celiac disease (Marget, 1971).

Cephradine

No data have been found on the pharmacokinetics of this specific antibiotic in newborns and infants. Children do show an absorption pattern similar to that seen in adults. After the administration of an oral suspension, peak concentrations are reached at 0.5 h. Doses of 125 mg and 250 mg give peak serum levels of 8.2 ± 0.89 and 15.6 ± 1.84 µg/ml, respectively (Neiss, 1973; Zaki et al., 1974).

AMINOGLYCOSIDES

The compounds discussed in this section share the same general range of antibacterial activity and the same pharmacologic behavior. Two of them, kanamycin (KNM) and gentamicin (GTM) are the most commonly used and well known, both from a pharmacokinetic point of view and in pediatric practice. Comparative studies have been made with amikacin (AMK) and tobramycin (TBM), respectively. Kinetic data will be summarized in the same tables, to allow a rapid assessment of their few differences and many similarities. With this class of compounds, it is known that there exists the possibility of damage to one or the other of the branches of the 8th nerve. Renal toxicity has also been frequently reported, especially in those disease states where altered kidney function is already present, or when other potentially nephrotoxic drugs are used at the same time.

Cross-resistance among these compounds does exist, but varies in different hospital situations depending primarily on the extent to which the aminoglycosides are used, therefore, an evaluation of the individual situation is needed. For example, the resistance to GTM is still rare, however, its wide use could lead, possibly, to serious problems in the near future (Franco et al., 1973). Topical use, especially, should be avoided because of the increased risk of inducing resistance (Snelling et al., 1971; Hamilton-Miller et al., 1974; Lacey, 1975). A recent survey has shown 50% of *Pseudomonas aeruginosa* strains resistant to KNM, 18.6 to GTM, 1.6 to TBM (Holmes et al., 1974). The introduction of new molecules is considered useful to avoid the emergent trend toward bacteriological resistance by increasing the number of drugs available for rotation (Kaplan et al., 1973; Klastersky et al., 1973a, b; Jaffe et al., 1974; Klastersky et al., 1975b).

Table 14. Kanamycin (K) and Amikacin (A) Disposition in Adult Volunteers

		Peak Time (h)	Peak Serum Level (μg/ml)	Steady State (μg/ml)	Half-Life (h)
Intravenous infusion					
Clarke et al., 1974					
(3.3 mg/kg/h loading dose	K		15.8 ± 1.4	12.0 ± 1.5	2.07 ± 0.21
1 mg/kg/h over 5 h)	A		15.0 ± 1.6	11.9 ± 0.7	2.30 ± 0.39
Intramuscular administration					
Cabana and Taggart, 1973					
250 mg	K	0.8	11.9	–	2.1
500 mg		1.0	20.6	–	2.3
250 mg	A	0.9	11.4	–	2.4
500 mg		1.15	20.4	–	2.2
Doluisio et al., 1973					
7.5 mg/kg	K	1-2	22 ± 4	–	2.4
2.0 g			92 ± 5		
Lumolthz et al., 1974					1.8 ± 0.5
500 mg	K				5.5 ± 2.5

Kanamycin

Different aspects of the clinical application and pharmacology of KNM were reviewed as early as ten years ago (Mann, 1966). However, in the last few years a more systematic approach has been developed. KNM was one of the first drugs for which nomograms and computer models were proposed (Cutler and Orme, 1969, Mawer et al., 1972, Tozer, 1974). This type of investigation was suggested by the clinical interest in avoiding accumulation phenomena and toxicity and was not difficult because of the rather simple kinetics of the drug. KNM is not protein-bound and is excreted unchanged, almost entirely in the urine. The relevant pharmacokinetic parameters have been summarized in Table 14, together with data on amikacin. Data obtained by different authors compare favorably both after i.m. administration, intravenous infusion or single bolus injection. A prolonged half-life is seen in elderly people (5.5 ± 2.5 h) (Lumholtz et al., 1974). This is in agreement with the strong correlation found between creatinine clearance and serum half-life (Mawer et al., 1972; Doluisio et al., 1973).

App. Vd (L)	(% BW)	Renal Clearance (ml/min/1.73 m²)	Serum Clearance (ml/min/1.73 m²)	Urinary Excretion (%)
21.0 ± 3.8	26.4 ± 5.5	84.2 ± 8.8	99.5 ± 12.8	–
23.5 ± 4.6	29.4 ± 5.8	82.9 ± 15.5	99.9 ± 8.6	–
0.22/kg	–	79.0	–	84 (0-24 h)
0.24/kg	–	71.3	–	
0.22/kg	–	70.0	–	84 (0-24 h)
0.22/kg	–	74.9	–	
19.6	–	77	95	81
–	16.7 ± 3.0	–	–	
–	23.1 ± 6.1	–	–	–

In contrast, serum creatinine could be misleading in determining dosage regimens. A difference between calculated and measured half-life has been noticed; with normal serum creatinine levels, lower values were obtained in the age group 20-50 years, and higher values were found in people older than 70 years. A similar change has been observed in the apparent Vd (20-50 years = 1.67 ± 3.0 liters, 51-70 = 16.0 ± 6.9; > 70 = 23.1 ± 6.1) (Lumholtz et al., 1974). The Vd suggests a distribution equivalent to the extracellular space. In dogs, whose kinetic behavior is similar to man's, a half-life of 6 min was measured for distribution into the tissues (Cabana and Taggart, 1973). Slow and poor KNM penetration into the CSF occurs when the meninges are not inflamed (Kunin, 1966). No significant absorption is seen when the drug is given by aerosol (Lifshitz and Denning, 1970).

The observed ratio of renal KNM clearance to creatinine clearance (0.62-0.76) suggests that about 30% of the administrered dose undergoes tubular resorption (Cutler and Orme, 1969; Clarke et al., 1974; Doluisio et al., 1973). A negligible amount of the drug is excreted in the bile and in pancreatic fluid;

Table 15. Kanamycin Disposition in Newborns

	Age	Peak Time (h)	Peak Level (μg/ml)	Half-Life (h)	Urinary Excretion (% of dose)
Simon and Axline, 1966					
Premature					
0.8-2.5 mg/kg/	48 h	1	17.5	18	20 (0-12 h)
7.5 mg/kg	5-22 days			6	60 (0-12 h)
Eichenwald, 1966					
Premature and full-term					
10-mg/kg	0-4 days	0.7-1	28 ± 7	3.69	
	5-8 days	0.7-1	26 ± 7	3.08	
7.5 mg/kg	0-4 days	0.7-1	19 ± 3	5.04	
	5-9 days	0.7-1	18 ± 4	3.60	
	10-14 days	0.7-1	16 ± 3	3.71	
	15-30 days	0.7-1	17 ± 4	3.03	
McCracken, 1974					
7.5 mg/kg					
Premature			4.7-27.8		
Full-term			6.7-29.0		

this very small extrarenal clearance increases slightly in severe renal insufficiency (Mawer et al., 1972). The urinary excretion of KNM is nearly complete after 8 h. A smaller percentage of excretion has been reported by other investigators, ranging from 40 to 80% (Kunin, 1966). Differences in absorption from the injection site, and the wide variability that occurs in assaying the high concentration of urine specimens, might be the reasons behind these discrepancies (Doluisio et al., 1973).

Data referring to the disposition of kanamicin in the neonatal period are summarized in Table 15. Limited correlation with creatinine clearance has been found in a small series of seven premature infants at least 2 days of age. With clearance values from 7 to 10% of those seen in normal adults, the apparent serum half-life ranged from 15.7 to 23.1 h; values of 3.1-4.8 h were found in those infants with higher clearances. Under these conditions, accumulation may occur after multiple-dosing (every 12 h). Maturation of renal function, however, tends to compensate for this trend by decreasing serum half-life (Simon and Axline, 1966). No correlation seems to exist between drug disposition and birth weight or gestational age (Eichenwald, 1966). Concentrations ranging from 1/10 to 1/5 of the peak serum levels were demonstrated in the spinal fluid 3 to 6 h following intramuscular injection in infants with normal meninges and a concentration approximately twice as high is reached in bacterial meningitis (Eichenwald, 1966). Similar values were reported by McCracken (1974), with peak concentrations ranging from 2.4 µg/ml to 12 µg/ml 4 h after a single intramuscular administration. A prospective study to determine long-term effects on hearing and development showed no signs of toxicity in a series of 225 newborn infants matched with 120 untreated controls. Duration of the therapy varied from 4 to 30 days (mean: 7.8 days). These results apply to both KNM (15 mg/kg/day), and to GTM (5 mg/kg/day) (McCracken and Chrane, 1972).

The emergence of resistant strains and the availability of new aminoglycoside compounds has led to a progressive decrease in the use of KNM (Franco et al., 1973).

Gentamicin

Gentamicin (GTM) has been discussed quite extensively with respect to plasma levels because of the importance given to this parameter and its potential relationship to toxicity. Specific attention has been given to the development of rapid and reliable analytical methods. At present, the enzymatic procedure seems to be the most accurate and to correlate more closely with the actual values (Andrews et al., 1974; Holmes and Sanford, 1974). In a recent survey, only 14 out of 88 laboratories tested (16%) gave good results; in the same series, 45 laboratories were considered highly misleading and 29 gave a poor response. Even those laboratories with the best results had accuracies of ± 15-20%. Moreover, the quality of these results did not change in two different circulations of GTM assays over a one-year period. The large majority of laboratories were using plate diffusion assays or broth dilution methods (Reeves, 1974b). *Most of the published information discussed in the following section has been obtained by similar methods,* a fact to be remembered when interpreting the data reported. The use of serum is recommended, as it permits the avoidance of heparin, which has been shown to interfere negatively on the measurement of GTM in blood (Regamey et al., 1972). Modification of the old methods and wider use of those based on enzymatic and RIA procedures make the effective monitoring of GTM levels feasible in routine hospital practice and in emergency situations (Sabath et al., 1971; Smith et al., 1972; Berk et al., 1974; Daigneault et al., 1974; Edmunds and Heddle, 1974; Noone et al., 1974a; Smith and Smith, 1974; Lund et al., 1973; Broughall and Reeves, 1975).

Pharmacokinetic data on GTM are reported in Table 16, together with those on tobramycin.

GTM is very poorly absorbed (0.2-0.5%) when given orally; only 1-2% of an orally administered dose is excreted in the urine. However, in some disease states, such as the acute phase of shigella dysentery, more than 10% of the dose

Table 16. Pharmacokinetic Data on Gentamicin (G) and Tobramicin (T) in Adults

		Serum Concentrations (μg/ml) Peak	Steady State	Half-Life (h)	Apparent Vd (L)	(% BW)	Renal Clearance (ml/min/1.73 m^2)	Plasma Clearance (ml/min/1.73 m^2)
Regamey et al., 1973								
Intravenous infusion*	G	4.86 ± 0.49	3.90 ± 0.18	2.00 ± 0.21	22.4 ± 3.3	30.8 ± 3.4	109.8 ± 16.2	117.5 ± 3.1
	T	4.61 ± 0.49	3.83 ± 0.38	2.15 ± 0.10	24.5 ± 3.0	33.5 ± 1.4	113.7 ± 4.5	120.1 ± 5.6
Intramuscular injection °	G	4.96 ± 0.42		2.04 ± 0.27	21.4 ± 2.6	27.9 ± 3.9		
	T	5.16 ± 0.56		2.11 ± 0.09	23.2 ± 3.4	30.6 ± 2.1		
Simon et al., 1973c								
Intravenous infusion**	G	1.06 ± 0.16	1.04 ± 0.06	1.73 ± 0.14	14.45 ± 1.7		81.80 ± 9.20	95.80 ± 7.00
	T		0.94 ± 0.10	1.59 ± 0.08	16.90 ± 1.6		87.90 ± 9.50	115.70 ± 9.50
Intramuscular injection°°	T	3.67 ± 0.26		2.14 ± 0.06				
				2.14 ± 0.06				
Geddes et al., 1974								
Intramuscular injection °°°	T	2.58 ± 0.38		1.80	16.55	21.8	–	
Naber et al., 1973								
Intravenous injection***	T	–	–	3.0 ± 1.1	11.7 ± 3.1	15.6 ± 2.7	31	43.5 ± 13.5

*Loading dose of 100 mg over 60 min; then 30 mg/h x 2 h.
**6.6 mg/h x 4 h.
° 100 mg (1.3-1.5 mg/kg/: Peak levels are reached between 0.5-1 h after i.m. administration.
°° 80 mg.
°°° 50 mg.
***1 mg/kg.

given p.o. can be found in the urine (Riley et al., 1971). Intramuscular administration is the route most commonly used. Peak levels are reported to occur between 20 min and 90 min after the dose is given, but there is a large degree of variability in the published data. Some investigators ascribe part of this variability to differences in the rate of absorption from the injection site, as is evident in the case of repeated injections in the same site (Winters et al., 1971b) or when previously unused, anatomically distinct sites are chosen (Reeves et al., 1974).

The hematocrit has also been recognized as a factor contributing to variations in peak GTM levels, since a difference of 5 points inversely raises or lowers the serum level by approximately 2 μg/ml. Patterns are obtained during maintenance therapy which differ from patient to patient. The curve is consistent during the treatment period for any given individual and seems independent of the site of injection, thus appearing to the overall result of a dynamic response (Riff and Jackson, 1971). The same authors underlined for the first time the occurrence of a pattern of responses, classified as normal, accelerated or damped, which have been documented recently in another study which failed to show any relationship between the administered dose and resulting serum levels. These same authors denied any substantial contribution of the hematocrit to such variability (Kaye et al., 1974).

The use of the intravenous route has been widely discussed and very recently reviewed (Editorial, 1974b). A retrospective analysis of the clinical implications of various regimens proposed, for patients with varying degrees of renal impairment, has been made by Schumacher (1975). Unanimous agreement does not exist on the safety of this method of administering the drug, even if a majority of the authors tend to deny any real danger of toxicity with high GTM serum levels of short duration (George et al., 1974; McGhie et al., 1974; Stratford et al., 1974; Van de Walle and Adriaensen, 1974). Slow continuous infusions over a 30-120 min period show a plasma disappearance pattern very similar to that observed after i.m. administration. Slightly higher levels are obtained in a shorter time with infusions, but the same pattern of disappearance can be seen after 2-3 h, and the same trough levels are observed (Regamey et al., 1973). Whether or not there exist any advantages in giving slow i.v. infusions is controversial (Bailey and Lynn, 1974). This method seems to be appropriate if no risk whatsoever is desired, and when the i.m. route is impractical, e.g., in bleeding disorders and in the case of shock or altered muscle consistency (McCracken et al., 1971a). A slow intravenous bolus injection over a 2½-3 min (Stratford et al., 1974) or a 10 min period (Reeves, 1974a) seems to be the preferred method of administration; however, no agreement exists about peak levels attainable in this way, and levels as high as 25 μg/ml, lasting 5-13 min, have been measured 2-3½ min after the start of the injection. Here, too, marked individual variations have been attributed to differences in the hematocrit (Michel et al., 1974). Significantly different levels are not obtained when the drug is given either in a fixed standard dose or by weight or on a body surface area basis (Winters et al., 1971b; Stratford et al., 1974; Michel et al., 1974). In patients subjected to a regimen of forced diuresis, an infusion of 40 mg/h of GTM has been shown to be necessary to maintain adequate blood levels. These data support the fact that substantial modifications in the disposition kinetics are found in abnormal conditions of hydration, most commonly seen in infants and in acutely ill patients (Daschner and Marget, 1973). No differences in GTM disposition have been reported when GTM was given in association with carbenicillin (Winters et al., 1971a).

Twenty to 30% of GTM has been reported to be protein-bound. This commonly accepted finding (Gyselynck et al., 1971) is now being questioned by recent data obtained under physiologic conditions, regarding temperature and pH, which show that no serum protein-binding of GTM occurs (Regamey et al., 1973). The same should be true for tobramycin (Naber et al., 1973). Binding to the blood cells accounts for 10% of the amount present in the blood. GTM distributes in a volume similar to the extracellular space (16-26.L or 15.2-30.8% B.W.) (Regamey et al., 1973), and this distribution tends to markedly increase in renal failure (Gyselynck et al., 1971), possibly indicating slow distribution in the intracellular space. Dialytic treatment reverses this trend, giving values of 28.1 ± 2.39 (Milman, 1974; Wilson et al., 1973b). It was demonstrated that blood cells were not a storage site for GTM in patients showing prolonged low serum concentrations (up to 8 days) and those with prolonged urinary excretion (up to 20 days) and no sign of renal impairment (Kahlmeter and Kamme, 1975). A marked increase of the Vd has been noted with increasing age (Lumholtz et al., 1974); the distribution volume of 0.275 L/kg/BW proposed in a nomogram recently (Mawer et al., 1974a,b) and based on a serum creatinine values increases by about 40% in individuals over age 70. In this study, serum creatinine was not a good measure of changing renal function; creatinine clearance and excretion were more reliable as indices.

The GTM penetration into the CSF is low, even when there are inflamed meninges. From one-sixteenth to one-half of the serum concentration has been found in the CSF, with serum concentrations in the range of 8-16 μg/ml (Riff and Jackson, 1971); interestingly, however, a higher ratio of CSF/serum levels, approaching unity, has been observed by other authors (Riley et al., 1971). Peak levels are reached between 2 and 6 h after GTM administration, and are dependent on the extension and gravity of the meningeal inflammation (Mc-Cracken et al., 1971a).

In specimens of bile collected from T-tube drainage, a GTM activity corresponding to one-fourth to one-half of the serum concentration was measured by Riff and Jackson (1971). In most cases of a large series of patients, GTM failed to reach levels considered to be in the therapeutic range of 5-10 μg/ml (Waitz and Weinstein, 1969). This finding has been confirmed in another study showing a scarce correlation between serum and bile levels; no evidence of accumulation was found following a repeated administration every 8 h (Mendelson et al., 1973). Good distribution has been observed in renal lymph, with concentrations approaching those present in plasma; the equilibration between these two fluids is prompt. A lymph/serum ratio between 0.7 and 0.8 has been observed in dogs (Gingell et al., 1969) and in man. As lymph levels are an index of tissue concentration, blood levels are a reliable indication of the drug present in renal tissue. High urinary concentrations do not influence distribution in kidney. The subject has recently been briefly reviewed (Chisholm, 1974). GTM also tends to be low, with a delayed peak, in pleural effusions (Riff and Jackson, 1971), in bronchial secretions and in sputum; no definite correlation seems to exist with corresponding serum concentrations. Inhalation of GTM allows higher levels to be reached in these fluids from the respiratory tract but does not improve the bactericidal power (Vogt, 1973). Different data have been very recently reported. Following endotracheal or aerosol administration of 40 mg/kg of GTM, levels $>$ 20 μg/ml were measured in the bronchial secretions of children with cystic fibrosis. No significant serum levels were detected (Baran and Klastersky, 1974). The risk of emergent resistance by this route has been confirmed (Klastersky et al., 1974b).

One-fifth of the peak activity measured in the mother has been reported present in her milk after a single i.m. administration of 40 mg of gentamycin (Ito, 1974). Concentrations 50% lower than in serum have been observed in experimental "tissue cages" following a single i.m. administration (Chisholm et al., 1973). This closed system is interesting as a possible model of the inner ear, a structure so critical for GTM toxicity (Reeves, 1974a). Measurements of GTM in human synovial fluid show a slow accumulation of the drug in this tissue. Concentrations corresponding to 55 and 300% of those in serum are found, respectively, 1-5 h and 8-11 h after the last administration (Fluerette et al., 1973). No significant amounts have been measured by these authors in the liver, in cardiac or osseous tissues.

GTM is not metabolized in the body and can be considered to be excreted completely, and unchanged, via the kidney, mainly by glomerular filtration. The existence of a tubular mechanism has been discussed which could account for the 0.85-0.95 ratio between renal and creatinine clearance (Gyselynck et al., 1971; Regamey et al., 1973). Administration of probenecid, however, does not modify either GTM blood levels or urinary excretion, suggesting that no tubular excretion occurs (Bergan et al., 1972). Extrarenal clearance accounts for 15% of GTM excretion (Simon et al., 1973c). High urinary concentrations of carbenicillin could inactivate GTM in the urinary tract when both drugs are given concurrently (Young et al., 1974).

The plasma half-life, calculated at steady state after continuous infusion or after two single i.m. injections, ranges between 93 and 216 min (Regamey et al., 1973) in patients with values of creatinine clearance between 125 and 29 ml/min (Lumholtz et al., 1974). These studies show a proportional relationship with creatinine clearance and a progressive increase of the T½ with age. Different data are proposed by other authors (Kaye et al., 1974) who confirm the above values only for those patients having a Ccr greater than 88 ml/min. When Ccr values drop below 50 ml/min, the T½ cannot be determined from Ccr or serum creatinine. In general, nomograms should be used as a guide and should be supplemented with GTM serum level measurements, especially in the presence of changing renal function (Noone et al., 1974a).

Between 80 and 96% of the administered dose of GTM is excreted in the urine within 24 h; 90% of this total amount is excreted within the first 9 h (Regamey et al., 1973; Simon et al., 1973b). According to Jackson (1967), only 40% of the first dose is found in urine, whereas 100% of the tenth dose is recovered. No further data have been presented to support the suggestion of a "saturation" process of a peripheral compartment. Moreover, variations in urinary pH between 5.4 and 7.8 after acid or alkaline loading do not seem to change the plasma and renal clearance of GTM (Mariet et al., 1972).

Newborns. It has been stated that the clinical pharmacology of GTM in the neonatal period is well-known (McCracken, 1974). The relevant and comparable kinetic data applicable to this age group are shown synoptically in Table 17. An attempt has been made to maintain the classification suggested in the original papers with regard to importance of weight and age. The results of a recent study have been reported separately as they refer to a homogeneous group of full-term newborns, where an interesting picture is given of an age-related change in half-life (Marzetti et al., 1974). Unfortunately, in the pertinent studies the variability of content is so great and the comparison so difficult that the proposed dosages and regimens should be regarded as only a rough index of standard therapy (McCracken, 1974; McCracken and Eichenwald, 1974b; Milner, 1974).

There is a large amount of data available for the first week of life, but in the various studies the complete clinical picture usually is not given for individual cases, thus there is not sufficient documentation to allow an adequate appreciation of the specific neonatal problem. Erratic absorption from the injection site, depending upon the changing conditions of vascularization and upon the patient's hydration, secondary to his underlying pathology, is one factor to be considered (McCracken and Eichenwald, 1974b; Andersen et al., 1972). GTM-binding to red blood cells does not seem to influence serum concentrations in the neonate, as in adult subjects, possibly due to a lower affinity of the neonatal erythrocyte for the antibiotic (McCrackent et al., 1971a). Preliminary results showing a displacing effect of GTM on bilirubin have not been confirmed and appear to be due to some unknown contaminant (Wenberg and Rasmussen, 1975; Odell et al., 1975). This is in agreement with the fact that GTM is not protein-bound (Regamey et al., 1973) and that no nervous system manifestation of kernicterus have been observed in a large series of newborns treated with aminoglycosides (McCracken, 1975).

No apparent correlation seems to exist between dosages and serum levels.

According to some investigators, gestational age does not play a role in determining serum concentration and half-life (Rosdahl and Andersen, 1973). The same serum concentration and apparent half-life has been observed after i.m. administration and after 120 min infusion in newborns during the first week of life, whereas a 20 min infusion of the same amount of the drug resulted in somewhat briefer, higher-serum levels and a shorter half-life. Mean values referring to serum concentrations and half-life, however, were within the range observed after i.m. administration of the same dose in the above-mentioned cases (McCracken et al., 1971a). In another series of infants, 0.75-1.3 mg/kg of GTM was given either by i.m. or by intravenous infusion over a 20-30 min period. Samples taken, starting 15-30 min after drug administration, showed very similar serum concentrations in both situations, indicating a quick distribution from tissue to circulation and vice versa (Paisley et al., 1973). Similar data have been reported, after i.v. injection of 0.6-0.8 mg/kg, in newborns less than 2 weeks old, who showed a relative Vd of 46% of BW with an elimination half-life of 2 h, 25 min (Rohwedder and Goll, 1970).

Such discrepancies are partially accounted for by differences in analytical methods, together with the understandable difficulties encountered in obtaining enough samples and data in newborn babies. A clearer picture could, perhaps, be obtained in the future by the pooling of cases from various centers, especially if collected and examined following standardized procedures as regards clinical data, analytical methods and kinetic parameters (for implications about effective dose/levels and toxicity, see below). According to Andersen et al. (1972), an apparent trend exists toward lower serum levels following repeated administration, even if not enough data are available to document such a claim. The same authors suggest that their data support the fact that GTM diffuses into the extracellular space, which in the newborn accounts for 40% of the body weight.

After i.m. administration, peak levels in the CSF are observed between 4-6 h and correlated with the degree of inflammation and the given dose. Intrathecal and i.m. administration can be usefully combined, and CSF levels as high as 24-40 μg have been observed 2½-3 h after the administration of 1 mg intrathecally (McCracken and Eichenwald, 1974b). However, much lower concentrations were reported by other authors (Newman and Holt, 1971). In their study, peak CSF levels increased following repeated intrathecal administration of 1 mg, suggesting a progressive accumulation of the drug (from 1 to 8.5 μg/ml after 5 days), with increasing trough levels between 0.5 and 4 μg/ml, 24 h after single doses. Intraventricular instillation of 0.5-1.0 mg gave levels of 4.3-60 μg/ml in infants who were also being treated by the i.m. route, cumulative effect has been observed after several days of administration with CSF levels of 120 μg/ml (Lorber et al., 1970; McCracken et al., 1971a; Zoumboulakis et al., 1973; McCracken and Eichenwald, 1974b, McAllister, 1974).

Measurable amounts (20 μg/ml) of GTM have been found for as long as 30 h after birth in the urine of newborns of mothers treated with GTM (Fleurette

Table 17. Gentamicin in Newborns

0.7 days	Dose (mg/kg)	Route	Peak Time (h)	Peak Level (µg/ml)	Trough Level (µg/ml)	B.W. (g)	T½ (h)	
McCracken et al., 1971a	1.5	i.m.	0.5-1	1.8-4.6	0.2-1.9	<1,500	11.5	
						1,500-2,000	8.0	Mean = 5.5
						>2,000	4.5-5	
McCracken et al., 1973	2.5	i.m.				<2,000	5.1-5.9	
						2,000-3,000	3.5-3.9	Mean = 4.1
						>3,000	3.8-4.2	
Andersen et al., 1972	1.0	i.m.	2	1.9-3.2		1,500-2,000	6.5	
						2,000-2,500	3.2-9.5	
Rosdahl and Andersen, 1973	2.0	i.m.	—	4.0-7.6	0-5.5	>2,500	3.5-8.7	
Ito, 1970	0.8	i.m.	1	3.9-13.2	2.4		5.5	
	2	i.m.	1.5	13.5-40			3.7	

1-4 weeks						
McCracken et al., 1971a	1.5	i.m.	0.5-1	1.8-7.2	n.d.	Mean = 3
	2.5	i.m.	0.5-1	1.3-6.4	0.3-0.8	Mean = 3.5
Andersen et al., 1972	1-1.4	i.m.	–	1.3-6.4	0-1	Mean = 5
Garfunkel, 1971	2.5	i.m.	1	1.2-4.9	0-2.5	
Marzetti et al., 1974	1	i.m.	1			
1 day			1.1	3.0 ± 1.4	0.5 ± 0.1	3,464 6.7
3-14 days	1		0.8	3.1 ± 1.2	1.0 ± 0.4*	2,790 4.9
15-30 days			0.5	3.5 ± 1.0	0.6 ± 0.2*	3,010 3.3

*at 8 hrs

Table 18. Gentamicin in Infants and Children

	Dose (mg/kg)	Route	Peak Time (h)	Peak Level (µg/ml)	Trough Level (µg/ml)	Vd (% B.W.)	T½ (h)
Rohwedder and Goll, 1970	0.6-0.8	i.v.	–	–	–		
1-12 mos	0.6-0.8	i.v.	–	–	–	50.9	M: 1.4
1-5 yrs	0.6-0.8	i.v.	–	–	–	34.9	M: 1.1
6-15 yrs	0.6-0.8	i.v.	–	–		21.5	M: 1.05
Riley et al., 1971							
3 mo-16 yrs	0.4	i.m.	0.5	1.9 ± 0.7	0.04-0.14	–	–
	1	i.m.	0.5	4-10	0.5-2.0	–	2.5-4.0
Vogt, 1973							
3 mo-7 yrs	1	i.m.	1	3-4	–	–	2.0
McCracken, 1972							
2-24 mos	1.5-2.5	i.m.	0.5-1	1.7-8.6	0.2-1 (at 8 h)	–	1.7-5.4
Simon et al., 1973b							
3-12 mos	0.4	i.m.	1	1.7 ± 0.1	0.3 ± 0.03	–	2.0 ± 0.1
1-5 yrs	0.8	i.m.	1	2.8 ± 0.1	0.5 ± 0.04		1.6 ± 0.1

M = mean

et al., 1973). A high correlation between Ccr and GTM excretion has been shown in newborn babies. The pattern of excretion in babies younger than 3 days of age is different from those 5-40 days of age, a mean of 10% administered dose being excreted by the neonates within 12 h (McCracken et al., 1971b). Similar data are reported by other authors, who underline the fact that no information is available about the fate of the GTM not excreted in the urine (Milner et al., 1972, Paisley et al., 1973). In the 5-to-40-day-old group, 50% of the dose is excreted within the first 4 h, showing a pattern similar to that seen in adults (McCracken et al., 1971b). Data based on 24 h collection periods confirm a similar distinction for babies younger than 3 days, who excrete only 34% and those older than 3 days, who excrete 50% of the dose (Ito, 1970).

Infants and children. Very little information is available about the disposition of GTM in this age group. Such data as exist are summarized in Table 18. It is evident that they are not complete enough to allow the construction of a comprehensive picture of age-related differences. Moreover, since they refer to different ages and dosages, the data do not give thorough enough documentation to support the opinion of several authors that no substantial differences exist in GTM disposition between infants older than 1 year of age and adults (Simon et al., 1973b). A dosage schedule 2-5 times higher than that for adults has been proposed in order to achieve therapeutic levels in severely ill children aged 3 days to 12 years (McAllister, 1974). Use of intravenous GTM proved to be successful in cystic fibrosis; the use of antibiotic aerosol plus systemic administration failed to add to GTM therapeutic efficacy (Mearns, 1974).

Serum levels vs. therapeutic efficacy and toxicity of GTM. Even if they are not specifically part of our discussion, these two points deserve a brief comment because of the role they have had, and still have, in directing research efforts and establishing models for correct dosage regimens. A few statements, such as the following, are sufficient to give an idea of the problem:

—No agreement exists about therapeutic and toxic ranges of GTM. Tentatively (Hewitt, 1973b; Reeves, 1974a), levels of 4-5 μg/ml can be considered therapeutically valid, and levels of 12-15 μg/ml potentially toxic. There is marked disagreement about the probability of attaining these levels. According to some investigators, they are reported to be very rare, yet these levels are cited as being curative and nontoxic in other cases. In one report, levels higher than 8 μg/ml were needed to cure life-threatening pneumonia, whereas 5 μg/ml were enough to cure other cases of life-threatening sepsis (Noone et al., 1974b).

—Killing power can also be obtained with levels as low as 1-2 μg/ml when the bactericidial power of the serum adds to that of the antibiotics (Discussion, 1971).

—No strict correlation exists between the MIC *in vivo* and *in vitro*. Moreover, different microorganisms and different strains of the same microorganism need different MICs for different periods of time (McCracken, 1974). Attainment of a more than adequate MIC is not enough to ensure sterilization if other appropriate measures (e.g., drainage of CSF) are not taken (McCracken et al., 1971a).

—No data are available which show that toxicity is dependent on high transient peaks. Trough levels are a better index of both efficacy and potential toxicity. A steady trough level of 1.5-2.0 μg/ml would be considered safe; an upward trend of this measure should be regarded with caution. No agreement, however, exists on where to put the dividing line between safety and toxicity (Mawer et al., 1974; Hewitt, 1974, and discussion following this paper).

—Toxicity manifests itself as a progressive damage. Repeated courses with GTM or a similarly toxic drug are more dangerous than giving a single treatment (Banck et al., 1973, Nordström et al., 1973, Galioto et al., 1974). Vestibular damage is more likely to appear when renal damage is present, thus favoring permanence of the drug in the body, and when there is something already wrong with the vestibular function (Tjernström et al., 1973).

—Vestibular damage is more common than auditory impairment, but its appearance is not self-evident in bedridden patients, nor in infants. Courses longer than a few days do not seem to be justified (Reeves, 1974a). Certainly, when large doses of GTM are given, determination of serum levels and timely analyses should be made.

—Otoxicity is often preclinical or asymptomatic (Jackson and Arcieri, 1971). It is more frequently reported in European literature (18% of the treated cases by Noone et al. [1974b]); nephrotoxicity is more a concern of American authors, who emphasize its rarity (Hewitt, 1974). A good, but not perfect, consensus exists about the increased risk of nephrotoxicity following combined cephalosporin and GTM treatment, whose advantages are not definitely established (Kleinknecht et al., 1973; Noone et al., 1974a; Klastersky et al., 1974c). Experimental data show that the same risk could be present also with concurrent diuretic treatment (Hewitt, 1973b).

—Too much concern in avoiding toxicity could lead to use of suboptimal doses of the drug, which, in turn, can be more dangerous. When clinical and bacteriological reasons clearly suggest the use of GTM, a high loading dosage should be the rule, whatever the renal conditions. Monitoring of levels and assessment of individual pharmacokinetic response must then follow (Holmes and Sanford, 1974; McAllister, 1974). even if not all authors agree about the actual feasibility of this approach in hospital practice (Hewitt, 1974).

Tobramycin

Tobramycin (TBM) is a relatively new antibiotic that is closely related to GTM and has been shown to be slightly more active than GTM against *Pseudomonas aeruginosa,* however, a higher MIC of TBM is needed against *E. coli* strains. Cross-resistance exists between the two molecules, thus strains resistant to GTM (3 μg/ml) show the same resistance against TBM. Both drugs exhibit synergistic activity with carbenicillin and related compounds in gram-negative infections (Klastersky et al., 1973a; Libke et al., 1973; Simon, 1973; Geddes et al., 1974). The same pattern of activity is observed with sisomycin (Henri et al., 1973; Klastersky et al., 1973b, 1974c). TBM can also be considered

Table 19. Disposition of TBM in Infants After i.m. Administration of 2 mg/kg/dose every 12 h

B. W. and Age	Peak Time (h)	Peak Levels (µg/ml)	Serum Half-Life (h)	Trough Levels (12 h) (µg/ml)	Urinary Excretion (%)
<1,500 (5)					
<3d	0.5	4.92 ± 1.33 (3.80-7.20)	8.71 ± 5.80 (3.54-17.10)	1.90 ± 0.36 (1.50-2.20)	25 (6-94)
>1 wk	1.0	5.02 ± 1.88 (2.90-7.20)	6.12 ± 2.19 (3.85-8.50)	2.16 ± 1.22 (0.94-4.06)	24 (14-39)
1,500-2,500					
<3d (8)	0.5-1	5.55 ± 1.22 (4.00-7.20)	8.08 ± 4.24 (3.68-16.67)	2.20 ± 0.95 (0.71-3.28)	15 (2-40)
>1 wk (7)		5.38 ± 2.22 (2.40-8.36)	5.99 ± 1.70 (4.08-8.16)	1.58 ± 0.59 (1.14-2.70)	24 (15-37)
>2,500 (7)					
<3d	0.5-1	4.94 ± 2.07 (1.84-7.4)	4.56 ± 1.20 (3.39-6.54)	1.11 ± 0.59 (0.23-1.84)	22 (9-30)
>1 wk		4.54 ± 2.55 (0.36-8.80)	3.87 ± 0.36 (3.34-4.32)	0.57 ± 0.09 (0.50-0.70)	37 (11-59)

( ): Number of infants and range of variability.
<3d: After 1 or 2 doses.
>1 wk: After 10-20 doses.
Adapted from Kaplan et al., 1973.

equivalent to GTM from a pharmacokinetic point of view. Comparative studies show an identical pattern of disposition (Table 19) (Regamey et al., 1973; Simon et al., 1973c; Lockwood and Bower, 1973; Geddes et al., 1974). Lower values of volume of distribution, a longer half-life (3.0 ± 1.1 h) and a lower plasma clearance (43.5 ± 13.5 ml/min/1.73 m^2) are reported following a single intravenous injection of 1 mg/kg (Naber et al., 1973). The data have been obtained in elderly patients and are in contrast with a distribtuion volume increasing with age observed by Lumholtz et al. (174) for KNM and GTM.

Low urinary excretion of TBM has been observed by some authors (8-37% in 24 h). Conceivably, this could be the result of differences in pH in different groups of patients which might influence both the excretion rate and the assay procedure (Geddes et al., 1974, see, however, Mariel et al., 1973). Extrarenal elimination has been calculated to account for 24% of the dose (Simon et al., 1973c). No significant penetration in sputum has been observed in patients with cystic fibrosis 2-24 years of age. Levels ranging from 0 to 0.82 µg/ml were measured which remained the same after repeated administration and did not change with either peak or trough serum levels (Hawley et al., 1974).

Newborns. To our knowledge, the only study which deals specifically with TBM use and disposition in this age group has been done by the same investigators who have extensively studied GTM (Kaplan et al., 1973). Their data are reported in Table 19. They confirm the strict similarity between TBM and GTM. It is worthwhile to emphasize certain features since they contribute to a better understanding of the handling of these two drugs in newborn infants.

Higher variability was observed at 3 days of age than after 1 week, in both serum concentration and half-life and in urinary excretion. No accumulation seemed to occur following the adopted dosage schedule. A small increase in dosage (5.0 mg/kg/day), however, gave serum concentrations suggesting accumulation of the antibiotic (trough levels of 2.0-3.5 µg/ml). It is apparent that even with the lower dosage schedule values approximating this range were reached. Urinary excretion 0-12 h after antibiotic administration is very low in many subjects. Since no TBM accumulation seems to occur, the question remains as to where the rest of the administered dose has been distributed. There are no available data on Vd to calculate possible differences. The unavoidable difficulties in urine collection suggest that incomplete specimens could partially account for the low excretion (see, however, the above-mentioned data from Geddes et al., 1974). After 1 week of age, the largest percentage of the administered dose was excreted in the first 4 h. Similar findings have been reported by Periti et al. (1974), in both premature and full-term newborns. A mean serum half-life of 1.5 ± 0.35 h has been measured in infants older than 1 month of age (range: 1-6 month, 1.6 ± 0.3 h, > 7 months, 1.4 ± 0.4) (Rosaschino, 1974).

Amikacin

This new molecule has been proposed as having higher activity than KNM against all strains of *Pseudomonas* and also as offering advantages over the other aminoglycosides against the common pathogens within the enterobacteriaceae. A major advantage of amikacin over GTM may be the absence of cross-resistance against some microorganisms. Detailed discussions of the clinical significance of this molecule have been published recently (Klastersky et al., 1975a; Marks, 1975).

TETRACYCLINES

The structural formulas of the major compounds of this class are reported in Fig. 2 (see Barringer et al., 1974, for a comparative presentation of their physicochemical properties). A critical review of their place in modern anti-

STRUCTURAL FORMULA

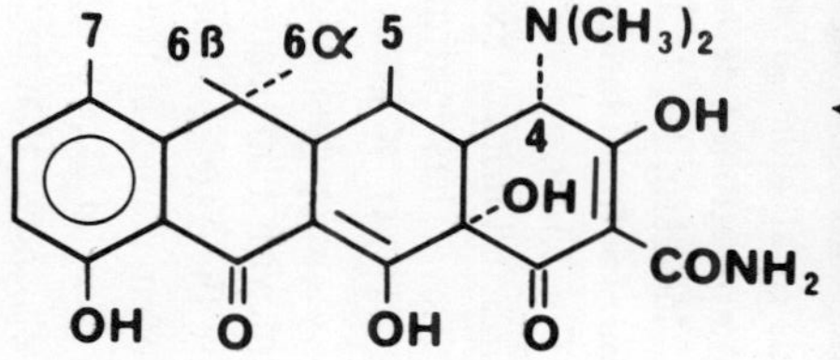

	TC	OTC	CTC	DMC	MC	DC	MN
7	H	H	Cl	Cl	H	H	N(CH$_3$)$_2$
6α	CH$_3$	CH$_3$	CH$_3$	H	(CH$_2$=)	CH$_3$	H
6β	OH	OH	OH	OH		H	H
5	H	OH	H	H	OH	OH	H

TC = Tetracycline ; OTC = Oxytetracycline ;
CTC = Chlortetracycline ; DMC = Demeclocycline ;
MC = Methacycline ; DC = Doxycycline ; MN = Minocycline

Fig. 2

microbial therapy was made on the occasion of the silver anniversary of the discovery of the first compound (Finland, 1974), and from the available data it can be concluded that they still have an important role to play in clinical practice. In this review, the validity of restriction on their use in infants and young children is confirmed due to the tendency of these compounds to fix in growing osseous tissues (Garrod et al., 1973). Recent studies have also focused on the interaction of tetracyclines with host-defense mechanisms, and on the relationship between resistance and degree of uptake by bacteria (Forsgren and Gnarpe, 1973a, Kuck and Forbes, 1973; Forsgren and Gnarpe, 1973b). Alternative analytical techniques to the traditional bioassays have been developed and compare favorably with microbiological methods, offering the advantages of more specificity and speed (Wilson et al., 1972; Tsuji and Robertson, 1973; Tsuji et al., 1974).

Oral absorption of tetracyclines takes place from all levels of the alimentary tract, being much less in the lower portion of the intestinal tract and negligible from the colon. Absorption is thought not to be complete for the older compounds. Demeclocyline appears to be better absorbed than chlortetracycline and oxytetracycline, whereas methacycline is the least absorbed compound of this class (Weinstein, 1970b; Notari, 1973). The newer molecules doxycycline and minocycline have been reported to be completely absorbed orally in comparison studies with intravenous administration (Leibowitz et al., 1972; MacDonald et al., 1973; Brogden et al., 1975b).

No concordant data have been found about bioequivalence of commercially available tetracycline products. Significant differences have been reported by Barr et al. (1972); the difference is already seen after single doses, and becomes greater after multiple-dosing. The clinical significance of these findings is stressed by these authors; noncompliance and occasional concomitant administration of medications containing antacids or alkaline substances enhance the risk of nontherapeutic levels after some preparations (see also Barr et al., 1971). These and other findings (Tuomisto and Männisto, 1973) have been discussed in a paper describing an extensive trial on 16 formulations of 250 mg capsules of tetracycline (Meyer et al., 1974a) in which no significant differences were found among the products tested: reported urinary excretion values ranged from 49% to 60%. A subsequent trial, however, has confirmed the existence of therapeutic nonequivalence (Barnett et al., 1974). A lower bioavailability has been shown for sugar-coated tablets of oxytetracycline dihydrate compared with preparations of the hydrochloride and with film-coated tablets of the dihydrate (Hart et al., 1975). The extent, not the rate, of absorption is changed, and consequently no differences have been found in the apparent serum half-life of the several brands of tetracycline (Barr et al., 1972). Analysis of variance applied to urinary data and to serum levels shows that individual variability could explain the differences reported in other studies (Meyer et al., 1974a; Hart et al., 1975).

Table 20. Tetracyclines

	Protein-Binding* (%)	Serum Half-Life° (h) Day 1	Steady State	Renal Clearance (ml/min/1.73 m²)
Tetracycline	64.6	6.1 ± 1.0	10.8	73.5
Demeclocycline	90.8	8.7 ± 1.5	13.6	36.5
Methacycline	80.0[a]	7.4 ± 2.3	14.3	29.0[b]
Doxycycline	93.0	8.1 ± 2.2	16.6	16.0
Minocycline	76.0[b]	16.0[b] 13-15[c]	19.0[b] 24.6[c]	9.0[b]

*Kunin et al., 1973. °Doluisio and Dittert, 1969. [a]Weinstein, 1970. [b]MacDonald et al., 1973. [c]Brogden et al., 1975.

Decreased absorption due either to complexing with divalent and trivalent cations such as calcium, aluminum and magnesium, or to interference by food and milk, is a well-known phenomenon (see Notari, 1973, for a concise review). An inhibitory effect of various iron salts on the absorption of tetracycline has been also documented with both serum and urinary levels. Ferrous sulfate is the most active, followed successively, by the fumarate, the succinate and the gluconate, the tartrate, and ferric sodium edetate (Neuvonen and Turakka, 1974). The same interaction has been shown to occur between ferrous sulfate and doxycycline. From 20 to 45% lower serum levels are found even when the iron salt is given 3 to 11 h after the oral dose of the antibiotic. Similarly, the half-life of intravenous doxycycline is shortened from 16.6 ± 0.7 h to 11.0 ± 0.4 h by concomitant oral therapy with iron salts, suggesting that the interaction takes place during the long enterohepatic circulation of this tetracycline derivative (Neuvonen and Penttilä, 1974). An equivalent effect on the absorption process most likely also occurs with minocycline, which is reported to be less affected by food and milk; however, the comparative data on serum levels of doxycyline and minocycline are not conclusive (Brogden et al., 1975b). Recent studies have shown that tetracycline can inhibit the absorption of iron salts (Neuvonen et al., 1975).

Data on protein-binding, serum half-life and renal clearance of the most frequently used tetracyclines are summarized in Table 20. The prolongation of serum half-life after repeated dosing has been noted following both intravenous and oral administration and has been confirmed for all tetracyclines. The intervals for the administration of maintenance doses should take into account these findings which have proved useful to predict and maintain desired therapeutic levels (Doluisio and Dittert, 1969). The topic is reviewed by Notari (1973), who underlines the fact that data obtained after multiple-dosing represent the true half-life, as they correspond to the steady-state values.

Demeclocyline and methacycline do not undergo appreciable biologic transformation, 91.9% and 82.2%, respectively, of the administered doses are excreted in the active form in urine and feces. Both minocycline and doxycycline are partially metabolized to inactive substances, 23-38.5% and 61.1-81.3%, respectively, of the dose are excreted over 96 h in urine and feces (MacDonald et al., 1973). Values similar to those of democlocycline and methacycline are reported for tetracycline (Weinstein, 1970b; Brogden et al., 1975b). The fecal excretion is due both to the nonabsorbed drug and the enterohepatic circulation, which is particularly important for chlortetracycline, doxycycline and methacycline. Biliary levels of tetracyclines reach concentrations 5 to 10 times higher than those of serum (Acocella et al., 1968).

The degree of renal clearance of the various tetracyclines has been correlated with the percentage of the free drug available for glomerular filtration (Notari, 1973), and to the extent of tubular reabsorption (Weinstein, 1970b). The findings of Jaffe et al. (1973) fit well with this second hypothesis, since they show a significant increase in urinary excretion following alkaline treatment which correlates with the lower lipid solubility of tetracycline and doxycycline at a urinary pH higher than 6. Urinary excretion decreases proportionally to the degree of filtration. It is claimed that doxycycline and minocycline are safe in severely impaired renal function and in anephric subjects because of their low urinary excretion. A recent study, however, gave half-life values for doxycycline which are higher than those usually reported (24.8 h as assessed by microbiological methods, 32.5 h as measured with a radiolabeled compound), and a proportional decrease or urinary recovery was noted with decreasing renal function. An interesting hypothesis is proposed for the elimination of doxycycline via the g.i. tract. Biliary excretion would account for only a small part of the elimination, transmucosal diffusion from the blood into the intestinal lumen, and intraluminal chelation with consequent impaired resorption would be the major route of excretion (Whelton et al., 1974). On the other hand, doxycycline is claimed to be free of the antianabolic effect that leads to increased urea production (Porpaczy, 1970; Whelton et al., 1974). The question as to whether minocycline can be safely used in the presence of moderate or severe renal impairment is still open to discussion. There are conflicting data both about half-life and about exacerbation of renal failure due to increased urea production (Brogden et al., 1975b). A recent report suggests a high degree of safety, but points to the potential risk of high serum levels; close monitoring of renal function would seem advisable (Carney et al., 1974).

Oxytetracycline has been recently proposed as a suitable compound for urinary tract infections, due to the extent of its urinary excretion compared with other tetracyclines (Stamey et al., 1974; Villani et al., 1975); Its safety has been stressed (Taneja et al., 1974) despite earlier reports on its antianabolic and renal damaging effects (Korkeila, 1971; Stott et al., 1971). A selective inhibition of human tubular function of demeclocycline has been reported, suggesting a potential clinical use of this tetracycline when a potentiation of ADH activity is desired (Wildon et al., 1973a).

The distribution of the tetracyclines into body tissues is proportional to their degree of lipid solubility, rather than to their degree of protein-binding (Notari, 1973). Doxycycline (Eneroth et al., 1975; Gartmann, 1975) and minocycline (MacCulloch et al., 1974) are reported to be well distributed in poorly perfused areas and secretions. Minocycline diffuses more easily than other tetracyclines into the CSF, reaching 25-30% of the serum concentration, and has been suggested as a potential compound for treating meningococcal carriers (Carney et al., 1974; Brogden et al., 1975b). The data reported above can be usefully applied to pediatric practice in older children where the tetracyclines are still widely used (Herz and Gfeller, 1975). No significant differences from adult values were found in the disposition of doxycycline in two groups of children, 10-23 months old and more than 24 months old, respectively (Ceccarelli et al., 1971). Older data for the 1-methylenelysine-tetracycline derivative show a prolonged half-life in newborns 1-2 days old, with a reduced plasma clearance and a smaller volume of distribution. Decreased plasma clearance is reported to persist up to 7 months of age (Sereni et al., 1965).

ANTITUBERCULAR AGENTS

Streptomycin

Over the last few years, the use of this antibiotic has been constantly decreasing in clinical practice (see Shapiro and Levy, 1975, for a quantitative evaluation), and consequently no further data have been produced besides those reported in the classical textbooks (Garrod et al., 1973; Weinstein, 1970b). Following intramuscular administration, peak plasma levels are reached after 0.5-1.5 h in adults, and after 2 h in premature infants. About 30% of the drug is protein-bound, while the rest of the streptomycin dose diffuses readily in the extracellular space and is cleared from the body solely by glomerular filtration (30-70 ml/min). Therapeutic levels being aroudn 10 μg/ml, peak concentrations of 16-42 μg/ml and 25-50 μg/ml are reached after i.m. doses of 0.5 and 1 g, respectively, in adults, 17-42 μg/ml are obtained in prematures after administration of 10 mg/kg.

An apparent serum half-life of 2.4-2.7 h has been measured in adults, which can increase up to 9 h in older subjects with diminished renal function. On the other hand, renal immaturity is mainly responsible for the long half-life (7.0 h) that has been measured in premature newborns in their first 3 days of life (Simon and Yaffe, 1969). Excretion in adults is usually almost complete within 24 h. Infants 1 to 3 days of age excreted 29% of the administered dose in 12 h (Simon and Yaffe, 1969).

Isoniazid

After many years of clinical use, this drug still remains one of the most important agents in the treatment of tuberculosis. Furthermore, it has roused the interest of the geneticists, as well as that of clinicians and pharmacologists, because of its metabolic pathway. The compound is degraded in the liver by acetylation, the rate of this process is genetically controlled, and a distinction can be made between slow and fast acetylators. The percentage of a given population who can be categorized as fast acetylators might range from 6.3 to 80%, depending upon the group's ethnic make-up, a high percent of fast acetylators being found among black and Eskimo populations. Simplified screening procedures are available to separate individuals into either of the two genetically distinct groups, however, rigid classification often is not possible due to the high degree of variability observed in the individual patient (Eidus and Hodgkin, 1973; Eidus et al., 1974a; Vessell, 1975). In 1973, Mitchison presented a brief review of the therapeutic implications of isoniazid disposition.

Isoniazid can be given either orally or parenterally, but the oral route is most widely used. Peak plasma concentrations are reached 1-2 h after administration slightly earlier in fast than in slow inactivators. No differences in bioavailability have been noted among the currently available commercial preparations (Gelber et al., 1969). The plasma half-life and the AUC are 2.4 times higher in slow than in fast phenotypes; special slow-release preparations have been proposed as a therapeutic advantage for fast inactivators (Eidus et al., 1974b). Half-life values of 1.1-5.2 h have been reported in normal individuals, as compared to values of 1.3-10.7 h in patients with impaired renal function (Bowersox et al., 1973). Following intravenous administration, a plasma half-life of less than 80 min was observed in fast, and of more than 140 min in slow inactivators (Gelber et al., 1969).

Optimal peak concentrations are considered to be about 5 μg/ml in order to ensure a coverage period (not less than 0.2 μg/ml) of 14-15 h in fast, and of 29-31 h in slow inactivators. Higher concentrations are useless because mutant strains of M. tuberculosis are resistant to much higher concentrations and, therefore, need a combined-therapy approach (Mitchison, 1973, Øvreberg and Bjartveit, 1974). Isoniazid diffuses into both the extracellular and the intracellular spaces and is able to penetrate into the CSF even when inflammation is not present. From 50-70% of the drug is excreted within 24 h. Impaired renal function is usually not a risk factor, however, abnormally high, prolonged and potentially toxic serum levels can be reached when a marked degree of renal impairment is combined with a slow inactivator status (Bowersox et al., 1973). Slow inactivators also seem to be more susceptible to hepatic damage (Lal et al., 1972). This finding was observed in children 1-18 years of age who were phenotyped after showing SGOT elevation (Beaudry et al., 1974).

Interaction between rifampicin and isoniazid, possibly leading to additive toxicity, has been described. Hypothetically, it has been proposed that toxicity due to the acetyl metabolite of isoniazid might explain these findings. In experiments conducted to investigate isoniazid metabolism, a large amount of covalent binding of acetylisoniazid was found in rat liver. This binding was increased by hepatic exposure to inducing agents, and, by the same mechanism, PAS, a microsomal inhibitor, appeared to reduce isoniazid toxicity (Mitchell and Jollow, 1974, and corresponding quotations). Interestingly, recent clinical studies do not support this hypothesis. In tuberculosis patients, only a small increase in the serum levels of isoniazid was seen after 7 days of combined therapy, and no changes in bilirubin or in hepatic function were observed (Acocella et al., 1972a; Boman, 1974). These studies, however, do not represent the typical chronic treatment situation where an accumulation of the metabolite conceivably could take place.

Rifampicin

This drug has been greeted as a major step forward in the therapeutic control of tuberculosis (Editorial, 1969; Koch-Weser, 1970). Because of its high lipid solubility, rifampicin diffuses easily through cell membranes, thus killing bacteria intracellularly and offering a definite therapeutic advantage in both the tubercular and nontubercular diseases (Mandel, 1973; Mattson, 1973; Ezer and Soothill, 1974). A comprehensive review of the drug's pharmacological and clinical properties was published a few years ago (Binda et al., 1971), and an excellent monograph about side effects was presented even more recently (Mattson, 1973). For the purpose of this discussion, a few recently published papers have been considered in depth, as they supplement the older data by giving more specific information on some kinetic patterns. All of the authors have emphasized the occurrence of high variability in kinetic data, and, certainly, the available analytical procedures are partially responsible since they do not distinguish between the drug and its metabolites, adding to the individual differences in disposition patterns. Data are, therefore, always expressed as mean values, accompanied by ranges. Less variability in kinetic values is seen in studies of patients under chronic therapy than in those cases where rifampicin is used in acute treatment.

The complete absorption of the antibiotic from the gastrointestinal tract following oral administration was confirmed by the comparison with urinary data following intravenous injection (Riess et al., 1969). In one study, the influence of food on oral absorption seemed only a delaying factor and, consequently, did not appear to modify the antibacterial activity of sera (Dans et al., 1970). Other authors have found both delayed and decreased oral rifampicin absorption, with as much as 50% of the dose unabsorbed, depending possibly on the quality and quantity of food present (Riess et al., 1969). Recent data do confirm a significantly slower and lower absorption in concomitance with meals, as seen both from serum and from urinary concentrations. The results are not consistent, however, in different experiments even in the same subjects, and because the levels usually obtained are much higher than therapeutically useful MIC, the clinical significance of these findings has come under discussion (Siegler et al., 1974).

Following lower doses of the antibiotic (300 mg vs. 600 and 900 mg), an earlier serum peak is seen (Acocella et al., 1971), and proportionally higher serum levels are reached with higher doses, yet no substantial increase of the AUC is seen with dosages higher than 15 mg/kg (Iwainsky et al., 1974). After repeated treatment over a 4-7 day period, a significant increase can be measured in the transfer constant from intestine to blood (Acocella et al., 1972b). Diarrhea does not seem to influence the absorption process (Naveh and Friedman, 1973), and among the other antitubercular drugs only PAS has been shown to decrease the absorption of rifampicin. This effect is not seen, however, when PAS is given parenterally and 12 h before or 2 h after, oral rifampicin (Boman, 1974). Peak serum levels can be measured any time between 2-5 h after antibiotic administration. The corresponding ranges of concentrations are wider after acute than after chronic administration, so that 1 h after taking a 450 mg tablet acute vs. chronic serum levels of 1.5-16.0 and 3.4-9.6, respectively, were found (Virtanen and Tala, 1974).

In healthy subjects, from 87-91% of the drug is bound to plasma proteins, with somewhat lower binding (83.6-88.4%) seen in chronically treated, tuberculous patients. Concomitant antitubercular therapy does not influence the degree of binding, according to Boman and Ringberger (1974), who also review other works which give different, usually lower values. A significant amount of rifampicin is nonspecifically bound to fractions of plasma other than albumin, such as fibrinogen and the gamma globulins. The complex of rifampicin with gamma globulin is possibly related to the side effects seen in high-dosage, intermittent rifampicin therapy, but the immunological basis of these adverse reactions is open to further investigation (Mattson, 1973; Mattson et al., 1974).

The free portion of the drug is readily available for equilibration with body tissues. From 20 to 25% of serum levels have been found in bronchial secretions (Riess et al., 1969), while slow penetration (peak time: 5-11 h) and slow removal is seen in pleural fluids. Individual patterns of distribution into this compartment are highly variable and unpredictable, depending, perhaps, on the underlying pathological changes of the bronchopulmonary system. Drug concentrations higher than those in the plasma can be detected in the pleural fluid

24 h after dosing (Boman and Malmborg, 1974). Animal data with possible clinical relevance show that in lactating ewes there is a serum-milk ratio near to unity, supporting the concept of passive diffusion (Ziv and Sulman, 1974).

Rifampicin is extensively metabolized in the liver, mainly through a desacetylation process which results in a compound less active bactericidally (60% as active as the intact drug). Both the intact drug and its metabolite undergo a long enterohepatic circulation. The passage from portal blood into the bile is due to an active process of secretion, through which drug concentrations many times higher than those in blood are attained in the bile over a period of time (Acocella et al., 1971; Mattson, 1973). The desacetyl derivative accounts for all the activity present in the bile about 5 h after rifampicin administration (Acocella et al., 1972b). Other substances excreted in the bile may influence the kinetics of rifampicin and, in turn, have their own kinetics affected by the antibiotic. Earlier, higher and more prolonged rifampicin serum levels are seen after probenecid administration, the inhibition of antibiotic uptake by the hepatic cell is hypothesized as the responsible mechanism diminishing the metabolic degradation of the drug and increasing its availability for other tissues where it diffuses through a passive process (Kenwright and Levi, 1973). Serum levels and apparent plasma half-life are increased in patients with chronically impaired liver function (Acocella et al., 1972a); this fact is more evident in the obstructive diseases (Mattson, 1973).

Following repeated administration, after only 3 days (Boman, 1974) or a week (Curci et al., 1973; Acocella et al., 1971), and in patients being chronically treated (Virtanen and Tala, 1974), decreased serum levels and a shorter drug half-life are observed; greater reduction is seen in those patients with initially longer half-lives. No correlation has been found with the patterns of slow and fast isoniazid acetylation in patients treated with both drugs (Boman, 1974; Acocella et al., 1972a). These changes in serum half-life from acute to chronic treatment are not observed in patients with impaired liver function (Curci et al., 1973) or in patients who have been chronically treated with other antitubercular agents (Virtanen and Tala, 1974; Boman, 1974).

Dose-dependent kinetics, resulting in more than proportionally increased half-life values, have been seen after acute but not chronic treatment (Curci et al., 1972); the highly variable half-life values were also less scattered after chronic repeated treatment (Boman, 1974). Precise quantification of these metabolic variations has not been possible due to the lack of analytical methods capable of distinguishing rifampicin from its metabolites, but an increased rate of biliary excretion, following enhanced metabolic degradation due to enzymatic induction, is postulated to account for the phenomenon (Acocella et al., 1971; 1972b). This suggestion is further supported by data showing increased microsomal activity in human and guinea pig hepatocytes that have been exposed to rifampicin *in vivo* and *in vitro* (Jezequel et al., 1971), a decrease in the serum levels of rifampicin after phenobarbital treatment (De Rautlin de la Roy et al.,

1971; Radner, 1973) and the apparent capacity of rifampicin to induce the metabolism of drugs such as tolbutamide (Syvälathy et al., 1974), cortisol (Edwards et al., 1974; Maisey et al., 1974), digitoxin (Peters et al., 1974) and ethinyloestradiol (Bolt et al., 1974). The induction process was found to be more regular following continuous daily treatment than in intermittent regimens (Iwainsky et al., 1974; Acocella et al., 1971).

It is unlikely, however, that the induction hypothesis can be fully responsible for the alteration in serum level and half-life values observed by Boman (1974) in studies comprised of very short periods, and the development of an increased drug secretion in the bile has been postulated (Binda et al., 1971). A substantially higher bile recovery has been observed when comparing the 1st day (20.9 mg/12 h) with the 7th day (57.0 mg/12 h) of treatment accompanied by a statistically insignificant decline in urinary excretion of the antibiotic (Acocella et al., 1972b). Some authors have reported higher serum levels in women than in men (Scotti, 1973), but this is not a constant finding (Iwainsky et al., 1974), and comparable half-life values have been obtained in males and females. When they are present, these differences in serum values perhaps can be atrributed to sex-related differences in absorption and tissue distribution (Boman, 1974; Goble, 1975).

In healthy subjects, 20-50% of the administered dose is excreted in the urine, and the remainder in stools, as a sum of rifampicin and metabolites (Riess et al., 1969; Mattson, 1973). There appears to be no age-related differences in this pattern of elimination, as the urinary excretion of rifampicin and its metabolites is similar in both children and adults (Acocella et al., 1969).

Rifampicin disposition during development. A single study has been found where rifampicin was given to newborn infants, 1-3 days old and weighing not less than 3.2 kg (Acocella et al., 1969). Unfortunately, not much more data are available for infants and children (Acocclla et al., 1969; De Rautlin de la Roy et al., 1974). Serum levels were lower than those seen in adults in both pediatric age groups; however, it should be noted that, whereas infants and children demonstrated the adult pattern, with from 1/10 to 1/3 of adult serum levels, newborn babies showed a much later peak (at about 8 h) with a longer elimination phase. Therapeutic serum levels were still present in newborns 24 h after a single oral dose, suggesting the probability of an accumulation phenomenon in chronic treatment (Acocella et al., 1969). The lower profile of the serum concentration curve in infants and children (from 2 months up to 5 years) has been attributed to the larger volumes of distribution in children, but no quantitative data were given (Acocella et al., 1969). On the other hand, De Rautlin de la Roy et al. (1974) suggest a 50% lower absorption in this age group, which according to these authors is rather impaired by concomitant administration of ethambutol. Although no qualitative differences in rifampicin have been reported in children, data obtained in newborn infants suggest a lower biliary excretion (Acocella et al., 1969).

As has been observed in adults, in newborns repeated administration modifies some of the features that were found after acute dosing. Among these changes, a higher and earlier absorption peak and a correspondent increase in the urinary concentration of the desacetyl metabolite have been measured in the same group of newborns (Acocella et al., 1969). Strangely, the rifampicin serum levels, decreasing with chronic therapy, tended to increase again after 20 days of treatment in this study. No explanation was given for this finding and no possible underlying pathological effects on the liver were mentioned. Rifampicin concentrations in the CSF follow the serum patterns. Penetration is good even without inflamed meninges, however, the absorption peak in this fluid is delayed from 3 to 6 h, with an increase in the CSF/serum ratio from 0.111 to 0.150 (De Rautlin de la Roy et al., 1974). The urinary excretion of rifampicin and its metabolites is equivalent in all ages and reflects the negligible involvement of the renal system in the elimination processes of this drug (Acocella et al., 1969). The measurement of the desacetylated metabolite shows that the desacetylation is not a limiting factor in the disposal of the drug in the newborn. *In vitro* experiments with newborn plasma have shown that the binding of bilirubin is slightly decreased by rifampicin (11-25%) (Malaka-Zafiriu and Strates, 1969).

OTHERS

Chloramphenicol (CAP) and Thiamphenicol (TAP)

The use of CAP has been discouraged and is now considered contraindicated outside of very specific situations, due its dose-related effect of bone marrow depression and its capacity of provoking a dose-unrelated, and fatal, aplastic anemia. Its use has been declining steadily from 1966 to 1972 (Shapiro and Levy, 1975), yet is worth mentioning that in many countries CAP is still fairly widely and uncritically prescribed (Erill et al., 1974a,b; Schreier and Berger, 1974; Bertele and Marget, 1974). Twenty-nine percent of the ambulatory population of pediatric patients admitted to the hospital have been taking CAP during the previous six months (Masera et al., 1976). Extensive research has been made over the last few years in an attempt to understand the mechanisms underlying the two types of adverse reaction and, more generally, the immunosuppressive capacity of CAP. The topic has been very recently reviewed (Dimitrov and Nodine, 1974; Girdwood, 1973; PMJ, 1974). Epidemiological data have been collected documenting the dimensions of the problem, (Keiser, 1974b; Meyer et al., 1974b; Bottiger, 1974; Hausmann and Skrandies, 1974; Hellriegel and Gross, 1974; Weingartner and Exadaktylos, 1974). Data are beginning to become available that allow comparison with TAP, with which depression of bone marrow activity has also been described. However, with the latter drug not a single case of aplastic anemia has been described up to now, suggesting a possible role of

CAP's nitro group in inducing aplastic anemia (Krishna and Bonanomi, 1974; Yunis, 1974; Yunis et al., 1974; Keiser, 1974a,b; Tisnè, 1974; Van Cauwenberge, 1974; Frigerio, 1974).

CAP is usually given orally, and absorption is complete, as can be seen from comparison with i.v. infusion of the antibiotic (Betzien and Vomel, 1969). Pharmaceutical preparation, however, would seem to play a major role in determining the efficacy of absorption. Many studies have been made showing marked variations following either commercial preparations or brand products. Differences exist not only in the time of peak serum concentration but also in the absolute amount of drug absorbed, as seen from the AUC and the amount of drug excreted in the urine (Aguiar et al., 1967; Glazko et al., 1968; Chiou, 1971); moreover, this finding holds true not only for capsules but also for tablets and suspensions (Bell et al., 1971). Dissolution of particles of different size and the hydrolysis of the esteric bond in the gut appear to be the limiting steps in CAP absorption.

Less variability is observed after intramuscular administration, peak levels are delayed by this route and the plasma half-life is slightly prolonged (from 2-5 h to 4-6 h) (Garrod et al., 1973). Peak levels occur 1.5-3 h after oral administration; 60% of the drug is bound to plasma proteins. The drug diffuses freely into the tissues, so that from 20-30% of the plasma concentration is found in other body fluids, including CSF, which corresponds to the unbound portion of the drug (Betzien and Vomel, 1969). CAP is metabolized in the liver through two main pathways, namely, glucuronation and the formation of inactive arylamines. Only 5-10% of the dose is excreted unchanged and in active form by glomerular filtration; inactive metabolic products are excreted via tubular secretion. Glucuronidation in the liver is the critical step in the disposition of CAP (Kunin et al., 1959).

Only very small changes in serum concentrations of the active form are seen with impaired renal function (Lindberg et al., 1966). However, a low glucuronidating capacity, as seen in premature and very young, full-term infants, causes a markedly prolonged half-life. The combination of high dosages of CAP with an insufficient glucuronidizing ability and inadequate renal mechanism for excretion has been related to the "gray baby" syndrome noted in this age group (Weiss et al., 1960). T½ values of 1.5-5 h are measured in adults and children, while half-lives of 24-28 h or 15-22 h have been demonstrated in prematures, 1-2 days old, and 8-15 h in prematures 13-23 days old (Sereni and Principi, 1968; Garrod et al., 1973). After intramuscular administration, CAP half-life is 5.6 h in full-term newborns of 5-6 days of age (Albores et al., 1974). CAP markedly inhibits the hepatic enzymatic system (see Skovsted et al., 1974, for a recent review). Animal data suggest that inducing agents accelerate the hepatic inactivation of CAP (Remmer, 1974). CAP binds the intracellular liver protein Y, whose amount varies with age, and the same covalent binding can be established with bone marrow macromolecules. TAP show a lesser degree of this type of binding (Krishna, 1974; Weber and Cohen, 1975). The significance of these findings in explaining CAP toxicity is still a matter of discussion.

TAP disposition has been reviewed recently, with special emphasis on its dependence on renal function (PMJ, 1974). The GLC analytical procedure for this determination in biological specimens is now available which will permit more precise data to be obtained (Cattabeni and Gazzaniga, 1974); unfortunately, information on the antibiotic is not complete as yet. Preliminary data of protein-binding give values of about 10% (Ferrari and Della Bella, 1974). TAP has an apparent volume of distribution of 15 liters, the renal clearance ranges between 60-106 mg/min and the drug is not metabolized to any great extent. Between 70 and 90% of the administered dose is excreted as the active form by glomerular filtration. TAP half-life values range between 0.5 and 3.5 h in normal individuals, and in patients with various degrees of hepatic impairment, independently of the dose. In renal insufficiency, an increase in serum half-life is seen which correlates with the clearance of creatinine (Dettli and Spring, 1974; Tacquet et al., 1974; Monafo et al., 1974; Oldershausen et al., 1974). Only one study has been found which deals with TAP disposition in the neonate, using premature and full-term infants (the protocol of the study is questionable as it appears that a single experimental dose of CAP and TAP is given to healthy subjects) (Albores et al., 1974). Peak plasma levels are reached 1 h after an intramuscular administration of TAP in all the groups tested (group I, premature infants, aged 11 to 24 hours; group II, full-term newborns, aged 40 minutes to 36 hours; group III, full-term newborns, aged 7 to 9 days). Mean peak concentrations are slightly higher in group I and lower in group III. An average of 35.4% of the administered dose is excreted in urine over a 24 h period by newborns in group I, compared with 42.8 and 49%, respectively, in groups II and III. From the given data, values of half-life are 5.45 h, 4.82 h and 3.70 h in the three groups.

Erythromycin

This is the most commonly used compound of the related class. Other molecules do not offer any definite advantages; however, a steroid-sparing effect of troleandromycin in the treatment of asthma and bronchitis has been confirmed recently (Spector et al., 1974). Only a few comments need be added to the data available from the classical textbooks (Weinstein, 1970; Garrod et al., 1973). Considerable attention has been given to the preparation of different pharmaceutical forms that are capable of avoiding degradation in gastric juice and assure good absorption. Available data are summarized in Table 21. Efforts to obtain a palatable compound to be used in pediatric practice have led to the development of new esters which have proved in animal studies to compare favorably in therapeutically effectiveness with the existing ones (Sinkula, 1974). Analytical methods do not distinguish between the base and its esters, and therefore it is

Table 21. Erythromycin Serum Levels in Man
(Following Single Dose of 500 mg)

Preparation	Route	Peak Time (h)	Peak Level (μg/ml)	Half-Life (h)
Base	Oral	2-4	0.9-1.4	2-4
Stearate	Oral	2-4	0.4-1.8	–
Propionate	Oral	2-4	0.4-1.9	3-5
Estolate	Oral	1-2	1.4-5.0	2-4
Lactobionate	i.v.	–	11.5-30.0	1-2

Adapted from Garrod et al., 1973, p. 172. The absorption of the estolate is not affected by food, whereas the propionate and the stearate show a lower peak.

fairly difficult to obtain precise data on the kinetics of the active compound. *In vitro* hydrolysis during bioassay can also occur at different rates according to the pH (0.5 h at pH 8, 5.0 h at pH 5). Furthermore, several rate processes affect the time course of the drug and pro-drug in the plasma, making it difficult to define the exact amount of drug present in the body at each moment (Notari, 1973; Meland, 1972).

A few points should be kept in mind when evaluating data on erythromycin kinetics. According to one study, 73.4% of the erythromycin base and 92.6% of the propionate, the free base of the estolate, is bound to serum protein (Gordon et al., 1973). Different values are reported by other authors, who give 10% and 1.6%, respectively, of free drug available for diffusion in tissues. In the latter study, serum half-lifes of 1.18 h and 2.15 h, respectively, have been calculated (Wiegand and Chun, 1972). Similar values for binding have been found in children with cystic fibrosis, aged 5 months to 16 years (Valman and Evans, 1970).

There is good diffusion of erythromycin into all tissues, with from 1/8 to 1/64 of serum concentration found in the CSF after oral administration; higher amounts are found in the CSF following intravenous injection (Weinstein, 1970b). From 10% to 100% of the serum concentration has been found in middle ear exudates of children (5 months to 9 years) treated orally (Bass et al., 1971). High amounts are excreted into the bile, reaching concentrations 4 and 30 times greater than in serum, for the propionyl ester and the base, respectively (Garrod et al., 1973). From 2-5% of the dose is found in the urine as the intact compound following oral administration, and 12-15% can be recovered after i.v. infusion (Weinstein, 1970b). Alkalinization of the urine increases the antimicrobial activity (Zinner et al., 1971). From the very few data specifically reported on disposition during development and from the metabolic and excretory patterns, no substantial changes from the adult pattern are to be expected in the pediatric age group (see also Sereni and Principi, 1968).

Clindamycin

This compound will probably replace the parent compound, lincomycin, in clinical practice, due to its properties of better oral absorption and higher activity against gram-positive aerobes and both gram-positive and gram-negative anaerobes. It is commonly used as a second choice for the penicillins against many pathogens, one important exception being its low activity against *Haemophilus* (Bartlett et al., 1972; Carr, 1973; Feigin et al., 1973; Jackson, 1973; Ledger et al., 1974; Randolph et al., 1975; Cherubin et al., 1975). Compared with clindamycin, lincomycin has a twofold longer half-life (mean: 5.20, range: 2.44-13.8 h) (Wagner et al., 1968).

Analytical methods currently in use do not distinguish between clindamycin and its bioactive metabolites. It has been shown, however, that N-demethylclindamycin and clindamycin sulfoxide (respectively, 3 times more active and 7 times less active than clindamycin) should not contribute substantially to the activity measured in the serum. On the contrary, they account for most of the activity present in the bile and urine (De Haan et al., 1973).

The available data on disposition have been collected in Table 22. A specific discussion about the fate of the drug and of its phosphate ester, when they are given parenterally, has been published recently (De Haan et al., 1973; Sinkula and Yalkowsky, 1975). Intramuscular absorption is reported to be regular (20% of variation within different groups) and to occur faster in physically active subjects and in children (Kauffmann et al., 1973). After the absorption phase, the pattern of distribution and elimination are similar with i.v. or i.m. dosing. Eighty-seven percent of the orally administered dose is estimated to be absorbed. The hydrochloride salt and the palmitate ester (the latter being mostly used in pediatrics) show substantially the same pattern of absorption. A lower, delayed peak with a reduced AUC is seen when the hexadecylcarbonate ester is given (Forist et al., 1973).

Food delays, but does not reduce, the extent of oral absorption. No significant differences are seen between acute and chronic treatment, or between clindamycin given as capsules and tablets (Wagner et al., 1968). Children show approximately the same absorption pattern as adults when the drug is given orally (De Haan et al., 1973). The lower peak serum concentrations seen in children given the same dose per kg as adults have been attributed to the faster elimination rate (De Haan et al., 1972), but the data are incomplete and too few to allow any conclusion. No discussion is made, for instance, of the notable differences between the apparent volumes of distribution.

Table 22. Clindamycin Disposition in Man

Age	Dose (mg)	Peak Time (h)	Peak Level (μg/ml)	Ka (h^{-1})	Ke (h^{-1})	T½ (h)	Vd (L/m²/1.73)	Urinary Excretion (%)
Adults (i.m. adm.)								
Novak et al., 1970	116/m²	2.0	2.88			4.76	58.8	6-10
	173/m²	2.6				4.5	59.8	(2-24 h)
De Haan et al., 1973	300	1.5-2.0	4.36-6.56		0.138-0.345	2.01-50.2		
	300	2-3	3.17-4.77		0.309-0.646	1.07-2.24		
	600	1.5-2.0	4.49-6.71		0.431-0.887	0.78-1.61		
Adults (oral adm.)								
De Haan et al., 1972	150	1.06 ± 0.37	2.84 ± 0.65	3.73 ± 1.59	0.281 ± 0.099	2.82 ± 1.13	43.9 ± 7.4	14.3 (24 h)
	300	0.91 ± 0.38	3.44 ± 0.87	6.41 ± 3.55	0.223 ± 0.050	3.23 ± 0.67	78.9 ± 15.9	
	450	0.76 ± 0.31	5.58 ± 1.26	8.20 ± 4.55	0.197 ± 0.063	3.78 ± 0.98	74.3 ± 14.2	17.1 (48 h)
Forist et al., 1973	150	1.16 ± 0.24*	2.05 ± 0.66*	2.81 ± 0.92*	0.25 ± 0.07*	2.94 ± 0.83*	—	7*
		0.86 ± 0.53°	2.80 ± 1.26°	7.65 ± 7.56°	0.26 ± 0.07°	2.84 ± 0.76°	—	8.68
Eastwood and Gower, 1974	150	0.7-2	1.55-2.32	—	—	—	—	—

Study	Age	Dose							
Children (i.m. adm.)									
Kauffmann et al., 1973	2 mo-11 yrs	117/m²	1	9	—		2.41	21.49	19
		150/m²	1	9			3.43	19.90	8.749 (0-8 h)
Children (oral adm.)									
Shibata et al., 1973	2 mo	4/Kg	4	5.4					—
Unertl et al., 1974	3-14 mo	30/Kg	1.5	6.1	—	—		—	—
De Haan et al., 1972	8-11 yrs	2/Kg	0.56 ± 0.25	2.26 ± 0.77	8.64 ± 3.36	0.440 ± 0.205	1.89 ± 0.82	30.4 ± 10.0	5.7 ± 2.52 (0-6 h)

*Palmitate ester.
°Hcl.

Contradictory data are available about the changes in clindamycin half-life values. Higher values are given in one study following higher doses (De Haan et al., 1972), while the contrary is seen in a successive report (De Haan et al., 1973). More generally, the antibiotic's half-life seems to be longer following parenteral administration. Dose-dependent kinetics with a saturation effect of the liver have been hypothesized but not documented (Kauffman et al., 1973). The wide variability of results reported in different studies plus the possible role of varying amounts of metabolites, following different routes, on the measured antibiotic activity preclude any further speculations. From data on chronic treatment by any route, there is no indication either of accumulation or a speed-up in drug metabolism (Wagner et al., 1968; De Haan and Schellenberg, 1972; De Haan et al., 1972, 1973). Impairment of hepatic function does not modify clindamycin half-life even if higher concentrations are found at longer intervals after drug administration in subjects with abnormal liver function. Higher values of urinary excretion have also been observed in this situation. The inability to measure single metabolites does not allow precise calculations to be made (Williams et al., 1975).

Renal function should not influence the kinetic behavior of clindamycin to a great extent, as its clearance is mainly extrarenal. In support of this assumption, it has been shown that renal failure does not alter the serum half-life of the drug given orally (Eastwood and Gower, 1974). In contrast, a prolonged half-life has been calculated following intravenous administration of the drug to uremic patients (Joshi and Stein, 1974). Complete information is not given about the clinical conditions and the kinetic calculations in this study. Reported serum levels higher than in a control group suggest a change in the volume of distribution (Gibaldi and Perrier, 1972). A prolonged half-life has been measured in elderly people (mean age = 79.3 years, T½ = 4.46 h) with slightly delayed peak levels and with urinary excretion values comparable to younger adults (Campbell et al., 1973). Low urinary excretion was reported in immature babies (0.83% of the dose over 24 h; no age specified), whereas other infants (less than 1 year) gave values which approximate those of older children and adults (Nakamura et al., 1973).

Depending on the study, 60% (Eastwood and Gower, 1974) or 93.6% (Gordon et al., 1973) of the drug is reported to be bound to serum protein. Clindamycin diffuses easily and rapidly from serum to tissues, from where it diffuses back slowly (De Haan et al., 1973; Ishiyama et al., 1973). Very high antibiotic activity is found in bile, after i.v. infusion, with a pattern of elimination which is parallel to that of serum. Similarly, very high levels are measured in saliva up to 8 h after either i.m. or i.v. administrations, a finding which could have therapeutic implications (De Haan et al., 1973). Clincally useful MIC's are reached in normal and septic joints following oral administration (Deodhar et al., 1972). High concentrations are observed in sebaceous secretions. No drug is found in the leukocytes (Panzer et al., 1972).

Vancomycin

Vancomycin has a spectrum of activity which is restricted to those staphylococci or streptococci resistant to other antibiotics. No information on its disposition and kinetics in pediatric age has been found. Its use in treating bacterial meningitis has proved successful in cases where strains resistant to methicillin and CAP were present. According to the circumstances with meningeal disease, a combined systemic and intrathecal administration may be advisable (Bradford Hawley and Gump, 1973). A recent review on this antibiotic has been published (Alexander, 1974b).

CONCLUSIONS

The points made in introducing this chapter should be stressed once more in closing it. The pharmacokinetic data which have become available in the last few years will possibly contribute to a change in the attitude of doctors in prescribing antibiotics in their practice: from a mostly empirical approach to a more quantitative evaluation of the chosen regimens. A very close multidisciplinary interaction is needed to fully exploit the information produced in laboratories and wards, and by research groups. Pediatric age has been shown to need specific attention because of the paucity of data, the frequently ill-defined boundaries of diseases for which antibiotics are given, and the highly variable response of a developing organism. The critical application and the active development of data given above should already be in practice in clinical routine. What has been described by Jusko (1974) as a comprehensive approach to the pharmacokinetic management of antibiotic therapy could be usefully applied especially to groups of pediatric patients for whom a careful control of therapy is advisable. Optimization of dosage regimens, problems of bioavailability, monitoring of antibiotic effectiveness and pharmacokinetic studies in disease states represent a stimulating challenge for clinical pharmacologists, pharmacists and clinicians. The application of these data to daily hospital practice should favor the diffusion of appropriate information also to outpatient departments and community health-care centers, where antibiotics are most widely used.

Acknowledgment

This work has been partially supported by SAGO, S.p.A., Florence, Italy, through the research project S.I.F. (Sistema Informativo sui Farmaci—Drug Information System).

REFERENCES

Acocella, G., Bonollo, L., Garimoldi, M., Mainardi, M., Tenconi, L.T. and Nicolis, F.B. (1972a): Kinetics of rifampicin and isoniazid administered alone and in combination to normal subjects and patients with liver disease. *Gut, 13:* 47-53.

Acocella, G., Buniva, G., Flauto, U. and Nicolis, F.B. (1969): Absorption and elimination of the antibiotic rifampicin in newborns and children. In: *Progress in Antimicrobial and Anticancer Chemotherapy*, pp. 755-760, University of Tokyo.

Acocella, G., Lamarina, A., Nicolis, F.B., Pagani, V. and Segre, G. (1972b): Kinetic studies on rifampicin. II. Multicompartmental analysis of the serum, urine and bile concentrations in subjects treated for one week. *European Journal of Clinical Pharmacology, 5:* 111-115.

Acocella, G., Mattiussi, R., Nicolis, F.B., Pallanza, R. and Tenconi, L.T. (1968): Biliary excretion of antibiotics in man. *Gut, 9:* 536-545.

Acocella, G., Pagani, V. Marchetti, M., Baroni, G.C. and Nicolis, F.B. (1971): Kinetics studies on rifampicin. I. Serum concentration analysis in subjects treated with different oral doses over a period of two weeks. *Chemotherapy, 16:* 356-370.

Aerenlund Jensen, H., Halveg, A.B. and Saunamäki, K.I. (1971): Permanent impairment of renal function after methicillin nephropathy. *British Medical Journal, 4:* 406.

Aguiar, A.J., Krc, J., Jr., Kinkel, A.W. and Samyn, J.C. (1967): Effect of polymorphism on the absorption of chloramphenicol from chloramphenicol palmitate. *Journal of Pharmaceutical Sciences, 56:* 847-853.

Albores, J.M., Cammarota, H.E., Cosin, J.M., Gandolfi, A.F., Casares, M.S., Senet, O.J. and Correa de Araujo, E. (1974): Plasma levels and urinary excretion of thiamphenicol in premature and full-term newborn infants. *Postgraduate Medical Journal, 50*, suppl. 5: 46-49.

Alexander, J.W. (1974a): Emerging concepts in the control of surgical infections. *Surgery, 75:* 934-946.

Alexander, M.R. (1974b): A review of Vancomycin after 15 years of use. *Drug Intelligence and Clinical Pharmacy, 8:* 520-525.

Anders, M.W., Cooper, M.J., Rolewicz, T.F. and Mirkin, N.L. (1975): Application of high-pressure liquid chromatography in pediatric pharmacology: pharmacokinetics of cephalothin in man. In: *Basic and Therapeutic Aspects of Perinatal Pharmacology*, edited by P.L. Morselli, S. Garattini and F. Sereni, pp. 405-409, Raven Press, New York.

Andersen, J.B., Rosdahl, N. and Vejlsgaard, R. (1972): Aspects of pharmacology of gentamicin in newborn infants. *Acta Paediatrica Scandinavica, 61:* 343-349.

Andrews, J., Gillette, P., Williams, J.D. and Mitchard, M. (1974): Analysis of gentamicin in plasma: a comparative study of four methods. *Postgraduate Medical Journal, 50*, suppl. 7: 17-20.

Axelsson, A. and Brorson, J.-E. (1974): The concentration of antibiotics in sinus secretions. Ampicillin, cephradine and erythromycinestolate. *Annals of Otology, Rhinology and Laryngology, 83:* 323-331.

Axline, S.G., Yaffe, S.J. and Simon, H.J.. (1967): Clinical pharmacology of antimicrobials in premature infants. II. Ampicillin, methicillin, oxacillin, neomycin and colistin. *Pediatrics, 39:* 97-107.

Babb, R.R. (1975): The use of antibiotics in biliary tract disease. *American Journal of Gastroenterology, 63:* 37-39.

Baciocco, E.A. and Iles, R.L. (1971): Ampicillin and kanamycin concentrations in joint fluid. *Clinical Pharmacology and Therapeutics, 12:* 858-863.

Bailey, R.R. and Lynn, K.L. (1974): Serum levels of gentamicin after intravenous bolus injection. *Lancet, 1:* 730.

Banck, G., Belfrage, S., Johlin, I., Nordström, L., Tjernström, O. and Toremalm, N.G. (1973): Retrospective study of the ototoxicity of gentamicin. *Acta Pathologica et Microbiologica Scandinavia*, section B, *81:* 54-57.

Baran, D. and Klastersky, J. (1974): Concentration of gentamicin in bronchial secretions of children with cystic fibrosis or tracheostomy. *European Working Group for Cystic Fibrosis*, 5th Annual Meeting, Verona, 22-23, April 1974.

Barnett, H.L., McNammara, H., Schultz, S. and Tompsett, R. (1949): Renal clearances of sodium penicillin G. procaine penicillin G, and inulin in infants and children. *Pediatrics, 3:* 418-422.

Barnett, D.B., Smith, R.N., Greenwood, N.D. and Hetherington, C. (1974): Bioavailability of commercial tetracycline products. *British Journal of Clinical Pharmacology, 1:* 319-323.

Barr, W.H., Adir, J. and Garrettson, L. (1971): Decrease of tetracycline absorption in man by sodium bicarbonate. *Clinical Pharmacology and Therapeutics, 12:* 779-784.

Barr, W.H., Gerbracht, L.M., Letcher, K., Plaut, M. and Strahl, N. (1972): Assessment of the biological availability of tetracycline products in man. *Clinical Pharmacology and Therapeutics, 13:* 97-108.

Barringer, W.C., Schultz, W., Sieger, G.M., and Nash, R.A. (1974): Minocycline hydrochloride and its relationship to other tetracycline antibiotics. *American Journal of Pharmacy, 146:* 179-191.

Bartlett, J.G. and Finegold, S.M. (1974): Anaerobic infections of the lung and pleural space. *American Review of Respiratory Diseases, 110:* 56-77.

Bartlett, J.G., Sutter, V.L. and Finegold, S.M. (1972): Treatment of anaerobic infections with lincomycin and clindamycin. *New England Journal of Medicine, 287:* 1006-1010.

Barza, M., Samuelson, T. and Weinstein, L. (1974a): Penetration of antibiotics into fibrin loci in vivo. II. Comparison of nine antibiotics: effect of dose and degree of protein binding. *Journal of Infectious Diseases, 129:* 66-72.

Barza, M., Brusch, J., Bergeron, M.G. and Weinstein, L. (1974b): Penetration of antibiotics into fibrin loci in vivo. III. Intermittent vs. continuous infusion and the effect of probenecid. *Journal of Infectious Diseases, 129:* 73-78.

Barza, M. and Weinstein, L. (1974a): Penetration of antibiotics into fibrin loci in vivo. I. Comparison of penetration of ampicillin into fibrin clots, abscesses, and "interstitial fluid." *Journal of Infectious Diseases, 129:* 59-65.

Barza, M. and Weinstein, L. (1974b): Some determinants of the distribution of penicillins and cephalosporins in the body. Practical and theoretical considerations. *Annals of the New York Academy of Sciences, 235:* 613-620.

Bass, J.W., Crowley, D.M., Steele, R.W., Young, F.S.H. and Harden, L.B. (1974): Ampicillin blood levels as related to graded oral schedules. *Clinical Pediatrics, 13:* 273-279.

Bass, J.W., Steele, R.W. and Wiebe, R.A. (1971): Erythromycin concentrations in middle ear exudates. *Pediatrics, 48:* 417-422.

Beaudry, P.H., Brickman, H.F., Wise, M.B. and MacDougall, D. (1974): Liver enzyme disturbances during isoniazid chemoprophylaxis in children. *American Review of Respiratory Diseases, 110:* 581-584.

Bechtol, L.D. (1741): Therapy with cephaloridine in renal impairment. *Current Therapeutic Research, 14:* 790-800.

Bell, H., Johansen, H., Lunde, P.K.M., Andersgaard, H.A., Finholt, P., Midtvedt, T., Holum, E., Martinussen, B. and Aarnes, E.D. (1971): Absorption and dissolution characteristics of 14 different oral chloramphenicol preparations tested on healthy human male subjects. *Pharmacology, 5:* 108-120.

Bergan, T. and Øydvin, B. (1974): Cross-over study of penicillin pharmacokinetics after intravenous infusions. *Chemotherapy, 20:* 263-279.

Bergan, T., Westlie, L. and Brodwall, E.K. (1972): Influence of probenecid on gentamycin pharmacokinetics. *Acta Medica Scandinavica, 191:* 221-224.

Bergeron, M.G., Brusch, J.L., Barza, M. and Weinstein, L. (1973): Bacterial activity and pharmacology of cefazolin. *Antimicrobial Agents and Chemotherapy, 4:* 396-401.
Berk, L.S., Lewis, J.L. and Nelson, J.C. (1974): One-hour radioimmunoassay of serum drug concentrations, as exemplified by digoxin and gentamicin. *Clinical Chemistry, 20:* 1159-1164.
Bertele, R.M. and Marget, W. (1974): Observations made in selected cases on the reversible toxic effects and therapeutic value of chloramphenicol compared with ampicillin and penicilin-G. *Postgraduate Medical Journal, 50,* suppl. 5: 136.
Betzien, G. and Vömel, W. (1969): Pharmacokinetic studies on chloramphenicol. In: *Progress in Antimicrobial and Anticancer Chemotherapy,* pp. 914-924, University of Tokyo.
Binda, G., Domenichini, E., Gottardi, A., Ordandi, B., Ortelli, E., Pacini, B. and Fowst, G. (1971): Rifampicin, a general review. *Arzneimittel-Forschung, 21:* 1907-1977.
Bobrow, S.N., Jaffe, E. and Young, R.C. (1972): Anuria and acute tubular neurosis associated with gentamicin and cephalothin. *Journal of the American Medical Association, 222:* 1546-1547.
Bodey, G.P. (1974): Microbiologic aspects in patients with leukemia. *Human Pathology, 5:* 687-698.
Bodey, G.P., Vallejos, C. and Stewart, D. (1972): Flucloxacillin: a new semisynthetic isoxazolyl penicillin. *Clinical Pharmacology and Therapeutics, 13:* 512-515.
Boe, R.W., Williams, C.P.S., Bennett, J.V. and Oliver, T.K., Jr. (1967): Serum levels of methicillin and ampicillin in newborn and premature infants in relation to postnatal age. *Pediatrics, 39:* 194-201.
Bolt, H.M. (1974): Rifampicin and oral contraception. *Lancet, 1:* 1280.
Boman, G. (1974): Serum concentration and half-life of rifampicin after simultaneous oral administration of aminosalicylic acid or isoniazid. *European Journal of Clinical Pharmacology, 7:* 217-225.
Boman, G. and Malmborg, A.-S. (1974): Rifampicin in plasma and pleural fluid after single oral doses. *European Journal of Clinical Pharmacology, 7:* 51-58.
Boman, G. and Ringberger, V.-A. (1974): Binding of rifampicin by human plasma proteins. *European Journal of Clinical Pharmacology, 7:* 369-373.
Boothman, R., Kerr, M.M., Marshall, M.J. and Burland, W.L. (1973): Absorption and excretion of cephalexin by the newborn infant. *Archives of Disease in Childhood, 48:* 147-150.
Border, W.A., Lehman, D.H., Egan, J.D., Sass, H.J., Glode, J.E. and Wilson, C.B. (1974): Antitubular basement-membrane antibodies in methicillin-associated interstitial nephritis. *New England Journal of Medicine, 291:* 381-384.
Böttiger, L.E. (1974): Drug-induced aplastic anaemia in Sweden with special reference to chloramphenicol. *Postgraduate Medical Journal, 50,* suppl. 5: 127-131.
Bowersox, D.W., Winterbauer, R.H., Stewart, G.L., Orme, B. and Barron, E. (1973): Isoniazid dosage in patients with renal failure. *New England Journal of Medicine, 289:* 84-87.
Bradford Hawley, H. and Cump, D.W. (1973): Vancomycin therapy of bacterial meningitis. *American Journal of Diseases of Children, 126:* 261-264.
Breese, B.B. and Disney, F.A. (1958): Penicillin in the treatment of streptococcal infections: comparison of effectiveness of five different oral and one parenteral form. *New England Journal of Medicine, 259:* 57-62.
Broberger, U. (1973): Determination of glomerular filtration rate in the newborn. *Acta Paediatrica Scandinavica, 62:* 625-629.
Brogard, J.M., Kuntzmann, F., Lavillaureix, J. and Stahl, J. (1970): La céphalexine, nouvelle céphalosporine orale. Résultats d'une étude de pharmacologie humaine. *Thérapeutique, 46:* 315-323.

Brogard, J.M., Haegele, P., Dorner, M. and Lavillaureux, J. (1973): Biliary excretion of a new semisynthetic cephalosporin, cephacetrile. *Antimicrobial Agents and Chemotherapy, 3:* 19-23.
Brogden, R.N., Speight, T.M. and Avery, G.S. (1975a): Amoxycillin: a review of its antibacterial and pharmacokinetic properties and therapeutic use. *Drugs, 9:* 88-140.
Brogden, R.N., Speight, T.M. and Avery, G.S. (1975b): Minocycline: a review of its antibacterial and pharmacokinetic properties and therapeutic use. *Drugs, 9:* 251-291.
Broughall, J.M. and Reeves, D.S. (1975): The acetyltransferase enzyme method for the assay of serum gentamicin concentrations and a comparison with other methods. *Journal of Clinical Pathology, 28:* 140-145.
Brown, J.D., Mathies, A.W., Jr., Ivler, D., Warren, W.S. and Leedom, J.M. (1970): Variable results of cephalothin therapy for meningococcal meningitis. *Antimicrobial Agents and Chemotherapy, 1969:* 432-440.
Bulger, R.J., Lindholm, D.D., Murray, J.S. and Kirby, W.M.M. (1964): Effect of uremia on methicillin and oxacillin blood levels. *Journal of the American Medical Association, 187:* 319-322.
Burton, J.R., Lichtenstein, N.S., Colvin, R.B. and Hyslop, N.E., Jr. (1974): Acute renal failure during cephalothin therapy. *Journal of the American Medical Association, 229:* 679-682.
Cabana, B.E. and Taggart, J.G. (1973): Comparative pharmacokinetics of BB-K8 and kanamycin in dogs and humans. *Antimicrobial Agents and Chemotherapy, 3:* 478-483.
Cahn, M.M., Levy, E.J., Actor, P. and Pauls, J.F. (1974): Comparative serum levels and urinary recovery of cefazolin, cephaloridine, and cephalothin in man. *Journal of Clinical Pharmacology, 14:* 61-66.
Campbell, I.W., Hossack, D.J.N. and Munro, J.F. (1973): Absorption and urinary excretion clindamycin palmitate in the elderly. *Current Medical Research and Opinion, 1:* 369-375.
Carney, S., Butcher, R.A., Dawborn, J.K. and Pattison, G. (1974): Minocycline excretion and distribution in relation to renal function in man. *Clinical Experimental Pharmacology and Physiology, 1:* 299-308.
Carr, W.G.L. (1973): Clindamycin palmitate hydrochloride: a clinical trial in a pediatric office practice. *Current Therapeutic Research, 15:* 630-640.
Carrizosa, J., Levison, M.E. and Kaye, D. (1974): Double-blind comparison of phlebitis produced by cephalothin infusions with buffered and unbuffered diluents. *Antimicrobial Agents and Chemotherapy, 5:* 192-193.
Cattabeni, F. and Gazzaniga, A. (1974: Identification of thiamphenicol excretion products in rat urine using gaschromatography-mass spectometry. *Postgraduate Medical Journal, 50,* suppl. 5: 23-27.
Cattell, W.R. (1974): The management of urinary-tract infection. *The Practitioner, 212:* 27-36.
Cauwenberge, H. Van (1974): Thiamphenicol—clinical and haematological observations. *Postgraduate Medical Journal, 50,* suppl. 5: 142-143.
Ceccarelli, G., Rossoni, R., Romita, F. and Naddeo, A. (1971): Pharmacokinetic study of doxyxycline in children. *Chemotherapy, 16:* 1-10.
Cherubin, C.E., Magazine, D., Hargrove, C., Klopman, A., Stern, L., Purpura, D. and Zapiach, L. (1975): A comparative study of the treatment of presumed pneumococcal pneumonia: parenteral penicillin and clindamycin with continuation on oral therapy. *Current Therapeutic Research, 17:* 88-94.
Chiou, W.L. (1971): Mechanism of increased rates of dissolution and oral absorption of chloramphenicol from chloramphenicol. Urea solid dispersion system. *Journal of Pharmaceutical Sciences, 60:* 1406-1408.

Chisholm, G.D. (1974): The use of gentamicin in urinary tract infections with special reference to drug levels in complicated urological infections. *Postgraduate Medical Journal, 50,* suppl. 7: 23-30.

Chisholm, G.D., Waterworth, P.M., Calnan, J.S. and Garrod, L.P. (1973): Concentration of antibacterial agents in interstitial tissue fluid. *British Medical Journal, 1:* 569-573.

Cimmino, P.T. and Garaci, E. (1973): Livelli tessutali di cefazolina nell 'uomo dopo somministrazione per via parenterale. *Antibiotica, 11:* 31-44.

Clarke, J.T., Libke, R.D., Regamey, C. and Kirby, W.M.M. (1974): Comparative pharmacokinetics of amikacin and kanamycin. *Clinical Pharmacology and Therapeutics, 15:* 610-616.

Cockburn, F., Raeburn, J.A. and MacMillan, G. (1972): Cephalexin and the newborn human infant. *Advances in Antimicrobial and Antineoplastic Chemotherapy, 1:* 103-106.

Cohen, M.D., Raeburn, J.A., Devine, J., Kirkwood, J., Elliott, B., Cockburn, F. and Forfar, J.O. (1975): Pharmacology of some oral penicillins in the newborn infant. *Archives of Disease in Childhood, 50:* 230-234.

Cole, M., Kenig, M.D. and Hewitt, V.A. (1973): Metabolism of penicillins to penicilloic acids and 6-aminopenicillanic acid in man and its significance in assessing penicillin absorption. *Antimicrobial Agents and Chemotherapy, 3:* 463-468.

Cooper, M.J., Anders, M.W. and Mirkin, B.L. (1973): Ion-pair extraction and high-speed liquid chromatography of cephalothin and deacetylcephalothin in human serum and urine. *Drug Metabolism and Disposition, 1:* 659-662.

Cox, C.E. (1973): Pharmacology of carbenicillin indanyl sodium in renal insufficiency. In: *Indanyl Carbenicillin* Proc. Symp. Royal Society of Medicine, pp. 36-42. Excerpta Medica, Amsterdam.

Craig, W.A., Welling, P.G., Jackson, T.C. and Kunin, C.M. (1973): Pharmacology of cefazolin and other cephalosporins in patients with renal insufficiency. *Journal of Infectious Diseases, 128,* suppl.: S347-S353.

Crosson, F.J. (1975): Warning about using cephalothin with central nervous system infections. *Journal of Pediatrics, 86:* 316.

Curci, G., Bergamini, N., Delli Veneri, F., Ninni, A. and Nitti, V. (1972): Half-life of rifampicin after repeated administration of different doses in humans. *Chemotherapy 17:* 373-381.

Curci, G., Claar, E., Bergamini, N., Ninni, A., Claar, G.M., Ascione, A. and Nitti, V. (1973): Studies on blood serum levels of rifampicin in patients with normal and impaired liver function. *Chemotherapy, 19:* 197-205.

Cutler, R.E. and Orme, B.M. (1969): Correlation of serum creatinine concentration and kanamycin half-life. Therapeutic implications. *Journal of the American Medical Association, 209:* 539-542.

Dacey, R.G. and Sande, M.A. (1974): Effect of probenecid on cerebrospinal fluid concentrations of penicillin and cephalosporin derivatives. *Antimicrobial Agents and Chemotherapy, 6:* 437-441.

Daigneault, R., Gagné, M. and Brazeau, M. (1974): A comparison of two methods of gentamicin assay: an enzymatic procedure and an agar diffusion technique. *Journal of Infectious Diseases, 130:* 642-645.

Dans, P.E., McGehee, R.F., J.R., Wilcox, C. and Finland, M. (1970): Rifampicin: antibacterial activity in vitro and absorption and excretion in normal young men. *American Journal of the Medical Sciences, 259:* 120-132.

Daschner, F. and Marget, W. (1973): Erfordert die Intensivpflegestation eine spezielle Chemotherapie? *Klinische Pediatrie,* suppl. 70: 108-109.

Dawes, G.S. (1973): Antibiotic levels in tissue fluid. *British Medical Journal, 1:* 798.

DeHaan, R.M., Metzler, C.M., Schellenberg, D. and Vandenborsch, W.D. (1973): Pharmacokinetic studies of clindamycin phosphate. *Journal of Clinical Pharmacology and New Drugs, 13:* 190-209.
DeHaan, R.M., Metzler, C.M., Schellenberg, D., Vandenbosch, W.D. and Masson, E.L. (1972): Pharmacokinetic studies of clindamycin hydrochloride in humans. *International Journal of Clinical Pharmacology, 6:* 105-119.
DeHaan, R.M. and Schellenberg, D. (1972): Clindamycin palmitate flavored granules. Multidose tolerance, absorption, and urinary excretion. *Journal of Clinical Pharmacology and New Drugs, 12:* 74-83.
Deodhar, S.D., Russel, F., Carson Dick, W., Nuki, G. and Watson Buchanan, W. (1972): Penetration of lincomycin ("Lindocin") and clindamycin ("Dalacin C"). In the synovial cavity in rheumatoid arthritis. *Current Medical Research and Opinion, 1:* 108-115.
De Rautlin de la Roy, Y., Beauchant, G. and Brenil, K. (1971): Diminution du taux sérique de rifampicine par le phénobarbital. *Presse Medicale, 79:* 350.
De Raulin de la Roy, Y., Hoppeler, A., Creuset, G. and Brault, A.M. (1974): Taux de rifampicine dans le serum et le liquide cephalo-rachidien chez l'enfant. *Archives Francaises de Pediatrie, 31:* 477-488.
Dettli, L. and Spring, P. (1974): The dosage regimen of thiamphenicol in patients with kidney disease. *Postgraduate Medical Journal, 50,* suppl. 5: 32-35.
Diamant, M. and Diamant, B. (1974): Abuse and timing of use of antibiotics in acute otitis media. *Archives of Otolaryngology, 100:* 226-232.
Dimitrov, N.V. and Nodine, J.H. (eds) (1974): *Drugs and Hematologic Reactions,* the 29th Hahnemann Symposium, Grune & Stratton, New York.
Discussion (1971): *Journal of Infectious Diseases, 124,* suppl.: S259-S263.
Dittert, L.W., Griffen, W.O., Jr., LaPiana, J.C., Shainfeld, F.J. and Doluisio, J.T. (1970): Pharmacokinetic interpretation of penicillin levels in serum and urine after intravenous administration. *Antimicrobial Agents and Chemotherapy, 1969:* 42-48.
Dixon, R.L., Owens, E.S. and Rall, D.P. (1969): Evidence of active transport of benzyl-^{14}C-penicillin from cerebrospinal fluid to blood. *Journal of Pharmaceutical Sciences, 58:* 1106-1109.
Doluisio, J.T., Dittert, L.W. and LaPiana, J.C. (1973): Pharmacokinetics of kanamycin following intramuscular administration. *Journal of Pharmacokinetics and Biopharmaceutics, 1:* 253-265.
Doluisio, J.T. and Dittert, L.W. (1969): Influence of repetitive dosing of tetracyclines on biologic half-life in serum. *Clinical Pharmacology and Therapeutics, 10:* 690-701.
Doluisio, J.T., LaPiana, J.C., Wilkinson, G.R. and Dittert, L.W. (1970): Pharmacokinetic interpretation of dicloxacillin levels in serum after extravascular administration. *Antimicrobial Agents and Chemotherapy, 1969:* 49-55.
Donnison, A.B. and Davison, C.E. (1970): Cephalexin in paediatric infections. *Postgraduate Medical Journal, 46,* suppl: 93-95.
Driessen, J.H. (1975): A computer study of bacterial resistance patterns to antibiotics. *Chemotherapy, 21,* suppl. 1: 36-46.
Dugal, R., Brodeur, J. and Caillé, G. (1974): Ampicillin systemic bioavailability: the influence of dosage form. *Journal of Clinical Pharmacology, 14:* 513-519.
Eastwood, J.B. and Gower, P.E. (1974): A study of the pharmacokinetics of clindamycin in normal subjects and patients with chronic renal failure. *Postgraduate Medical Journal, 50:* 710-712.
Editorial (1974a); Antibiotics for disease. *Lancet, 2:* 1054-1055.
Editorial (1973): Cephalosporins, present and future. *Lancet, 2:* 364-365.
Editorial (1969): New drugs against tuberculosis. *Lancet, 1:* 1081-1082.
Editorial (1974b): Serum-gentamicin. *Lancet, 2:* 1185.

Edmunds, P.N. and Heddle, A.C. (1974): Rapid assay of gentamicin. *Lancet, 2:* 526-527.
Edwards, O.M., Courtenay-Evans, R.J., Galley, J.M., Hunter, J. and Tait, A.D. (1974); Changes in cortisol metabolism following rifampicin therapy. *Lancet, 2:* 549-551.
Ehrnebo, M., Agurell, S., Jalling, B. and Boréus, L.O. (1971): Age differences in drug binding by plasma proteins: studies on human foetuses, neonates and adults. *European Journal of Clinical Pharmacology, 3:* 189-193.
Eichenwald, H.F. (1966): Some observations on dosage and toxicity of kanamycin in premature and full-term infants. *Annals of the New York Academy of Sciences, 132:* 984-991.
Eidus, L. and Hodgkins, M.M. (1973): Screening of isoniazid inactivators. *Antimicrobial Agents and Chemotherapy, 3:* 130-133.
Eidus, l., Hodgkin, M.M., Hsu, A.H.E. and Schaefer, O. (1974b): Pharmacokinetic studies with an isoniazid slow-releasing matrix preparation. *American Review of Respiratory Diseases, 110:* 34-42.
Eidus, L., Pollak, B., Haragoz, A. and Hodgkin, M.M. (1974a): La chimiothérapie intermittente de la tuberculose: une étude des problèmes impliqués et compte rendu des contributions faites récemment au Canada. *L'Union Medicale du Canada, 103:* 1271-1274.
Eneroth, C.M., Lundberg, C. and Wretlind, B. (1975): Antibiotic conentrations in maxillary sinus secretions and in the sinus mucosa. *Chemotherapy, 21,* suppl. 1: 1-7.
Ericsson, H. and Malmborg, A.-S. (1973): A micromethod for determination of antibiotic concentrations in body fluids. *Acta Pathologica et Microbiologica Scandinavica,* suppl. 241: 107-109.
Erill, S., Du Souich, P. and Garcia-Sevilla, J.A. (1974a): Chloramphenicol. *Lancet, 1:* 1281.
Erill, S., Du Souich, P. and Garcia-Sevilla, J.A. (1974b): Chloramphenicol-containing drugs. *Journal of Clinical Pharmacology and New Drugs, 14:* 172-175.
Ezer, G. and Soothill, J.F. (1974): Intracellular bactericidal effects of rifampicin in both normal and chronic granulomatous disease polymorphs. *Archives of Disease in Childhood, 49:* 463-466.
Feigin, R.D., Keeney, R.E., Nusrala, J., Shackelford, P.G. and Lins, R.D. (1973): Efficacy of clindamycin therapy for otitis media. *Archives of Otolaryngology, 98:* 27-31.
Ferrari, V. and Dela Bella, D. (1974): Comparison of chloramphenicol and thiamphenicol metabolism. *Postgraduate Medical Journal, 50,* suppl. 5: 17-22.
Fiedelman, W. (1974). Sensitivity of "pseudomonas aeruginosa" to carbenicillin: an evaluation and susceptibility testing after four years of clinical usage. *Current Therapeutic Research, 16:* 1287-1295.
Finland, M. (1973): Superinfections in the antibiotic era. *Postgraduate Medicine, 54:* 175-182.
Finland, M. (1974): Twenty-fifth anniversary of the discovery of aureomycin: the place of the tetracyclines in antimicrobial therapy. *Clinical Pharmacology and Therapeutics, 15:* 3-8.
Flax, M.H. (1974): Drug-induced autoimmunity. *New England Journal of Medicine, 291:* 414-415.
Fleurette, J., Renaud, F. and Flandrois, J.-P. (1973): Diffusion de la gentamicine dans l'organisme. *Gazette Médicale de France,* special issues, 95-102.
Forist, A.A., DeHaan, R.M. and Metzler, C.M. (1973): Clindamycin bioavailability from clindamycin-2-palmitate and clindamycin-2-hexadecylcarbonate in man. *Journal of Pharmacokinetics and Biopharmaceutics, 1:* 89-98.
Forsgren, A. and Gnarpe, H. (1973a): Tetracycline interference with the bactericidal effect of serum. *Nature/New Biology, 244:* 82-83.
Forsgren, A. and Gnarpe, H. (1973b): Tetracyclines and host-defense mechanisms. *Antimicrobial Agents and Chemotherapy, 3:* 711-715.

Fossieck, B., Jr. and Parker, R.H. (1974): Neurotoxicity during intravenous infusion of penicillin. A review. *Journal of Clinical Pharmacology, 14:* 504-512.
Franco, J.A., Eitzman, D.V. and Baer, H. (1973): Antibiotic usage and microbial resistance in an intensive care nursery. *American Journal of Diseases of Children, 126:* 381-321.
Frigerio, G. (1974): Thiamphenicol in the treatment of typhoid fever. A controlled doubleblind trial in comparison with chloramphenicol. *Postgraduate Medical Journal, 50,* suppl. 5: 146.
Galioto, G.B., Grassi, C., Manara, G. and Santarelli, P. (1974): Studies on tolerance and blood levels of gentamicin in old subjects. *International Journal of Clinical Pharmacology, 10:* 95-100.
Ganshorn, A. and Kurz, H. (1968): Unterschiede zwischen der Proteinbindung Neugeborener und Erwachsener und ihre Bedeutung für die pharmakologische Wirkung. *Naunyn-Schmiedeberg's Archiv für Pharmakologie und Experimentelle Pathologie, 260:* 117-118.
Garcia de Olarte, D., Trujillo, H., Agudelo, N., Nelson, J.D. and Haltalin, K.C. (1974): Treatment of diarrhea in malnourished infants and children. A double-blind study comparing ampicillin and placebo. *American Journal of Diseases of Children, 127:* 379-388.
Gardner, P. (1974): Antimicrobial drug therapy in pediatric practice. *Pediatric Clinics of North America, 21:* 617-648.
Garfield, E. (1974): Journal citation studies. IX. Highly cited pediatric journals and articles. *Current Contents, 17:* n. 29, 5.
Garfunkel, J.M. (1971): Use of gentamicin in newborn infants. *Journal of Infectious Diseases, 124,* suppl.: S247-S248.
Garrod, L.P. (1974): Choice among penicillins and cephalosporins. *British Medical Journal, 3:* 96-100.
Garrod, L.P., Lambert, H.P., and O'Grady, F. (1973): *Antibiotic and Chemotherapy,* 4th ed. Churchill Livingstone, Edinburgh.
Garrod, L.P. and Waterworth, P.M. (1971): A study of antibiotic sensitivity testing with proposals for simple uniform methods. *Journal of Clinical Pathology, 24:* 779-789.
Gartmann, J. (1975): Doxycycline concentrations in lung tissue, bronchial wall, and bronchial secretions. *Chemotherapy, 21,* suppl. 1: 19-26.
Gavan, T.L. (1974): In vitro antimicrobial susceptibility testing. Clinical implications and limitations. *Medical Clinics of North America, 58:* 493-503.
Geddes, A.M., Goodall, J.A.D., Speirs, C.F., Gillett, A.P., Andrews, J. and Williams, J.D. (1974): Clinical and laboratory studies with tobramycin. *Chemotherapy, 20:* 245-256.
Geddes, A.M. and Williams, J.D. (eds.) (1973): *Current Antibiotic Therapy,* Churchill Livingstone, Edinburgh.
Gelber, R., Jacobsen, P. and Levy, L. (1969): A study of the availability of six commercial formulations of isoniazid. *Clinical Pharmacology and Therapeutics, 10:* 841-848.
George, R.H., Bint, A.J. and Prangnell, D.R. (1974): Serum gentamicin levels after intravenous bolus injection. *Lancet, 1:* 576-577.
Gibaldi, M. and Perrier, D. (1972): Drug distribution and renal failure. *Journal of Clinical Pharmacology, 12:* 201-204.
Gibaldi, M. and Schwartz, M.A. (1968): Apparent effect of probenecid on the distribution of penicillins in man. *Clinical Pharmacology and Therapeutics, 9:* 345-349.
Gingell, J.C., Chisholm, G.D., Calnan, J.S. and Waterworth, P.M. (1969): The dose, distribution and excretion of gentamicin with special reference to renal failure. *Journal of Infectious Diseases, 119:* 396-401.
Girdwood, R.H. (ed.) (1973): *Blood Disorders due to Drugs and Other Agents.* Excerpta Medica, Amsterdam.

Giusti, D.L. (1973): A review of the clinical use of antimicrobial agents in patients with renal and hepatic insufficiency. I. The penicillins. *Drug Intelligence and Clinical Pharmacy, 7:* 62-74.

Glazko, A.J., Kinkel, A.W., Alegnani, W.C. and Holmes, E.L. (1968): An evaluation of the absorption characteristics of different chloramphenicol preparations in normal human subjects. *Clinical Pharmacology and Therapeutics, 9:* 472-483.

Goble, F.C. (1975): Sex as a factor in metabolism, toxicity, and efficacy of pharmacodynamic and chemotherapeutic agents. *Advances in Pharmacology and Chemotherapy,* in press.

Gold, J.A., McKee, J.J. and Ziv, D.S. (1973): Experience with cefazolin: an overall summary of pharmacologic and clinical trials in man. *Journal of Infectious Diseases, 128,* suppl.: S415-S421.

Gorbach, S.L. and Bartlett, J.G. (1974): Anaerobic infections: old myths and new realities. *Journal of Infectious Diseases, 130:* 307-310.

Gordon, R.C., Regamey, C. and Kirby, W.M.M. (1973): Serum protein binding of erythromycin, lincomycin, and clindamycin. *Journal of Pharmaceutical Sciences, 62:* 1074-1077.

Gower, P.E. and Dash, C.H. (1969): Cephalexin: human studies of absorption and excretion of a new cephalosporin antibiotic. *British Journal of Pharmacology, 37:* 738-747.

Gravenkemper, C.F., Bennett, J.V., Brodie, J.L. and Kirby, W.M.M. (1965): Dicloxacillin. In vitro and pharmacologic comparisons with oxacillin and cloxacillin. *Archives of Internal Medicine, 116:* 340-345.

Griffith, R.S. (1974): Ten years of cephalosporins. *International Journal of Clinical Pharmacology, 8:* 6-20.

Griffith, R.S. and Black, H.R. (1970): Cephalexin. *Medical Clinics of North America, 54:* 1229-1244.

Griffith, R.S. and Black, H.R. (1971): Blood, urine and tissue concentrations of the cephalosporin antibiotics in normal subjects. *Postgraduate Medical Journal,* suppl.: 32-40.

Grossman, M. and Ticknor, W. (1966): Serum levels of ampicillin, cephalothin, cloxacillin, and nafcillin in the newborn infant. *American Society for Microbiology, 1965:* 214-219.

Gyselynck, A.-M., Forrey, A. and Cutler, R. (1971): Pharmacokinetics of gentamicin: distribution and plasma and renal clearance. *Journal of Infectious Diseases, 124,* suppl.: S70-S76.

Halprin, G.M. and McMahon, S.M. (1973): Cephalexin concentrations in sputum during acute respiratory infections. *Antimicrobial Agents in Chemotherapy, 3:* 703-707.

Hamilton-Miller, J.M.T. and Brumfitt, W. (1974): Whither the cephalosporins? *Journal of Infectious Diseases, 130:* 81-84.

Hamilton-Miller, J.M.T., Reynolds, A.V. and Brumfitt, W. (1974): Apparent emergence of gentamicin-resistant providencia stuartii during therapy with gentamicin. *Lancet, 2:* 527.

Hansen, I., Jacobsen, E. and Weis, J. (1975): Pharmacokinetics of sulbenicillin, a new broad-spectrum semisynthetic penicillin. *Clinical Pharmacology and Therapeutics, 17:* 339-347.

Harnack, G.A. Von (1971): Probleme der Antibiotica-Dosierung. *Monatsschrift für Kinderheilkunde, 119:* 120-123.

Harrod, J.R. and Stevens, D.A. (1974): Anaerobic infections in the newborn infant. *Journal of Pediatrics, 85:* 399-402.

Hart, A., Barber, H.E. and Calvey, T.N. (1975): Bioavailability and dissolution of different formulations of oxytetracycline preparations. *British Journal of Clinical Pharmacology, 2:* 277-280.

Hausmann, K. and Skrandies, G. (1974): Aplastic anaemia following chloramphenicol therapy in Hamburg and surrounding districts. *Postgraduate Medical Journal, 50,* suppl. 5: 131-136.

Hawley, H.B., Lewis, R.M., Schwartz, D.R. and Gump, D.W. (1974): Tobramycin therapy of pulmonary infections in patients with cystic fibrosis. *Current Therapeutic Research, 16:* 414-418.
Hellriegel, K.P. and Gross, R. (1974): Follow-up studies in chloramphenicol-induced aplastic anaemia. *Postgraduate Medical Journal, 50,* suppl. 5: 136-142.
Hellström, K., Rosén, A. and Swahn, Å. (1974a): Absorption and decomposition of potassium-35S-phenoxymethyl penicillin. *Clinical Pharmacology and Therapeutics, 16:* 826-833.
Helström, K., Rosén, A. and Swahn, Å. (1974b): Fate of oral 35S-cloxacillin in man. *European Journal of Clinical Pharmacology, 7:* 125-131.
Helwig, H., Kunz, H. and Hueppchen, Ch. (1972): Effectiveness and tolerance of cephalexin in children. *Zeitschrift für Kinderheilkunde, 111:* 307-314.
Henri, A., Daneau, A. and Klastersky, J. (1973): Emergence of bacteria resistant to gentamicin. *International Journal of Clinical Pharmacology, 8:* 216-221.
Herz, G. and Gfeller, J. (1975): Vibramycin in paediatrics. An evaluation of the onset of action and efficacy. *Chemotherapy, 21,* suppl. 1: 58-67.
Hewitt, W.L. (1973a): The cephalosporins—1973. *Journal of Infectious Diseases, 128,* suppl.: S312-S319.
Hewitt, W.L. (1973b): Reflections on the clinical pharmacology of gentamicin. *Acta Pathologica et Microbiologica Scandinavica,* section B, *81,* suppl. 241: 151-156.
Hewitt, W.L. (1974): Gentamicin: toxicity in perspective. *Postgraduate Medical Journal, 50,* suppl. 7: 55-59.
Hierholzer, G., Linzenmeier, G., Kleining, R. and Hörster, G. (1974): Vergleichende Untersuchungen über die Konzentration von Cephacetril und Cephalotin im normalen und chronisch entzüdeten Knochengewebe. *Arzneimittel Forschung, 24:* 1501-1504.
Hodges, G.R. and Perkins, R.L. (1973): Carbenicillin indanyl sodium oral therapy of urinary tract infections. *Archives of Internal Medicine, 131:* 679-681.
Hodson, A.H. and Holloway, W.J. (1974): Cephacetrile. A new cephalosporin antibiotic. *Arzneimittel Forschung, 24:* 1507-1510.
Höffler, D., Koeppe, P., Fiegel, P., Hölzel, D., Ringelmann, R., Goeschel, U. and Palmer, W.-W.-R. (1974): Zur Pharmakokinetik des Carbenicillins bei hoher Dosierung. *Deutsche Medizinische Wochenschrift, 99:* 399-403.
Hoffman, T.A., Cestero, R. and Bullock, W.E. (1970): Pharmacokinetics of carbenicillin in patients with hepatic and renal failure. *Journal of Infectious Diseases, 122,* suppl.: S75-S77.
Holloway, W.J. and Taylor, W.A. (1973): Long-term oral carbenicillin therapy in complicated urinary-tracts infections. *Journal of Infectious Diseases, 127,* suppl.: S143-S145.
Holmes, R.K., Minshew, B.H. and Sanford, J.P. (1974): Resistance of pseudomonas aeruginosa to aminoglycoside antibiotics. *Journal of Infectious Diseases, 130,* suppl.: S163-S165.
Holmes, R.K. and Sanford, J.P. (1974): Enzymatic assay for gentamicin and related aminoglycoside antibiotics. *Journal of Infectious Diseases, 129:* 519-527.
Howell, A., Sutherland, R. and Rolinson, G.N. (1972): Effect of protein binding on levels of ampicillin and cloxacillin in synovial fluid. *Clinical Pharmacology and Therapeutics, 13:* 724-732.
Huang, N.N. and High, R.H. (1953): Comparison of serum levels following the administration of oral and parenteral preparations of penicillin to infants and children of various age group. *Journal of Pediatrics, 42:* 667-668.
Ironside, A.G. (1974): Gastroenteritis of infancy. In: *A New Look at Infectious Diseases,* British Medical Association, London.
Ishiyama, S., Nakayama, I., Iwamoto, H., Iwai, S., Takatori, M., Kawabe, T., Sakata, I., Natsuno, T. and Akieda, Y. (1973): Clindamycin-2-palmitate: absorption and excretion, and clinical use in surgery. *Japanese Journal of Antibiotics, 26:* 381-388.

Ito, T. (1970): Studies on the absorption and excretion of gentamicin in newborn infants. *Japanese Journal of Antibiotics, 23:* 298-311.
Iwainsky, H., Winsel, K., Werner, E. and Eule, H. (1974): On the pharmacokinetics of rifampicin. I. Influence of dosage and duration of treatment with intermittent administration. *Scandinavian Journal of Respiratory Diseases, 55:* 229-236.
Jackson, G.G. (1967): Gentamycin. *Practitioner, 198:* 855-866.
Jackson, G.G. and Arcieri, G. (1971): Ototoxicity of gentamicin in man: a survey and controlled analysis of clinical experience in the United States. *Journal of Infectious Diseases, 124,* suppl.: S130-S137.
Jackson, G.G., Lolans, V.T. and Gallegos, B.G. (1973): Comparative activity of bacterial lactamases on penicillins and cephalosporins. *Journal of Infectious Diseases, 128,* suppl.: S327-S334.
Jackson, H. (1973): Prevention of rheumatic fever. A comparative study of clindamycin palmitate and ampicillin in the treatment of group A Beta hemolytic streptococcal pharyngitis. *Clinical Pediatrics, 12:* 501-503.
Jaffe, G., Ravreby, W., Meyers, B.R. and Hirschman, S.Z. (1974): Clinical study of the use of the new aminoglycoside tobramycin for therapy of infections due to gram-negative bacteria. *Antimicrobial Agents in Chemotherapy, 5:* 75-81.
Jaffe, J.M., Colaizzi, J.L., Poust, R.I. and McDonald, R.H., Jr. (1973): Effect of altered urinary pH on tetracycline and doxycycline excretion in humans. *Journal of Pharmacokinetics and Biopharmaceutics, 1:* 267-282.
Jalling, B., Malmborg, A.-S., Lindman, A. and Boréus, L.O. (1972): Evaluation of a micromethod for determination of antibiotic concentrations in plasma. *European Journal of Clinical Pharmacology, 4:* 150-157.
Jawetz, E. (1975): Combined actions of antimicrobial drugs. In: *Concepts in Biochemical Pharmacology,* edited by J.R. Gillette and J.R. Mitchell, pp. 343-358, Handbook of Experimental Pharmacology, V. 28, pt. III, Springer-Verlag, Berlin.
Jezequel, A.M., Orlandi, F. and Tenconi, L.T. (1971): Changes of the smooth endoplasmic reticulum induced by rifampicin in human and guinea-pig hepatocytes. *Gut, 12:* 984-987.
Johnson, B.L., Jr., Mandiola, S. and Dahlgren, J. (1974): Effects of administration of hydrocortisone on the renal and biliary excretion of ampicillin in the dog. *Journal of Infectious Diseases, 129:* 37-44.
Joshi, A.M. and Stein, R.M. (1974): Altered serum clearances of intravenously administered clindamycin phosphate in patients with uremia. *Journal of Clinical Pharmacology, 14:* 140-144.
Jusko, W.J. and Lewis, G.P. (1973): Comparison of ampicillin and hetacillin pharmacokinetics in man. *Journal of Pharmaceutical Sciences, 62:* 69-76.
Jusko, W.J. and Lewis, G.P. (1975): Pharmacokinetics of ampicillin in cirrhotic subjects. *Clinical Pharmacology and Therapeutics, 17:* 237.
Jusko, W.J., Lewis, G.P. and Schmitt, G.W. (1973): Ampicillin and hetacillin pharmacokinetics in normal and anephric subjects. *Clinical Pharmacology and Therapeutics, 14:* 90-99.
Kahlmeter, G. and Kamme, C. (1975): Prolonged excretion of gentamicin in a patient with unimpaired renal function. *Lancet, 1:* 286.
Kampmann, J., Mølholm Hansen, J. Siersbaek-Nielsen, K. and Laursen, H. (1972): Effect of some drugs on penicillin half-life in blood. *Clinical Pharmacology and Therapeutics, 13:* 516-519.
Kampmann, J., Lindahl, F., Mølholm Hansen, J. and Sierbaek-Nielsen, K. (1973): Effect of probenecid on the excretion of ampicillin in human bile. *British Journal of Pharmacology, 47:* 782-786.

Kaplan, J.M. and McCracken, G.H., Jr. (1973): Clinical pharmacology of benzathine penicillin G in neonates with regard to its recommended use in congenital syphilis. *Journal of Pediatrics, 82:* 1069-1072.
Kaplan, J.M., McCracken, G.H., Jr., Thomas, M.L., Horton, L.J. and Davis, N. (1973): Clinical pharmacology of tobramycin in newborns. *American Journal of Diseases of Children, 125:* 656-660.
Kaplan, J.M., McCracken, G.H., Jr., Horton, L.J., Thomas, M.L. and Davis, N. (1974a): Pharmacologic studies in neonates given large doses of ampicillin. *Journal of Pediatrics, 84:* 571-577.
Kaplan, J.M., McCracken, G.H., Jr. and Culbertson, M.C. (1974b): Penicillin and erythromycin concentrations in tonsils. *American Journal of Diseases of Children, 127:* 206-211.
Karney, W.W., Turck, M. and Holmes, K.K. (1974): Comparative therapeutic and pharmacological evaluation of amoxicillin and ampicillin plus probenecid for the treatment of gonorrhea. *Antimicrobial Agents and Chemotherapy, 5:* 114-118.
Kauffman, R.E., Shoeman, D.W., Han Wan, S. and Azarnoff, D.L. (1973): Absorption and excretion of clindamycin-2-phosphate in children after intramuscular injection. *Clinical Pharmacology and Therapeutics, 13:* 704-709.
Kaye, D., Levison, M.E. and Labovitz, E.D. (1974): The unpredictability of serum concentrations of gentamicin: pharmacokinetics of gentamicin in patients with normal and abnormal renal function. *Journal of Infectious Diseases, 130:* 150-154.
Kazemi, M., Gumpert, T.G. and Marks, M.I. (1973): A controlled trial comparing sulfamethoxazole-trimethoprim, ampicillin, and no therapy in the treatment of salmonella gastroenteritis in children. *Journal of Pediatrics, 83:* 646-650.
Keay, A.J., Syme, J. and Barnes, P.M. (1967): Cephaloridine in the treatment of prophylaxis of infection in the newborn. *Postgraduate Medicine, 43,* suppl.: 105-109.
Keiser, G. (1974a): Introduction. *Postgraduate Medical Journal, 50,* suppl. 5: 13-15.
Keiser, G. (1974b): Cooperative study of patients treated with thiamphenicol. Comparative study of patients treated with chloramphenicol and thiamphenicol. *Postgraduate Medical Journal, 50,* suppl. 5: 143-145.
Kenwright, S. and Levi, A.J. (1973): Impairment of hepatic uptake of rifamycin antibiotics by probenecid, and its therapeutic implications. *Lancet, 2:* 1401-1405.
Khan, A.J. (1973): Clinical and laboratory evaluation of cefazolin: a new celphalosporin antibiotic in pediatrics patients. *Current Therapeutic Research, 15:* 727-733.
Kind, A.C., Tupasi, T.E., Standiford, H.C. and Kriby, W.M.M. (1970): Mechanisms responsible for plasma levels of nafcillin lower than those of oxacillin. *Archives of Internal Medicine, 125:* 685-690.
Kirby, W.M.M. and Kind, A.C. (1967): Clinical pharmacology of ampicillin and hetacillin. *Annals of the New York Academy of Sciences, 145:* 291-297.
Kirby, W.M.M. and Regamey, C. (1973): Pharmacokinetics of cefazolin compared with four other cephalosporins. *Journal of Infectious Diseases, 128,* suppl.: S341-S346.
Klastersky, J., Daneau, D. and de Maertelaer, V. (1973a): Comparative study of tobramycin and gentamicin with special reference to anti-pseudomonas activity. *Clinical Pharmacology and Therapeutics, 14:* 104-111.
Klastersky, J., Daneau, D., Swings, G. and Weerts, D. (1974a): Antibacterial activity in serum and urine as a therapeutic guide in bacterial infections. *Journal of Infectious Diseases, 129:* 187-193.
Klastersky, J., Henri, A., Hensgens, C., Vandenborre, L. and Daneau, D. (1973b): Antipseudomonal drugs: comparative study of gentamicin, sisomicin and tobramycin "in vitro" and in human volunteers. *European Journal of Cancer, 9:* 641-648.
Klastersky, J., Hengrens, C., Gerard, M. and Daneau, D. (1975b): Sisomicin: bacteriological and clinical evaluation. *Journal of Clinical Pharmacology, 15:* 252-261.

Klastersky, J., Huymans, E., Weerts, D., Hensgens, C. and Daneau, D. (1974b): Endotracheally administered gentamicin for the prevention of infections of the respiratory tract in patients with tracheostomy: a double-blind study. *Chest, 65:* 650-654.
Klastersky, J., Nyamubeya, B. and Vanderborre, L. (1974c): Antimicrobial effectiveness of kanamycin, aminosidin, BB-K8, sisomicin, gentamicin and tobramycin combined with carbenicillin or cephalothin against gram-negative rods. *Journal of Medical Microbiology, 7:* 465-472.
Klastersky, J., Odio, W. and Hensgens, C. (1975a): Comparison of amikacin and gentamicin. *Clinical Pharmacology and Therapeutics, 17:* 348-354.
Klein, J.O. (1974): Current usage of antimicrobial combinations in pediatrics. *Pediatric Clinics of North America, 21:* 443-456.
Klein, J.O., Schaberg, M.J., Buncin, M. and Gezon, H.M. (1973): Levels of penicillin in serum of newborn infants after single intramuscular doses of benzathine penicillin G. *Journal of Pediatrics, 82:* 1065-1068.
Kleinknecht, D., Ganeval, D. and Droz, D. (1973): Acute renal failure after high doses of gentamicin and cephalothin. *Lancet, 1:* 1129.
Knirsch, A.K., Hobbs, D.C. and Korst, J.J. (1973): Pharmacokinetics, toleration, and safety of indanyl carbenicillin in man. *Journal of Infectious Diseases, 127,* suppl.: S105-S108.
Knittle, M.A., Eitzman, D.V. and Baer, H. (1975): Role of hand contamination of personnel in the epidemiology of gram-negative nosocomial infections. *Journal of Pediatrics, 86:* 433-437.
Kobayashi, Y., Akaishi, K., Tamura, T., Nishio, T., Kanenari, S., Kobayashi, Y., Ito, H. and Kono, A. (1970): Clinical studies on cefazolin in pediatric field. *Chemotherapy, 18:* 695-702.
Koch-Weser, D. (1970): Rifampicin. New hope in the fight against tuberculosis. *New England Journal of Medicine, 283:* 655-656.
Korkeila, J. (1971): Antianabolic effect of tetracyclines. *Lancet, 1,:* 974-975.
Kosmidis, J., Williams, J.D., Andrews, J., Goodall, J.A.D. and Geddes, A.M. (1972): Amoxycillin-pharmacology, bacteriology and clinical studies. *British Journal of Clinical Practice, 26:* 341-346.
Kretchmer, N. (1975): Perinatal pharmacology: an introduction. In: *Basic and Therapeutic Aspects of Perinatal Pharmacology,* edited by P.L. Morselli, S. Garattini and F. Sereni, pp. 1-6, Raven Press, New York.
Krishna, G. (1974): Covalent binding of drugs to tissue macromolecules as a biochemical mechanism of drug toxicities with special emphasis on chloramphenicol and thiamphenicol. *Postgraduate Medical Journal, 50,* suppl. 5: 73-77.
Krishna, G. and Bonanomi, L. (1974): Covalent binding of chloramphenicol as a biochemical basis for chloramphenicol-induced bone marrow damage. In: *Drug Interactions,* edited by P.L. Morselli, S. Garattini, and S.N. Cohen, pp. 173-180, Raven Press, New York.
Kuck, N.A. and Forbes, M. (1973): Uptake of minocycline and tetracycline by tetracycline-susceptible and resistant bacteria. *Antimicrobial Agents and Chemotherapy, 3:* 662-664.
Kunin, C.M. (1966): Absorption, distribution, excretion and fate of kanamycin. *Annals of the New York Academy of Sciences, 132:* 811-818.
Kunin, C.M. (1967): Clinical significance of protein binding of the pencillins. *Annals of the New York Academy of Sciences, 145:* 282-290.
Kunin, C.M. (1974): Blood level measurements and antimicrobial agents. *Clinical Pharmacology and Therapeutics, 16:* 251-256.
Kunin, C.M. (1975): Urinary tract infections in infancy. *Journal of Pediatrics, 87:* 483-484.
Kuning, C.M., Craig, W.A., Kornguth, M. and Monson, R. (1973): Influence of binding on the pharmacologic activity of antibiotics. *Annals of the New York Academy of Sciences, 226:* 214-224.

Kunin, C.M. and Finland, M. (1959): Persistence of antibiotics in blood of patients with acute renal failure. III. Penicillin, streptomycin, ethromycin and kanamycin. *Journal of Clinical Investigation, 38:* 1509-1519.

Kunin, C.M., Glazko, A.J. and Finland, M. (1959): Persistence of antibiotics in the blood of patients with acute and renal failure. II. *Journal of Clinical Investigation, 38:* 1498-1508.

Kuwahara, S., Mine, Y. and Nishida, M. (1970): Immunogenicity of cefazolin. *Antimicrobial Agents and Chemotherapy, 10:* 374-379.

Lacey, R.W. (1975): Antibiotic resistance plasmids of "staphylococcus aureus" and their clinical importance. *Bacteriological Reviews, 39:* 1-32.

Lal, S., Singhal, S.N., Burley, D.M. and Crossley, G. (1972): Effect of rifampicin and isoniazid on liver function. *British Medical Journal, 1:* 148-150.

Ledger, W.J., Kriewall, T.J., Sweet, R.L. and Fekety, F.R., Jr. (1974): The use of parenteral clindamycin in the treatment of obstetric-gynecologic patients with severe infections. *Obstetrics and Gynecology, 43:* 490-497.

Leibowitz, B.J., Hakes, J.L., Cahn, M.M. and Levy, E.J. (1972): Doxycycline blood levels in normal subjects after intravenous and oral administration. *Current Therapeutic Research, 14:* 820-832.

Levison, M.E., Levison, S.P., Ries, K. and Kaye, D. (1973): Pharmacology of cefazolin in patients with normal and abnormal renal function. *Journal of Infectious Diseases, 128,* suppl.: S354-S357.

Levy, G. (1967): Effect of bed rest on distribution and elimination of drugs. *Journal of Pharmaceutical Sciences, 56:* 928-929.

Libke, R.D., Clarke, J.T., Ralph, E.D., Luthy, R.P. and Kirby, W.M.M. (1975): Ticarcillin vs. carbenicillin: clinical pharmacokinetics. *Clinical Pharmacology and Therapeutics, 17:* 441-446.

Libke, R.D., Regamey, C., Clarke, J.T. and Kirby, W.M.M. 1973): Synergism of carbenicillin and gentamicin against enterococci. *Antimicrobial Agents and Chemotherapy, 4:* 564-568.

Lifschitz, M.I. and Denning, C.R. (1970): Safety of kanamycin aerosol. *Clinical Pharmacology and Therapeutics, 12:* 91-95.

Lindberg, A.A., Nilsson, L.H., Bucht, H. and Kallings, L.O. (1966): Concentration of chloramphenicol in the urine and blood in relation to renal function. *British Medical Journal, 2:* 724-728.

Lockwood, W.R. and Bower, J.D. (1973): Tobramycin and gentamicin concentrations in the serum of normal and anephric patients. *Antimicrobial Agents and Chemotherapy, 3:* 125-129.

Lode, H., Gebert, S. and Hendrischk, A. (1975): Comparative pharmacokinetics and clinical experience with a new cephalosporins derivative: cefazolin. *Chemotherapy, 21:* 19-32.

Lode, H., Janisch, P., Küpper, G. and Weuta, H. (1974): Comparative clinical pharmacology of three ampicillins and amoxicillin administered orally. *Journal of Infectious Diseases, 129,* suppl.: S156-S168.

Loo, J.C.K., Foliz, E.L., Wallick, H. and Kwan, K.C. (1974): Pharmacokinetics, of pivampicillin and ampicillin in man. *Clinical Pharmacology and Therapeutics, 16:* 34-43.

Lorber, J., Kalhan, S.C. and Mahgrefte, B. (1970): Treatment of ventriculitis with gentamicin and cloxacillin in infants born with spina bifada. *Archives of Diseases in Childhood, 45:* 178-185.

Lorian, V. and Topf, B. (1972): Microbiology of nosocomial infections. *Archives of Internal Medicine, 130:* 104-110.

Lumholtz, B., Kampmann, J., Siersbaek-Nielsen, K. and Hansen, J.M. (1974): Dose regimen of kanamycin and gentamicin. *Acta Medica Scandinavica, 196:* 521-524.

Lund, B., Morgensen, C. Mølholm-Hansen, J., Kampmann, J. and Siersbaek-Nielsen, K. (1974): Ampicillin in portal and peripheral blood and bile after oral administration of ampicillin and pivampicillin. *European Journal of Clinical Pharmacology, 7:* 133-135.

Lund, M.E., Blazevic, D.J. and Matsen, J.M. (1973): Rapid gentamicin bioassay using a multiple-antibiotic-resistant strain of "klebsiella pneumoniae." *Antimicrobial Agents and Chemotherapy, 4:* 569-573.

Lykkegaard Nielsen, M., Justesen, T. and Asnaes, S. (1974): Anaerobic bacteriological study of the human liver—with a critical review of the literature. *Scandinavian Journal of Gastroenterology,* 671-677.

Macaraes, P.V.J., Lasagna, L. and Bianchine, J.R. (1971): A study of hospital staff attitudes concerning the comparative merits of antibiotics. *Clinical Pharmacology and Therapeutics, 12:* 1-12.

MacCulloch, D., Richardson, R.A. and Allwood, G.K. (1974): The penetration of doxycycline, oxytetracycline and minocycline into sputum. *New Zealand Medical Journal, 80:* 300-302.

MacDonald, H., Kelly, R.G., Allen, E.S., Noble, J.F. and Kanegis, L.A. (1973): Pharmacokinetic studies on minocycline in man. *Clinical Pharmacology and Therapeutics, 14:* 852-861.

MacGregor, R.R. and Beaty, H.N. (1972): Evaluation of positive blood cultures. *Archives of Internal Medicine, 130:* 84-87.

MacMillan, M.G. (1971): Neonatal bacteraemia. *Archives of Diseases in Childhood, 46:* 739.

Maisey, D.N., Brown, R.C. and Day, J.L. (1974): Rifampicin and cortisone replacement therapy. *Lancet, 2:* 896-897.

Maki, D.G., Goldman, D.A., and Rhame, F.S. (1973a): Infection control in intravenous therapy. Clinical review. *Annals of Internal Medicine, 79:* 867-887.

Maki, D.G., Hennekens, C.G., Phillips, C.W., Shaw, W.V. and Bennett, J.V. (1973b): Nosocomial urinary tract infection with "serratia marcescens": an epidemiologic study. *Journal of Infectious Diseases, 128:* 579-587.

Malaka-Zafirin, K. and Strates, B.S. (1969): The effect of antimicrobial agents on the binding of bilirubin by albumin. *Acta Paediatrica Scandinavica, 58:* 281-286.

Mandell, G.L. (1973): Interaction of intraleukocytic bacteria and antibiotics. *Journal of Clinical Investigation, 52:* 1673-1679.

Mann, C.H. (ed.) (1966): Kanamycin: appraisal after eight years of clinical application. *Annals of the New York Academy of Sciences, 132,* n. 2.

Marget, W. (1971): Special aspects of cephalosporin therapy in infants and children. *Post graduate Medical Journal, 47,* suppl.: 54-57.

Marget, W. and Daschner, E. (1969): Untersuchungen zur Anwendung von Cephalexin im Kindesalter. *Arzneimittel Forschung, 19:* 1956-1958.

Marget, W. and Wagner, M. (1967): Orale Anwendung von Propicillin, Ampicillin und Dicloxacillin im Säuglingsalter. *Medizinische Klinik, 62:* 300-305.

Mariel, C., Veyssier, P., Pechere, J-C. and De Cerner, E. (1972): Urinary pH and excretion of gentamicin. *British Medical Journal, 2:* 406.

Marks, M.I. (1975): In vitro antibacterial activity of amikacin, a new aminoglycoside, against clinical bacterial isolates from children. *Journal of Clinical Pharmacology, 15:* 246-251.

Marzetti, G., Panero, A., Conca, L. and Orzalesi, M. (1974): Il dosaggio della gentamicina nel neonato. *Minerva Pediatrica, 26:* 1185-1190.

Masera, G., Uderzo, C., Brecher, A., Tognoni, G. (1976): Il chloramfenicolo oggi. *Prospettive in Pediatria, 6:* 245-255.

Mattson, K. (1973): *Side Effects of Rifampicin. A Clinical Study.* Printaco, Helsinki.

Mattson, K., Riska, H., Forsstrom, J. and Kock, B. (1974): Acute renal failure following rifampicin administration. *Scandinavian Journal of Respiratory Diseases, 55:* 291-297.

Maurice, P.N., Riess, W., Welke, A. and Amson, K. (1973): Celospor (C 36278-Ba), ein neues Antibiotikum aus der Cephalosporinreihe: Pharmacokinetik und Klinische prüfung. *Schweizerische Medizinische Wochenschrift, 103:* 817-824.
Mawer, G.E., Ahmad, R., Dobbs, S.M., McGough, J.G., Lucas, S.B. and Tooth, J.A. (1974a): Prescribing aids for gentamicin. *British Journal of Clinical Pharmacology, 1:* 45-52.
Mawer, G.E., Ahmad, R., Dobbs, S.M. and Tooth, J.A. (1974b): Experience with a gentamicin nomogram. *Postgraduate Medical Journal, 50,* suppl. 7: 31-32.
Mawler, G.E., Lucas, S.B., Knowles, B.R., Stirland, R.M. and Tooth, J.A. (1972): Computer-assisted prescribing of kanamycin for patients with renal insufficiency. *Lancet, 1:* 12-15.
May, F.E., Stewart, R.B. and Cluff, L.E. (1974): Drug use in the hospital: evaluation of determinants. *Clinical Pharmacology and Therapeutics, 16:* 834-845.
May, J.R. and Ingold, A. (1974): Amoxicillin in the treatment of infections of the lower respiratory tract. *Journal of Infectious Diseases, 129,* suppl.: S189-S193.
Mayersohn, M. and Endrenyi, L. (1973): Relative bioavailability of commercial ampicillin formulations in man. *Canadian Medical Association Journal, 109:* 989-993.
McAllister, T.A. (1974): Gentamicin in paediatrics. *Postgraduate Medical Journal, 50,* suppl. 7: 45-52.
McCracken, G.H., Jr. (1972): Clinical pharmacology of gentamicin in infants 2 to 24 months of age. *American Journal of Diseases of Children, 124:* 884-887.
McCracken, G.H., Jr. (1974): Pharmacological basis for antimicrobial therapy in newborn infants. *American Journal of Diseases of Children, 128:* 407-419.
McCracken, G.H., Jr. (1975): Commentary. *Journal of Pediatrics, 86:* 615-616.
McCracken, G.H., Jr. and Chrane, D.F. (1972): Evaluation of hearing and development one year following gentamicin therapy of neonates. In: *Abstracts, Proc. 12th. Interscience Conference on Antimicrobial Agents and Chemotherapy,* Atlantic City, N.J., Sept. 1972, p. 100.
McCracken, G.H., Jr., Chrane, D.F. and Thomas, M.L. (1971a): Pharmacologic evaluation of gentamicin in newborn infants. *Journal of Infectious Diseases, 124,* suppl.: S214-S223.
McCracken, G.H., Jr. and Eichenwald, H.F. (1974a): Antimicrobial therapy: therapeutic recommendations and a review of the newer drugs. I. Therapy of infectious conditions. *Journal of Pediatrics, 85:* 297-312.
McCracken, G.H., Jr. and Eichenwald, H.F. (1974b): Antimicrobial therapy: therapeutic recommendations and a review of the newer drugs. II. The clinical pharmacology of the newer antimicrobial agents. *Journal of Pediatrics, 85:* 451-456.
McCracken, G.H., Jr., Ginsberg, C., Chrane, D.F., Thomas, M.L. and Horton, L.J. (1973): Clinical pharmacology of penicillin in newborn infants. *Journal of Pediatrics, 82:* 692-698.
McCracken, G.H., Jr. and Kaplan, J.M. (1974): Penicillin treatment for congenital syphilis: a critical reappraisal. *Journal of the American Medical Association, 228:* 855-858.
McCracken, G.H., Jr., West, N.R. and Horton, L.J. (1971b): Urinary excretion of gentamicin in the neonatal period. *Journal of Infectious Diseases, 123:* 257-262.
McGhie, D., Hutchison, J.G.P. and Geddes, A.M. (1974): Serum-gentamicin. *Lancet, 2:* 1463-1464.
McGowan, J.E., Jr. and Finland, M. (1974): Usage of antibiotics in a general hospital: effect of requiring justification. *Journal of Infectious Diseases, 130:* 165-168.
McGowan, J.E., Jr., Garner, C., Wilcox, C. and Finland, M. (1974): Antibiotic susceptibility of gram-negative bacilli isolated from blood cultures. *American Journal of Medicine, 57:* 225-238.
Mearns, M. (1974): Discussion following McAllister article. Gentamicin in paediatrics. *Postgraduate Medical Journal, 50,* suppl.: 53.

Meland, M. (1972): Erythromycin in the middle ear: further information. *Pediatrics, 4:* 784.
Mendelson, J., Portnoy, J. and Sigman, H. (1973): Pharmacology of gentamicin in the biliary tract of humans. *Antimicrobial Agents and Chemotherapy, 4:* 538-541.
Meyer, M.C., Dann, R.E., Whyatt, P.L., and Slywka, G.W.A. (1974): The bioavailability of sixteen tetracycline products. *Journal of Pharmacokinetics and Biopharmaceutics, 2:* 287-297.
Meyer, L., Polak, B.C.P., Wesseling, H., Schut, D. and Herxheimer, A. (1974): Blood dyscrasias attributed to chloramphenicol. *Postgraduate Medical Journal, 50,* suppl. 5: 123-126.
Michel, J., Sacks, T., Stessman, J. and Licht, A. (1974): Serum gentamicin levels after intravenous bolus injection. *Lancet, 2:* 525-526.
Milman, N. (1974): Renal failure associated with gentamicin therapy. *Acta Medica Scandinavica, 196:* 87-91.
Milner, R.D.G. (1974): Gentamicin in the newborn. *Postgraduate Medical Journal, 50,* suppl. 7: 40-44.
Milner, R.D.G., Ross, J., Froud, D.J.R. and Davis, J.A. (1972): Clinical pharmacology of gentamicin in the newborn infant. *Archives of Disease in Childhood, 47:* 927-932.
Mitchell, J.R. and Jollow, D.J. (1974): Metabolic activation of acetaminophen, furosemide and isoniazid to hepatotoxic substances. In: *Drug Interactions,* edited by P.L. Morselli, S. Garattini, and S.N. Cohen, pp. 65-79, Raven Press, New York.
Mitchison, D.A. (1973): Plasma concentrations of isoniazid in the treatment of tuberculosis. In: *Biological Effects of Drugs in Relation to Their Plasma Concentrations,* edited by D.S. Davies and B.N.C. Prichard, pp. 169-182, Macmillan, London.
Monafo, V., Azzolini, F., Gazzaniga, A. and Lodola, E. (1974): Thiamphenicol elimination in renal insufficiency. *Postgraduate Medical Journal, 50,* suppl. 5: 41-43.
Morehead, C.D., Shelton, S., Kusmiesz, H. and Nelson, J.D. (1972): Pharmacokinetics of carbenicillin in neonates of normal and low birth weight. *Antimicrobial Agents and Chemotherapy, 2:* 267-271.
Mulholland, S.G., Bruun, J.N., Coriell, L.L. and Blakemore, W.S. (1973): Experience with intensive surveillance of urinary tract infection. *Surgery, 137:* 789-793.
Naber, K.G., Westenfelder, S.R. and Madsen, P.O. (1973): Pharmacokinetics of the aminoglycoside antibiotic tobramycin in humans. *Antimicrobial Agents and Chemotherapy, 3:* 469-473.
Nakamura, T., Hachimori, K. and Sugimori, S. (1973): Clinical studies on clindamycin-2-palmitate hydrochloride in the field of pediatrics. *Japanese Journal of Antibiotics, 26:* 342-349.
Nakazawa, S., Sato, H. and Nakji, Y. (1972): Studies on cefazolin. A new semi-synthetic cephalosporin, in the field of pediatrics. *Advances in Antimicrobial and Antineoplastic Chemotherapy, 1:* 1067-1068.
Naumann, P. (1966): Laboratory and clinical evaluation of dicloxacillin. *Antimicrobial Agents and Chemotherapy, 1965:* 937-946.
Naumann, P. and Reintjens, E. (1974): Antibacterial activity and pharmacokinetic behaviour of cefazolin as compared with five other cephalosporin antibiotics. *Infection, 2:* 19-24.
Naumann, P. and Rosin, H. (1973): Zur oralen Carbenicillintherapie mit Carindacillin. *Deutsche Medizinische Wochenschrift, 98:* 2200-2205.
Nauta, E.H. and Mattie, H. (1975): Pharmacokinetics of flucloxacillin and cloxacillin in healthy subjects and patients on chronic intermittent haemodialysis. *British Journal of Clinical Pharmacology, 2:* 111-121.
Naveh, Y. and Fridman, A. (1973): Rifampicin therapy in gram-negative bacteraemia in infancy. *Archives of Disease in Childhood, 48:* 967-969.

Neiss, E.S. (1973): Cephradine. A summary of preclinical studies and clinical pharmacology. *Journal of the Irish Medical Association, 66,* suppl.: 1-12.

Nelson, J.D. (1970): Carbenicillin therapy of infections due to "pseudomonas" in children. *Journal of Infectious Diseases, 122,* suppl.: 48-58.

Nelson, J.D. (1971): Antibiotic concentrations in septic joint effusions. *New England Journal of Medicine, 284:* 349-353.

Nelson, J.D. and Haltalin, K.C. (1974): Amoxicillin less effective than ampicillin against shigella in vitro and in vivo: relationship of efficacy to activity in serum. *Journal of Infectious Diseases, 129,* suppl.: 222-227.

Nelson, J.D. and McCracken, G.H., Jr. (1973): Clinical pharmacology of carbenicillin and gentamicin in the neonate and comparative efficacy with ampicillin and gentamicin. *Pediatrics, 52:* 801-812.

Nelson, J.D., Shelton, S., Kusmiesz, H.T. and Haltalin, K.C. (1972): Absorption of ampicillin and nalidixic acid by infants and children with acute shigellosis. *Clinical Pharmacology and Therapeutics, 13:* 879-886.

Neu, H.C. (1974): Antimicrobial activity and human pharmacology of amoxicillin. *Journal of Infectious Diseases, 129,* suppl.: 123-131.

Neu, H.C. (1975): New broad-spectrum penicillins. *Drugs, 9:* 81-87.

Neuvonen, P.J., Pentikainen, P.J. and Gothoni, G. (1975): Inhibition of iron absorption by tetracycline. *British Journal of Clinical Pharmacology, 2:* 94-96.

Neuvonen, P.J. and Penttilä, O. (1974): Effect of oral ferrous sulphate on the half-life of doxycyline in man. *European Journal of Clinical Pharmacology, 7:* 361-363.

Neuvonen, P.J. and Turakka, H. (1974): Inhibitory effect of various iron salts on the absorption of tetracycline in man. *European Journal of Clinical Pharmacology, 7:* 357-360.

Neussel, H. and Olbing, H. (1972): Zur Pharmakokinetic von Carbenicillin bei Kindern nach intramuskularer Injektion. *International Journal of Clinical Pharmacology, 5:* 444-449.

Newman, R.L. and Holt, R.J. (1971): Gentamicin in pediatrics. I. Report on intrathecal gentamicin. *Journal of Infectious Diseases, 124,* suppl.: 254-256.

Nishimura, T., Kotani, Y., Yoshida, R. and Asatani, Y. (1973): The laboratory and clinical studies of amoxycillin in pediatric field. *Chemotherapy* (Tokyo), *21:* 1597-1600.

Nissenson, A.R., Levin, N.W. and Parker, R.H. (1972): Effect of renal failure and hemodialysis on cephacetrile pharmacokinetics. *Clinical Pharmacology and Therapeutics, 13:* 887-894.

Noone, P. (1973): A rapid assay method for cephalosporins. *Journal of Clinical Pathology, 26:* 506-510.

Noone, P., Parsons, T.M.C., Pattison, J.R., Slack, R.C.B., Garfield-Davies, D. and Hughes, K. (1974a): Experience in monitoring gentamicin therapy during treatment of serious gram-negative sepsis. *British Medical Journal, 1:* 447-481.

Noone, P., Pattison, J.R. and Davies, D.G. (1974b): The effective use of gentamicin in life-threatening sepsis. *Postgraduate Medical Journal, 50,* suppl. 7: 9-16.

Noone, P. and Shafi, M.S. (1973): Controlling infection in a district general hospital. *Journal of Clinical Pathology, 26:* 140-145.

Nordström, L., Banck, G., Belfrage, S., Juhlin, I., Tjernström, O. and Toremalm, N.G. (1973): Prospective study of the ototoxicity of gentamicin. *Acta Pathologica et Microbiologica Scandinavica,* Section B, *81:* 58-61.

Notari, R.E. (1973): Pharmacokinetics and molecular modification: implications in drug design and evaluation. *Journal of Pharmaceutical Sciences, 62:* 865-881.

Novak, E., Vitti, T.G., Gove, R.S., Hunt, J., Ko, H. and Lummis, W.L. (1969): The absorption and excretion of penicillin G and triple sulfas in four pediatric preparations in normal children. *Current Therapeutic Research, 11:* 384-389.

Novak, E., Vitti, T.G., Panzer, J.D., Schlagel, C. and Hearron, M.S. (1971): Antibiotic tolerance and serum levels after intravenous administration of multiple large doses of lincomycin. *Clinical Pharmacology and Therapeutics, 12:* 793-797.

Noval, E., Wagner, T.G., and Lamb, D.J. (1970): Local and systemic tolerance, absorption and excretion of clindamycin hydrochloride after intramuscular administration. *International Zeitschrift für Klinische Pharmakologie, Therapie und Toxikologie, 3:* 201-208.

O'Callaghan, C.H., Tootill, J.P.R. and Robinson, W.D. (1971): A new approach to the study of serum concentrations of orally administered cephalexin. *Journal of Pharmacy and Pharmacology, 23:* 50-57.

O'Connell and Plaut, M.E. (1969): Fibrin penetration by penicillin: in vitro simulation of intravenous therapy. *Journal of Laboratory and Clinical Medicine, 73:* 258-265.

O'Connor, W.J., Warrne, G.H., Edrada, E.S., Mandala, P.S., and Rosenman, S.B. (1966): Serum concentrations of sodium nafcillin in infants during the perinatal period. *Antimicrobial Agents and Chemotherapy, 1965:* 220-222.

Odell, G.B., Cukier, J.O., and Maglalang, A.C. (1975): Commentary. *Journal of Pediatrics, 86:* 614.

O'Grady, F. and Lambert, H.P. (1973): Antibiotics in perspective. In: *Current Antibiotic Therapy,* edited by A.M. Geddes and J.D. Williams, pp. 1-14. Churchill Livingstone, Edinburgh.

Oldershausen, H.F. Von, Menz, H.P., Hartmann, I., Bezler, H.J., Ilg, R. and Burck, G.C. (1974): Serum levels and elimination of thiamphenicol in patients with impaired liver function and with renal failure on dialysis. *Postgraduate Medical Journal, 50,* suppl. 5: 44-46.

Orsolini, P. (1970): Tissue distribution and serum levels of cephalexin in man. *Postgraduate Medical Journal, 46,* suppl.: 13-16.

Orzalesi, M. (1975): Problems of drug therapy in the newborn period. In *Basic and Therapeutic Aspects of Perinatal Pharmacology,* edited by P.L. Morselli, S. Garattini and F. Sereni, pp. 13-20, Raven Press, New York.

Øvreberg, K. and Bjartveit, K. (1974): A national therapy project for drug resistant pulmonary tuberculosis. *Scandinavian Journal of Respiratory Diseases, 55:* 218-228.

Owens, D.R., Luscombe, D.K., Russell, A.D. and Nicholls, P.J. (1975): The cephalosporin group of antibiotics. *Advances in Pharmacology and Chemotherapy, 13:* 83-172.

Paisley, J.W., Smith, A.L. and Smith, D.H. (1973): Gentamicin in newborn infants. Comparison of intramuscular and intravenous administration. *American Journal of Diseases of Children, 126:* 473-477.

Panzer, J.D., Brown, D.C., Epstein, W.L., Lipson, R.L., Mahaffey, H.W. and Atkinson, W.D. (1972): Clindamycin levels in various body tissues and fluids. *Journal of Clinical Pharmacology, 12:* 259-262.

Pearson, R.E. (1974): Amoxicillin—a comparison with ampicillin. *Drug Intelligence and Clinical Pharmacy, 8:* 542-547.

Periti, P., Giusti, M. and Lamanna, A. (1974): Clinical pharmacology of tobramycin in newborns. In: *Future Trends in Chemotherapy,* edited by A. Bertelli, M. Neuman and J.R. Prous, pp. 135-140, Drugs of Today, Barcelona.

Pesnel, G., Geslin, P., Borderon, J.-C., Reinert, Ph., Canet, J., Fabre, A., Bouhana, A. and Lajouanine, P. (1973): Apport pratique d'un laboratoire spécialisé en antibiothérapie dans un service de pédiatrie génerale. *Annales de Pédiatrie, 20:* 239-244.

Peters, U., Hausamen, T-U. and Grosse-Brockhoff, F. (1974): Einfluss von Tuberkulostatika auf die Pharmakokinetik des Digitoxins. *Deutsche Medizinische Wochenschrift, 99:* 2381-2386.

Pickering, L.K., O'Connor, D.M., Anderson, D., Bairan, A.C., Feigin, R.D. and Cherry, J.D. (1973): Clinical and pharmacologic evaluation of cefazolin in children. *Journal of Infectious Diseases, 128,* suppl.: 407-414.

Pickering, L.K., O'Connor, D.M., Anderson, D., Bairan, A.C., Feigin, R.D. and Cherry, J.D. (1974): Comparative evaluation of cefazolin and cephalothin in children. *Journal of Pediatrics, 85:* 842-847.
Plaut, M.E., O'Connell, C.J., Pabico, R.C. and Davidson, D. (1969): Penicillin handling in normal and azotemic patients. *Journal of Laboratory and Clinical Medicine, 74:* 12-18.
Porpaczy, P. (1970): Doxycyline (Vibramycin®) bei eingeschränkter Nierenfunktion. *Wiener Klinische Wochenschrift, 82:* 710-714.
Postgraduate Medical Journal, 50, suppl. 5. (1974): Chloramphenicol thiamphenicol: known and unknown aspects of drug-host interactions.
Prescott, L.F. (1975): Pathological and physiological factors affecting drug absorption, distribution, elimination, and response in man. In: *Concepts in Biochemical Pharmacology,* edited by J.R. Gillette and J.R. Mitchell, Handbook of Experimental Pharmacology, V. 28, pt. 3, pp. 234-257, Springer-Verlag, Berlin.
Radner, D.B. (1973): Toxicologic and pharmacologic aspects of rifampicin. *Chest, 64:* 213-216.
Ram, M.D. and Watanatittan, S. (1974): Cephalothin levels in human bile. *Archives of Surgery, 108:* 187-189.
Randolph, M.F., Reyds, J.J., Cope, J.B. and Morris, K.E. (1975): Streptococcal pharyngitis: posttreatment carrier prevalence and clinical relapse in children treated with clindamycin palmitate or phenoxymethyl penicillin. *Clinical Pediatrics, 14:* 119-122.
Ratzan, K.R., Ruiz, C. and Irivin, G.L. III (1974): Biliary tract excretion of cefazolin, cephalothin, and cephaloridine in the presence of biliary tract disease. *Antimicrobial Agents and Chemotherapy, 6:* 426-431.
Reeves, D.S. (1974a): Gentamin therapy. *British Journal of Hospital Medicine, 12:* 837-850.
Reeves, D.S. (1974b): Accuracy of gentamicin assays. *Postgraduate Medical Journal, 50:* 20-21.
Reeves, D.S., Bywater, M.J., Wise, R. and Whitmarsh, V.B. (1974): Availability of three antibiotics after intramuscular injection into thigh and buttock. *Lancet, 2:* 1421-1422.
Regamey, C., Gordon, R.C. and Kirby, W.M.M. (1973): Comparative pharmacokinetics of tobramycin and gentamicin. *Clinical Pharmacology and Therapeutics, 14:* 396-403.
Regamey, C., Gordon, R.C. and Kirby, W.M.M. (1974): Cefazolin vs. cephalothin and cephaloridine. A comparison of their clinical pharmacology. *Archives of Internal Medicine, 133:* 407-410.
Regamey, C., Schaberg, D. and Kirby, W.M.M. (1972): Inhibitory effect of heparin on gentamicin concentrations in blood. *Antimicrobial Agents and Chemotherapy, 1972:* 329-332.
Reller, R.B., Karney, W.W., Beaty, H.N., Holmes, K.K. and Turck, M. (1973): Evaluation of cefazolin, a new cephalosporin antibiotic. *Antimicrobial Agents and Chemotherapy, 3:* 488-497.
Remmer, H. (1974): The inhibition and stimulation of chloramphenicol conjugation by drugs. *Postgraduate Medical Journal, 50,* suppl. 5: 28-32.
Riess, W., Schmid, K., Keberle, H., Dettli, L. and Spring, P.: (1969): Pharmacokinetic studies in the field of rifamycins. In: *Progress in Antimicrobial and Anticancer Chemotherapy,* pp. 905-913, University of Tokyo.
Riff, L.J. and Jackson, G.G. (1971): Pharmacology of gentamicin in man. *Journal of Infectious Diseases, 124,* suppl.: 98-105.
Riley, H.D., Jr., Rbio, T., Hinz, W., Nunnery, A.W. and Englund, J. (1971): Clinical and laboratory evaluation of gentamicin in infants and children. *Journal of Infectious Diseases, 124,* suppl.: 236-246.
Rohwedder, H.-J. and Goll, U. (1970): Untersuchungen über die Pharmakokinetik von Gentamycin bei Kindern. *Deutsche Medizinische Wochenschrift, 95:* 1171-1174.

Rolinson, G.N. (1973a): Plasma concentrations of penicillin in relation to the antibacterial effect. In: *Biological Effects of Drugs in Relation to Their Plasma Concentrations*, edited by D.S. Davies and B.N.C. Prichard, pp. 183-189, Macmillan, London.
Rolinson, G.N. (1973b): Assessment of resistance. In: *Current Antibiotic Therapy*, edited by A.M. Geddes and J.D. Williams, pp. 43-50, Churchill Livingstone, Edinburgh.
Rolinson, G.N. and Sutherland, R. (1973): Semisynthetic penicillins. *Advances in Pharmacology and Chemotherapy, 11:* 157-220.
Romankiewicz, J.A. (1974): Factors influencing renal distribution of antibiotics. A key to therapy of pyelonephritis. *Drug Intelligence and Clinical Pharmacy, 8:* 512-519.
Rosaschino, F. (1974): Microbiological and clinical evaluation of tobramycin in pediatrics In: *Future Trends in Chemotherapy*, edited by A. Bertelli, M. Neuman and J.R. Prous, pp. 141-147, Drugs of Today, Barcelona.
Rosdahl, N. and Andersen, J.B. (1973): Aspects of the pharmacology of gentamicin during the neonatal period. *Acta Pathologica et Microbiologica Scandinavica*, Section B, *81*, suppl. 241: 119-123.
Rosenblatt, J.E., Kind, A.C., Brodie, J.L. and Kirby, W.M.M. (1968): Mechanisms responsible for the blood level differences of isoxazolyl penicillins: oxacillin, cloxacillin, and dicloxacillin. *Archives of Internal Medicine, 121:* 345-348.
Ross, S., Kuraybill, E.N. and Kahn, W. (1970): Treatment of proteus meningitis with carbenicillin: a report of four cases. *Journal of Infectious Diseases, 122*, suppl.: 62-70.
Sabath, L.D., Casey, J.I., Ruch, P.A., Stumpf, L.L. and Finland, M. (1971): Rapid microassay of gentamicin, kanamycin, neomycin, streptomycin, and vancomycin in serum or plasma. *Journal of Laboratory and Clinical Medicine, 78:* 457-463.
Sabra, A., Metrau, F., Feitosa, N., Mendes Santi, J. and Trabulsi, L.R. (1973): Serum levels of anhydrous ampicillin administered orally in normal infants. *Current Therapeutic Research, 15:* 866-870.
Sanders, W.E., Jr., Johnson, J.E., III and Taggart, J.G. (1974): Adverse reactions to cephalothin and cephaprin. Uniform occurrence on prolonged intravenous administration of high doses. *New England Medical Journal, 290:* 424-429.
Saslaw, S. (1970): Cefalosporin. *Medical Clinics of North America, 54:* 1217-1228.
Schreier, H.A. and Berger, L. (1974): On medical imperialism. *Lancet, 1:* 1161.
Schumacher, G.E. (1975): Practical pharmacokinetic techniques for drug consultation and evaluation. IV: Gentamicin blood level versus time profiles of various dosage regimens recommended for renal impairment. *American Journal of Hospital Pharmacy, 32:* 299-308.
Scotti, R. (1973): Sex difference in blood levels of some antibiotics. *Chemotherapy, 18:* 205-211.
Sereni, F., Perletti, L., Manfredi, N. and Marini, A. (1965): Tissue distribution and urinary excretion of a tetracycline derivative in newborn and older infants. *Journal of Pediatrics, 67:* 299-305.
Sereni, F. and Principi, N. (1968): Developmental pharmacology. *Annual Review of Pharmacology, 8:* 453-466.
Shapiro, S. and Levy, M. (1975): Use of antimicrobials in medical inpatients. *Clinical Pharmacology and Therapeutics, 17:* 244.
Shibata, K. and Fujii, M. (1970): Clinical studies of cefazolin in the surgical field. *Antimicrobial Agents and Chemotherapy, 10:* 467-472.
Shibata, K., Itoh, T., Fujii, M., Shinagawa, N., Nishi, H. and Muramatsu, T. (1973): Laboratory and clinical studies of clindamycin-2-palmitate in surgical practice. *Japanese Journal of Antibiotics, 26:* 389-392.
Shoji, K.T., Axnick, K. and Rytel, M.W. (1974): Infections and antibiotic use in a large municipal hospital, 1970-1972: a prospective analysis of the effectiveness of a continuous surveillance program. *Health Laboratory Science, 11:* 283-292.

Siegler, D.I., Burley, D.M., Bryant, M., Citron, K.M., Standen, S.M. (1974): Effect of meals on rifampicin absorption. *Lancet, 2:* 197-198.

Silverio, J. and Poole, J.W. (1973): Serum concentrations of ampicillin in newborn infants after oral administration. *Pediatrics, 51:* 578-580.

Simmons, H.E. and Stolley, P.D. (1974): This is medical progress? Trends and consequences of antibiotic use in the United States. *Journal of the American Medical Association, 227:* 1023-1028.

Simon, C. (1973): Tobramycin, ein neues Pyocyaneus-Antibiotikum. *Medizinische Welt, 24:* 1852-1853.

Simon, C., Hamacher, A., Malerczyk and Rohwedder, J. (1971): Zur Blutspiegelkinetik von Carbenicillin. *Arzneimittel-Forschung, 21:* 78-85.

Simon, C., Malerczyk, E. Brahmstaedt and Toeller, W. (1973a): Cefazolin ein neues Bretspektrum-Antibiotikum. *Deutsche Medizinische Wochenschrift, 98:* 2448-2450.

Simon, C. Malerczyk, V., Zierott, G., Lehmann, K. and Thiesen, U. (1975): Blut-Harn-, und Gallespiegel von Ampicillin bei intravenöser Dauerinfusion. *Arzneimittel-Forschung, 25:* 654-656.

Simon, C., Schmitt, E., Malerczyk, V. and Arkenau, C. (1973b): Zur Pharmakokinetik von Gentamycin bei Erwachsenen und Kindern verschiedenen Alters. *Medizinische Welt, 24:* 626-630.

Simon, C., Sievers, G., Rohwedder, V. and Malerczyk, V. (1970): Zur Pharmakokinetik von Cephalexin bei Erwachsenen und Kindern. *Deutsche Medizinische Wochenschrift, 95:* 2103-2108.

Simon, C. and Toeller, W. (1974): Amoxycillin ein neues Aminobensylpenicillin. *Arzneimittel-Forschung, 24:* 181-184.

Simon, H.J. and Axline, S.G. (1966): Clinical pharmacology of kanamycin in premature infants. *Annals of the New York Academy of Sciences, 132:* 1020-1025.

Simon, V.K., Mösinger, E.U. and Malerczy, V. (1973c): Pharmacokinetic studies of tobramycin and gentamicin. *Antimicrobial Agents and Chemotherapy, 3:* 445-450.

Simon, H.J. and Yaffe, S.J. (1969): Clinical pharmacologic studies in premature infants: penicillins, aminoglycosides and colistin. In: *Progress in Antimicrobial and Anticancer Chemotherapy*, pp. 761-767, University of Tokyo.

Sinkula, A.A. (1974): Chemical modification of erythromycin: synthesis and preliminary bioactivity of selected amides and esters. *Journal of Pharmaceutical Sciences, 63:* 842-848.

Sinkula, A.A. and Yalkowsky, S.H. (1975): Rationale for design of biologically reversible drug derivatives: prodrugs. *Journal of Pharmaceutical Sciences, 64:* 181-210.

Skovsted, L., Hansen, J.M., Kristensen, M. and Christensen, L.K. (1974): Inhibition of drug metabolism in man. In: *Drug Interactions*, edited by P.L. Morselli, S. Garattini and S.N. Cohen, pp. 81-90, Raven Press, New York.

Smith, A.L. and Smith, D.H. (1974): Gentamicin: adenine mononucleotide transferase: partial purification, characterization, and use in the clinical quantitation of gentamicin. *Journal of Infectious Diseases, 129:* 391-401.

Smith, D.H., Van Otto, B and Smith, A.L. (1972): A rapid chemical assay for gentamicin. *New England Journal of Medicine, 286:* 583-586.

Smith, H. (1973): Opportunistic infection. *British Medical Journal, 2:* 107-110.

Smith, H. (1975): Microbial interference with host defense mechanisms. *Monographs in Allergy, 9:* 13-38.

Snelling. C.F.T., Ronald, A.R., Cates, C.Y. and Forsythe, W.C. (1971): Resistance of gram-negative bacilli to gentamicin. *Journal of Infectious Diseases, 124*, suppl.: S264-S270.

Søgaard, H., Zimmermann-Nielsen, C. and Siboni, K. (1974): Antibiotic-resistant gram-negative bacilli in a urological ward for male patients during a nine-year period: relationship to antibiotic consumption. *Journal of Infectious Diseases, 130:* 646-650.

Solberg, C.O., Schreiner, A., Hamre, E. and Digranes, A. (1973): Therapy of infections with parenteral cephalexin. *Chemotherapy, 19:* 215-220.
Spector, S.L., Katz, F.H. and Farr, R.S. (1974): Troleadomycin: effectiveness in steroid-dependent asthma and bronchitis. *Journal of Allergy and Clinical Immunology, 54:* 367-379.
Sprunt, K., Redman, W. and Leidy, G. (1973): Antibacterial effectiveness of routine hand washing. *Pediatrics, 52:* 264-271.
Stamey, T.A., Fair, W.R., Timothy, M.M., Millar, M.A., Mihara, G. and Lowery, Y.C. (1974): Serum versus urinary antimicrobial concentrations in cure of urinary-tract infections. *New England Journal of Medicine, 291:* 1159-1163.
Stevenson, J. (1974): Bacterial meningitis and tuberculous meningitis. In: *A New Look at Infectious Diseases,* pp. 152-163, British Medical Association, London.
Stewart, D.A. and Moghadam, H. (1972): Are antibiotic drugs needed for the treatment of upper respiratory tract infections in infants? *Canadian Medical Association Journal, 107:* 1082-1084.
Stokes, E.J. and Whitby, J.L. (1971): Quality control in bacteriology: preliminary trials. *Journal of Clinical Pathology, 24:* 790-797.
Stott, R.B., Cameron, J.S., Ogg, C.S. and Toseland, P. (1971): Tetracyclines and impaired renal function? *Lancet, 2:* 1378-1379.
Stratford, B.C., Dixson, S. and Concroft, A.J. (1974): Serum levels of gentamicin and tobramycin after slow intravenous bolus injection. *Lancet, 1:* 378-379.
Symposium on infectious disease. (1974): *Pediatric Clinics of North America, 21:* n.3.
Syvälahti, E.K.G., Pihlajamäki, K.K., and Ilsalo, E.J. (1974): Rifampicin and drug metabolism. *Lancet, 2:* 232-233.
Taber, L.H., Yow, M.D. and Nieberg, F.G. (1967): The penetration of broad-spectrum antibiotics into the cerebrospinal fluid. *Annals of the New York Academy of Sciences, 145:* 473-481.
Tacquet, A., Devulver, B., Curvelier, D. and Legros, J. (1974): Pharmacokinetic aspects of thiamphenicol in subjects with normal renal function and in patients with chronic renal insufficiency, with or without haemodialysis. *Postgraduate Medical Journal, 50,* suppl. 5: 36-38.
Tager, I. and Speizer, F.E. (1975): Role of infection in chronic bronchitis. *New England Journal of Medicine, 292:* 563-571.
Tan, J.S., Bannister, T. and Phair, J.P. (1974): Levels of amoxicillin and ampicillin in human serum and interstitial fluid. *Journal of Infectious Diseases, 129,* suppl: S146-S148.
Taneja, O.P., Grover, N.K., Thakur, L.C. and Bhatia, V.N. (1974): Effects of blood levels of tetracycline and oxytetracycline on hepatic and renal functions in normal subjects. *Chemotherapy, 20:* 201-211.
Thrupp, L.D. (1974): Newer cephalosporins and "expanded-spectrum" penicillins. *Annual Review of Pharmacology, 14:* 435-467.
Thrupp, L.D., Leedom, J.M., Ivler, D., Wehrle, P.E., Portnoy, B. and Mathies, A.W. (1966): Ampicillin levels in the cerebrospinal fluid during treatment of bacterial meningitis. *Antimicrobial Agents and Chemotherapy, 1965:* 206-213.
Tice, A.D., Barza, M., Bergeron, M.G., Brusch, J.L. and Weinstein, L. (1975): Effect of diuretics on urinary excretion of cephalothin in humans. *Antimicrobial Agents and Chemotherapy, 7:* 168-171.
Tisné, M. (1974): Ten years of clinical experience with thiamphenicol in France. *Postgraduate Medical Journal, 50,* suppl. 5: 142.
Tjernström, O., Banck, G., Belgrage, S., Juhlin, I., Nordström, L. and Toremalm, N.G. (1973): The ototoxicity of gentamicin. *Acta Pathologica et Microbiologica Scandinavica,* Section B, *81,* suppl. 241: 73-78.

Tognoni, G., Morselli, P.L. and Sereni, F. (1975): Ethical and methodological challenges in research in perinatal pharmacology. In: *Basic and Therapeutic Aspects of Perinatal Pharmacology*, edited by P.L. Morselli, S. Garattini and F. Sereni, pp. 413-430. Raven Press, New York.

Tozer, T.N. (1974): Nomogram for modification of dosage regimens in patients with chronic renal function impairment. *Journal of Pharmacokinetics and Biopharmaceutics*, 2: 13-28.

Tsuji, K. and Robertson, J.H. (1973): Formation of trimethylsilyl derivatives of tetracyclines for separation and quantitation by gas-liquid chromatography. *Analytical Chemistry, 45:* 2136-2140.

Tsuji, K., Robertson, J.H. and Beyer, W.F. (1974): High pressure liquid chromatographic determination of tetracyclines. *Analytical Chemistry, 46:* 539-542.

Tuomisto, J. and Männisto, P. (1973): Cross-over study of ten tetracycline preparations. *European Journal of Clinical Pharmacology, 6:* 64-68.

Unertl, K., Daschner, F.D. and Marget, W. (1974): A semiautomatic microtube dilution method for determining antibiotic blood concentrations. *Chemotherapy, 20:* 331-338.

Valman, H.B. and Evans, K.E. (1970): Serum unbound levels of cloxacillin and erythromycin in cystic fibrosis. *Archives of Disease in Childhood, 45:* 686-689.

Van de Walle, J. and Adriaensen, H. (1974): Serum-gentamicin levels after intravenous bolus injection. *Lancet, 2:* 525.

Veale, D.R., Smith, H. and Witt, K. (1975): Penetration of penicillin into human phagocytes containing gonococci. *Lancet, 1:* 306-308.

Vesell, E.S. (1975): Gentically determined variations in drug disposition and response in man. In: *Concepts in Biochemical Pharmacology*, edited by J.R. Gillette and J.R. Mitchell, Handbook of Experimental Pharmacology, V. 28, pt. 3, pp. 169-212, Springer-Verlag, Berlin.

Vianna, N.J. and Kaye, D. (1967): Penetration of cephalothin into the spinal fluid. *American Journal of Medicinal Chemistry, 254:* 261-220.

Vietor, K.W., Simon, C., Malerczyk, V., Pandel, E. and Dumke, E. (1974): Ampicillin-clearance bei Kindern mit angeboren Herzfehlern und Herzinsuffizienz. *Zeitschrift für Kinderheilkunde, 117:* 175-182.

Villani, F., Bonhet, A., Sakellaridès, E. and Schelling, J.L. (1975): Concentration urinaire et effet antibactérien de tétracyclines à courte et longue durée d'action. *Schweizerische Medizinische Wochenschrift, 105:* 341-344.

Virtanen, S. and Tala, E. (1974): Serum concentration of rifampicin after oral administration. *Clinical Pharmacology and Therapeutics, 16:* 817-820.

Vogt, E. (1973): Bronchialsekret-und Serumspiegel bei mit Gentamicin behandelten Mucoviscidose-Kindern. *Praxis, 62:* 444-447.

Vukovich, R.A., Brannick, L.J., Sugerman, A.A. and Neiss, E.S. (1975): Sex differences in the intramuscular absorption rate and bioavailability of cephradine. *Clinical Pharmacology and Therapeutics, 17:* 246-247.

Wagner, J.G. (1974): Relevant pharmacokinetics of antimicrobial drugs. *Medical Clinics of North America, 58:* 470-492.

Wagner, J.G., Novak, E., Patel, N.C., Chidester, C.G. and Lummis, W.L. (1968): Absorption, excretion and half-life of clinimycin in normal adult males. *American Journal of Medicinal Sciences, 256:* 25-37.

Waitz, J.A. and Weinstein, M.J. (1969): Recent microbiological studies with gentamicin. *Journal of Infectious Diseases, 119:* 355-360.

Walker, S.H. and Gonzales, E.P. (1971): Cephalexin: effective oral antibiotic for coccal infections. *Maryland State Medical Journal, 20:* 63-65.

Walker, S.H. and Maisog, V.T. (1969): Cephaloridine dosage in infants and children. *Maryland State Medical Journal, 18:* 65-82.

Weber, W.W. and Cohen, S.N. (1975): Aging effects and drugs in man. I. Introduction. In: *Concepts in Biochemical Pharmacology*, edited by J.R. Gillette and J.R. Mitchell. Handbook of Experimental Pharmacology, V. 28, pt. 3, pp. 213-233, Springer-Verlag, Berlin.

Weingärtner, L. and Exadaktylos, P. (1974): Panmyelopathien nach Chloramphenicolgabe. *Klinische Paedriatrie, 186:* 394-407.

Weinstein, L. (1970a): Chemotherapy of microbial diseases. General considerations. In: *The Pharmacological Basis of Therapeutics*, edited by L.S. Goodman and A. Gilman, pp. 1150-1176, 4th ed., Macmillan, London.

Weinstein, L. (1970b): Antibiotics, IV. Miscellaneous antimicrobial, antifungal and antiviral agents. In: *The Pharmacological Basis of Therapeutics*, edited by L.S. Goodman and A. Gilman, pp. 1269-1310, 4th ed., Macmillan, London.

Weiss, C.F., Glazko, A.J. and Westein, J.K. (1960): Chloramphenicol in the newborn infant: a physiologic explanation of its toxicity when given in excessive doses. *New England Journal of Medicine, 262:* 787-794.

Weitzman, S. and Berger, S. (1974): Clinical trial design in studies of corticosteroids for bacterical infections. *Annals of Internal Medicine, 81:* 36-42.

Welling, P.G., Craig, W.A., Amidon, G.L. and Kunin, C.M. (1974): Pharmacokinetics of cefazolin in normal and uremic subjects. *Clinical Pharmacology and Therapeutics, 15:* 344-353.

Wennberg, R.P. and Rasmussen, L.F. (1975): Effects of gentamicin on albumin binding of bilirubin. *Journal of Pediatrics, 86:* 611-613.

Westenfelder, S.R., Naber, K.G. and Madsen, P.O. (1973): Pharmacokinetics of a new cephalosporin, cephacetrile, in patients with normal and impaired renal function. *Infection, 1:* 157-162.

Whelton, A., Carter, G.G., Bryant, H.H., Porteous, L.A. and Walker, W.G. (1974): Carbenicillin concentrations in normal and diseased kidneys. *Annals of Internal Medicine, 78:* 659-662.

Whelton, A., Schach Von Witenau, M., Twomey, T.M., Gordon Walker, W. and Bianchine, J.R. (1974): Doxycycline pharmacokinetics in the absence of renal function. *Kidney International, 5:* 365-371.

Wiegand, R.G. and Chun, A.H.C. (1972): Serum protein binding of erythromycin and erythromycin 2'-propionate ester. *Journal of Pharmaceutical Sciences, 61:* 425-429.

Wilkinson, P.J., Reeves, D.S., Wise, R. and Allen, J.T. (1975): Volunteer and clinical studies with carfecillin: a new orally administered ester of carbenicillin. *British Medical Journal, 2:* 250-252.

Wilcox, R.R. (1974): Effective treatment of gonorrhoea in London, with two oral doses of amoxycillin. *British Journal of Venereal Diseases, 50:* 120-124.

Williams, D.N., Crossley, K., Hoffman, C. and Sabath, L.D. (1975): Parenteral clindamycin phosphate: pharmacology with normal and abnormal liver function and effect on nasal staphylococci. *Antimicrobial Agents and Chemotherapy, 7:* 153-158.

Williams, J.D. and Andrews, J. (1974): Sensitivity of haemophilus influenzae to antibiotics. *British Medical Journal, 1:* 134-137.

Williams, J.D. and Geddes, A.M. (1973): Advertising of antibiotics. *British Medical Journal, 2:* 613.

Wilson, D.M., Lever, M., Brosnon, E.A. and Stilwell, A. (1972): A simplified tetracycline assay. *Clinica Chimica Acta, 236:* 260-261.

Wilson, D.M., Perry, H.O., Sans, M.W., Jr. and Dousa, T.P. (1973): Selective inhibition of human distal tubular function by demeclocycline. *Current Therapeutic Research, 15:* 734-740.

Wilson, H.D. and Haltalin, K.C. (1975): Ampicillin in haemophilus influenzae meningitis. *American Journal of Diseases of Children, 129:* 208-215.

Wilson, T.W., Mahon, W.A., Inaba, T., Johnson, G.E. and Kadar, D. (1973a): Elimination of tritiated gentamicin in normal human subjects and in patients with severely impaired renal function. *Clinical Pharmacology and Therapeutics, 14:* 815-822.

Winters, R.E., Chow, A.W., Hecht, R.H. and Hewitt, W.L. (1971a): Combined use of gentamicin and carbenicillin. *Annals of Internal Medicine, 75:* 925-927.

Winters, R.E., Litwack, K.D. and Hewitt, W.L. (1971b): Relation between dose and levels of gentamicin in blood. *Journal of Infectious Diseases, 127,* suppl.: S90-S95.

Wise, R. (1974): A guide of the cephalosporin antibiotics. *British Journal of Hospital Medicine, 11:* 583-589.

Wise, R. and Reeves, D.S. (1974): Pharmacological studies on cephacetrile in human volunteers. *Current Medical Research and Opinion, 2:* 249-255.

Wolff, S.M. (1974): Some challenges for future investigation in infectious diseases and clinical immunology. *Journal of Infectious Diseases, 130:* 85-88.

Yaffe, S.J. and Juchau, M.R. (1974): Perinatal pharmacology. *Annual Review of Pharmacology, 14:* 219-238.

Young, L.S., Decker, G. and Hewitt, W.L. (1974): Inactivation of gentamicin by carbenicillin in the urinary tract. *Chemotherapy, 20:* 212-200.

Yunis, A.A. (1974): Effects of chloramphenicol on erythropoiesis. In: *Drugs and Haematologic Reactions,* edited by N.V. Dimitrov and J.H. Nodine, pp. 133-140, Grune & Stratton, New York.

Yunis, A.A., Manyan, D.R. and Arimura, G.K. (1974): Comparative metabolic effects of chloramphenicol and thiamphenicol in mammalian cells. *Postgraduate Medical Journal, 50,* suppl. 5: 60-65.

Zaki, A., Schreiber, E.C., Weliky, I., Knill, J.R. and Hubsher, J.A. (1974): Clinical pharmacology of oral cephradine. *Journal of Clinical Pharmacology, 14:* 118-126.

Zarowny, D., Ogilvie, R., Tamblyn, D., MacLeod, C. and Ruedy, J. (1974): Pharmacokinetics of amoxicillin. *Clinical Pharmacology and Therapeutics, 16:* 1045-1051.

Zeman, B.T., Pike, M. and Samet, Ct. (1974): The antibiotic utilization committee. *Hospitals, 48:* 73-76.

Zinner, S.H., Casey, J.I., Sabath, L.D. and Finland, M. (1971): Erythromycin and alkalinisation of the urine in the treatment of urinary-tract infections due to gram-negative bacilli. *Lancet, 1:* 1267-1268.

Ziv, G. and Sulman, F.G. (1974): Evaluation of rifamycin SV and rifampin kinetics in lactating ewes. *Antimicrobial Agents and Chemotherapy, 5:* 139-142.

Zoumboulakis, D., Anagnostakis, D., Arseni, A., Nicolopoulos, D. and Matsaniotis, N. (1973): Gentamicin in the treatment of purulent meningitis in neonates and infants. *Acta Pediatrics Scandinavica, 62:* 55-58.

8

Sulfonamides Cotrimoxazole and Urinary Antiseptics

MARINELLA MANDELLI AND GIANNI TOGNONI

The choice of the drugs discussed in this chapter has been dictated by two main criteria: the first is their clinical use in pediatric practice, the second, the availability of reliable kinetic data. Antifungal and antiparasitic agents have been therefore omitted, together with older sulfonamides and some other minor compounds which have proven to be clinically useful but which do not seem as yet to merit specific attention for use in our age group. Fusidic acid and some urinary antiseptics whose use is sometimes recommended in adults, e.g., as oxolinic acid, methenamine, nifuratel and cinoxacin, are some of these. For data on their spectrum of action, clinical pharmacology and kinetics, the reader is referred to classical textbooks and some very recent synthetic reviews (Garrod et al., 1973; Weinstein, 1975; Ball et al., 1975).

SULFONAMIDES

The clinical importance of this group of drugs has been decreasing both because of the appearance of the new classes of antibiotics (see Chapter 7) and because of the reported high incidence of side effects. In fact, the introduction of long-acting sulfonamides with low rate of excretion, the use of highly soluble compounds and a better knowledge of the properties of their disposition and metabolism has greatly decreased the risks of toxic effects. (Garrod et al., 1973). Sulfonamides can still be considered a first choice in some urinary tract infections due to gram-negative bacteria, in the prophylactic treatment of carriers of meningitis infections and in some rare infections such as nocardiosis (Weinstein, 1973). The use of sulfonamides in pediatric practice has been particularly marked by the problem of side effects. The high degree of protein-binding and the capability of displacing bilirubin from the binding site have been extensively studied both to elucidate the mechanisms of adverse reactions and as a useful tool for pharmacological research on drug actions and interactions (see Chapter 3, also, Chignell et al., 1971; Wardell, 1973).

The above indications can be considered valid for clinical use in pediatric age (Barnett, 1972). The sulfonamide compounds reviewed in the following in more detail can be usefully considered as representative of different classes, as they have been classified by Williams (1975) according to the length of half-life and the recommended dosage:

—those with half-lives of less than 6 h; 4 doses daily (sulfisoxazole)
—those with half-lives up to 20 h; 2 doses daily (sulfadioazine)
—those with half-lives up to 40 h; 1 dose daily (sulfametoxypyridazine)
—those with half-lives over 40 h; 1 dose weekly (sulfamethopyrazine)

The structural formulas of the four compounds are given in Fig. 1.

Sulfamethoxazole is discussed separately with trimethoprom since it is used clinically in this combination. Sulfasalazine is also considered separately because of its very specific indications.

Sulfadimethoxine is not presented here, despite the large amount of data published in the literature, since it was withdrawn from the market because of its teratogenic potential.

Fig. 2 reviews the basic metabolic steps of sulfonamides.

Sulfisoxazole

Adults. Sulfisoxazole (SSX) is still one of the most widely used sulfonamides. Oral preparations of this drug are usually employed because absorption from the g.i. tract is complete. In comparing the oral with the intramuscular and intravenous administration of 2 g of SSX in adult volunteers, the following values were obtained. AUC i.m./AUC i.v. = 1.03-1.3, AUC p.o./AUC i.v. = 0.94-1.3 (Kaplan et al., 1972). Peak plasma levels are reached 2 h after i.m. and after oral administration, but the variability present following oral ingestion (44-185 μg/ml free SSX), is more marked than that seen after i.m. injection (121-158 μg/ml free SSX). An earlier peak absorption time of 30 min has been observed when the drug is given in solution, however, no differences in plasma levels are evident 2 h after administration of either tablets or solution (Van Petten et al., 1971).

About 84% of the drug present in plasma is protein-bound (Anton, 1973).

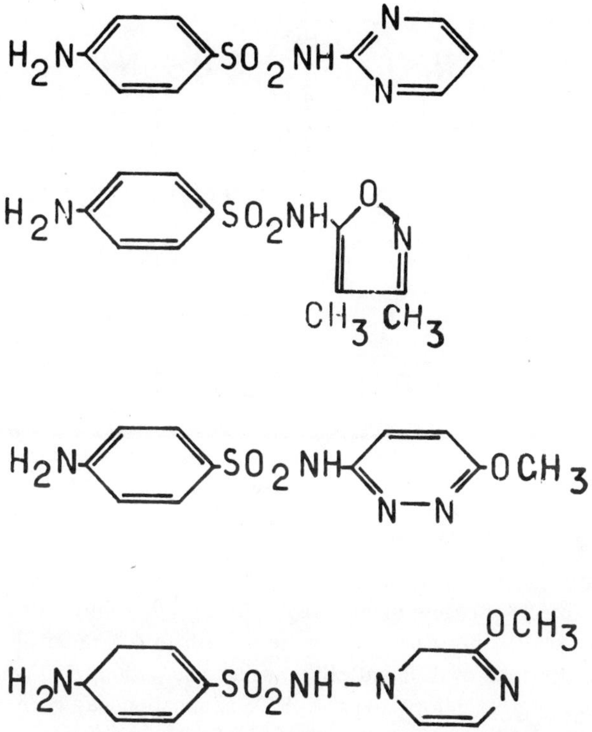

Fig. 1: I. Sulfadiazine; II. Sulfisoxazole; III. Sulfamethoxypyrydazine; IV. Sulfamethopyrazine

The apparent volume of distribution of SSX is approximately 0.16 L/kg. Its distribution, limited to the extracellular compartment, explains the resulting plasma levels which are twice as high as those obtained with the same dose of sulfadiazine. CSF levels are about one-third of those reached in the plasma (Weinstein, 1975). The apparent plasma half-life is practically identical regardless of the route of administration, and ranges from 4.6 to 7.8 h (Kaplan et al., 1972). From 39 to 65% of the dose is excreted unchanged over a 48-h interval. When metabolites are included, all the administered drug is excreted over the same period of time, with no differences consequent to the various routes of administration. The acetylated form accounts for 30% of the total SSX urinary

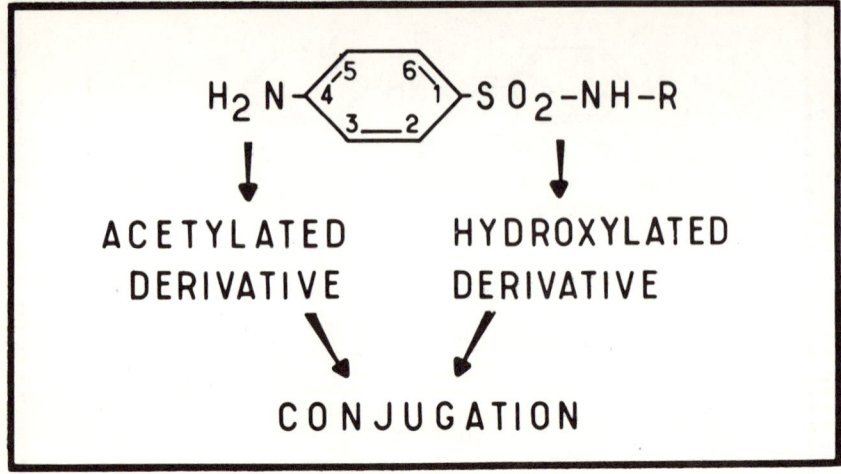

Fig. 2: Metabolic pathway of sulfonamides

excretion (Weinstein, 1975). Variations of the urinary pH can markedly modify the half-life of SSX; because of the drug's pK_a of 4.9, a shift in the urine from pH 5 to pH 8 may shorten T½ values from 9.5 h to 4.7 h (Dettli and Spring, 1968). The influence of different physiological and pathological conditions on the metabolic and excretory steps of SSX elimination has been studied by Reidenberg et al. (1969), following the i.v. administration of 2 g of the drug. Results of this study indicated that lower doses are needed in azotemic patients because both the metabolic rate constant and the excretion rate constant are significantly reduced under these conditions. In starved obese patients, a reduced urinary elimination rate constant was found, in agreement with the concomitant acidification of urine present in this clinical situation.

Newborns, Infants and Children. Krauer et al. (1968) investigated the pharmacokinetics of sulfisoxazole in 52 infants. They found that the gastrointestinal absorption constant was 0.99 ± 0.72 (h^{-1}), indicating high speed of absorption. In the first 10 days of life, the apparent half-life was about twice as long as comparative values reported in adults (11.26 h vs. 5.89); from 1 to 3 months, it was equal to adult values (5.83 h vs. 5.89), and from 3 months to 1 year of age it decreased, with a mean value of 4.02 h. The relative volume of distribution decreases to a much lesser extent with increasing age. It changes from 0.431 L/kg in the first 10 days of life to 0.341 at 1 year, but is always higher than in adults (0.16L/kg).

In a recent report, Krauer (1975) studied the influence of urinary pH on the biological half-life of sulfisoxazole in the pediatric patient. In children who have

Table 1. Effect of Age on Pharmacokinetic Parameters of Sulfisoxazole

Age	Mean Apparent Half-Life (h)	Mean Apparent Volume of Distribution (L/Kg)
5-10 days	11.26	0.431
12-26 days	7.73	0.335
1-3 months	5.83	0.382
3-12 months	4.02	0.341
Adults	5.6-5.89	0.164

Data are derived from Krauer et al., 1968; Kaplan et al., 1972; Reidenberg et al., 1969.

developed a distinct biphasic, diurnal periodicity of their urine pH, the elimination rate of sulfisoxazole is more than 100% lower at night. The ratio ($Q = \frac{t\frac{1}{2} \text{ night}}{t\frac{1}{2} \text{ day}}$) between half-life of sulfisoxazole during the night and during the day ranges from 1.2 to 2.7. In newborns, the elimination rate is about equal during the day and at night, and in young infants (under 1 year of age) it is only slightly lower at night than during the day, since no significant diurnal variations of the urine pH were observed in these age groups. Not unexpectedly, the apparent volume of distribution increases in infants and in children during sleep as a result of the enhanced diffusion of neutral drug molecules from the extracellular into the intracellular compartment. Table 1 summarizes the principal kinetic data for different age groups.

Sulfadiazine

Sulfadiazine, or 2-sulfanilamido-pyrimidine (SDZ), is well absorbed from the g.i. tract when given orally. Peak plasma levels of 160-200 µg/ml are reached within 3-4 h after an oral dose of 4 g, but marked variability has been reported to exist among different commercial preparations (Van Petten et al., 1971a). Similar values for peak time, but lower values for peak levels, have been measured following administration of SDZ suppositories (Finland, 1972).

About 50% of the drug present in plasma is protein-bound, with a β-value (app. maximum binding capacity) of 31.5 µmoles/g of albumin, according to Deetli and Spring (1973). Anton and Corey (1917), however, reported protein-binding of only 29-36% of the drug. After i.v. sulfadiazine injection, an apparent relative Vd of 0.33 ± 0.06 L/kg was observed, both in normal and nephropathic patients, by Ohnhaus and Spring (1975). Even higher values (0.6-1.6 L/kg) were reported by Bunger et al. (1961) and Reider (1963), following oral administration. Therapeutic concentrations in the CSF are already reached 4 h after a single dose of 60 mg/kg p.o. Following i.v. administration, mean apparent plasma half-lives of 8-14 h have been measured in patients with normal kidneys and of 12-40 h in patients with compromised renal function (Ohnhaus and Spring 1975; Dettli, 1974). Higher values of up to 17 h in subjects with normal renal function were reported by Rieder (1963) and Bunger et al. (1961) after oral administration.

In the body, SDZ is partially acetylated and is then excreted by the kidney, both as such (about 54%) and as the acetylated derivative. The amount excreted as the acetyl derivative increases progressively with renal impairment (Ohnhaus and Spring, 1975). More than 70% of the drug filtered by the glomeruli undergoes tubular reabsorption (Ohnhaus and Spring, 1975). A linear relationship has been found between the elimination rate constant of SDZ and the endogenous CrCl (ml/min), with a renal plasma water clearance of 27 ml/min. With the drug having a pK_a of 6.4, SDZ excretion is quite sensitive to variations of urinary pH. Dettli and Spring (1968) have shown that even slight acidosis during sleep is capable of increasing the tubular reabsorption, thus enhancing the mean plasma half-life of the drug (from 9.7 h to 13.9 h). Similar mean values (9.0 h during daytime; 11.4 h during the nighttime) have been reported in a more recent study by Ornhaus and Spring (1975). However, when the creatinine clearance is below 30 ml/min, this shift is no longer evident. As would be expected, alkalinization of the urine increases SDZ excretion. The same result is reached when an adequate fluid intake is maintained. In children, a water intake of at least 700 ml/m^2/day is recommended to avoid the risk of crystalluria and anuria (Winterborn and Mann, 1973). In the rare instances when therapy with SDZ is indicated, children (over 2 months of age) should receive half of a calculated daily dose to initiate therapy followed by 65 to 150 mg/kg daily in four to six divided doses (Weinstein, 1975).

Sulfamethoxypyridazine

Sulfamethoxypyridazine (3-sulfanilamido-6-methoxypyridazine, SMD) is classified among those sulfonamides which are rapidly absorbed and slowly excreted (Weinstein, 1975). The compound is no longer available in the United States but is still in use in other countries. In fasting adults, serum levels of 110-180 µg/ml are reached 5 h after an oral dose of 4 g. These levels are maintained for 3 h, thereafter declining very slowly, so that even after 4 days 20-50 µg/ml are still measurable in the serum (Seneca, 1966). From 83 to 85% of the drug is protein-bound, with an apparent maximum binding capacity of human plasma albumin that ranges from 23.2 to 29.7 µmoles/g (Anton, 1960; Seydel, 1969; Dettli and Spring, 1973). SMD has an apparent volume of distribution of 0.19-0.20 L/kg (Bunger et al., 1961; Seydel, 1969; Dettli and Spring, 1973; Chow and Ronfeld,

1975), and an apparent plasma half-life of 34-36 h, as reported by various authors (Seneca, 1966, Dettli and Spring, 1973, Chow and Ronfeld, 1975). The drug reaches concentrations in the CSF that are about 5-10% of plasma levels when no meningeal inflammation is present. 10% to 15% of SMD is acetylated in the liver. A low incidence of genetic polymorphism has been reported for this drug in respect to other sulfonamides, e.g., sulfamethiazine. The "slow acetylator" status, therefore, does not influence the risk of toxicity (White and Price-Evans, 1967). Approximately 25% of the administered dose is excreted within the first 24 h, a further 20% being eliminated in the subsequent 24 h. The non acetylated form undergoes extensive tubular reabsorption, but the acetylated form is excreted more rapidly and accounts for 70-80% of the total drug in the urine. Lower values (50.65 ± 1.66 in "fast acetylators"; 44.76 ± 1.9 in "slow acetylators") have been reported by White and Price-Evans (1967). Alkalinization of the urine favors elimination of the drug.

Pediatric use. The use of SMD is not recommended in the pediatric age group due to the high risk of causing the Stevens-Johnson syndrome. Some older data on its use during the last days of pregnancy indicate that 22-26 h following the administration of 2 g of SMD, the maternal plasma levels did not differ substantially from cord serum levels (86 μg/ml vs. 90 μg/ml). In addition, 4 days after the dose was given (3 days after delivery), plasma levels of 2 μg/ml and 38 μg/ml were measured in the mother and in the newborn, respectively, thus indicating an impaired ability to dispose of the drug in the newborn (Sparr and Pritchard, 1958). When SMD was given to lactating mothers, low levels were found in the milk, and negligible amount found in their newborns (maternal plasma levels, 75-125 μg/ml; milk levels, 10-27 μg/ml, newborns, 0-3 μg/ml) (Sparr and Pritchard, 1958).

Sulfamethopyrazine

Sulfamethopyrazine (2-sulfanilamide-3-methopyrazine, SMP) is one of the ultra-long-acting sulfonamides. A summary overview of the kinetic disposition of SMP is given in Table 2. SMP is well absorbed from the g.i. tract, and after 2-4 h plasma levels of 80-60 μg/ml are achieved with a 2 g dose. About 63-70% of the drug is bound to plasma proteins, with the maximal binding capacity of human plasma albumin being 29.7 μmoles/g (Dettli and Spring, 1973), yet Sereni et al. (1968), observed a reduction in protein-binding in people over 70 years of age. The drug has an apparent volume of distribution of 0.18-0.20 L/kg in adults, which becomes 0.15-0.32 L/kg in the elderly. The apparent plasma half-life may range from 50 to 72 h in adults, and from 69 to 123 h in the elderly subject (Sereni et al., 1968; Berlin, 1969). Furthermore, in the individual patient this parameter varies in a circadian rhythm; a "night" plasma half-life of 110.6 h compared to a "day" plasma half-life of 49.1 h was measured by Dettli and Spring (1968).

Table 2. Effect of Age on Pharmacokinetic Parameters of Sulfamethopyrazine

Age	Mean Apparent Half-Life (h)	Plasma Protein-Binding (%)	Mean Apparent Volume of Distribution (L/Kg)
1-10 days	135-280	–	0.36-0.47
11-30 days	136	57	0.47
1-11 months	53-68	63	0.28-0.36
3-12 months	44-47	–	0.25-0.28
1-4 years	44	–	0.21
4-9 years	50	79	0.20
Adult	62-63	63	0.22-0.25
Elderly	97	62	0.26

Data are derived from Sereni et al., 1968; Gladtke, 1971; Dettli and Spring, 1973.

SMP undergoes extensive acetylation, which is followed by glucuronization; 66% of the drug recovered in the urine is in the acetylated form (Reeves, 1975; Krüger-Thiemer and Bünger, 1965). The drug undergoes extensive tubular reabsorption since, having a pK_a value of 6.1, 55-80% of the SMP is normally present in the distal tubule in the unionized form. Alkalinization of the urine does not affect the excretion of the acetylated form, whereas it does increase the urinary concentration of the free form, thus decreasing the risk of crystalluria, which is dependent on the less-soluble acetylated form. These results, although theoretically of clinical use, are difficult to attain in actual practice, due to poor patient compliance in taking the quantities of alkali needed (Reeves, 1975). A single dose of 2 g allows therapeutic levels to be maintained for 1 week (Garrod et al., 1973). Higher and/or more frequent dosages do not significantly improve the therapeutic efficacy of this drug, while they do increase the risk of crystalluria. Mean plasma following various therapeutic regimens may range from 20 to 107 $\mu g/ml$ after a 2 g dose and from 47 to 184 $\mu g/ml$ for 4 g given once a week. The same therapeutic regimen allows urinary concentrations ($\mu g/ml$) of 15-59 and 34-107, respectively, over a 7-day period.

Newborns, infants and children. Some relevant pharmacokinetic parameters in the pediatric patient were reported by Sereni et al. (1968). Dost and Gladtke (1971) and Gladtke (1971). The apparent plasma half-life changes from 280 h in the first 10 days of life to 136 h in the first month, and decreases to about 44.7-47 h at the end of the first year. As would be expected, an inverse trend was observed when the apparent volume of distribution was considered.

When compared with adult values, the drug concentration in plasma water at

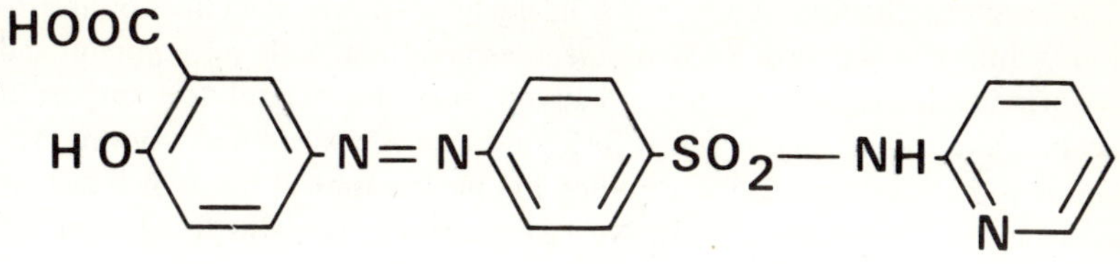

Fig 3: Structural formula of sulfasalazine

half-saturation binding is higher in newborns (K = 513.25 μgmole/l), while it is rather low in infants (K = 293.76) and in children (K = 199.74). This difference could be attributed to the lower concentration of plasma proteins and/or to the higher bilirubin values in newborns. In 1971, Gladtke proposed a different dosage regimen to be used with infants and children. The calculation of this dosage schedule includes a tenfold safety measure and takes into account the different plasma water levels observed in infants (9.6 mg%) and in children (12.5 mg%).

Sulfasalazine

Sulfasalazine (salicylazosulfapyridine, SASP) is composed of 5-aminosalicylate (5-ASA) in azo-kinkage with sulfapyridine (SP) (Fig. 3). Its use has been limited almost exclusively to the treatment of ulcerative colitis, either alone or in combination with corticosteroids, and its value in Crohn's disease is currently being investigated (Ament, 1975). Comprehensive reviews on this drug have been recently published (Anthonisen et al., 1974; Goldman and Peppercorn, 1975; Eastwood and Das, 1975). The place of SASP in the therapy of ulcerative colitis during infancy and childhood has also been reviewed. The drug appears particularly suited for those forms of the disease which can be treated medically, as it does not interfere with growth processes. No data are available on its disposition in infants and children because of the low specific morbidity in this age group. Less than 1% of the reported cases is related to infants younger than 2 years (Ament, 1975).

The drug's mechanism of action is still largely unknown. Main lines of investigation include the action of SASP on the intestinal flora, both in its amount and in its organizational patterns, the effects on fluid and electrolyte transport in the colon, and the inhibition which SASP has been shown to exert on the synthesis of some prostaglandins controlling the mechanisms of mucosal transport (Goldman and Peppercorn, 1975). No agreement yet exists as to whether the pharmacological action should be attributed to SASP, or to the respective actions of SP and 5-aminosalicylate (Goldman, 1973). The combined formulation, however, allows both SP and 5-ASA to be delivered to the site of disease. The two drugs, given separately, do not reach the site of inflammation because of proximal gastrointestinal absorption.

Over the last few years, careful studies have been done to elucidate the complex kinetic behavior of SASP itself, of the two basic molecules, and of the respective metabolites. The sequence of metabolic degradation is shown in Fig. 4. Some relevant pharmacokinetic data are presented in Table 3. SASP is rapidly absorbed in the upper g.i. tract, detectable blood levels (12-50 μg/ml) are reached within 1-2 h after a first dose of 4 g. Marked individual variability in SASP serum concentrations has been noted and it is independent of the dose-related variation in concentration (Schroder and Campbell, 1972); presumably gastric emptying time plays a major role. Intestinal transit time and character of the intestinal flora are responsible for the amount of the intact SASP found in feces. Most of the intact molecule is returned to the g.i. tract due to biliary excretion. Between 2-10% of the administered dose is excreted unchanged in the urine.

The cleavage of the azo-bound (main compounds: SP and 5-ASA) occurs in the colon. In rats, it has been shown to depend exclusively on those intestinal bacteria which are also present in man. When intestinal flora are abolished or greatly modified, a very large amount of the intact compound (53%) is recovered in the feces (Peppercorn and Goldman, 1972). In man, total colectomy does not affect the urinary excretion of intact SASP. Neither colitis nor phenobarbital influences this metabolic step. Phenobarbital pre-treatment, however, decreases urinary excretion of SASP, probably by increasing its biliary excretion (Schroder et al., 1973). Ferrous sulfate decreases blood levels of SASP, presumably through a chelation process within the intestinal lumen, but does not affect the formation of SP (Das and Eastwood, 1973). Antibiotic pre-treatment or different dietary habits modify the pattern of intestinal flora and could contribute to the marked variation of intra- and intersubject metabolic disposition of SASP and its metabolites (Goldman et al., 1974).

SP is well absorbed in the caecum and undergoes extensive hepatic metabolism (Weinstein, 1975). The appearance of SP in the blood starts 5 h after oral

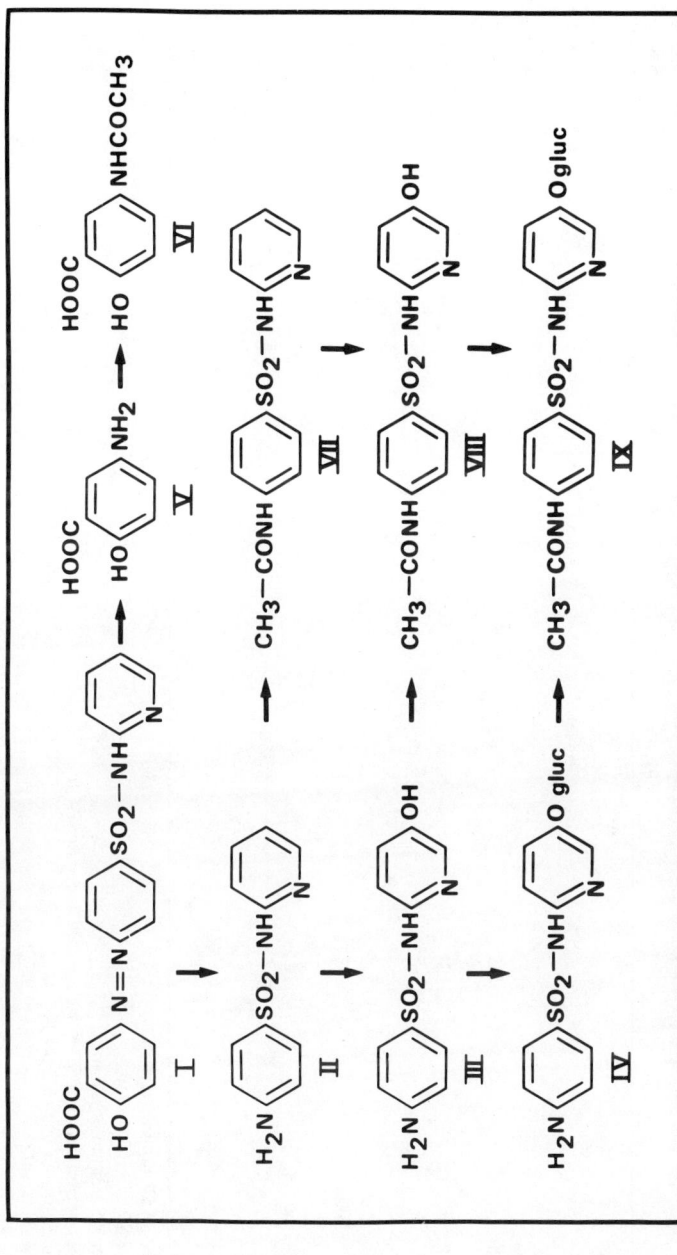

Fig. 4: Metabolic pathway of sulfasalazine. I. Sulfasalazine; II. Sulfapyridine; III. 5-OH-sulfapyridine; IV. 5′-OH-sulfapyridine-O-glucuronide; V. 5-amino salicyclic acid; VI. Acetyl 5-amino salicyclic acid; VII. N-acetyl sulfapyridine; VIII. N-acetyl 5′OH sulfapyridine; IX. N-acetyl 5′OH sulfapyridine-O-glucuronide

Table 3. Mean Pharmacokinetic Parameters of Sulfasalazine

	Peak Time (h)	Peak Level (µg/ml)	T½ (h)	Renal Clearance (ml/min)	Urinary Excretion (% of dose)
SASP	3-5	26 (acute adm.) 18 (st. state)	5.7 ± 0.7 (ac.) 7.6 ± 1.0 (chr.)	7.3 ± 1.7	84*
SP a	12*	33*	10.4 ± 5.3*	9.9 ± 1.9	81 ± 7*
b	3-5*	35-60	8.4 ± 2.1*		
AC SP a	12*	33*		30.4 ± 5.2	81 ± 7*
b	3-5*	35-60			
SP-Gluc a	12*	33*		258 ± 71	81 ± 7*
b	3-5*	35-60*			
AcSP-Gluc a	12*	33*		61.1 ± 10.5	81 ± 7*
b	3-5*	35-60*			
5-ASA + Ac5-ASA a		< 2			34.0 ± 8
c					73 ± 14 (0-48 h)

[a] After SASP administration.
[b] After SP administration.
[c] After ASA administration.
*Total concentration of SP + AcSP + SP-Gluc + AcSP-Gluc.
From Schroder and Campbell, 1972.

administration of 4 g of SASP, and a steady-state concentration is achieved at least 5 days after continuous therapy. SP is subject to ring hydroxylation, followed by conjugation to glucuronic acid and to N-acetylation. This step occurs following the same pattern which has been shown for isoniazid, sulfadimidine, hydralazine and dapsone; these drugs are subject to genetic polymorphism governed by alleles at a single locus. In a group of healthy volunteers (H) and of colitis patients (P), total acetylation of SP has been shown to account for 81.3(H)-85.5(P) and 48.8(H)-47.2(P) of the urinary excretion in "rapid" and "slow" acetylators, respectively.

Highly significant differences in serum levels at steady state (after 5 and 10 days, equally) of SP and its acetyl metabolites are found in two types of population. Phenobarbital pre-treatment causes a significant decrease in the urinary excretion of AcSP metabolites and a more highly significant increase of total glucuronide metabolites. Hydroxylation is increased at the cost of the acetylation, and not of unchanged SP. No influence of urinary pH on the total urinary excretion has been demonstrated. The proportion of AcSP-Gluc shows a slightly significant increase in alkaline conditions (Schroder et al., 1973).

Very low amounts of 5-ASA plus Ac-5-ASA are found in the serum, after either acute or chronic treatment (< 2 µg/ml); one-third of the amount formed through the cleavage of the azo-bound is excreted in the urine as the acetyl derivative. Twice as much is found following 5-ASA administration. This suggests that a major portion of the 5-ASA moiety of SASP is excreted in feces (Schroder and Campbell, 1972; Goldman, 1973).

SASP serum concentration does not correlate with therapeutic success, but serum concentrations of SP appear to be a more reliable index. Levels higher than 20 µg/ml are usually associated with remission, the major exception being those patients who have so-called "constipated" colitis. In this situation, it is suggested that SASP, SP and 5-ASA do not reach the diseased tissue because of spasm (Eastwood and Das, 1975). Between 5 and 55% of patients treated with SASP have shown adverse reactions to the drug. Nausea, vomiting, maculopapular skin rashes, drug fever, "cyanosis," hemolysis, reticulocytosis and leukopenia have all been reported to occur. A high rate of toxic symptoms is found with serum levels of total SP higher than 50 µg/ml. About 85% of these patients have been shown to be "slow" acetylator phenotypes (Das and Eastwood, 1973).

COTRIMOXAZOLE

Adults. Extensive data have been published about cotrimoxazole (trimethoprim-sulfamethoxazole; TMP-SMZ) (Fig. 5), and, together with a lively discussion about its advantages, this subject has been recently and authoritatively reviewed (Brumfitt et al., 1973; Wardell, 1973; Finland, 1974; Kaplan and Abruzzo, in press). Trimethoprim (TMP) selectively inhibits dihydrofolic

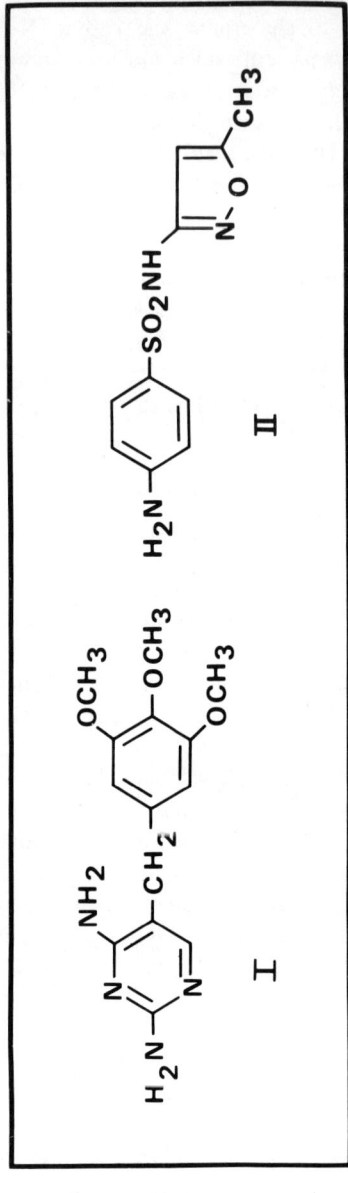

Fig. 5: Structural formula of cotrimoxazole, I. Trimethoprim; II. Sulfamethoxazole

acid reductase, and sulfamethoxazole (SMZ) blocks the synthesis of dihydrofolic acid from p-aminobenzoic acid. In bacteria, the affinity of trimethoprim for the enzyme is many thousand times that in man (Burchall, 1973). Synergism has been shown to occur *in vitro* with concentration ratios of TMP and SMZ between 1:10 and 1:40. The dosage combination proposed for *in vivo* administration, in order to reproduce this condition, is 1:5. Clinical studies have shown that this formulation gives satisfactory results. Both molecules are rapidly, almost completely absorbed from the gastrointestinal tract (Schwartz and Ziegler, 1969). Some delay and impairment of SMZ absorption has been shown to exist when hepatic impairment is present (Rieder and Schwartz, 1975). In adults, routine dosages of 160 mg TMP and 800 mg SMZ every 12 h produce blood levels in the optimal synergy range. Kaplan et al. (1973) reported mean peak levels of 3.13 μg/ml (range from 1.82 to 4.49) with 2-3 h of ingestion for TMP, and 53.3 μg/ml (range from 27.0-70.5) within 3-4 h for free SMZ, after the first standard dosage. In patients with Crohn's disease, signficantly lower plasma levels of TMP at 2 h, and significantly higher levels of SMZ over a 24 h period, have been measured (Parson et al., 1975).

A mean of 63.5-73% of the total sulfonamide content of serum has been calculated to be in the active form between 0 and 12 h, this percentage decreases to 45.7-51% in the period between 24-36 h (Rieder and Schwartz, 1975). At steady-state plasma levels, 65% of SMZ is in the active form (Nolte and Buttner, 1974). Trimethoprim is 44% protein-bound and has a wider distribution than SMZ, which is 65.9% protein-bound in normal sera but only 41.7% bound in uremic sera (Craig, 1975). The respective serum half-lives are 14.5 h (8.3-31.9) for TMP and 11.0 h (6.1-22.5) for SMZ (Kaplan et al., 1973). Highly variable and prolonged half-life values (17.5-215.0 h for TMP; 79.2-273.6 h for total SMZ) have been measured in patients with severe renal impairment (CrCl < 10 ml/min) (Bergan and Brodwall, 1972). Similar data are reported by Welling et al. (1973) and Craig and Kunin (1975). In these patients, the standard dosage ratio is no longer optimal and may need to be changed in order to maintain optimal synergistic serum concentrations.

It has been demonstrated that 24.9% of the dose of SMZ is metabolized to form an inactive compound within 4 h and about 48% is metabolized in 24 h (Fig. 6). TMP is metabolized to a lesser extent than SMZ as 76 ± 10% of its measurable activity is represented by the intact molecule. Small amounts of metabolites of TMP have been identified in the urine (Fig. 7); unconjugated TMP metabolites are also active (Siegel et al., 1975). Hepatic impairment, regardless of degree, does not influence the metabolic disposition of SZM (Rieder and Schwartz, 1975). Both drugs are excreted in the kidneys by glomerular filtration and, to a lesser extent, by tubular secretion (Sharpstone, 1969; Garrod et al., 1973). Acid urines tend to increase TMP excretion and decrease SMZ excretion, but neither drug seems to influence the excretion of the other (Welling et al., 1973). In renal failure, the TMP clearance appears to fall very little (Sharpstone,

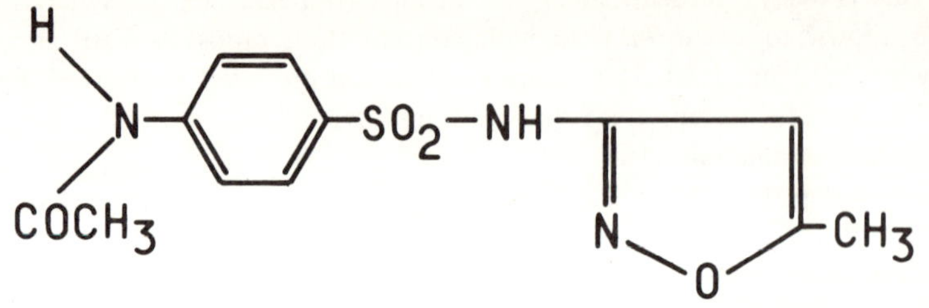

Fig. 6: N-acetyl-sulfamethoxazole (major metabolite of sulfamethoxazole)

1969), and the SMZ clearance is affected only when CRCL falls below 10 ml/min (Welling et al., 1973). No change in the metabolic disposition of these two antibiotics is seen during chronic treatment (Kaplan et al., 1973; Sigel et al., 1975).

Ratios of intact TMP to active SMZ have been calculated as 1:23.8-1:29.1 over a 1-36 h period, ratios of the free drugs have been reported to be 1:14.7-1:18 (Rieder and Schwartz, 1975). Unfortunately, the optimal ratio for synergistic activity is not maintained in the tissues, since TMP diffuses more freely due to its greater lipid solubility. Particularly favorable concentrations of TMP are found in bronchial secretions, lung, saliva, bone, seminal fluid and the prostate (Hansen and Nielsen, 1973; Hansen et al., 1973, 1975; Meares, 1973; Hughes, 1973; Mamborg et al., 1975). In infections involving these tissues, TMP is mainly responsible for therapeutic success. Considering the minor role played by SMZ under these circumstances, combinations with an alkaline sulfonamide, such as sulfadimidine, have been suggested for the treatment of prostatitis. Similarly, TMP alone accounts for therapeutic activity in the bile, since SMZ does not reach significant concentrations in these tissues (Brumfitt et al., 1973). Therapeutic concentrations of both drugs have been measured in the aqueous humor (Pohjanpelto et al., 1974; Salmon et al., 1975). Levels of TMP are very low in brain tissue and CSF (Brumfitt et al., 1973), but therapeutic levels are attainable in the CSF in the presence of meningeal inflammation (Morzaria et al., 1969; Kirwan 1974; Sabel and Brandber, 1975). The presence of very high levels of both compounds possibly compensates for the nonsynergistic concentrations obtained in urine (active SMZ; TMP ration between 1-1.5) (Baethke et al., 1972; Bergan and Brodwall, 1972; Kremers et al., 1974).

In a group of women treated with cotrimoxazole and undergoing therapeutic

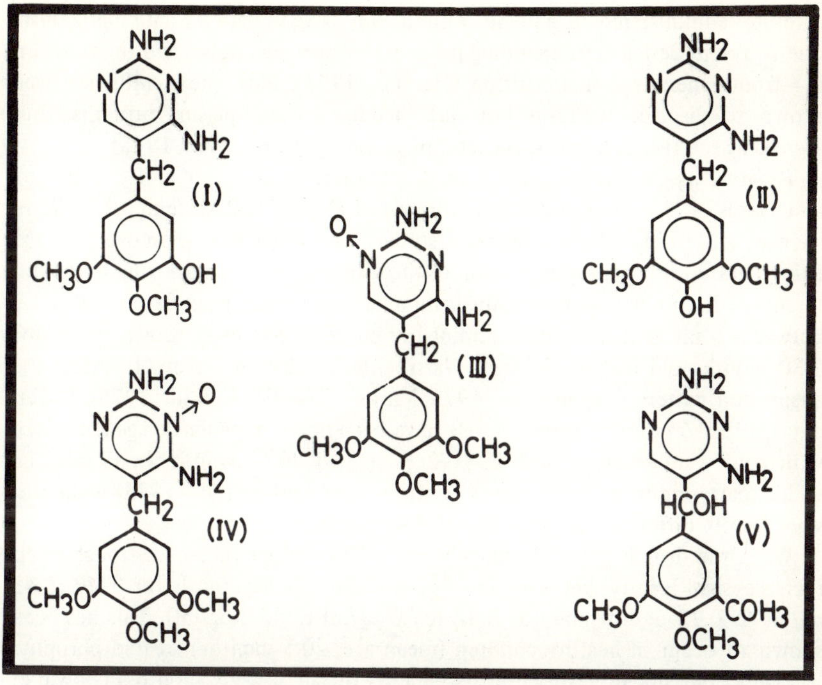

Fig. 7: Metabolic pathway of trimethoprim, I. 2,4-diamino-5(3-hydroxy-4, 5-dimethoxybenzyl)pyrimidine; II. 2,4-diamino-5(4-hydroxy-3,5-dimethoxybenzyl)pyrimidine; III. 2,4-diamino-5(3,4,5-trimethoxybenzyl) pyrimidine-N-oxide; 2,4-diamino-5(3,4,5-trimethoxybenzyl) pyrimidine-3-oxide; V. 2,4-diamino-5(alpha hydroxyl-3,4,5-trimethoxylbenzyl) pyrimidine

abortion, SMZ levels were significantly lower ($P < 0.05$) in amniotic fluid than in maternal serum (18-16 µg/ml vs 40.10 µg/ml); on the contrary, TMP levels in fetal and maternal sera, and in amniotic fluid, were similar. Concentration ratios of TMP to SMZ in this condition appear to be much higher than in normal adults, both in maternal (1:87) and in fetal (1:97) serum. This finding is possibly due to the different tissue distribution of TMP and SMZ, as it has been documented by the concentration ratios in placenta (1:9), amniotic fluid (1:8), fetal liver (1:10) and fetal lung (1:5) (Reid et al., 1975).

The reported frequency of side effects varies but is considered acceptable, since the most common symptoms are related to transient gastrointestinal disturbances. Careful control of hematologic parameters is useful, mainly in patients with abnormal bone marrow function (Bernstein Hahn and Barclay, 1975); instances of deterioration in renal function in association with cotrimoxazole therapy suggest that these drugs should be used with extreme caution in patients with impaired renal function. The antibiotic combination should be carefully administered to patients who already have impaired folate metabolism due to folate deficiency, including pregnant women, alcoholics and those suffering from generalized malnutrition (Herbert, 1973). SMZ (not TMP) has been shown to displace warfarin but not dicumarol from plasma proteins, thus increasing the risk of hemorrhagic complications (Tilstone et al., 1975).

Pediatric age. Cotrimoxazole is used extensively in pediatric patients (Fernex and Havas, 1972; Bose et al., 1974; Fowle et al., 1975; Bernstein, 1975; Bernstein et al., 1975). Pharmacokinetic studies have been rare, moreover, the existing data do not permit evaluation of the disposal patterns occurring in the different pediatric age groups. Absorption is rapid with peak levels occurring between 2 and 4 h after oral administration. This has been shown in infants 1-30 months old and in children. Gastroenteritis does not seem to affect the absorption pattern (Lewin et al., 1973; Marks, 1975; Fowle et al., 1975). Different TMP-SMZ ratios in plasma levels have been noted in pediatric age compared with adult values: range of 1:22-1:72 vs. 1:16-1:20 (Lewin et al., 1975). The wider scattering in pediatric age is confirmed by Fowle et al. (1975) while not significantly different ratios are reported by Marks (1975).

When the drug is given chronically, on a 12 h dosage schedule, trough levels increase significantly between the 3rd and the 6th day, both for TMP (0.43 μg/ml to 0.72 μg/ml) and for SMZ (37.0 μg/ml to 47.2 μg/ml). This has been shown to occur in healthy children (mean age, 20.5 months) treated phrophylactically, but not in gastroenteritis patients (mean age, 9.2 months) (Fowle et al., 1975). Data obtained by Lenox-Smith (quoted by Brumfitt, 1973) in different age groups suggest a pattern of T½ values for SMZ which has been shown to occur also for other groups of drugs: the very long half-life (unspecified values) in neonates less than 10 days old, sharp decreases from 3 weeks to 1 year (from 9 h to 4-5 h), to rise to adult values after 6-8 years. Values of 7.1 h are reported for a mixed group of infants and children (Vest et al., 1974). Higher values have been found by Lewin et al. (1975) in three mixed groups with mean age of 13 months (range 1 month-5 years: T½ 14.0 h), 4.7 years (range 2-8 years: T½ 10.0 h), 3.9 years (range 1 month-14 years: T½ 14.0 h), respectively. These same authors for the same age groups report data for TMP half-life of 7.6 h, 5.5 h and 8.4 h respecitvely. In a similarly mixed group of infants and children, the half-life of TMP was found to be 6.4 h (Vest et al., 1974).

URINARY ANTISEPTICS

Nitrofurantoin

Among the various nitrofurans, nitrofurantoin is the most commonly used compound (Fig. 8). The place of nitrofurantoin in the management of urinary

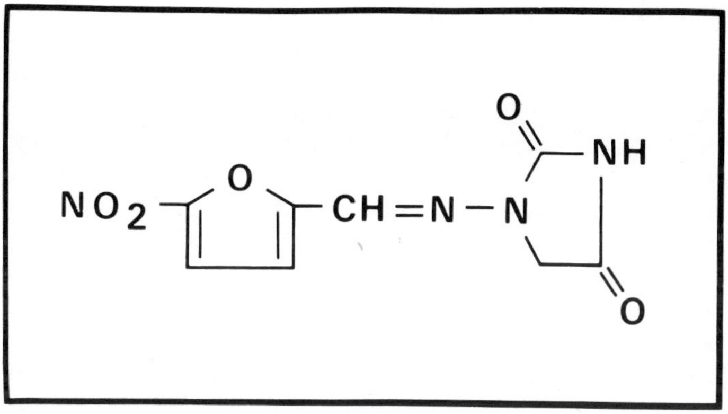

Fig. 8: Structural formula of nitrofurantoin

tract infections (UTI) is discussed extensively in several manual and textbooks (Williams et al., 1973; Kunin, 1974; Garrod et al., 1973). Nitrofurantoin is usually administered by the oral route, but parenteral administration may be required when UTI has been shown to be resistant to alternate drugs in *in vitro* sensitivity testing (Kunin, 1974). Nitrofurantoin is well absorbed by mouth, and doses of 100 mg give rise to peak plasma levels of 0.8-1.5 µg/ml within 1-3 h (Conklin, 1972; Garrod et al., 1973; Albert et al., 1974). Peak levels are followed by a very rapid decay of plasma concentrations, which fall below analytical sensitivity within a few hours. Consistent differences in bioavailability have been shown among the various pharmaceutical preparations with different particle size, however, no useful correlation could be established between the amount of the drug recoverable in the urine and the *in vitro* test for disintegration and dissolution (Paul et al., 1967; McGilveray et al., 1971; Meyer et al., 1974; Albert et al., 1974). The improved availability that the microcrystalline form shows does not appear to reach the significance level, and, on the other hand, the incidence of side effect e.g., nausea and emesis, observed with the macrocrystalline form is minor (Paul et al., 1967; Conklin, 1972; Schwartlander and Eulenhofer, 1972; Meyer et al., 1974).

Recently, Bates et al. (1974) showed that, by administering nitrofurantoin concomitantly with food, there is a delay in absorption, however, this disadvantage is compensated for by an increased bioavailability with an increase in peak body levels (more pronounced for the macrocrystalline form) and by a prolonged (2 h) therapeutic urinary concentration. Following intramuscular administration of 180 mg of nitrofurantoin sodium, Cox et al. (1971) observed peak plasma levels of 1.8-6.4 µg/ml 1 h after the injection. According to Reckendorf et al. (1963) and Conklin (1972), the apparent plasma half-life is about 20-30 min, while McGilverary et al. (1971) and Meyer et al. (1974) reported a T½ of about 1 h. About one-half of an oral dose is metabolized, mainly in the liver, and the remainder is rapidly excreted in the urine (Garrod et al., 1973; Ball et al., 1975). Nitrofuratoin is excreted by both glomerular filtration and tubular secretion (Garrod et al., 1973). Drugs excreted by the same route can markedly reduce nitrofurantoin excretion. This has been shown to occur with ASA (Hüller et al., 1975). Since the compound is a weak acid, at favorable pH, a consistent part of the filtrate may be reabsorbed by noninomic back-diffusion in the distal tubule. This may result in a peritubular concentration of nitrofurantoin as high as 12-48 µg/ml (Garrod et al., 1973). Direct assay of renal lymph has revealed concentrations about twofold higher than those in the plasma (Garrod et al., 1973).

Maximal urinary concentrations are usually achieved within 2-4 h after oral drug intake, and peak concentrations after a standard dose are about 80-250 µg/ml (Paul et al., 1967; Ball et al., 1971; Kalowsky et al., 1974). Following intramuscular administration, urinary levels of 180-264 µg/ml can be achieved within 1 h (Cox et al., 1971). Approximately 20-50% of the administered dose is excreted within 4-6 h (Paul, 1967; Conklin and Hailey, 1969; Albert, 1974; Mayer et al., 1974), and therapeutic urinary concentrations of 30-50 µg/ml are detectable for about 6-8 h (Garrod et al., 1973; Bates et al., 1974). These concentrations are usually higher than the MIC for most sensitive urinary tract pathogens, however, resistant strains require concentrations higher than 75 µg/ml. Bailey et al. (1971) reported that a single daily oral dose of 50 mg at night should be effective in preventing urinary tract infection and should result in a very low rate of side effects.

It is important to remember that in cases with seriously compromised renal function effective antimicrobial levels cannot be achieved using reduced dosages, yet severe neurological side effects may occur if customary or higher doses are used (Sachs et al., 1968; Felts et al., 1971; Garrod et al., 1973; Ballet et al., 1975). Consequently, nitrofurantoin is contraindicated in renal failure. The overall incidence of severe or disturbing side effects in the course of nitrofurantoin treatment is 3.5-9% according to various reports (Koch-Weser et al., 1971; Garrod et al., 1973; Kalowsky et al., 1974). Less severe side effects consist of gastric disturbances such as nausea and emesis, which can be partially avoided by administering the drug with food and in macrocrystalline forms (Kean and Hoskins, 1972). More severe side effects include peripheral neuropathy and pulmonary reactions, such as acute and subacute pneumonitis. Peripheral neuropathy is often associated either with overdosage or with impairment of kidney function, and in these instances clearly appears to be linked to toxic plasma concentrations, as shown by the work of Toole et al. (1968) in normal volunteers. These side effects are particularly severe since, both with the neuropathy and the pulmonary reactions, complete recovery is not always the rule, even after immediate drug withdrawal (Rosenow et al., 1968; Felts et al., 1971; Garrod et al., 1973; Back et al., 1974; Ball et al., 1975). Hemolytic anemia, most common in those subjects with G6PD deficiency and with megaloblastic anemia, has also been reported (Pritchard et al., 1965; Garrod et al., 1973; Ball et al., 1975). Occurrence of cholestasis and hepatocellular injury is a relatively rare event, it does not seem to be related to toxic plasma levels but probably is due to hypersensitivity reactions (Ernaelsteen and Williams, 1961; Goldstein et al., 1974).

Kinetic data on pediatric patients are practically nonexistent. This scarcity of data contrasts not only with the widespread attention that the problem of treating or not treating pediatric bacteriuria has received but also with the extensive use of nitrofurantoin in pediatric practice (McCracken et al., 1969a,b; McCracken and Eichenwald, 1974). It has been reported that, following conventional oral doses, the concentration in cord blood is generally less than the maternal levels (Perry and Leblanc, 1967; Garrod et al., 1973), and thus, there is little danger of fetal toxicity. On the other hand, drug intake by the mother in the hours immediately preceding delivery could result in measurable amounts in the newborn, whose abilities to eliminate the drug via the kidney are very poor, hence the possibility of toxicity does exist. The same holds true for breast-fed newborns. Although Hosbach and Foster (1967) found the concentrations of nitrofurantoin in human milk significant, it is true that detectable amounts occasionally can be measured in the milk of a mother who has been given relatively high amounts (200 mg) 2 h before sampling (Varsano et al., 1973). This possibility should be kept in mind for the potential risk it presents in populations with high incidence of G6PD deficiency. In such a case, in fact, even a very small amount of nitrofurantoin may be sufficient to trigger a hemolytic reaction. A case of benign intracranial hypertension associated with nitrofurantoin therapy has been recently reported in a 10-month-old boy receiving 25 mg t.i.d. for 7 days (Sharma and James, 1974). Discontinuation of therapy led to normal conditions only after 6 days. According to Faigle and Ziment (1968), infants below 1 month of age should not be treated with the drug at all, and older children should not recieve more than 9 mg/kg daily. Even lower dosages, 1.5 mg/kg in infants and 5-7 mg/kg in children, are recommended by Silver et al. (1975) and by *AMA Drug Evaluations* (1973).

Nalidixic Acid

Nalidixic acid, a derivative of 1.8 napththylpyridine, is a synthetic chemotherapeutic agent which, like nitrofurantoin, finds its main indication in oral treatment of urinary tract infections (Garrod et al., 1973). The structural formula and the metabolic pathway are given in Figs. 9 and 10.

Adults. In adults, nalidixic acid given by mouth is rapidly and nearly completely absorbed. Doses of 1 g give rise to peak plasma levels of 15-30 μg/ml

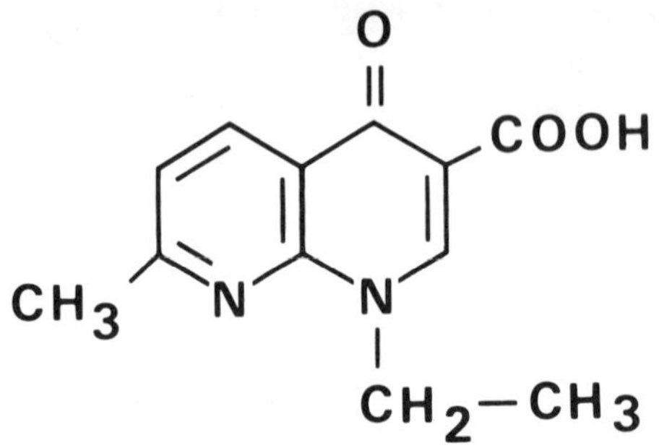

Fig. 9: Structural formula of nalidixic acid

within 60-150 min (Moore et al., 1965; Portmann et al., 1966a,b; Harrison and Cox, 1970; Brühl et al., 1973). Peak levels ranging from 70 to 120 μg/ml were obtained by Rohwedder et al. (1970) following a 2 g dose. The sodium-salt form is absorbed faster and to a greater extent than the acid form (Portmann et al., 1966a). Administration of the drug with an alkali may increase its rate of absorption, but, more importantly, it may permit less tubular reabsorption of the drug, thus leading to higher urinary levels. Nalidixic acid is strongly bound to plasma proteins (93%) and has an apparent volume of distribution of 0.25-0.55 L/kg (Moore et al., 1965; Portmann et al., 1966a,b; Rohwedder et al., 1970). The drug does not cross the blood-brain barrier in any appreciable amount (Finegold and Ziment, 1968), and its apparent plasma half-life is about 1-1.5 h (Portmann et al., 1966a; Brühl et al., 1973).

Nalidixic acid is rapidly metabolized to an active derivative, hydroxynalidixic acid, and both compounds are readily conjugated with glucuronic acid; a minor metabolic pathway leads to the formation of dicarboxylic derivatives, including 3,7-dicarboxylic acid (Moore et al., 1965). The ratio of nalidixic acid to its hydroxy derivative is < 1 during chronic treatment (McChesney et al., 1967), and the hydroxyderivative can be detected in measurable amounts as soon as 8 min after administration of nalidixic acid (Portmann et al., 1966a). About 94% of the administered dose can be recovered in the 24 h urine, but urinary

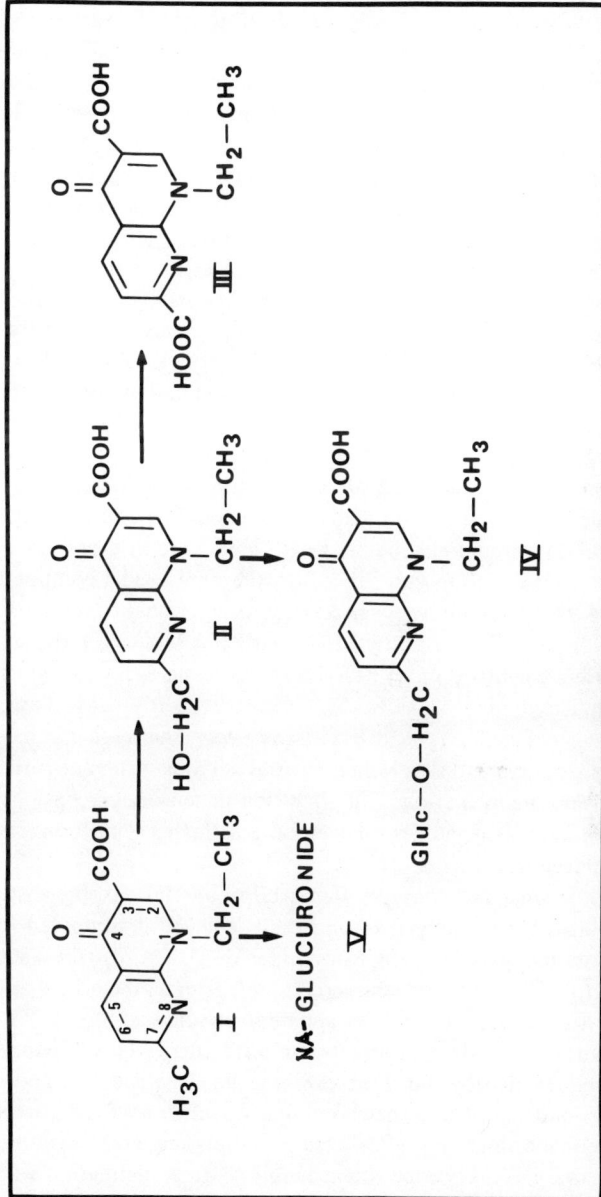

Fig. 10: Metabolic pathway of nalidixic acid, I. Nalidixic acid; II. 7-OH-nalidixic acid; III. 3-7-dicarboxylic acid

excretion of the drug is maximal 3 h after dosing, and more than 50% of the total dose is excreted during the first 5 h (Moore et al., 1965; Portmann, 1966a; Brühl et al., 1973). Only 1-3% of the excreted material is due to unchanged nalidixic acid; 13% is represented by the free hydroxy metabolite, the rest being due to inactive glucuronides (76%) and dicarboxylic derivatives (4.3%) (Portmann et al., 1966b; McChesney et al., 1967). The biologically effective plasma and urinary levels are a function of the sum of the free nalidixic and free hydroxynalidixic acid concentrations (McChesney et al., 1967). Following a dose of 1 g, concentrations higher than 100 μg/ml of the drug are maintained in the urine 4-8 h, and concentrations over 50 μg/ml may be present for up to 24 h (Brühl et al., 1973). The urinary excretion of nalidixic acid is very sensitive to variation in the pH and alkalinization may considerably increase the drug's concentration in urine (Portmann et al., 1966b; Garrod et al., 1973).

In agreement with its apparent plasma half-life value, the drug does not seem to accumulate in plasma when it is given at 6 h intervals in the course of chronic treatment (Buchbinder et al., 1962). Since the drug is extensively metabolized before being excreted through the kidney, no accumulation of nalidixic acid is to be expected in renal failure cases, however, there is little or no sense at all in administering nalidixic acid to patients with impaired renal function, as very little probability exists that adequate amounts of the active compounds will be present in the urine. The use of nalidixic acid should be avoided in patients with hepatic failure. It should also be used with great care in those cases where the drug is given in association with other highly bound, acidic compounds. An increase of 64 to 160% in free warfarin, with consequent increased danger of hemorrhage, has been reported by Seller and Kock-Weser (1970), and the same displacing effect might occur with oral hypoglycemic agents, anti-inflammatory drugs and diphenylhydantoin.

The toxicity of nalidixic acid is relatively low; the most common reported side effects are nausea and skin rashes. Central nervous system disturbances, such as blurred vision, hallucinations and alteration of sensory perceptions, as well as seizures, have been associated with overdosages. Such a symptomatology is fully reversible on drug withdrawal.

Newborns, infants and children. In newborns and infants, the absorption rate of nalidixic acid given orally is considerably delayed if compared to values of children or adults. According to Rohwedder et al. (1970) (see Table 4), peak levels of 71 to 110 μg/ml are achieved 3 to 4 h after a 20 mg/kg dose. The elimination rate is also reduced, with an apparent plasma half-life of 3.8 ± 1.3 h in newborns and of 2.6 ± 0.6 h in infants. No differences were observed for the apparent volume of distribution. Furthermore, the same authors reported that in 2 prematures and 8 full-term newborns the calculation of the elimination rate could not be made since, 8 h after dosing, the plasma levels were still very high (in plateau). As a consequence, the possibility of accumulation with resulting toxic plasma levels is likely, and therefore nalidixic acid should not be

Table 4. Pharmacokinetics of Nalidixic Acid in Different Age Groups

Age Groups	App. Vd (L/Kg)	Peak Levels (μg/ml)	App. T½ (h)	Invasion Constant (h^{-1})	Elimination Constant (h^{-1})
Newborns	0.22 ± 0.13	85 ± 16	3.86 ± 1.33	0.648 ± 0.178	0.199 ± 0.066
Infants (> 3 mo)	0.25 ± 0.06	49 ± 16	2.68 ± 0.64	0.715 ± 0.221	0.278 ± 0.091
Children (1-3 yrs)	0.26 ± 0.11	53 ± 16	1.81 ± 0.61	0.949 ± 0.403	0.433 ± 0.178
> 3 yrs	0.19 ± 0.05	65 ± 13	1.82 ± 0.69	1.757 ± 0.468	0.415 ± 0.106

Adapted from Rohwedder et al., 1970.

administered to infants below 3 months of age. If it is absolutely necessary to use the drug, doses should be in the range of 10 mg/kg b.i.d.

In children, the disappearance rate is similar (app. plasma half-life, 1.8 ± 0.7 h) to that observed in adults, but the absorption rate is reduced with peak levels of 50-60 μg/ml at 1.5-2.5 h. Similar apparent plasma half-lives in children were reported by Nelson et al. (1972) in their observations on the kinetics of nalidixic acid during the course of acute shigellosis. With regard to the absorption rate, two distinct patterns were noticed. A group of patients defined as "prompt" absorbers were shown to have peak levels of 24-73 μg/ml 1 h after drug intake, while a second group of "delayed" absorbers had peak levels of 16-31 μg/ml at about 4 h after the dose. Furthermore, in the acute phase of the disease in all patients, there seemed to be an impairment in the metabolic breakdown of the drug, with a low percentage of conjugated nalidixic acid (4%) and hydroxynalidixic acid (22%) found in the plasma. During convalescence, the metabolic rate increased to normal values, both for nalidixic gulucuronide (17%) and the hydroxy derivatives (56%). These data tend to suggest that in the acute phase of the disease the metabolism of nalidixic acid is altered, while the absorption rate appears to be variably influenced. No significant differences in clinical response were observed between "prompt" and "delayed" absorbers, nor could such differences as did exist be related to the degree of dehydration or to the blood urea nitrogen. Toxic reactions to nalidixic acid are most likely to occur in infants and are often associated with overdosages. The severe side effects that may be seen include acute intracranial hypertension (which may appear after only the first 2-3 doses), tachydyspnea, metabolic acidosis and cardiocirculatory collapse (Boreus and Sundstrom, 1967; Fisher, 1967; Guran et al., 1972; Deonna and Guignard, 1974). Cases of hemolytic anemia purportedly caused by the drug have also been reported (Mandal and Stevenson, 1970).

REFERENCES

Albert, K.S., Sedman, A.J., Wilkinson, P., Stoll, R.G., Murray, W.J. and Wagner, J.G. (1974): Bioavailability studies of acetaminophen and nitrofurantoin. *Journal of Clinical Pharmacology, 14:* 264-270.
Ament, M.E. (1975): Inflammatory disease of the colon: ulcerative colitis and Crohn's colitis. *Journal of Pediatrics, 86:* 322-334.
American Medical Association (1973): *AMA Drug Evaluations,* 2nd ed., Ch. 56, American Medical Association, Chicago.
Anthoninsen, P., Barany, F. and Folkenborg, O. (1974): The clinical effect of salazosulphapyridine in Crohn's disease. *Scandinavian Journal of Gastroenterology, 9:* 549-554.
Anton, A.H. (1960): The relation between the binding of sulfonamides to albumin and their antibacterial efficacy. *Journal of Pharmacology and Experimental Therapeutics, 129:* 282-290.
Anton, A.H. and Corey, W.T. (1971): Interindividual differences in the protein binding of sulfonamides: the effect of disease and drugs. *Acta Pharmacologica et Toxicologica, 29:* suppl. 3: 134-151.
Bäck, O., Lundgren, R. and Winan, L.-G. (1974): Nitrofurantoin-induced pulmonary fibrosis and lupus syndrome. *Lancet, 1:* 930.
Baethke, R., Golde, G. and Gahl, G. (1972): Sulphamethoxazole/trimethoprim: pharmacokinetic studies in patients with chronic renal failure. *European Journal of Clinical Pharmacology, 4:* 233-240.
Bailey, R.R., Roberts, A.P., Gower, P.E. and de Wardener, H.E. (1971): Prevention of urinary-tract infection with low-dose nitrofurantoin. *Lancet, 2:* 1112-1114.
Ball, A.P., Gray, J.A. and Murdoch, J.McC. (1975): Antibacterial drugs today, Pt. I. *Drugs, 10:* 1-55.
Barnett, H. (1972): *Pediatrics,* 15th ed., Appleton Century Croft, New York.
Bates, T.R., Sequeira, J.A. and Tembo, A.V. (1974): Effect of food on nitrofurantoin absorption. *Clinical Pharmacology and Therapeutics, 16:* 63-68.
Bergan, T. and Brodwall, E.K. (1972): Human pharmacokinetics of a sulfamethoxazole-trimethoprim combination. *Acta Medica Scandinavica, 192:* 483-492.
Berlin, H. (1969): Protein binding of sulfonamides. In: *Farmitalia, Simposio Internazionale sulla Sulfametopirazina,* pp. 48-57, Minerva Medica, Torino.
Bernstein, L.S. (1975). Adverse reactions to trimethoprimsulfamethoxazole, with particular reference to long-term therapy. *Canadian Medical Association Journal, 112:* 96S-98S.
Bernstein Hanh L. and Barclay, C.A. (1975): Long-term treatment with the combination SMZ/TMP in children with urinary tract infections. In: *Abstracts, 9th International Congress of Chemotherapy,* London, July 13-18, 1975, Abstr. M633, Garden City Press, Letchworth.
Boréus, L.O. and Sundström, B. (1967): Intracranial hypertension in a child during treatment with nalidixic acid. *British Medical Journal, 2:* 744-745.
Böse, W., Karama, A., Linzenmeier, G., Olbing, H. and Wellmann, P. (1974): Controlled trial of co-trimoxazole in children with urinary-tract infection. Bacteriological efficacy and haematological toxicity. *Lancet, 2:* 614-616.
Brühl, P., Gundlach, G., Wintjes, K., Eichner, W. and Bastian, H.P. (1973): Neue untersuchungen zur pharmakokinetik der Nalidixinsäure. I. Serum-und urinspiegel bei normaler nierenfunktion. *Arzneimittel-Forschung, 23:* 1311-1313.
Brumfitt, W., Hamilton-Miller, J.M.T. and Kosmidis, J. (1973): Trimethoprim-sulfamethoxazole: the present position. *Journal of Infectious Diseases, 128,* suppl.: S778-S791.
Buchbinder, M., Webb, J.C., La Verne Aderson and McCabe, W.R. (1962): Laboratory studies and clinical pharmacology of nalidixic acid (WIN 18,320). *Antimicrobial Agents and Chemotherapy,* 308-317.

Bünger, P., Diller, W., Führ, J. and Krüger-Thiemer, E. (1961): Vergleichende Untersuchungen an neueren Sulfanilamiden. *Arzneimittel-Forschung, 11:* 247-255.
Burchall, J.J. (1973): Mechanism of action of trimethoprimsulphamethoxazole. II. *Journal of Infectious Diseases, 128,* suppl.: 437-441.
Chignell, C.F., Vesell, E.S., Starkweather, D.K. and Berlin, C.M. (1971): The binding of sulfaphenazole to fetal-neonatal and adult human plasma albumin. *Clinical Pharmacology and Therapeutics, 12:* 897-901.
Chow, M.S.S. and Ronfeld, R.A. (1975): Pharmacokinetic data and drug monitoring. I. Antibiotics and antiarrhythmics. *Journal of Clinical Pharmacology, 15:* 405-418.
Conklin, J.D. (1972): Biopharmaceutics of nitrofurantoin. *Pharmacology, 8:* 178-181.
Conklin, J.D. and Hailey, F.J. (1969): Urinary drug excretion in man during oral dosage of different nitrofurantoin formulations. *Clinical Pharmacology and Therapeutics, 10:* 534-539.
Cox, C.E., O'Connor, F.J. and Lacy, S.S. (1971): Clinical effectiveness of intramuscular sodium nitrofurantoin against urinary tract infections. *Journal of Urology, 105:* 113-118.
Craig, W.A. (1975): Further studies on the protein binding inhibitor of antimicrobials in uremic sera. In: *Abstracts of the 9th International Congress of Chemotherapy,* London, July 13-18, 1975, Abstr. M401, Garden City Press, Letchworth.
Craig, W.A. and Kunin, C.M. (1975): Trimethoprim/sulfamethoxazole: pharmacodynamic effects of urinary pH and impaired renal function. In: Wellcome Med. Educational Service. *Trimethoprim/Sulfamethoxazole (Septra),* pp. 6-12, Science Medicine.
Crawford, J.S. and Hodi, H.W.Y. (1968): Binding of salicylic acid and sulphanilamide in serum from pregnant patients, cord blood and subjects taking oral contraceptives. *British Journal of Anaesthesiology, 40:* 825-833.
Das, K.M. and Eastwood, M.A. (1973): Effect of iron and calcium on salicylazosulphapyridine metabolism. *Scottish Medical Journal, 18:* 45-50.
Deonna, T. and Guignard, P. (174): Acute intracranial hypertension after nalidixic acid administration. *Archives of Disease in Childhood, 49:* 743.
Dettli, L.C. (1974): Drug dosage in patients with renal disease. *Clinical Pharmacology and Therapeutics, 16:* 274-280.
Dettli, L. and Spring, P. (1968): In: *Proceedings, 3rd International Pharmacological Meeting, Sao Paulo, 1966, 7:* 5.
Dettli, L. and Spring, P. (1973): Krüger-Thiemer's theory on drug dosage: a simplified presentation. In: *Biological Effects of Drugs in Relation to Their Plasma Concentrations,* edited by D.S. Davies and B.N.C. Prichard, pp. 157-168, Macmillan, London.
Dost, F.H. and Gladtke, E. (1969): Pharmakokinetik des 2-Sulfanilamido-3-methoxypyrazin beim kind (Elimination, enterale Absoprtion,'Verteilung und Dosierung). *Arzneimittel-Forschung, 19:* 1304-1307.
Eastwood, M.A. and Das, K.M. (1975): The treatment of ulcerative colitis with sulphasalzine. *British Journal of Hospital Medicine, 13:* 142-149.
Ernaelsteen, D. and Williams, R. (1961): Jaundice due to nitrofurantoin. *Gastroenterology, 41:* 590-593.
Felts, J.H., Hayes, D.M., Gergen, J.A. and Toole, J.F. (1971): Neural, hematologic and bacteriologic effects of nitrofurantoin in renal insufficiency. *American Journal of Medicine, 51:* 331-339.
Fernex, M. and Havas, L. (1972): Clinical experience with trimethoprim and sulfamethoxazole with special reference to its use in 867 children. In: Proceedings, 10th SEAMEO-TROPMED Seminar. *Symposium on Chemotherapy in Tropical Medicine of Southeast Asia and the Far East,* Bangkok, Oct. 1971, edited by T. Harinasuta, pp. 129-148.
Finegold, S.M. and Ziment, I. (1968): Sulfonamide, nitrofurans and nalidixic acid. *Pediatric Clinics of North America, 15:* 95-105.

Finland, M. (1972): Adventures with antibacterial drugs. *Clinical Pharmacology and Therapeutics, 13:* 469-511.
Finland, M. (1974): Combinations of antimicrobial drugs: trimethoprim/sulfamethoxazole. *New England Journal of Medicine, 291:* 624-627.
Fisher, O.D. (1967): Nalidixic acid and intracranial hypertension. *British Medical Journal, 3:* 370.
Fowle, A.S.E., Bye, A., Hariri, F. Middlemiss, D. and Naficy, K. (1975): The dosage of co-trimoxazole in childhood. *European Journal of Clinical Pharmacology, 8:* 217-222.
Garrod, L.P., Lambert, H.P. and O'Grady, F. (1973): *Antibiotic and Chemotherapy*, 4th ed., Churchill Livingstone, Edinburgh.
Gladtke, E. (1971): Pharmacokinetics of 2-sulfanilamido-3-methoxypyrazin in children. In: *Progress in Antimicrobial and Anticancer Chemotherapy*, pp. 633-636. University of Tokyo Press, Tokyo.
Goldman, P. (1973): Therapeutic implications of the intestinal microflora. *New England Journal of Medicine, 289:* 623-628.
Goldman, P., Peppercorn, M.A. and Goldin, B.R. (1974): Drugs metabolized by intestinal microflora. In: *Drug Interactions*, edited by P.L. Morselli, S. Garattini and S.N. Cohen, pp. 91-102, Raven Press, New York.
Goldman, P. and Peppercorn, M.A. (1975): Sulfasalazine. *New England Journal of Medicine, 292:* 20-23.
Goldstein, L.I., Eshak, K.G. and Burns, W. (1974): Hepatic injury associated with nitrofurantoin therapy. *American Journal of Digestive Diseases, 19:* 987-998.
Gurau, P., Monette, G. and Blanc, A. (1972): Hypertension intracranienne aigüe et transitoire chez une enfant de 9 ans traitée par l'acide nalidixique. *Archives Franaises de Pediatrie, 29:* 1107-1115.
Hansen, I., Nielsen, M.L. and Bertelsen, S. (1973): Trimethoprim in human saliva, bronchial secretion and lung tissue. *Acta Pharmacologica et Toxicologica, 32:* 337-344.
Hansen, I., Nielsen, M.L., Heerfordt, L., Henriksen, B. and Bertelsen, S. (1973): Trimetroprim in normal and pathological human lung tissue. *Chemotherapy, 19:* 221-234.
Hansen, I., Nielsen, M.L. and Nielsen, J.B. (1975): A new method for homogenization of bone exemplified by measurement of trimethoprim in human bone tissue. *Acta Pharmacologica et Toxicologica, 37:* 33-42.
Harrison, L.H. and Cox, C.E. (1970): Bacteriologic and pharmacodynamics aspects of nalidixic acid. *Journal of Urology, 104:* 908-913.
Herbert, V. (1973): Metabolism of folic acid in man. *Journal of Infectious Diseases, 128*, suppl.: 601-606.
Hosbach, R.H. and Foster, R.B. (1967): Absence of nitrofurantoin from human milk. *Journal of the American Medical Association, 202:* 1057.
Hughes, D.T.D. (1973): Use of combinations of trimethoprim and sulfamethoxazole in the treatment of chest infections. *Medical Journal, 1*, suppl.: 58-61.
Hüller, H., Amon, I. and Amon, K. (1975): Interactions of nitrofurantoin with other drugs in the human organism. In: *Abstracts of 9th International Congress of Chemotherapy*, London, July 13-18, abstr. M. 163, Garden City Press, Letchworth.
Kalowski, S., Radford, N. and Kincard-Smith, P. (1974): Crystalline and macrocrystalline nitrofurantoin in the treatment of urinary-tract infection. *New England Journal of Medicine, 290:* 385-387.
Kaplan, S.A. and Abruzzo, C.W. (1976): Clinical pharmacokinetics of cotrimoxazole. Presented at the "International Symposium on Clinical Pharmacy and Pharmacology," Boston, Mass., 17-19 September 1975, in press.
Kaplan, S.A., Weinfeld, R.E. Abruzzo, C.W. and Lewis, M. (1972): Pharmacokinetic profile of sulfisoxazole following intravenous, intramuscular and oral administration to man. *Journal of Pharmaceutical Sciences, 61:* 773-778.

Kaplan, S.A., Weinfeld, R.E., Abruzzo, C.W., McFaden, K., Jack, M.L. and Weissman, L. (1973): Pharmacokinetic profile of trimethoprim-sulfamethoxazole in man. *Journal of Infectious Diseases, 128*, suppl.: S547-S555.

Kean, B.H. and Hoskins, D.W. (1972): Drugs for intestinal parasitism. In: *Drugs of Choice, 1972-1973,* edited by W. Modell, pp. 331-342, Mosby, St. Louis.

Kirwan, W.O. (1974): Cerebrospinal fluid cotrimoxazole levels. *Journal of Irish Medical Association, 67:* 76-77.

Koch Weser, J., Sidel, V.W., Dexter, M., Parish, C., Finer, D.C. and Kanarek, P. (1971): Adverse reactions to sulfosoxazole sulfamethoxazole, nitrofurantoin. *Archives of Internal Medicine, 128:* 399-404.

Krauer, B. (1975): The development of diurnal variation in drug kinetics in the human infant. In: *Basic and Therapeutic Aspects of Perinatal Pharamcology,* edited by P.L. Morselli, S. Garattini and F. Sereni, pp. 347-356, Raven Press, New York.

Krauer, B., Spring, P. and Dettli, L. (1968): Zur Pharmakokinetik der Sulfonamide im ersten Lebensjahr. *Pharmacologia Clinica, 1:* 47-53.

Kremers, P. Duvivier, J. and Heusghem, C. (1974): Pharmacokinetic studies of co-trimoxazole in man after single and repeated doses. *Journal of Clinical Pharmacology, 14:* 112-117.

Krüger-Thiemer, E. and Bünger, P. (1965): Evaluation of the risk of crystalluria with sulpha drugs. In: Proceedings of the European Society for the Study of Drug Toxicity, V. 6, *Experimental Studies and Clinical Experience–The Assessment of Risk,* pp. 185-207, Excerpta Medica, Amsterdam.

Kunin, C.M. (1974): *Detection Prevention and Management of Urinary Tract Infections,* 2nd ed., Lea-Febiger, Philadelphia.

Lewin, E.B., Fralonardo, S.A., Colaiace, J.D. and Klein, J.O. (1975): Pharmacology of co-trimoxazole in infants and children. In: *Abstracts of 9th International Congress of Chemotherapy,* London, July 13-18, Abstr. M417, Garden City Press, Letchworth.

Lewin, E.B., Klein, J.O. and Finland, M. (1973): Trimethoprim-sulfamethoxazole: absorption, excretion, and toxicity in six children. *Journal of Infectious Diseases, 128,* suppl.: S618-S621.

McChesney, E.W., Portmann, G.A. and Koss, R.F. (1967): Pharmacokinetic model for nalidixic acid in man. III. *Journal of Pharmaceutical Sciences, 56:* 594-599.

McCracken, J.H., Jr. and Eichenwald, H.F. (1974): Antimicrobial therapy: therapeutic recommendations and a review of newer drugs. I. *Journal of Pediatrics, 85:* 297-312.

McCracken, G.H., Jr., Eichenwald, H.F. and Nelson, J.D. (1969a): Antimicrobial therapy in theory and practice. I. Clinical Pharmacology. *Journal of Pediatrics, 75:* 742-757.

McCracken, G.H., Jr., Eichenwald, H.F. and Nelson, J.D. (1969b): Antimicrobial therapy in theory and practice. II. Clinical approach to antimicrobial therapy. *Journal of Pediatrics, 75:* 923-936.

McGilveray, I.J., Mattok, G.L. and Hossie, R.D. (1971): A study of bioavailability and dissolution rates of commercial tablets of nitrofurantoin. *Journal of Pharmacy and Pharmacology, 23:* 246S.

Malmborg, A.-S., Dornbusch, K., Elias-Son, R. and Lindholmer, C. (1975): Concentrations of various antibacterials in human seminal plasma. In: *Abstracts, 9th International Congress of Chemotherapy,* Abstr. M683, Garden City Press, Letchworth.

Mandal, B.K. and Stevenson, J. (1970): Haemolytic crisis produced by nalidixic acid. *Lancet, 1:* 614.

Marks, M.I. (1975): Pharmacokinetics and efficacy of trimethoprimsulfamethoxazole in the treatment of gastroenteritis in children. *Canadian Medical Association Journal, 112:* 33S-34S.

Meares, E.M. (1973): Observations on activity of trimethoprimsulfamethoxazole on the prostate. *Journal of Infectious Diseases, 128,* suppl.: 679-685.

Meyer, M.C., Slywka, G.W.A., Dann, R.E. and Whyatt, P.L. (1974): Bioavailability of 14 nitrofurantoin products. *Journal of Pharmaceutical Sciences, 63:* 1693-1698.

Moore, W.E., Portmann, G.A., Stander, H. and McChesney, E.W. (1965): Biopharmaceutical investigation of nalidixic acid in man. *Journal of Pharmaecutical Sciences, 54:* 36-41.

Morzaria, R.N., Walton, I.G. and Pickering, D. (1969): Neonatal meningitis treated with trimethoprim and sulfamethoxazole. *British Medical Journal, 2:* 511-512.

Nelson, J.D., Shelton, S., Kusmiesz, H.T. and Haltalin, K.C. (1972): Absorption of ampicillin and nalidixic acid by infants and children with acute shigellosis. *Clinical Pharmacology and Therapeutics, 13:* 879-886.

Nolte, H. and Büttner, H. (1974): Investigations on plasma levels of sulfamethoxazole in man after single and chronic oral administration alone and in combination with trimethoprim. *Chemotherapy, 20:* 321-330.

Ohnhaus, E.E. and Spring, P. (1975): Elimination kinetics of sulfadiazine in patients with normal and impaired renal function. *Journal of Pharmacokinetics and Biopharmaceutics, 3:* 171-179.

Parsons, R.L., Paddock, G.M., Hossack, G.M. and Hailey, D.M. (1975): Antibiotic absorption in Crohn's disease. In: *Abstracts of 9th International Congress of Chemotherapy,* London, July 13-18, 1975, abstr. M611, Garden City Press, Letchworth.

Paul, H.E., Hayes, K.J., Paul, M.F. and Russell Borgmann, A. (1967): Laboratory studies with nitrofurantoin. *Journal of Pharmaceutical Sciences, 56:* 882-885.

Peppercorn, M.A. and Goldman, P. (1972): The role of intestinal bacteria in the metabolism of salicylazosulfapyridine. *Journal of Pharmacology and Experimental Therapeutics, 181:* 555-562.

Perry, J.E. and Leblanc, A.L. (1967): Transfer of nitrofurantoin across the human placenta. *Texas Report of Biological Medicine, 25:* 265-269.

Pohjanpelto, P.E.J., Sarmela, T.J. and Raines, T. (1974): Penetration of trimethoprim and sulphamethoxazole into the aqueous humour. *British Journal of Ophthamology, 58:* 606-608.

Portmann, G.A., McChesney, E.W., Stander, H. and Moore, W.E. (1966a): Pharmacokinetic model for nalidixic acid in man. I. *Journal of Pharmaceutical Sciences, 55:* 59-62.

Portmann, G.A., McChesney, E.W., Stander, H. and Moore, W.E. (1966b): Pharmacokinetic model for nalidixic acid in man. II. *Journal of Pharmaceutical Sciences, 55:* 72-78.

Pritchard, J.A., Scott, D.E. and Mason, R.A. (1965): Severe anemia with hemolysis and megaloblastic erythropoiesis. *Journal of the American Medical Association, 194:* 457-459.

Reckendorf, H.K., Castringius, R.G. and Spingler, H.K. (1963): Comparative pharmacodynamics, urinary excretion, and half-life determinations of nitrofurantoin sodium. *Antimicrobial Agents and Chemotherapy,* pp. 531-537.

Reeves, D.S. (1975): Laboratory and clinical studies with sulfametopyrazine as a treatment for bacteriuria in pregnancy. *Journal of Antimicrobial Chemotherapy, 1:* 171-186.

Reid, D.W.J., Caillé, G. and Kaufmann, N.R. (1975): Maternal and trasplacental kinetics of trimethoprim and sulfamethoxazole, separately and in combination. *Canadian Medical Association Journal, 112:* 67S-72S.

Reidenberg, M.M., Kostenbauder, H. and Adams, W.P. (1969): Rate of drug metabolism in obese volunteers before and during starvation and in azotemic patients. *Metabolism, 18:* 209-213.

Rieder, J. (1963): Physikalisch-chemische und biologische Untersuchungen au Sulfonamiden. I, II, III. *Arzneimittel-Forschung, 13:* 81-103.

Rieder, J. and Schwartz, D.E. (1975): Pharmakokinetik der Wirkstoffkombination Trimethoprim + Sulfamethoxazol bei Leberkranken im vergleich zu Gesunden. *Arzneimittel-Forschung, 25:* 656-666.

Rohwedder, H.-J., Simon, C., Kübler, W. and Hohnfnauer, M. (1970): Untersuchungen über die Pharmakokinetik von Nalidixinsäure bei kindern Verschiedenen Alters. *Zeitschrift für Kinderheilkunde, 109:* 124-134.
Rosenow, E.C. III, De Remee, R.A. and Dines, D.E. (1968): Chronic nitrofurantoin pulmonary reaction. Report of five cases. *New England Journal of Medicine, 279:* 1258-1262.
Sabel, K.G. and Brandberg, A. (1975): Treatment of meningitis and septicemia in infancy with a sulphamethoxazole/trimethoprim combination. *Acta Paediatrica Scandinavica, 64:* 25-32.
Sachs, J., Geer, T., Noell, P. and Kunin, C.M. (1968): Effect of renal function on urinary recovery of orally administered nitrofurantoin. *New England Journal of Medicine, 278:* 1032-1035.
Salmon, J.D., Fowle, A.S.E. and Bye, A. (1975): Concentrations of trimethoprim and sulphamethoxazole in aqueous humour and plasma from regimens of co-trimoxazole in man. *Journal of Antimicrobial Chemotherapy, 1:* 205-211.
Schröder, H. and Campbell, D.E.S. (1972): Absorption, metabolism and excretion of salicylazosulfapyridine in man. *Clinical Pharmacology and Therapeutics, 13:* 539-551.
Schroder, H., Lewkonia, R.M. and Price-Evans, D.A. (1973): Metabolism of salicylazosulfapyridine in healthy subjects and in patients with ulcerative colitis. Effects of colectomy and of phenobarbital. *Clinical Pharmacology and Therapeutics, 14:* 802-809.
Schwartländer, D. and Eulenhöfer, H.G. (1972): Experimentelle Untersuchungen zur Ausscheidung von Nitrofurantoin im Harn gesunder versuchspersonen. *Arzneimittel-Forschung, 22:* 877-881.
Schwartz, D.E. and Ziegler, W.M. (1969): Assay and pharmacokinetics of Trimethoprim in man and animals. *Postgraduate Medical Journal, 45,* suppl.: 32-37.
Sellers, E.M. and Koch-Weser, J. (1970): Displacement of warfarin from human albumin by diazoxide and ethacrynic, mefanamic and nalidixic acids. *Clinical Pharamcology and Therapeutics, 11:* 524-529.
Seneca, H. (1966): Long-acting sulfonamides in urinary tract infections. *Journal of the American Medical Association, 198:* 975-980.
Sereni, F., Perletti, L., Marubini, E. and Mars, G. (1968): Pharmacokinetic studies with a long-acting sulfonamide in subjects of different ages. *Pediatric Research, 2:* 29-37.
Seydel, J.K. (1969): The relationship of pharmacokinetic properties of some sulfonamides to certain physicochemical parameters. In: *International Congress of Chemotherapy,* Tokyo, 1969.
Sharma, D.B. and James, A. (1974): Benign intracranial hypertension associated with nitrofurantoin therapy. *British Medical Journal, 4:* 771.
Sharpstone, P. (1969): The renal handling of trimethoprim and sulfamethoxazole in man. *Postgraduate Medical Journal, 45,* suppl.: 32-37.
Sigel, C.W., Grace, M.E. and Nichol, C.A. (1975): Trimethoprim metabolism in man during repeated treatment with septrin. In *Abstracts of 9th International Congress of Chemotherapy,* London, July 13-18, 1975, Abstr. M621, Garden City Press, Letchworth.
Silver, H.K., Kempe, C.H. and Bruyn, H.B. (1975): *Handbook of Pediatrics,* 11th ed., Lange Medical Publ., Los Altos, California.
Sparr, R.A. and Pritchard, J.A. (1958): Maternal and newborn distribution and excretion of sulfamethoxypyridazine (Kynex). *Obstetrics and Gynecology, 12:* 131-134.
Tilstone, W.J., Nimmo-Smitg, R.H., Gray, J.M.B., Lawson, D.M. and Welch, R.M. (1975): Interaction between warfarin and sulphamethoxazole. In: *Abstracts, 9th International Congress of Chemotherapy,* London, July 13-18, Abstr. M165, Garden City Press, Letchworth.
Toole, J.F., Gergem, J.A., Hayes, D.M. and Felts, (1968): Neural effects of nitrofurantoin. *Archives of Neurology, 18:* 680-687.

Van Petten, G.R., Becking, G.C., Withey, R.J. and Lettau, H.F. (1971a): Studies on the physiological availability and metabolism of sulfonamides. I. Sulfadiazine. *Journal of Clinical Pharmacology, 11:* 27-34.
Van Petten, G.R., Becking, G.C., Withey, R.J. and Lettau, H.F. (1971b): Studies on the physiological availability and metabolism of sulfonamides. II. Sulfisoxazole. *Journal of Clinical Pharmacology, 11:* 35-41.
Varsano, I., Fischl, J. and Schochet, S.B. (1973): The excretion of orally ingested nitrofurantoin in human milk. *Journal of Pediatrics, 82:* 886-887.
Vest, M., Olefsson, A. Rieder, J. and Schwartz, D.E. (1974): Pharmakokinetik von Bactrim-Sirup bei Seinglingen und Kindern. *Helvetical Paediatrica Acta,* suppl. 33: 24.
Wardell, W.M. (1973): British usage and American awareness of some new therapeutic drugs. *Clinical Pharmacology and Therapeutics, 14:* 1022-1034.
Wardell, W.M. (1974): Redistributional drug interactions: a critical examination of putative clinical examples. In: *Drug Interactions,* edited by P.L. Morselli, S. Garattini and S.N. Cohen, pp. 123-134, Raven Press, New York.
Weinstein, L. (1975): Chemotherapy of microbial diseases. In: *The Pharmacologial Basis of Therapeutics,* edited by L.S. Goodman and A. Gilman, 5th ed., pp. 1113-1129, Macmillan, New York.
Welling, P.G., Craig, W.A., Amidon, G.L. and Kunin, C.M. (1973): Pharmacokinetics of trimethoprim and sulfamethoxazole in normal subjects and in patients with renal failure. *Journal of Infectious Diseases, 128,* suppl.: 556-566.
White, T.A. and Price-Evans, D.A. (1967): The acetylation of sulfamethazine and sulfamethoxypyridazine by human subjects. *Clinical Pharamcology and Therapeutics, 9:* 80-88.
Williams, J.D. (1974): The sulphonamides. *British Journal of Hospital Medicine, 12:* 722-730.
Winterborn, M.H. and Mann, J.R. (1973): Anuria due to sulphadiazine. *Archives of Disease in Childhood, 48:* 915-917.

9

Anticoagulants

GIOVANNI DE GAETANO
AND
MARIA-BENEDETTA DONATI

The drugs considered in this chapter are heparin, warfarin, bishydroxycoumarin, acenocoumarol, ethylbiscoumacetate and fluorophenindione. They have in common the property to impair the blood coagulation mechanism. Heparin is active both *in vitro* and *in vivo,* whereas the other drugs are active exclusively *in vivo.* Heparin has to be administered either intravenously or subcutaneously, whereas indirect anticoagulants are usually given per os (they are also known as "oral anticoagulants"). Heparin is a direct anticoagulant (acting mainly as an antithrombin), whereas the other drugs act through an indirect mechanism, i.e., by inhibiting the hepatic synthesis of four factors essential for normal blood coagulation to occur. The effect of heparin is, therefore, immediate and can be instantaneously blocked by injection of antagonists such as protamine sulfate. In contrast, the effect of oral anticoagulants (even if administered intravenously) becomes apparent after many hours (or days) and cannot be rapidly counteracted even by intravenous injection of vitamin K, the fat-soluble vitamin essential for the biosynthesis of the four clotting factors depressed by oral anticoagulants. Heparin is used in clinical practice as a first antithrombotic defense until the effects of the oral anticoagulants are established.

Heparin has its main use in established thromboembolic disease (coronary artery disease, deep vein thrombosis, pulmonary embolism, peripheral arterial disease) (McNicol, 1975), in extracorporeal circulation and dialysis (Nyman et al., 1975) and in the therapy of diffuse intravascular coagulation (Verstraete et al., 1965; Lasch and Heene, 1975; Straub, 1975). The evidence in favor of the

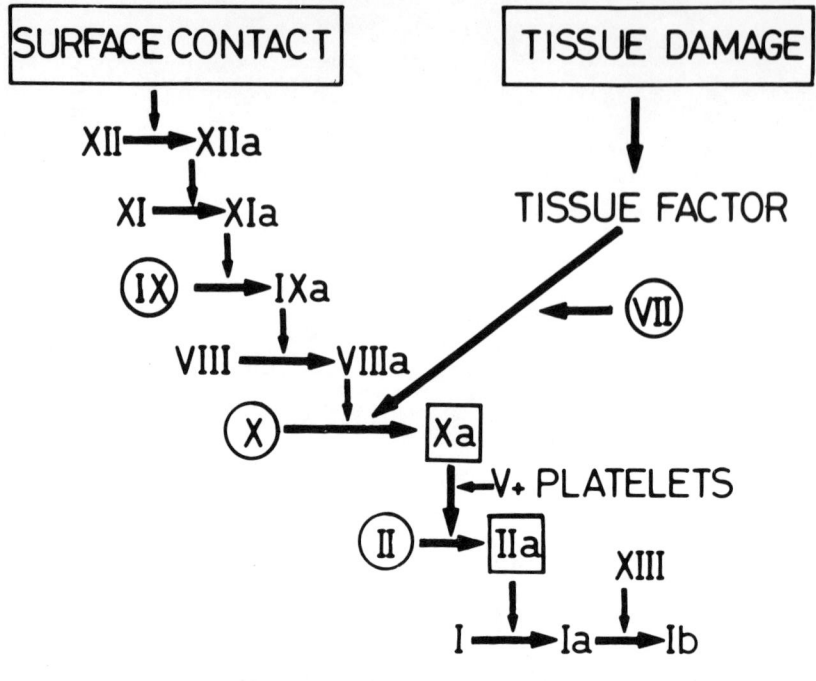

Fig. 1: Blood coagulation scheme showing the intrinsic (left) and extrinsic (right) pathways leading to the activation of factor X (common pathway). Factor I is fibrinogen, Ia is fibrin and Ib is stabilized fibrin; factor IIa is thrombin. "a" indicates the activated factor. The vitamin K-dependent factors are encircled, whereas the two main activated factors inhibited by heparin are inserted in a square.

use of heparin in conventional doses for established thromboembolic disease is largely presumptive, and there is an almost total absence of rigorously designed, controlled clinical trials with modern diagnostic criteria (McNicol, 1975). Recently, it has been shown that small quantities of heparin greatly increase the rate of neutralization of activated clotting factor X (see Fig. 1) by a naturally occurring inhibitor (antithrombin III, heparin cofactor) (Yin et al., 1971). The latter would be reduced in cases of "hypercoagulability," occurring, for instance, in patients undergoing major surgical operations; small amounts of heparin, given prior to the development of hypercoagulability could, therefore, prevent postoperative venous thromboembolism (Wessler and Yin, 1973). Indeed, published evidence presently available indicates that low-dose heparin (10,000-

20,000 i.u. daily subcutaneously, starting two h prior to surgery and continuing during the first postoperative week) effectively prevents venous thromboembolism and does not produce excessive surgical bleeding (Wessler, 1975; Kakkar, 1975). Since low-dose subcutaneous heparin usually does not prolong conventional clotting tests, no data are yet available on the kinetics of the drug given on this therapeutic regimen.

Oral anticoagulants have been recommended for cardiac, cerebral and peripheral arterial lesions and for venous and pulmonary arterial lesions. They have also been used in several categories of patients who are at special risk from thromboembolism (atrial fibrillation with rheumatic heart disease, heart valve prosthesis, hip fracture, congestive heart failure, etc.). Despite interest in oral anticoagulant therapy over 30 years, it is impossible to be dogmatic about the current role of these drugs in the prevention or treatment of thromboembolic disease, particularly in the arterial system. A critical, detailed appraisal of the therapeutic value of oral anticoagulants has been recently given by Douglas and McNicol (1973).

HEPARIN

Heparin is a highly sulfated mucopolysaccharide with a molecular weight of about 20,000. When administered by oral route, it is very poorly absorbed and enters the general circulation only to a very small extent, thus having no effect on blood coagulation (Windsor and Freena, 1964; Ehrlich and Stivala, 1973). It is therefore administered intravenously or subcutaneously. Very few studies have been performed on the disposition of heparin, mainly due to the lack of an adequate method for the direct chemical assay of heparin in biological fluids. The available data pertain to the kinetics of its anticoagulant effect. In adults, Estes et al. (1969) found that in a wide range of doses the apparent half-life of heparin anticoagulant activity (after i.v. administration) is approximately 90 min and that the relative volume of distribution corresponds to the plasma volume (0.057 ± 0.001 L/kg).

The kinetics of heparin's disappearance from plasma appear to follow a first-order process of elimination. It is not yet known whether heparin is metabolized or otherwise biotransformed. It is unlikely, however, that a molecule as large as that of heparin, possibly bound to plasma proteins (mainly fibrinogen and globulins) (Estes and Poulin, 1975) by large electronegative charges, is excreted rapidly or in unchanged form in significant amounts. It has been suggested that heparin may leave the plasmatic compartment by uptake into the reticuloendothelial system (Estes et al., 1969). The minimum dose of heparin which produces a clinically useful prolongation of the clotting time has been calculated to be about 35 units/kg body weight (Estes and Poulin, 1975).

According to Estes (1971), due to its very short biological half-life heparin should be given by continuous intravenous infusion in order to provide continuous and adequate anticoagulation. Heparin does not cross placenta and can therefore be used during pregnancy. Its administration should be discontinued when labor is established, to avoid hemorrhagic complications (Noble, 1974). It is always possible to reverse the action of heparin with intravenous protamine sulfate, but it is better to avoid this procedure in pregnancy because complete neutralization may be difficult to achieve (Noble, 1974). Twenty-four hours after delivery, heparin can be restored in low dosages (Noble, 1974). To our knowledge, no data are available concerning the disposition of heparin during development. Indeed, experience in the treatment of the hemorrhagic or thrombotic manifestations in neonates is extremely limited. The use of heparinized blood for exchange transfusion in cases of diffuse intravascular coagulation in neonates has not prevented a fatal outcome (Edson et al., 1968; Leissring and Vorlicky, 1968; Skyberg and Jacobsen, 1969). However, treatment with heparin (50 units/kg every 3 h for 2½ days) did result in a marked improvement in the abnormal coagulation of a postmature infant with evidence of fetal distress (Markarian et al., 1971). Therefore, further investigation on the use of heparin in neonates, appears warranted. Heparin has seldom been used in children, except in some cases of hemolytic uremic syndrome (Lieberman, 1972), of microangiopathic hemolytic anemia (Brain et al., 1968) and of thrombotic thrombocytopenic purpura (Berberich et al., 1974). The dose of heparin usually required to prolong the clotting time 2-3 fold is 200 u/Kg every 4-6 h. Regulation of heparin dosage has proved difficult, especially in young infants with marked variations in the clotting time (Lieberman, 1972). Notwithstanding some successes, data are not available which prove conclusively that heparin has altered the case-fatality rate. Brain et al. (1968) pointed out that the different response to heparin (or other drugs) might well depend upon the relative pathophysiological contribution of the vascular, platelet and fibrin components of the above-mentioned conditions. Although this explanation may be true, possible differences in the pharmacokinetic properties of heparin in relation to its pharmacological actions should also be taken into account.

ORAL ANTICOAGULANTS

Oral anticoagulants are widely used in the prevention and management of thromboembolic diseases. The therapeutic effect of these drugs is derived from their ability to inhibit the action of vitamin K, a fat-soluble vitamin; for this reason they are also known as "vitamin K antagonists." Vitamin K is essential for the hepatic synthesis of four plasma clotting factors: factor VII (serum prothrombin conversion accelerator or stable factor); factor IX (plasma thromboplastin component or Christmas factor); factor X (or Stuart factor) and factor II (or prothrombin). The place of these factors in the coagulation cascade and their half-lives are reported in Fig. 1 and Table 1, respectively.

Table 1. Biological Half-Life of the Four Clotting Factors
Whose Synthesis is Vitamin K-Dependent

Factor	Half-Life (h)
Factor VII	3-5
Factor IX	20-30
Factor X	20-30
Factor II	100-120

From Deykin, 1970.

After an oral "loading" dose of anticoagulant, the prolongation of the "prothrombin time" that follows primarily reflects the depression of factor VII; factors IX and X are depressed more slowly, and prothrombin (factor II) itself does not decrease appreciably during this initial period. Since the depression of factor VII seems to be a major cause of the hemorrhagic complications of anticoagulant therapy, the traditional "loading dose" technique has been criticized and substituted for by some authors with a continuous administration of small doses of the anticoagulant (Deykin, 1970). In any case, full anticoagulant effect is reached after several days of therapy. For this reason, when anticoagulation has to be urgently instituted, heparin is given concurrently with vitamin K antagonists until the effect of the latter is fully developed.

After administration of a vitamin K antagonist, plasma contains (at least) three anamalous proteins which are immunologically identical to factor IX, X and II, respectively (Hemker et al., 1963; Reeker et al., 1973); these proteins differ from the corresponding normal coagulation factors not only because they lack biological activity, but also because they possess anticoagulant activity. The latter effect can influence some of the test systems used for monitoring anticoagulant therapy (Hemker and Muller, 1968). The nature of the interaction between vitamin K, synthesis of clotting factors and coumarin anticoagulants has not been definitely established.

The vitamin K antagonists most frequently used in current practice are listed in Figs. 2 and 3. It can be seen that they derive from two parent molecules: 4-hydroxycoumarin and indane-1:3-dione. A primary consideration in the use of these drugs is the appreciation that serious and, sometimes, fatal sensitivity reactions to the indanedione derivatives can occur, while the coumarin drugs appear to be almost free from these complications (Douglas and McNicol, 1972). Although the safest anticoagulant drug is the one with which the clinician has the most experience, the case for using coumarin drugs in preference to indane-

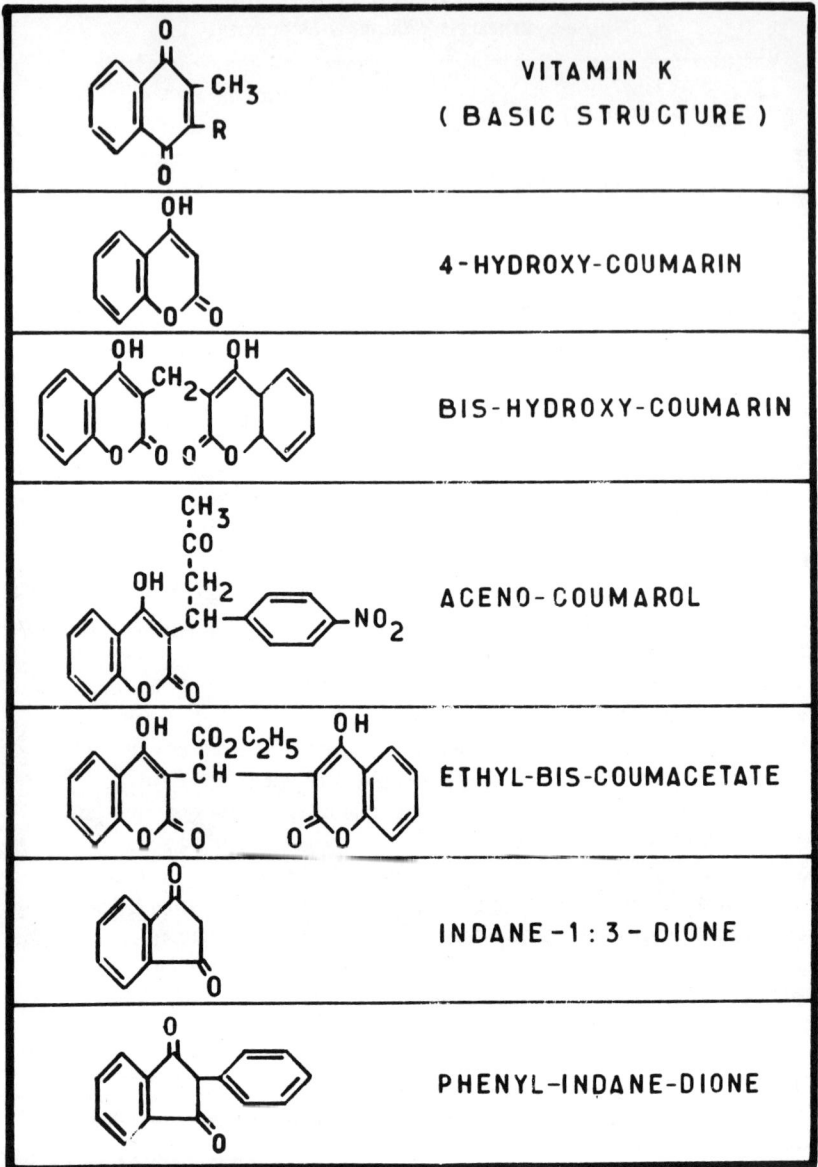

Fig. 2: Structural formulae of the most commonly used anticoagulant drugs.

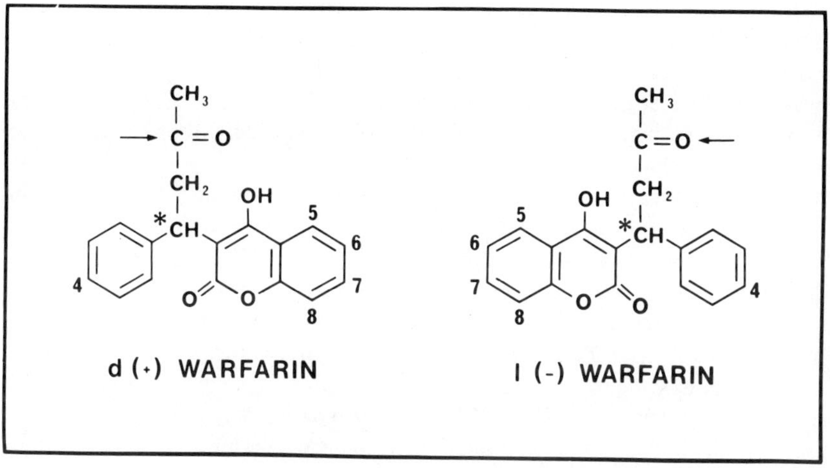

d (+) WARFARIN   **l (−) WARFARIN**

Fig. 3: Structural formulae of R [d(+)] and S [l (−)] warfarin. The asterisk indicates the asymmetrical carbon that gives rise to the two naturally occurring optical enantiomers present in all commercial sodium warfarin. The arrow indicates the position where metabolic insertion of a hydroxyl group gives rise to the warfarin alcohols. The numbers indicate the positions of hydroxyl groups inserted during metabolism to form the metabolic products of warfarin.

dione derivatives is strong. The most common side effect encountered with this class of drugs is hemorrhage (hematuria, epistaxis, rectal bleeding, gum oozing, hemoptysis, hematemesis, melena, intracranial bleeding). It is commonly believed, however, that the occurrence of hemorrhage is mainly due to inappropriate treatment and/or to the concomitant administration of other drugs which potentiate the action of oral anticoagulants (Douglas and McNicol, 1973). Several cases of skin necrosis with coumarin-type drugs (warfarin and bishydroxycoumarin) have also been reported (see Lacy and Godin, 1975).

Warfarin

In adults, the gastrointestingal absorption of warfarin is very rapid. Peak plasma levels of about 0.6 µg/ml are attained within 4 h after a single-dose oral administration of 7.5 mg (Kaisen and Martin, 1974). With higher doses of warfarin (0.5-1.5 mg/kg), peak plasma levels ranging between 4 and 14 µg/ml are obtained (Nagashima et al., 1969; Breckenridge and Orme, 1973; Ambre and Fischer, 1973; Lewis et al., 1974). According to Breckenridge and Orme (1973), peak drug concentrations in plasma are reached by 25 to 60 min after oral dosing (0.5 mg/kg). Between 77% and 100% of the administered dose is apparently absorbed (Breckenridge and Orme, 1973).

Cholestyramine decreases warfarin absorption by binding the drug in the intestine (Robinson et al., 1971), whereas antacids (aluminum and magnesium hydroxides) have no effect (Ambre and Fischer, 1973). The apparent volume of distribution varies from 6.4% to 18.7% body weight (0.03-0.12 L/kg) and does not seem to be related to the dose or to the route (oral or intravenous) of warfarin administration (O'Reilly et al., 1963, 1971; Breckenridge and Orme, 1973).

Warfarin is strongly bound to plasma proteins, namely to albumin, both *in vitro* and *in vivo* (O'Reilly, 1967). In *in vitro* experiments, the amount of the drug bound to albumin is remarkably dependent on the relative concentrations of drug and protein present (O'Reilly, 1973). The binding capacity of normal human plasma for warfarin is about 200 µg drug/ml, but since the plasma levels of warfarin rarely exceed 20 µg/ml in clinical practice, the drug in the plasma is almost entirely bound to plasma albumin (Solomon and Schrogie, 1967). In fact, it has been reported that warfarin is 97% bound *in vivo* (O'Reilly et al., 1962); *in vitro*, at albumin concentrations of 0.15 and 0.45 mM, approximately 94% and 97% of the drug, respectively, is bound (Solomon and Schrogie, 1967).

Following intravenous administration of warfarin (1.5-3.0 mg/kg), the apparent half-life ranges between 29 and 37 h (O'Reilly et al., 1963). At doses ranging from 50 to 600 mg, the average apparent half-life is 35.6 h (range: 17.3-44.9 h) (O'Reilly et al., 1971). After a single oral dose of warfarin (1.5 mg/Kg or 75 mg total), the apparent half-life is 43 ± 10 and 32 ± 4 h, respectively (O'Reilly and Aggeler, 1968; Ambre and Fischer, 1973). In patients receiving chronic oral administration of warfarin (0.04-0.22 mg/kg/day), the apparent half-life varies for 20.2 h to 87.3 h with a good correlation (r = +0.78) with the steady-state plasma warfarin concentration (Breckenridge and Orme, 1973). No evident relationship between steady-state plasma levels and the daily dose (0.04-0.40 mg/kg) of warfarin could be found by Breckenridge and Orme (1973), who also described a fivefold interindividual difference (0.6-3.1 µg/ml) in warfarin steady-state plasma levels during chronic treatment in patients suffering from cardiovascular disease.

As far as the correlation of the blood levels of the drug and its anticoagulant effect is concerned, the higher the drug levels or the more prolonged the half-life of warfarin, the greater is the area under the curve for the anticoagulant effect. Usually, the maximum anticoagulant effect is reached with 48-72 h and lasts 7-10 days (O'Reilly, 1972). There is therefore no direct relationship between the inhibition of prothrombin-complex activity at a given time and the plasma warfarin concentration at the same time. The reason for this delay is that the anticoagulant, as already mentioned, inhibits the synthesis of certain clotting factors and thus affects the prothrombin activity only indirectly. However, when the anticoagulant effect of warfarin is expressed in terms of the inhibition of prothrombin-complex activity synthesis rate, it directly correlates with the warfarin concentration in the plasma (Nagashima et al., 1969). The synthesis rate is inhibited by 50% per day at plasma concentrations of warfarin around 3 µg/ml (O'Reilly and Levy, 1970).

Warfarin is extensively metabolized (Fig. 3). Clinically available warfarin is a racemic mixture of two enantiomers, d (+) and l (-) warfarin (Eble et al., 1966). d (-) warfarin is 5 to 6 times more potent as an anticoagulant than l (+) warfarin (O'Reilly, 1974; Hewick and McEwen, 1973; Lewis et al., 1974), although the albumin-binding of the two enantiomers does not differ (O'Reilly, 1971). There are also no differences in the absorption of the isomers as indicated by the similarity in their peak plasma levels (average of 5.8 µg/ml and 6.4 µg/ml, respectively, for d and l enantiomers after a single oral dose of 0.75 mg/Kg) (Lewis et al., 1974). They differ, in contrast, in their metabolism; d (+) warfarin is mainly metabolized to 6-hydroxywarfarin and (d, l) warfarin alcohol (alcohol 1), whereas l (-) warfarin is primarily metabolized to 7-hydroxywarfarin, (l, l) warfarin alcohol (alcohol 2) and 6-hydroxywarfarin (Lewis and Trager, 1971; Lewis et al., 1973, 1974; Hewick and McEwen, 1973).

The average apparent half-life for d (+) and l (-) warfarin after a single oral dose (0.75 mg/Kg) of either enantiomer is 45 h (range: 33-81 h) and 28 h (range: 18-41 h), respectively (Lewis et al., 1974). Following a single oral administration of 100 mg of either d (+) or l (-) warfarin, the average apparent half-life is 45 h (range: 34-64 h) and 32 h (range: 23-51 h), respectively (Hewick and McEwen, 1973). These observations in man are the reverse of the situation found in the rat, where l (-) warfarin is the isomer more slowly metabolized (Breckenridge and Orme, 1972). The apparent volumes of distribution of the enantiomers range from about 8% to 12% of body weight, no significant differences being observed between the two compounds (Hewick and McEwen, 1973). After oral administration of 0.75 mg/kg of d (+) warfarin, the average maximum plasma concentration of alcohol 1 is 600 µg/L (range: 300-890 µg/L) and that of alcohol 2 is 32 µg/L (range: 23-50 µg/L) (Lewis et al., 1974). The peak plasma concentration is reached about 36 h after drug administration (Hewick and McEwen, 1973), and the average maximum plasma concentration of 7-hydroxywarfarin is 35 µg/L (range: 10-80 µg/L) (Lewis et al., 1974). After an oral administration of 0.75 mg/kg of l (-) warfarin, the average maximum plasma concentration of alcohol 1 is 30 µg/L (range: 10-65 µg/L) and that of alcohol 2 is 89 µg/L (range: 42-170 µg/L (Lewis et al., 1974). The peak plasma concentration is reached about 28 h after drug administration (Hewick and McEwen, 1973), and the average maximum plasma concentration of 7-hydroxywarfarin is 496 µg/L (range: 180-1,050 µg/L (Lewis et al., 1974).

Alcohol 1 is cleared at a rate similar to racemic warfarin, whereas alcohol 2 is eliminated about 2.5 times more rapidly. The apparent half-lives of alcohol 1 and alcohol 2 in a normal subject were 33 h and 12 h, respectively, the half-life of racemic warfarin in the same subject being 35 h (Lewis and Trager, 1971). The apparent volume of distribution of both alcohols ranges between 10 and 13% of body weight, a range similar to that reported for warfarin (Lewis et al., 1973). Both alcohols induce a similar anticoagulant response, but the action of alcohol 1 is more sustained (Lewis et al., 1973).

After administration of the racemic warfarin to normal humans, seven fluorescent compounds have been chromatographically separated from extracts of their urine. Some of these substances have been identified as unchanged warfarin, two oxidized derivatives (6-hydroxywarfarin and 7-hydroxywarfarin) and two reduced derivatives (alcohol 1 and alcohol 2) (Lewis and Trager, 1970). After 7-10 days' urine collection, from 33 to 55% of the administered dose of racemic warfarin is recovered in the urine; when d (+) warfarin is given, the recovery in urine is relatively poor (from 20 to 31% of the dose), whereas after l (-) warfarin administration from 48 to 71% of the dose is found in the urine. In all cases, unchanged warfarin constitutes less than 5% of the total compounds recovered in the urine (Lewis et al., 1974). Primarily alcohol 1 and 6-hydroxywarfarin are excreted after oral administration of d (+) warfarin, while 7-hydroxywarfarin followed by 6-hydroxywarfarin and alcohol 2 are the main metabolites found in urine after ingestion of l (-) warfarin (Lewis et al., 1974). After oral administration of alcohol 1, 60% of the dose is recovered in urine whereas alcohol 2 is totally excreted (Lewis et al., 1973).

The two isomers of warfarin also differ in their interaction with other drugs. The clearance of l (-) warfarin is indeed inhibited by phenlybutazone (from 31 to 44 h and from 22 to 62 h), although that of d (+) warfarin is stimulated (from 45 to 24 h and from 81 to 45 h). As expected, phenylbutazone does not modify the half-life of the racemate; in contrast, it increases the concentration of 7-hydroxywarfarin (Lewis et al., 1974). The above-mentioned results indicate that the impairment in the metabolism of the potent l (-) isomer provides a mechanism by which the anticoagulant effect of warfarin would be augmented by phenlybutazone, despite the fact that the clearance of the racemate is not altered (Lewis et al., 1974). This observation opens new perspectives in the study of drug interactions.

The rate of plasma clearance of racemic warfarin is almost doubled when 100 mg/day (for 3 days) of pentobarbital are administered concomitantly (Lewis et al., 1973). This effect is not unexpected since an increased drug-oxidizing enzymatic activity is a well-documented response to barbiturate administration. No data are available, to our knowledge, on the effect of pentobarbital on the two warfarin isomers. In contrast, Lewis et al. (1973) have reported that neither the anticoagulant effect nor plasma levels of the two warfarin alcohols were altered during 5 days of pentobarbital administration (200 mg/day). A delayed effect of pentobarbital, however, could have been missed; nevertheless, the availability of a coumarin anticoagulant not susceptible to the induction of drug metabolizing enzymes would be of great clinical interest.

No data are available on warfarin disposition in newborns, infants and children.

Bishydroxycoumarin (Dicoumarol)

In adults, the gastrointestinal absorption of bishydroxycoumarin (BHC) is rapid. According to Ambre and Fischer (1973), peak plasma levels of about 15 µg/ml are attained within 8 h after a single oral dose of 300 mg, in individual subjects, peak plasma levels are also obtained 2 h after the administration of the drug. Co-administration of BHC with magnesium hydroxide produces higher (about 30 µg/ml) and earlier (4 h) peak plasma levels of BHC than those reported above. Co-administration of BHC with aluminum hydroxide has no effect on the mean plasma levels of BHC.

As already mentioned, the co-administration of these antacids with warfarin in the same experimental conditions has no effect on warfarin plasma levels (Ambre and Fischer, 1973). Barbiturates decrease the absorption of BHC and lead to increased levels of unchanged BHC in the stool, decreased blood levels (from 60 to 40 µg/ml), decreased anticoagulant response and increased plasma disappearance rate. When BHC is given intravenously, no unchanged BHC appears in the stool (Aggeler and O'Reilly, 1969). In both *in vivo* and *in vitro* experiments, BHC is almost totally bound to proteins, namely, albumin; according to O'Reilly et al. (1962), 100% of BHC is protein-bound *in vivo*, and 99% binding was reported *in vitro* by Weiner et al. (1950). Garten and Wozilait (1971) have found that BHC is bound to human serum albumin (9 moles per mole of protein) to a greater extent than the other coumarin anticoagulants (the stoichiometry of warfarin was about 2 moles/mole of protein). The volume of distribution of BHC has been calculated following intravenous administration of the drug and has been found to range between 0.13 and 0.20 L/kg, independently of the dose administered (from 2.1 to 8.6 mg/kg) (Weiner et al., 1950; O'Reilly et al., 1964b).

Characteristically, the apparent half-life of BHC increases as the dose (administered either i.v. or p.o.) of drug is increased. O'Reilly et al. (1964b) reported a half-life of 10 and 32 h after i.v. administration of 2.1 or 8.6 mg/kg BHC, respectively. After oral administration of 100, 150 or 300 mg BHC, the respective half-lives were 22 ± 6.32 ± 7 and 42 ± 5 h (Schrogie and Solomon, 1967; Ambre and Fischer, 1973). In a subject sensitive to the drug, single oral doses of 50, 100 or 150 mg resulted in half-lives of 38, 54 and 82 h, respectively (Solomon, 1968). Vesell and Page (1968) have reported half-lives of 24.4 and 48.3 h in normal adults receiving 2 or 4 mg BHC/kg on two different occasions. In some of these individuals, the half-life was approximately 82 h after 5 days of a daily dose of 2 mg/kg. The explanation for the dose-dependence of BHC plasma half-life is still being discussed (Nagashima and Levy, 1969). Vesell and Page (1968) have also reported data indicating that for a given dose of BHC, the half-life is under genetic control; interestingly, the half-life is remarkably similar in pairs of identical twins but varies in pairs of fraternal twins and varies even more (from 7 to 74 h) among unrelated subjects. Co-administration of antacids slightly prolongs the half-life of BHC (from 42 ± 5 h to 55 ± 7 h) in normal subjects (Ambre and Fischer, 1973).

While the maximum plasma concentrations of BHC after oral administration may occur within 2-12 h, the maximum inhibition of prothrombin-complex activity occurs only after about 38 h (O'Reilly et al., 1966). As was also demonstrated for warfarin (Nagashima et al., 1969), a distinct relationship exists between the anticoagulant effect of BHC, when expressed in terms of inhibition of prothrombin-complex activity synthesis rate, and its concentration in the plasma. The synthesis rate (percent per day) is inhibited by 50% at plasma BHC concentrations around 20 µg/ml (O'Reilly and Levy, 1970). BHC is extensively metabolized by hepatic microsomal enzymes, the major metabolites in the rat are ring hydroxylated compounds (Christensen, 1966). To our knowledge, the metabolites of BHC in man have not been characterized.

As was the case for warfarin, no information on BHC kinetics in newborns, infants and children is available.

Acenocoumarol

In adults, the gastrointestinal absorption of acenocoumarol is rapid. According to Blatrix et al. (1968), peak plasma levels of about 2, 2.5 and 5 µg/ml are attained within 6-12 h after a single oral administration of 16, 24 or 36 mg, respectively. Very often, the first plasma peak of the drug is followed (within 24-48 h) by one or two additional peaks which makes it difficult at the present time to evaluate the half-life and the volume of distribution after oral ingestion of the drug. It is conceivable that the drug enters an important enterohepatic circulation. After intravenous administration of 40 or 60 mg of acenocoumarol, the apparent half-life ranges between 20 and 30 h, being slightly longer after the higher dose, and the apparent volume of distribution is extremely variable (from 17 to 76% body weight). A rough correlation between the steady-state acenocoumarol concentration and its anticoagulant effect has been reported, the therapeutic range being between 1.5 and 2.0 µg/ml (Blatrix et al., 1968). Regardless of the oral dose of acenocoumarol used, the maximum anticoagulant effect is reached after 24 h and completely disappears within 96 h (Blatrix et al., 1968). *In vitro*, the binding capacity of acenocoumarol to human serum albumin is slightly higher than that of warfarin and lower than that of BHC and ethylbiscoumacetate, i.e., about 3 moles drug/mole of protein are bound (Garten and Wosilait, 1971). According to Tillement et al. (1974), *in vitro* acenoucoumarol at a concentration of 1.2 µg/ml is bound to human albumin to the extent of

81.0 ± 3.5%, while under the same experimental conditions warfarin is 78.8 ± 2.9% bound.

Urinary excretion of acenocoumarol results in about 25% of the administered dose recoverable in urine during the first 24 h; within 6 days, 35-50% of the administered dose can be found. The product(s) excreted in the urine has the same spectrophotometric characteristics as the parent molecule, suggesting that acenocoumarol is poorly metabolized.

No data are available on metabolism and disposition of the drug in newborns, infants and children.

Ethylbiscoumacetate

In adults, the gastrointestinal absorption of ethylbiscoumacetate is rapid. According to Blatrix et al. (1968), peak plasma concentrations of about 20 or 100 µg/ml are attained within 3 h of the single oral ingestion of 900 or 3,000 mg, respectively. *In vitro,* the binding affinity of ethylbiscoumacetate to human serum ablumin is lower than that of BHC and slightly higher than that of acenocoumarol and warfarin, the stoichiometry is, indeed, between 3 and 4 moles drug/mole of protein (Garten and Wosilait, 1971). According to Tillement et al. (1974), ethylbiscoumacetate at a concentration of 3.2 µg/ml *in vitro* is bound to human albumin 88.2 ± 5.0%. In the same experimental conditions, warfarin and acenocoumarol are 78.8 ± 2.9% and 81.0 ± 3.5% bound, respectively.

Plasma clearance of ethylbiscoumacetate is very rapid, the drug being hardly detectable 24 h after its administration, interindividual variations are, therefore, extremely high. Blatrix et al. (1968) maintain that calculations of both the half-life and the volume of distribution of ethylbiscoumacetate are of questionable validity. Regardless of the oral dose of ethylbiscoumacetate used, the maximum anticoagulant effect is observed after 24 h and completely disappears after 72-96 h (Blatrix et al., 1968). Urinary excretion of ethylbiscoumacetate is maximal during the first 24 h but never reaches 10% of the administered dose, this would indicate an extensive hepatic degradation resulting in metabolites that are not easily detectable (Blatrix et al., 1968). According to Burns et al. (1953), the main metabolite of ethylbiscoumacetate most likely is hydroxytromexane.

No data are available on the metabolism and disposition of the drug in newborns, infants and children.

Fluorophenindione

We have already briefly discussed the reasons why anticoagulant drugs of the coumarin-type are clinically preferred to those of the indanedione type. Recently, however, a new compound, fluorophenindione, has been introduced into therapeutics which is chemically related to phenindione but behaves like the coumarins (Rumeau et al., 1971; Faivre and Neimann, 1972). In recent studies, some pharmacokinetic data on this new drug were obtained following single oral doses (80 mg) in adults (Tillement et al., 1975).

Gastrointestinal absorption is rapid, and peak plasma concentrations of about 15 μg/ml are attained within 4 h. *In vivo,* 94.5 ± 2.3% of the drug is bound to plasma proteins, but Tillement et al. (1974) reported that *in vitro* fluorophenindione, at a concentration of 20 μg/ml, is bound to human albumin to the extent of 87.3 ± 1.7%. This figure is similar to that obtained under the same experimental conditions with ethylbiscoumacetate. It is of interest that chlorophenoxysobutyrate (the active form of clofibrate) does not modify the binding percentage of either fluorophenindione or phenindione, whereas it does inhibit the binding of courmarin-type anticoagulants (Tillement et al., 1974). These results suggest that coumarinic derivatives are bound to sites other than those of phenindione derivatives and that the two groups of compounds are not similarly susceptible to the displacement from albumin induced by other drugs.

The average apparent half-life of fluorophenindione is 31 h (range: 16-60 h), which is longer than that of phenindione (5 h, according to Schulert and Weiner 1954), but comparable to that of another deriviative of phenindione, phenyl-2-morpholinomethyl-2-indanedione (29 h, according to Blatrix et al., 1972). The mean of the apparent volumes of distribution of fluorophenindione is 9.4 ± 2.5% body weight, a figure similar to that of warfarin. After a single loading dose of fluorophenindione (80 mg, p.o.), the maximum anticoagulant effect is obtained after about 72 h and completely disappears after 120 h.

Only 33% of unchanged drug is found in urine within 6 days. The remainder seems likely to be excreted in the form of various, yet unidentified metabolites, similar to phenindione but in smaller proportions. This would confirm the relative stability of fluorophenindione as compared to the nonfluorinated derivative. Nevertheless, considerable interindividual differences have already been observed.

No data are yet available on the metabolism and disposition of the drug in newborns, infants and children.

CONCLUSIONS

According to Breckenridge and Orme (1973), in view of the precision with which the pharmacological effect (i.e., anticoagulation) of vitamin-K antagonists can be measured by laboratory tests and of the interindividual kinetic and dynamic variations observed especially with warfarin and BHC, there are few clinical situation in which measurement of plasma levels of anticoagulants are useful. Two situations worth of mention are the documentation of resistance to anticoagulants (O'Reilly et al., 1964a; O'Reilly, 1972) and of their surreptitious ingestion (O'Reilly and Aggeler, 1970). The main practical interest of measuring plasma anticoagulant concentration remains, however, the understanding of drug interactions with oral anticoagulants, particularly warfarin, whose complex metabolism is a continuous challenge to the clinical pharmacologist.

In prescribing oral anticoagulant therapy, one should take into account that vitamin K antagonists cross the placenta and do appear in mother's milk, in addition, several reports claim that warfarin possesses a teratogenic effect (Fillmore and McDevitt, 1970; Bloomfied, 1970; Shaul et al., 1975; Becker et al., 1975). Oral anticoagulant therapy should, therefore, be avoided during the first three months and the last two weeks of pregnancy, and during puerperium, if the mother is breast-feeding her baby. If anticoagulation is required in the above-mentioned conditions, heparin should be used. With the aid of reliable laboratory controls of their anticoagulant effect, coumarin drugs have been used without complications during the second and third trimesters of pregnancy (Noble, 1974). Some authors recommend the prophylactic administration of vitamin K_1 (1 mg intramuscularly) to newborn infants in view of the frequent vitamin K-dependent defects of clotting tests observed in apparently healthy children under 15 months of age (Lovric et al., 1971).

Vitamin K deficiency in infants has been attributed to oral antibiotic therapy and/or associated diarrhea, and to feeding with artificial milks low in vitamin K or with breast milk (the latter containing less vitamin K than cow's milk) (Nammacher et al., 1970). However, the reason(s) for vitamin K deficiency in normal neonates remain(s) obscure at present. A reduced activity of vitamin K-dependent clotting factors has been reported in several clinical conditions, such as hemorrhagic disease of the newborn, obstructive jaundice, intestinal malabsorption syndrome (idiopathic steatorrhea, kwashiorkor, infantile gastroenteritis, sprue, celiac disease), uremia and congenital cyanotic heart disease (Hazell and Baloch, 1970; Goldschmidt, 1970). Although the use of coumarin anticoagulants in the neonatal period and in the above-mentioned conditions is rare, the possibility of an increased sensitivity to these drugs should be considered. To the best of our knowledge, the disposition of vitamin K antagonists in subjects less than 20 years old thus far has not been systematically investigated.

REFERENCES

Aggeler, P.M. and O'Reilly, R.A. (1969): Effect of heptobarbital on the response to bishydroxycoumarin in man. *Journal of Laboratory and Clinical Medicine, 74:* 229-238.

Ambre, J.J. and Fischer, L.J. (1973): Effect of coadministration of aluminum and magnesium hydroxides on absorption of anticoagulants in man. *Clinical Pharmacology and Therapeutics, 14:* 231-237.

Becker, M.H., Genieser, N.B., Finegold, M., Miranda, D. and Spackman, T. (1975): Chondrodysplasia punctata—is maternal warfarin therapy a factor. *American Journal of Diseases of Children, 129:* 356-359.

Berberich, F.R., Cuene, S.A., Chard, R.L. and Hartmann, J.R. (1974): Thrombotic thrombocytopenic purpura. Three cases with platelet and fibrinogen survival studies. *Journal of Pediatrics, 84:* 503-509.

Blatrix, C., Charonnat, S., Tillement, J.P., Israel, J., Brevet, J.P., Debraux, J. and Merlin, M. (1968): Métabolisme chez l'homme du dérivé de la 4-hydroxycoumarine: 3(γ-acétonyl-p-nitrobenzyl)4-hydroxycoumarine (Sintrom). *Revue Francaise d'Etudes Cliniques et Biologiques, 13:* 948-995.

Blatrix, C., Tillement, J.-P. and Paquelin, A. (1972): Métabolisme et action thérapeutique d'un noveau dérivé de l'indane dione-1,3. Le phényl-2 morpholinométhyl-2 indane dione-1,3. *Gazette Médicale de France, 79:* 2564-2568.

Bloomfield, D.K. (1970): Fetal deaths and malformations associated with the use of coumarin derivatives in pregnancy. *American Journal of Obstetrics and Gynecology, 107:* 883-888.

Brain, M.C., Baker, L.R., McBride, J.A., Rubenberg, M.L. and Dacie, J.V. (1968): Treatment of patients with microangiopathic haemolytic anaemia with heparin. *British Journal of Haematology, 15:* 603-621.

Breckenridge, A. and Orme, M.L'E. (1972): The plasma half-lives and the pharmacological effect of the enantiomers of warfarin in rats. *Life Sciences, 11,* pt. 2: 337-345.

Breckenridge, A. and Orme, M.L'E. (1973): Measurement of plasma warfarin concentrations in clinical practice. In *Biological Effects of Drugs in Relation to Their Plasma Concentrations,* edited by D.S. Davies and B.N.C. Prichard, pp. 145-154, MacMillan, London.

Burns, J., Weiner, M., Simson, G. and Brodie, B.B. (1953): The biotransformation of ethylbiscoumacetate (Tromexan) in man, rabbit and dog. *Journal of Pharmacology and Experimental Therapeutics, 108:* 33-41.

Christensen, F. (1966): Crystallization and preliminary characterization of a dicoumarol metabolite in the faeces of dicoumarol-treated rats. *Acta Pharmacologica et Toxicologica, 24:* 232-242.

Deykin, D. (1970): Warfarin therapy. *New England Journal of Medicine, 283:* 691-694.

Douglas, A.S. and McNicol, G.P. (1972): Anticoagulant therapy. In: *Human Blood Coagulation, Haemostasis and Thrombosis,* edited by R. Biggs, pp. 497-542, Blackwell, Oxford.

Eble, J.N., West, B.D. and Link, K.P. (1966): A comparison of the isomers of warfarin. *Biochemical Pharmacology, 15:* 1003-1006.

Edson, J.R., Blaese, R.M., White, J.G. and Krivit, W. (1968): Defibrination syndrome in an infant born after abruptio placentae. *Journal of Pediatrics, 72:* 342-346.

Ehrlich, J. and Stivala, S.S. (1973): Chemistry and pharmacology of heparin. *Journal of Pharmaceutical Sciences, 62:* 517-544.

Estes, J.W. (1971): The kinetics of heparin. *Annals of the New York Academy of Sciences, 179:* 187-204.

Estes, J.W., Pelikan, E.W. and Kruger-Thiemer, E. (1969): A retrospective study of the pharmacokinetics of heparin. *Clinical Pharmacology and Therapeutics, 10:* 329-337.

Estes, J.W. and Poulin, P.F. (1975): Pharmacokinetics of heparin. Distribution and elimination. *Thrombosis et Diathesis Haemorrhagica, 33:* 26-37.

Faivre, G. and Neimann, J.L. (1972): Étude clinique d'un nouveau dérivé de l'indane dione: le Préviscan. *Annales Medicales de Nancy, 11:* 1055-1061.

Fillmore, S.J. and McDevitt, E. (1970): Effects of coumarin compounds on the fetus. *Annals of Internal Medicine, 73:* 731-735.

Garten, S. and Wosilait, W.D. (1971): Comparative study of the binding of coumarin anticoagulants and serum albumins. *Biochemical Pharmacology, 20:* 1661-1668.

Goldschmidt, B. (1970): Effect of vitamin K on clotting factors in children with congenital cyanotic heart disease. *Acta Paediatrica Academiae Scientiarium Hungaricae, 11:* 135-139.

Hazell, K. and Baloch, K.H. (1970): Vitamin K deficiency in the elderly. *Gerontologia Clinica, 12:* 10-17.

Hemker, H.C. and Muller, A.D. (1968): Kinetic aspects of the interaction of blood-clotting enzymes. VI. Localization of the site of blood-coagulation inhibition by the protein induced by vitamin K absence (PIVKA). *Thrombosis et Diathesis Haemorrhagica, 20:* 78-87.

Hemker, H.C., Veltkamp, J.J., Hensen, A. and Loeliger, E.A. (1963): Nature of prothrombin biosynthesis: preprothrombinaemia in Vitamin K-deficiency. *Nature* (London), *200:* 589-590.

Hewick, D.S. and McEwen, J. (1973): Plasma half-lives, plasma metabolites and anticoagulant efficacies of the enantiomers of warfarin in man. *Journal of Pharmacy and Pharmacology, 25:* 458-465.

Kaiser, D.G. and Martin, R.S. (1974): GLC determination of warfarin in human plasma. *Journal of Pharmaceutical Sciences, 63:* 1579-1581.

Kakkar, V.V. (1975): Low dose heparin in the prevention of venous thromboembolism. Rationale and results. *Thrombosis et Diathesis Haemorrhagica, 33:* 87-96.

Lacy, J.P. and Goodin, R.R. (1975): Warfarin-induced necrosis of skin. *Annals of Internal Medicine, 82:* 381-385.

Lasch, H.G. and Heene, D.H. (1975): Heparin therapy of diffuse intravascular coagulation (DIC). *Thrombosis et Diathesis Haemorrhagica, 33:* 105-106.

Leissring, J.C. and Vorlicky, L.N. (1968): Disseminated intravascular coagulation in a neonate. *American Journal of Diseases of Children, 115:* 100-106.

Lewis, R.J. and Trager, W.F. (1970): Warfarin metabolism in man: identification of metabolites in urine. *Journal of Clinical Investigation, 49:* 907-913.

Lewis, R.J. and Trager, W.F. (1971): The metabolic fate of warfarin: studies on the metabolites in plasma. *Annals of the New York Academy of Sciences, 179:* 205-212.

Lewis, R.J., Trager, W.F., Chan, K.K., Breckenridge, A., Orme, M., Roland, M. and Schary, W. (1974): Warfarin. Stereochemical aspects of its metabolism and the interaction with phenylbutazone. *Journal of Clinical Investigation, 53:* 1607-1617.

Lewis, R.J., Trager, W.F., Robinson, A.J. and Chan, K.H. (1973): Warfarin metabolites: the anticoagulant activity and pharmacology of warfarin alcohols. *Journal of Laboratory and Clinical Medicine, 81:* 925-931.

Lieberman, E. (1972): Hemolytic-uremic syndrome. *Journal of Pediatrics, 80:* 1-16.

Lovric, V.A., Glasson, M.J., Dey, D.L., Middleton, A.W. and Llewelyn, D.M. (1971): Vitamin K deficiency in apparently healthy children. *Australian and New Zealand Journal of Medicine, 1:* 35-38.

Markarian, M., Cohen, R.J. and Milbauer, B. (1971): Disseminated intravascular coagulation in a neonate treated with heparin. *Journal of Pediatrics, 78:* 74-77.

McNicol, G.P. (1975): Conventional uses of heparin. *Thrombosis et Diathesis Haemorrhagica, 33:* 97-101.

Nagashima, R. and Levy, G. (1969): Comparative pharmacokinetics of coumarin anticoagulants. V. Kinetics of warfarin elimination in the rat, dog, and rhesus monkey compared to man. *Journal of Pharmaceutical Sciences, 58:* 845-849.

Nagashima, R., O'Reilly, R.A. and Levy, G. (1969): Kinetics of pharmacologic effects in man: the anticoagulant action of warfarin. *Clinical Pharmacology and Therapeutics, 10:* 22-35.

Nammacher, M.A., Willemin, M., Harmann, J.R. and Gaston, L.W. (1970): Vitamin K deficiency in infants beyond the neonatal period. *Journal of Pediatrics, 76:* 549-554.

Noble, L.M. (1974): Prescribing in pregnancy. *Practitioner, 212:* 657-664.

Nyman, D., Thurnherr, N. and Duckert, F. (1975): Heparin dosage in extracorporeal circulation and its neutralization. *Thrombosis et Diathesis Haemorrhagica, 33:* 102-104.

O'Reilly, R.A. (1967): Studies on the coumarin anticoagulant drugs: interaction of human plasma albumin and warfarin sodium. *Journal of Clinical Investigation, 46:* 829-837.

O'Reilly, R.A. (1971): Interaction of several coumarin compounds with human and canine plasma albumin. *Molecular Pharmacology, 7:* 209-218.
O'Reilly, R.A. (1972): Sodium warfarin. *Pharmacology, 8:* 181-190.
O'Reilly, R.A. (1973): The binding of sodium warfarin to plasma albumin and its displacement by phenylbutazone. *Annals of the New York Academy of Sciences, 226:* 293-308.
O'Reilly, R.A. and Aggeler, P.M. (1968): Studies on coumarin anticoagulant drugs. Initiation of warfarin therapy without a loading dose. *Circulation, 38:* 169-177.
O'Reilly, R.A. and Aggeler, P.M. (1970): Determinants of the response to oral anticoagulant drugs in man. *Pharmacological Reviews, 22:* 35-96.
O'Reilly, R.A., Aggeler, P.M., Hoag, M.S. and Leong, L. (1962: Studies on the coumarin anticoagulant drugs: the assay of warfarin and its biologic application. *Thrombosis et Diathesis Haemorrhagica, 8:* 82-95.
O'Reilly, R.A., Aggeler, P.M., Hoag, M.S. and Leong, L.S. (1964a): Hereditary transmission of exceptional resistance to coumarin anticoagulant drugs. The first reported kindred. *New England Journal of Medicine, 271:* 809-815.
O'Reilly, R.A., Aggeler, P.M. and Leong, L.S. (1963): Studies on the coumarin anticoagulant drugs: the pharmacodynamics of warfarin in man. *Journal of Clinical Investigation, 42:* 1542-1551.
O'Reilly, R.A., Aggeler, P.M. and Leong, L.S. (1964b): Studies on the coumarin anticoagulant drugs: a comparison of the pharmacodynamics of dicumarol and warfarin in man. *Thrombosis et Diathesis Haemorrhagica, 11:* 1-22.
O'Reilly, R.A. and Levy, G. (1970): Kinetics of the anticoagulant effect of bishydroxycoumarin in man. *Clinical Pharmacology and Therapeutics, 11:* 378-384.
O'Reilly, R.A., Welling, P.G. and Wagner, J.G. (1971): Pharmacokinetics of warfarin following intravenous administration to man. *Thrombosis et Diathesis Haemorrhagica, 25:* 178-186.
Reekers, P.P.M., Lindhout, M.J., Kop-Klaassen, B.H.M. and Hemker, H.C. (1973): Demonstration of three anomalous plasma proteins induced by a vitamin K antagonist. *Biochimica et Biophysica Acta, 317:* 559-562.
Robinson, D.S., Benjamin, D.M. and McCormack, J.J. (1971): Interaction of warfarin and nonsystemic gastrointestingal drugs. *Clinical Pharmacology and Therapeutics, 12:* 491-495.
Rumeau, M., Durand, D., Fauvel, J.M. and Slavador, M. (1971): Résultats cliniques de l'utilisation d'un nouvel anticoagulant LM 123: Préviscan. *Revue Médicale de Toulouse, 7:* 1511S-1514S.
Schrogie, J.J. and Solomon, H.M. (1967): The anticoagulant response to bishydroxycoumarin. II. The effect of d-thyroxine, clofibrate, and norethandrolone. *Clinical Pharmacology and Therapeutics, 8:* 70-77.
Schulert, A.R. and Weiner, M. (1954): The physiologic disposition of phenylindanedione in man. *Journal of Pharmacology and Experimental Therapeutics, 110:* 451-457.
Shaul, W.L., Emery, H. and Hall, J.G. (1975): Chondrodysplasia punctata and maternal warfarin use during pregnancy. *American Journal of Diseases of Children, 129:* 360-362.
Skyberg, D. and Jacobsen, C.D. (1969): Defibrination syndrome in a newborn, and its treatment with exchange transfusion. *Acta Paediatrica Scandinavica, 58:* 83-86.
Solomon, H.M. (1968): Variations in metabolism of coumarin anticoagulant drugs. *Annals of the New York Academy of Sciences, 151:* 932-935.
Solomon, H.M. and Schrogie, J.J. (1967): The effect of various drugs on the binding of warfarin-^{14}C to human albumin. *Biochemical Pharmacology, 16:* 1219-1226.
Straub, P.W. (1975): A case against heparin therapy of intravascular coagulation. *Thrombosis et Diathesis Haemorrhagica, 33:* 107-112.

Tillement, J.-P., Mattei, C. and Zini, R. (1974): Effect of sodium chlorophenoxyisobutyrate on the binding of vitamin K antagonists to human albumin in vitro. *Experientia, 30:* 460-461.

Tillement, J.-P., Thébault, J.J., Mattei, C., D'Athis, P. and Blatrix, C. (1975): Anticoagulant effect and plasma kinetics of fluorophenindione after a single does in man. *European Journal of Clinical Pharmacology, 8:* 271-275.

Verstraete, M., Vermylen, C., Vermylen, J. and Vandenbroucke, J. (1975): Excessive consumption of blood coagulation components as cause of hemorrhagic diathesis. *American Journal of Medicine, 38:* 899-908.

Vessell, E.S. and Page, J.G. (1968): Genetic control of dicumarol levels in man. *Journal of Clinical Investigation, 47:* 2657-2663.

Weiner, M., Shapiro, S., Axelrod, J., Cooper, J.R. and Brodie, B.B. (1950): The physiological disposition of dicumarol in man. *Journal of Pharmacology and Experimental Therapeutics, 99:* 409-420.

Wessler, S. (1975): Small doses of heparin and a new concept of hypercoagulability. *Thrombosis et Diathesis Haemorrhagica, 33:* 81-86.

Wessler, S. and Yin, E.T. (1973): Theory and practice of minidose heparin in surgical patients. A status report. *Circulation, 47:* 671-676.

Windsor, E. and Freeman, L. (1964): An investigation of route of administration of heparin other than injection. *American Journal of Medicine, 37:* 408-416.

Yin, E.T., Wessler, S. and Stoll, P.J. (1971): Identity of plasma-activated factor X inhibitor with antithrombin III and heparin cofactor. *Journal of Biological Chemistry, 246:* 3712-3719.

10
Antipyretic and Nonsteroid Antiinflammatory Drugs

MARINELLA MANDELLI

AND PAOLO LUCIO MORSELLI

Most of the antipyretic and nonsteroid antiinflammatory drugs actually available are "old" drugs, which have been in the medical "armamentarium" for many years, and which are widely used both in children and adults. This class of drugs is probably the one for which, together with anticonvulsants, we have the most detailed information on disposition in the various age groups as well as in different pathological situations. The data available from the literature indicate that several important differences in various pharmacokinetic parameters are linked to age and, more important, that such differences may have a significant bearing on the toxicity of these agents. The agents reviewed in this chapter include salicylates, phenybutazone, indomethacin, pirazolone derivatives, phenacetin and acetaminophen.

SALICYLATES

Adults

Both in normal adults and in patients, the gastrointestinal absorption of salicylates is a very rapid process with an apparent half-life of 6–15 min. Peak levels of 40–60 µg/ml are, in fact, attained 30–60 min after an oral intake of 500–600 mg (Leonards, 1963; Levy and Leonards, 1966; Rowland et al., 1967, 1972; Davison and Mandel, 1971; Davison, 1971; Soren, 1975). The rate of absorption and the amount absorbed are dependent on numerous factors, such as gastric and intestinal pH, disintegration and dissolution time, gastric motility, pharmaceutical formulation, etc. (Levy et al., 1961; Levy and Leonards, 1966; Siurala et al., 1969; Chio and Onyenelukwe, 1974).

Leonards (1963) has shown that while with conventional buffered aspirin (640 mg) peak levels of 30–40 µg/ml are attained after 60 min, peak levels considerably higher (50–60 µg/ml) may be obtained within 20–30 min with an equivalent amount of effervescent aspirin or sodium salicylate. From a practical point of view, in addition to the characteristics of the formulation, other important factors that significantly influence the absorption of salicylates are gastric emptying time and the presence of food in the stomach. In fact, it has been shown that presence of food stuff in the stomach may more than double the absorption half-life of aspirin (Davison and Mandel, 1971). The higher absorption rate observed with effervescent preparations, particularly, may be explained as an effect on gastric motility mediated through a slight alkalinization of gastric fluids. The dose may also influence the rate of absorption and the amount absorbed, as reported by Levy and Leonards (1966). Concomitant administration of activated charcoal significantly reduces the amount absorbed (Levy and Tsuchiya, 1972b).

Absorption of sodium salicylate from the mouth is very slow and inefficient, and the same holds true for rectal preparations. Coldwell et al. (1969) and more recently Nowak et al. (1974) have shown that the absorption of aspirin from suppositories may be exceedingly slow (half-life = 3 h) and completely unreliable, with a urinary recovery which may vary from 26 to 80% of the administered dose. By oral route at doses not exceeding 2 gm, the urinary recovery is practically complete (98–99%). Following cutaneous applications, the absorption of salicylates given in various forms (acids, salts or esters) is very rapid, and dissolution of esters in ethanol or anhydrous lanolin may greatly increase the percutaneous absorption (Wurster and Kramer, 1961; Davison and Mandel, 1971).

Aspirin or other salicylates administered by oral or intravenous routes are rapidly hydrolized to salicylic acid (SA), which is further degraded to several metabolites. Menguy et al. demonstrated in 1972 that esterases in erythrocytes from females were less active than those of males in releasing salicylic acid from aspirin. This finding has recently been confirmed by Windorfer et al. (1974). It may be interesting to underline that while the area under the curve obtained after i.v. or oral administration of aspirin shows a complete equivalence of the plasma levels of SA, if we consider the aspirin concentrations the plasma curve obtained after oral intake is about 60% of the i.v. (Rowland et al., 1972). These data are indicative of the fact that a considerable hydrolysis may already have taken place during the absorption step and the first pass through the liver. According to the same authors, only 20% of aspirin hydrolysis occurs in blood (Rowland et al., 1967).

Salicylic acid is considerably bound (80–85%) to plasma proteins, mainly to the albumin fraction. This protein binding of SA, however, appears to be dose-dependent, while for concentrations in plasma of 10–20 mg/100 ml the free fraction is about 15–20%, for plasma concentration over 40 mg/100 ml the free fraction may be as high as 50% (Smith et al., 1946; Reynolds and Cluff, 1960; Davison and Smith, 1961; Davison, 1971; Kucera and Bullock, 1969; Kramer and Routh, 1973; Ali and Routh, 1969; Spector et al., 1972). This phenomenon may be even more evident, and have clinical consequences, in case of hypoalbuminemia, e.g., in patients suffering from rheumatoid arthritis (Bernstein and Allerhand, 1964). In cases of reduced binding, the amount of drug diffusing into the tissues may significantly increase with higher risk of severe toxicity.

In normal adults, the apparent SA association constant is 4×10^5 M^{-1}. Krasmer et al. (1973) have shown that a serum with an albumin content of 3.5 g/100 ml binds 7 mg of salicylates at the primary site. At higher concentrations exceeding the 1:1 molar ratio, secondary binding with a large number of weak interactions may occur. The binding of salicylates to plasma proteins may be reduced by several anions (Davison and Strautz, 1961), and salicylates may displace other drugs from plasma protein-binding (Davison, 1971; Kunin, 1964; APA, 1973; Morselli et al., 1974; Cohen and Armstrong, 1974). On the contrary, increased binding due to acetylsalicylate has been observed for acetrizoate (Pinckard et al., 1973). Salicylate may also interact at the binding level with endogenous body constituents such as thyroid hormone, bilirubin, urate and FFA (Oppenheimer, 1973; Larsen, 1972; Bluestone et al., 1969; Odell, 1973). A gradual reduction of the binding affinity has been noted in the course of pregnancy (Crawford and Hodi, 1968; Krasner and Jaffe, 1975). The apparent volume of distribution of salicylic acid, according to various authors, is around 0.13–0.20 L/kg, indicating that the drug is mainly distributed into extracellular water (Rowland and Riegelman, 1968; Levy and Hollister, 1964; Wiegand and Sanders, 1964; Hollister and Levy, 1965). However, in the case of salicylic acid the apparent volume of distribution is also a function of the dose, and a higher apparent volume of distribution (up to 0.4 L/kg) has been described with dosages of 10 g/day.

Salicylates are not evenly distributed in the body, and higher concentrations are found in the liver and kidneys. Brain levels are usually about 10% of those of the plasma, but this ratio may substantially change for pH variations. Higher brain levels may be reached in cases of hypercapnia, and this may be a relevant factor in salicylate toxicity (Davison, 1971; Levy and Leonards, 1966; Hill, 1970). Sholkoff et al. (1967) have demonstrated that total concentrations of salicylates in synovial fluids are 50% of the plasma ones but that unbound concentrations in plasma and joint fluids are essentially the same. The presence in the synovial fluid of esterases capable of hydrolyzing aspirin was also described by the same authors. In a recent study, Soren (1975) found that measurable amounts of salicylate appear in joint fluids within 12–20 min in cases of post-traumatic synovitis and synovitis in ostheoarthritis, while a significant delay may be present in patients with rheumatoid arthritis and recurrent effusions.

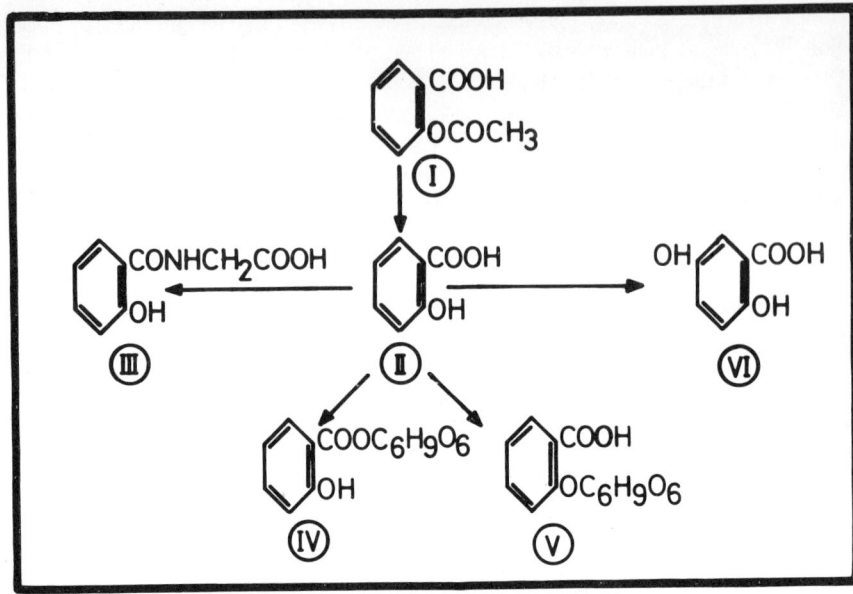

Fig. 1: Metabolism of salicylates; (I) acetylsalicylic acid; (II) salicylic acid; (III) salicyluric acid; (IV) salicylic acyl glucuronide; (V) salicylic phenolic glucuronide; (VI) gentisinic acid.

Following an oral dose of 600 mg, peak joint fluid levels were attained in about 2 h with concentrations of 11-17 µg/ml.

For dosages lower than 4 mg/kg, the plasma disappearance rate of salicylates follows first-order kinetics with an apparent plasma half-life of 2-4 h (Levy and Tsuchiya, 1972a; Levy, 1965a). For higher doses, the elimination proceeds according to zero-order kinetics, with an apparent half-life of 15-30 h until the total amount in the body is below 350-400 mg (Levy, 1965b; Levy et al., 1969). When this amount is reached, the elimination then proceeds according to first-order kinetics. The metabolism of salicylates in man is represented in Fig. 1. Starting with aspirin, the first step is the hydrolysis of acetylsalicylic acid to salicylic acid. This process is a very rapid one, with a K of 2.3 h^{-1} (Rowland and Riegelman, 1968). Salicylic acid is further degraded to salicyluric acid through conjunction with glycine, to salicyl acyl glucuronide and salicylphenolic glucuronide through conjugation with glucuronic acid, to gentisinic acid through a hydroxylation in the 5-position (Baldoni, 1915; Levy and Leonards, 1966; Davison, 1971).

The metabolic pathway which leads to the formation of salicyluric acid takes place mainly in the liver, according to Schachter and Manis (1958), while, according to recent data of Von Lehman et al. (1973), the synthesis of salicyl urate occurs primarily in the kidney. The metabolic steps leading to conjugation of salicylic acid with glycine (salicyluric acid) and glucuronic acid (salicyl phenolic glucuronide) are easily saturable in man (Levy and Leonards, 1971; Bedford et al., 1965; Elliott, 1966; Levy et al., 1969a,b; Tsuchiya and Levy, 1972) and are responsible for the Michaelis-Menten type of kinetics described for salicylates. According to Levy and Tsuchiya (1972a), the Vmax for salicyluric acid is 63.3 mg/h with a Km of 338 mg, while for the salicyl phenolic glucuronide the Vmax is 32.3/h and the Km is 629 mg. The rate of formation of salicyl acyl glucuronide and gentisinic acid are, respectively, 0.007 h^{-1} and 0.0023 h^{-1} (Levy et al., 1972), and for these two metabolites no saturation phenomena have as yet been described.

Co-administration of salicylamide may result in a decreased formation of salicylphenolic glucuronide (Levy and Procknal, 1968).

Generally, from 80 to 95% of the total administered dose is recovered in the urine, with the proportions of the various metabolites varying with the dose. For dosages of up to 1.5 g/day, in humans with normal liver and kidney function, about 50% of the administered dose is recovered as salicyluric acid and 15 to 40% as the glucuronide derivatives. Gentisinic acid usually accounts for about 1%, and salicylic acid may be present in amounts varying from 5 to 15% of the dose (Schachter and Manis, 1958; Bedford et al., 1965; Elliott, 1966; Levy and Leonards, 1966; Davison, 1971; Levy et al., 1972; Tsuchiya and Levy, 1972). Schachter and Manis (1958) have reported values of 444, 331 and 384 ml/min for renal clearance rates of salicyluric acid, salicyl acyl glucuronide, and salicyl phenolic glucuronide, respectively; these values imply that the urinary excretion of salicylates requires a combination of glomerular filtration and tubular secretion. When higher doses are administered, a considerable amount may be excreted as salicylic acid, for the saturation of the metabolic pathways leading to salicyluric acid and salicylphenolic glucuronide (Levy et al., 1969b; Gibson et al., 1975). In such a condition, even small variations of urinary pH may be very important since they may substantially modify the amount of SA reabsorbed at tubular levels (Miller and Melmon, 1972).

The salicylic acid clearance is around 10-15% of the creatinine clearance for a urinary pH of 6, but it may become considerably greater than creatinine values for pHs over 7.4. On the basis of these data, and given a situation in which plasma levels are between 15-18 mg/100 ml, the variation of urinary pH from 5 to 8 may increase the amount of salicylic acid excreted in the urine from 5 to 80% of the total amount excreted (MacPherson et al., 1955). It is thus apparent that routine monitoring of urinary pH may be useful in the course of chronic treatment. From all these observed phenomena, it is understandable that with chronic treatment even very small variations of the daily dose may lead to remarkable increases in salicylate plasma and tissue levels. As shown by Paulus et al. (1971), due to large variations in maximum concentrations obtained with the same daily dose, optimal therapy can be achieved only by individualization of therapy using serum levels as a guideline: large increases in serum levels were observed for small increments in dose, and increasing the aspirin dose by 50% tripled the serum salicylate level in two subjects.

Similarly, Levy and Tsuchiya (1972a) found that an increase from 1.5 to 3 g in the daily dose may increase the total salicylate content in the body sixfold. At variance with these data, in a more recent study Gibson et al. (1975) could not observe a wide individual variation of plasma salicylate levels in patients with rheumatoid arthritis, and the increase in plasma levels after a consistent dosage increment was minimal (30%) in three patients. The same authors showed that in the course of chronic treatment there does not appear to be clear correlation between salicylate plasma levels and the percentage of urine salicylate excreted as salicyluric acid or salicylic phenolic glucuronide. The possibility of individual variations in the metabolic thresholds is underlined, and this fact may be, according to Gibson et al. (1975), the main reason for variable plasma salicylate levels with high aspirin doses.

In the course of normal use of the salicylates as antipyretics, plasma levels are usually around a few μg/ml, while for the treatment of rheumatoid arthritis levels of about 250 μg/ml are needed. These levels are not too far from those which may induce symptoms of salicylism, and in certain cases salicylism may already be present at lower levels. The most frequent toxic signs present when levels are over 300 μg/ml are increased pulmonary ventilation, tinnitus, vomiting, hyperthermia, abdominal pain, hemorrhage and, in the most severe cases, acid base and electrolyte disturbances, delirium; hallucinations and coma (Brown et al., 1967; Miller and Melmon, 1972; Editorial, 1972; Hill, 1973). In such cases, the possibility of measuring the actual blood level may be of great help in deciding on the therapeutic intervention (Done, 1960; 1974).

Two effects which in the last few years have received considerable attention are the "anti-aggregating" effect of aspirin and related compounds on platelets with its implications for hemostasis, and the "hepatic toxicity" of salicylate. The effect of aspirin and related drugs on platelets seems to be linked to the inhibition of a cyclic endoperoxide intermediate necessary for the synthesis of prostaglandins (Willis, 1974; de Gaetano et al., 1975). As for the possible hepatotoxic effects of aspirin, these have been emphasized since 1956 by Manso et al., but only recently has the high incidence of this toxic effect been recognized by several authors (Russell et al., 1971; Rich and Johnson, 1973; Pinedo et al., 1973; Editorial, 1974; Seaman et al., 1974). The most common features appear to be elevation of SGOT and SGPT, fall in eosinophils and other evidence of hepatic dysfunction such as abnormalities of LDH, BSP retention and alkaline phosphatase. These effects are usually observed when serum levels rise above 25 mg/100 ml. The regular determination of routine liver function tests and serum salicylate levels in patients receiving salicylate therapy in high doses is strongly advisable.

Newborns

A consistent body of data has recently become available on salicylate kinetics in the newborn human, mainly through the studies of Levy's group (Levy, 1975). All the data available refer to cases where salicylate was transferred from the mother, either transplacentally or through breast-feeding. There is a very high possibility of the former occurring since, according to various reports, aspirin appears to be the drug most frequently used during pregnancy, with an incidence of use varying from 25% to 70% of the total pregnancies (Nora et al., 1963; Bleyer and Breckenridge, 1970; Bleyer et al., 1970; Hill et al., 1972; Lewis and Schulman, 1973; Collins and Turner, 1973; Levy and Garrettson, 1974; Garrettson et al., 1975). The possibility that a newborn from a mother taking aspirin has to be considered "at risk" is not a remote one. Palmisano and Cassady (1969) have reported that about 10% of consecutively delivered infants had serum salicylate concentrations over 1 mg/100 ml with individual values ranging from 1.2 to 10 mg/100 ml. Higher levels have been reported by Earle (1961), Garrettson et al. (1975) and Levy and Garrettson (1974).

The placental transfer of salicylate is very rapid, and 4–6 min after an intravenous administration to the mother the salicylate concentration in the cord serum may be 60–80% of that found in the mother (Boda et al., 1971). According to Noschel et al. (1972), the ratio between newborn and mother serum concentration approaches unity within 70 min, and continues to increase up to an average of 1.5 beyond 4 h after aspirin administration to the mother. The levels of salicylate usually found at birth in newborns are higher than those of the mother, this being indicative of the fact that the fetus acts as a "deep compartment" (Levy, 1975). Levy and Garrettson (1974) calculated that in cases where amounts of 350 to 996 mg of aspirin were ingested by the mother in the 24 h preceding the delivery, up to 2.3% of the dose was recovered in the newborn's urine. In cases of intake through breast-feeding, the amount absorbed is around 0.16–0.38% of the daily dose ingested by the mother (Giacoia et al., 1975).

Plasma protein-binding of salicylate in newborns is significantly reduced if compared to adult values (Behrman and Battaglia, 1967; Ganshorn and Kurz, 1968; Palmisano and Cassady, 1969; Krasner et al., 1973; Windorfer et al., 1974; Krasner and Yaffe, 1975). The apparent association constant in cord serum is $1.7 \times 10^5 \, M^{-1}$ against a value of $4 \times 10^5 \, M^{-1}$ in adults (Krasner et al., 1973), and, as observed in adults, the degree of binding is dependent on the salicylate serum levels. An increase in the free fraction is, in fact, observed for higher concentrations (Windorfer et al., 1974). In premature newborns, the binding is even lower than in full-term newborns, and, as found with other drugs, high levels of serum salicylate may significantly increase the free fraction of serum salicylate (Windorfer et al., 1974). Krasner and Yaffe (1975) have hypothesized that the reduced association constant of salicylate in the newborn may be due to the presence of a dialyzable factor which diminishes the protein affinity for salicylates. On the other hand, salicylate levels over 2–3 mg/100 ml in the newborn may decrease the mean reserve albumin-binding capacity (Palmisano and Cassady, 1969), and concentrations over 10 mg/100 ml may double the free fraction of bilirubin in neonatal plasma (Øie and Levy, 1975).

Theoretically, such a displacement should only occur for concentrations of salicylates 100 to 1,000 times greater than bilirubin, which itself has an association constant of 10^7 M^{-1} (Krasner and Yaffe, 1975). The presence of other mechanisms which might play a role in the salicylate-bilirubin-protein interactions, thus modifying the affinity of bilirubin for albumin, is a possible explanation for this discrepancy (see Chapter 3). In fact, the displacing effect of salicylate over bilirubin may be magnified by the presence of high concentrations of FFA (Odell, 1973; Windorfer et al., 1974). Odell demonstrated that a high-caloric, elevated FFA feeding for infants induced a reduction of the percentage of the bilirubin which was displaced by salicylate. Because of these mutual interactions, Levy (1975) recently stressed that it is very important to know, in evaluating bilirubin levels, if a newborn has been exposed to salicylate and to be able to predict within reasonable limits of accuracy the time course of elimination of the drug by the infant.

The apparent volume of distribution of salicylate in newborns, calculated on the available data, may range from 0.08 to 0.22 L/kg for plasma levels of about 1 to 10 mg/100 ml (Levy and Garrettson, 1974). On the average, it is higher than that recorded for similar salicylate levels in adults. In fact, for plasma or serum levels over 20 mg/100 ml apparent volumes as high as 0.30 and 0.35 L/kg have been observed (Earle, 1961; Garrettson et al., 1975).

The reduced plasma protein-binding and the consequently increased apparent volume of distribution may have some important, practical bearing. One should remember that, because of the expanded apparent Vd, a given plasma or serum level in the newborn reflects a larger amount of salicylate in the body than the same concentration in older children and adults (Garrettson et al., 1975; Levy, 1975; Levy and Yaffe, 1975). Another point which deserves mention is the fact that the relative hypoxemia of the newborn, and the lower blood pH, may contribute to increased salicylate tissue levels and, hence, the toxic risk. The activity of the blood esterases, responsible in part for the splitting of aspirin into salicylic acid and acetyl groups, has been found consistently reduced in premature and full-term newborns as compared to older children and adults (Windorfer et al., 1974).

The time course of salicylate elimination in the neonate is considerably slower than that observed in older children and normal adults (Earle, 1961; Levy and Garrettson, 1974; Garrettson et al., 1975; Levy, 1975). The process of salicylate elimination is, as mentioned before, "capacity-limited," and the apparent half-lives of the near-exponential phase found by Levy and Garrettson in newborns range from 4.5 to 11 h, with a mean of about 7 h. The corresponding values in children and adults are 2–3 h. In those cases where aspirin was taken by the mother in a single dose shortly before delivery, the apparent Km values were about 0.6 mg/kg (Vmax 0.08 mg/kg/h) with the near-exponential elimination occurring only at about 2 mg. These data suggest that under normal conditions there is a relative immaturity of the processes responsible for salicylate elimination. However, a recent report of Garrettson et al. (1975) describes one case of chronic exposure to salicylate during intrauterine life where the near-exponential elimination occurred at 10 mg. In this neonate, born with a plasma concentration of 25 mg/100 ml, the apparent Km was 3.9 mg/kg (Vmax 0.80 mg/kg/h), actually not very far from the value of 4.6 mg/kg recorded in adults.

In the first 40-48 h the excretion of salicylate in the newborn occurs mainly as salicyluric acid (50-86%) and salicyl phenolic glucuronide (10-25%), while salicylic acid and salicyl acyl glucuronide are present only in traces. Interestingly, salicylic acid excretion may then represent 20% of the urinary salicylates in the following hours. The increment of salicylic acid with time may be partially explained by the rise in urinary pH which usually occurs within the 2nd and 3rd day of life and with the maturation of renal function, as reflected by the increase in creatinine and urea clearance (Chapter 5). The immaturity of the renal excretory mechanism is well-illustrated by the case previously mentioned in which, despite the fact that the kinetics of salicylate formation were similar to adult values, the total drug elimination rate was considerably slower than in adults. As suggested by Garrettson et al. (1975), this finding raises the interesting possibility that prolonged exposure to salicylate during fetal life may induce a more rapid maturation of some of the mechanisms responsible for salicylate elimination (in this case, the conjugation of salicylic acid with glycine). From the same data, however, it appears that other processes are still significantly immature, namely, the glucuronidation process and the renal excretory pathway.

It is interesting to keep in mind that, while an exposure to phenobarbital seems to increase the possibility of conjugation of salicylamide, the increment in the glucuronide derivative of salicylates is minimal (Yaffe et al., 1966). As far as the possible toxic effect of transplacentally acquired salicylate is concerned, one should remember that, in addition to the already mentioned interaction with bilirubin, another important effect is the marked suppression of platelet aggregation in the newborn (Corby and Schulman, 1971; Casteels-Van Daele et al., 1972). The platelets of newborn infants are much more susceptible to the effects of anti-aggregating agents, but whether these observations are significant in the pathogenesis of hemorrhagic events in the neonate still remains to be clarified.

Infants and Children

Despite the large number of reports on the toxic effects of salicylates in infants and children (Done, 1960; Craig et al., 1966; Lamont et al., 1968; Segar, 1969; Brem et al., 1973; Reimold et al., 1973; Pierce, 1974; Rich and Johnson,

1973; Hill, 1973; Buchanan and Rabinowitz, 1974), the data available on salicylate kinetics in these two age groups are surprisingly scanty and fragmentary. From the available data on urinary recovery, sodium salicylate and aspirin are readily, and almost completely, absorbed in both groups when given by the oral route, whereas rectal absorption when using suppositories is very slow and unreliable (Yaffe et al., 1966; Nowak et al., 1974; Levy and Yaffe, 1968). The *in vitro* observations of Windorfer et al. (1974) seem to indicate that infants between 1 and 10 months of age have protein-binding values similar to those of older children and adults, with a free fraction of about 35% for serum concentrations of 10–13 mg/100 ml. According to a report of Buchanan and Rabinowitz (1974), however, the *in vivo* protein-binding may be markedly variable in intoxicated infants in the age range of from 3 weeks to 13 months. The bound fraction under these circumstances may vary from 40 to 80%, apparently without having any direct relationship to the total serum salicylate concentration. On the contrary, a consistent relationship seems to exist between the salicylate serum/CSF ratio and the actual serum bicarbonate, suggesting that, as previously observed in the experimental animal, the greater the arterial acidosis, the more salicylate is present in the CSF. These data clearly indicate that salicylate plasma protein-binding does not depend solely upon serum concentrations, but that other factors, such as arterial blood pCO_2 and blood pH, do play a significant role in determining both the percentage bound and the salicylate diffusion into the tissues. In the ten cases reported by Buchanan and Rabinowitz, the CSF salicylate concentrations ranged from 23 to 110 of those in the serum, without any evident relationship to the free fraction. A CSF concentration of salicylate as high as 52% of that in the serum was also reported by Brem et al. (1973) in a 9-month-old boy with a serum level of 34 mg/100 ml. In infants, the apparent volume of distribution may range from 0.13 L/kg to 0.18 L/kg (Levy and Yaffe, 1974), while the apparent near-exponential serum half-lives are on the order of 3 to 6 h (Levy and Yaffe, 1968, 1974). The urinary excretion pattern is similar to that of older children and adults, with 50 to 68% of the dose excreted as salicyluric acid (Yaffe et al., 1966; Levy and Yaffe, 1968). A reduced binding to plasma proteins and a decreased formation of salicyluric acid in Down's syndrome has been reported by Ebady and Kugel, 1970).

In older children, 3 to 13 years of age, the pharmacokinetic profile of salicylate is practically identical to that observed in adults. The compound is eliminated at a near-exponential rate when the amount of salicylate in the body is about 50 to 120 mg, with an apparent half-life of 2–3 h (Levy and Yaffe, 1968). In children from 2 to 13 years of age, according to Levy and Yaffe (1974), a clear relationship exists between the apparent volume of distribution and the dose, with values of 0.16 to 0.34 L/kg for dosages of 50 to over 300 mg/kg. In the same report, the authors stress the point that the apparent volume of distribution is obviously a function of the initial conditions (i.e., highest concentrations attained), and they give a rational explanation of the well-known normogram of Done (1960), which is based on the close connection between salicylate concentration and the severity of salicylate intoxication.

The fact that the Vd on an established dose does not change in the individual patient as salicylate concentration drops could be explained by hypothesizing the release from the tissues as the limiting step. If this is true, it indicates both the necessity of avoiding fluctuations in the blood pH in the control of salicylate acidosis and the reason for preferring steady control through bicarbonate infusion, as suggested by Done (1974).

The toxic effects in children and infants do not differ from those already mentioned for adults and consist essentially of direct stimulation of the CNS respiratory center, increased metabolic rate with consequent hyperpyrexia, interference with carbohydrate metabolism and interference with normal blood coagulation mechanisms (Pierce, 1974; Done, 1960; Craig et al., 1966; Segar, 1969; Brem et al., 1973). The factor "time" is a very important consideration in the treatment of the intoxicated child. It must be remembered that the actual level of plasma or serum salicylate may be meaningless if not related to the time of ingestion. One should never forget that, not infrequently, infants and children die because of either delay in hospitalization or incorrect diagnosis (Craig et al., 1966).

PHENYLBUTAZONE

Adults

According to the early study of Burns et al. (1953), phenylbutazone in normal adults is rapidly and well absorbed from the gastrointestinal tract, with peak plasma levels of about 90 µg/ml achieved within 2 h after administration of an 800 mg dose. More recently, after administering a 200 mg dose of different brands of phenylbutazone tablets, Van Petten et al. (1971) observed a remarkable interindividual variability including maximal concentrations ranging from 12 to 50 µg/ml and a "physiological availability" of 60 to 100%. Consolo et al. (1970) also reported, both in volunteers and in patients, peak levels of 20–40 µg/ml attained 4–6 h after an oral dose of 400 mg. Similarly, peak levels of 70–80 µg/ml, reached 6–8 h after an oral dose of 600 mg, were recently reported by Ober (1974). After intramuscular administration, the absorption is delayed, probably because of local precipitation of the drug at the site of injection (Burns, 1953; Rechenberg, 1962). The area-under-the-curve (AUC) values, are, however, of the same magnitude as those obtained with the corresponding oral dose. On the contrary, rectal absorption appears to be more erratic and unpredictable (Rechenber, 1962); with the suppositories, consistent differences may also be observed among the various brands (Morselli, unpublished data). The intravenous route has been abandoned because of the disturbing and severe side effects which may occur.

Phenylbutazone is highly bound to plasma proteins, particularly to albumin (Burns et al., 1953; Brodie et al., 1954; Wunderls, 1956), with an affinity constant for albumin of 1.17×10^5 M^{-1} (Solomon et al., 1968). At therapeutic concentrations (50–120 µg/ml) phenylbutazone is bound to the extent of 98%, but at plasma concentrations over 200 µg/ml the binding capacity of normal human plasma becomes saturated, resulting in a marked increase of the free fraction. With regard to binding, phenylbutazone may interact with several drugs and also with endogenous compounds. For a more detailed and comprehensive description, the reader is referred to the recent publications and reviews (Solomon et al., 1968; Anton, 1973; Cohen and Armstrong, 1974; O'Reilly, 1973; Dayton et al., 1973; Morselli et al., 1974; APA, 1973; Cluff and Petrie, 1974).

Concentrations of the drug in the tissues and other body fluids are usually lower by several-fold than those in the plasma (Rechenberg, 1962); however, increased tissue concentrations may be observed in the presence of inflammation. Consequently, levels as high as 100 µg/ml have been shown to exist in the synovial fluid of arthritis by Hunziker (1956). The apparent volume of distribution of phenylbutazone ranges from 0.13 to 0.15 L/kg (O'Malley et al., 1971). Elevated concentrations have been found in the bile (Rechenberg, 1962), indicating that the possibility of an extensive enterohepatic cycle is very likely. Phenylbutazone crosses the placenta very slowly, and only minimal traces were found in the milk of lactating women (Rechenberg, 1962).

The decay of plasma concentrations may vary considerably in different individuals, and apparent plasma half-lives ranging from 30 to 140 h have been reported by several authors (Burns et al., 1953, 1960; Herrmann, 1959; Vasell and Page, 1968; Vasell et al., 1971; O'Malley et al., 1971; Davies and Thorgeirsson, 1971; Whittaker and Price Evans, 1970; Hvidberg et al., 1974). The chronic administration of phenylbutazone may lead to considerable reduction in the apparent plasma half-life values, probably through an autoinduction of liver microsomal enzymes. At metabolic levels, phenylbutazone may also interact with several drugs, both inhibiting or inducing their metabolism or being induced or inhibited. For a more detailed description, see recent specialized publications on this topic (Cohen and Armstrong, 1974; Morselli et al., 1974; Cluff and Petrie, 1974; APA, 1973).

In the body, phenylbutazone is converted to oxyphenylbutazone and to a second compound with an alcoholic OH group in the 3-position of the butyl side chain (Burns et al., 1955) (Fig. 2). Oxyphenylbutazone maintains the same antirheumatic and sodium-retaining properties as the parent drug (Yu et al., 1958). The pharmacokinetic profile is also very similar as far as absorption, binding to plasma protein (98%) and disposition rate (T½ = 40–100 h) are concerned (Jakob, 1968; Rechenberg and Herman, 1961; Sir, 1964; Barcelo and

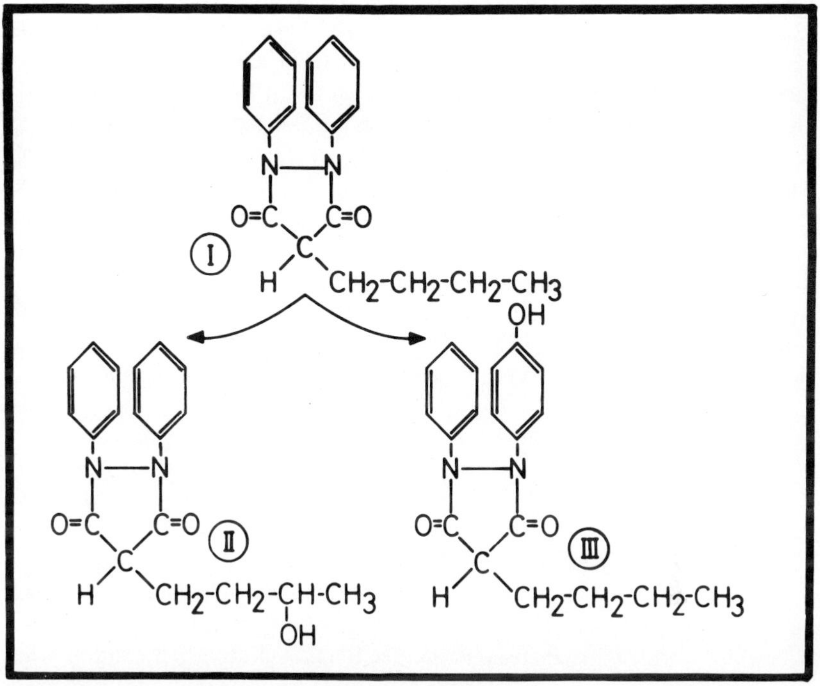

Fig. 2: Metabolism of phenylbutazone; (I) phenylbutazone; (II) 2-hydroxy butyl phenylbutazone; (III) oxyphenylbutazone.

Serra Peralba, 1964). The other derivative, on the contrary, has a marked uricosuric effect but is completely devoid of any antirheumatic and sodium-retaining activity (Yu et al., 1968). Its plasma disappearance rate is much shorter, with an apparent half-life of 10–12 h (Burns et al., 1960), and is 92–94% bound to plasma proteins (Dayton et al., 1973). The shorter half-life of the alcohol metabolite has been attributed by Dayton et al. (1973) to its higher acidity, resulting in a reduced passive resorption at the tubular level. Phenylbutazone and oxyphenylbutazone, being less acidic compounds, are reabsorbed to a higher extent.

After phenylbutazone administration, traces of the unchanged drug can be found in the urine, whereas oxyphenylbutazone is present in amounts ranging from 4 to 8% of the dose and the alcoholic metabolite from 14–18%. Other metabolites are presently unknown. In one study, about 60% of the administered radioactivity was recoverable in urine, and 15–18% in the feces, over 10 days' collection, after an oral dose of 200 mg of C^{14}phenylbutazone (Dayton et al.,

1973). Therapeutic levels are considered to be in the range of 50–120 μg/ml (Rechenberg, 1962; Currie, 1952; Bruch et al., 1954), and with levels over 120–150 μg/ml toxic effects are very likely to occur. Steady-state levels within the therapeutic range are usually attained in 3–6 days with 1–2 loading doses of 6–10 mg/kg followed by maintenance daily doses of 2–4 mg/kg. The usefulness of these agents is greatly limited by their potential activity. The most commonly reported side effects and adverse reactions include gastrointestinal disturbances (ranging from nausea, vomitus and epigastric discomforts to peptic ulcer and gastrointestinal bleeding), aphthous stomatitis and rashes, while the most serious side effects include bone marrow depression, hepatitis and anuria. Phenylbutazone should be used with great care in senile patients and in patients with liver, kidney and cardiovascular diseases. The possibility of interaction with coumarin-like anticoagulant and oral hypoglycemic agents must also be kept in mind.

Newborns, Infants and Children

In newborns, infants and children, the gastrointestinal absorption of phenylbutazone after oral administration may vary from 64 to 100% (mean: 84%) of the administered dose (Gladtke, 1968). Peak levels are reached within 2–8 h. By rectal route, as in adults the bioavailability is markedly reduced with a mean value of 54% of the dose. Oxyphenylbutazone plasma protein-binding is reduced in newborns, with a 40% increase in the free fraction (Kurz, 1968), and the same is probably true for phenylbutazone. The apparent volume of distribution is considerably greater in newborns, with values of 0.25–0.20 L/kg against values of 0.12–0.15 in older children and adults (Gladtke, 1968). Such a variation is in good agreement with the difference in extracellular water, which is considerably higher in newborns and young infants.

Apparent plasma half-lives after an i.v. administration of 10 mg/kg were found to range between 21 and 34 h in newborns (16–24 days of age), while in infants and younger children the average was around 17–18 h, with individual values ranging from 12 to 30 h (Table 1). In older children, the mean value was 21 h. Alvares et al. (1975), in a more recent study of 10 children from 1–8 years of age, reported an apparent plasma half-life of 40 ± 7 h, which is about 30% less than the corresponding value observed by the same authors in adults (75 h). Levels of oxyphenylbutazone ranging from 20 to 152 μg/ml were obtained by Sir (1964) in children with oral or rectal administration of 400–700 mg. Tissue concentrations (tonsils) were about 15–20% of those in serum. Steady-state plasma levels appeared to be dose-related. According to Gladtke, the therapeutic levels in children are in the same range as those observed in adults, and a single daily administration of 6–8 mg/kg was recommended on the basis of the kinetic findings. These drugs, however, should be used with great care in children below 14 years and restricted to those cases in which other antirheumatic compounds are either ineffective or poorly tolerated.

Table 1. Phenylbutazone
Pharmacokinetic Parameters During Development

Age Group	Plasma T½ (h)	Vd (L/kg)	Drug Clearance (1/h/kg)
Newborns (16-24 days)	26.5 ± 2.7	0.25 ± 0.02	7.03 ± 1.08
Infants (1-24 months)	17.9 ± 1.1	0.15 ± 0.08	6.53 ± 0.51
Children (2-7 years)	17.9 ± 1.1	0.12 ± 0.04	5.02 ± 0.33
Children	22.7 ± 2.15	0.13 ± 0.07	4.52 ± 0.31

Modified from Gladtke, 1968.

INDOMETHACIN

Adults

In adult volunteers and in patients undergoing chronic treatment, indomethacin, administered by oral route to subjects in a fasting state, is readily absorbed with peak plasma levels between 40 min and 3 h (Holt and Hawkins, 1965; Rothermich, 1966; Hucker et al., 1966; Hvidberg et al., 1972; Skeith et al., 1967; Champion et al., 1972; Rubin et al., 1973; Traeger et al., 1972, 1973; Palmer et al., 1974; Brooks et al., 1974). When it is administered in a postprandial state, the attainment of peak plasma concentrations of indomethacin may be delayed by 1 or 2 h (Champion et al., 1974; Rothermich, 1966). Peak levels are dose-dependent, and may range from 0.8 to 3 µg/ml for a dose of 25 mg, from 3 to 6 µg/ml for a dose of 50 mg and from 3 to 13 µg/ml for doses of 100 mg. Indomethacin is also absorbed satisfactorily by the rectal route, reaching a plasma peak 1-2 h after administration with levels that are about 75% of those obtained with an equivalent oral dose (Holt and Hawkins, 1965; Kerckhoffs and Huizinga, 1967; Rothermich, 1971). Concomitant oral administration of aspirin may induce a lower peak plasma level, but the area under the curve does not seem to be modified, and during chronic treatment this effect is minimal (Champion et al., 1972; Rubin et al., 1973). Very recently, Garnham et al. (1975) showed that the rate of indomethacin absorption may be significantly increased by pre-treatment with a concurrent administration of buffered aspirin. Indomethacin is about 90% bound to plasma proteins, mainly to albumin (Hucker et al., 1966; Skeith et al., 1967, Hvidberg et al., 1972), with an association constant for albumin of 0.86×10^3 M^{-1} (Hvidberg et al., 1972). Traces of the compound have been noted to be present in CSF (Hucker et al., 1966; Rothermich, 1971), and in the synovial fluid it has been found in concentrations about 20% of those in the plasma (Kunze et al., 1974).

The apparent Vd is 0.48-0.79 L/kg, according to the data of Duggan et al. (1972), while it is stated as 1.2-1.8 L/kg in the more recent data of Palmer et al. (1974). Several authors have assigned indomethacin an apparent plasma half-life of 1-3 h (Hucker et al., 1966; Champion, 1972; Traeger et al., 1972, 1973; Kunze, 1974). However, the urinary data of Skeith et al. (1967) indicate an apparent T½ of 10h, and Hvidberg (1972) mentions that the reported short half-life actually represents the initial alpha-phase of a biexponential decay. This finding has recently been confirmed by Palmer et al. (1974), who, using a more specific and sensitive method, demonstrated that in man the terminal β-phase of indomethacin plasma concentration has the apparent T½ of 7 h (4-11), while the T½ of the initial alpha-phase is 0.3-1.2 h. In the presence of probenecid (Skeith et al., 1967), or in cases of altered biliary flow (Traeger et al., 1972; Kunze et al., 1974), the disappearance rate of indomethacin may be considerably prolonged.

The compound undergoes catabolism, and Duggan et al. (1972) found the main metabolite to be the demethylated derivative (desmethyl indomethacin), which is further deacylated to desmethyldeschlorobenzoylindomethacin (DMBI). The formation of another product, deschlorobenzoyl indomethacin (DB), is a minor pathway. All the compounds are then further conjugated to glucuronide derivatives. There is evidence from several sources that indomethacin and its metabolites may undergo extensive enterohepatic recycling in humans (Hucker et al., 1966; Rothermich, 1971; Kunze et al., 1971) and that, in cases of reduced kidney function, the biliary excretion may represent the major pathway for the elimination of indomethacin derivatives (Traeger et al., 1972; Kunze et al., 1974).

About 40-60% of the administered dose of this compound is excreted in the urine within 24-48 h as indomethacin (50%), desmethyl indomethacin (25%) and deschlorobenzoyl indomethacin (15%); approximately 15-30% of the dose may be recovered in the feces as both conjugated indomethacin and desmethyl-deschlorobenzoyl indomethacin (Hucker et al., 1966; Duggan et al., 1972). Indomethacin is excreted through glomerular filtration and tubular secretion (Skeith et al., 1967; Traeger et al., 1973) with a renal clearance that in normal condition oscillates from 115 to 226 ml/min (Skeith et al., 1967). Probenecid and other organic acids can significantly reduce the urinary excretion of indomethacin (Skeith et al., 1967, Traeger et al., 1973; Brooks et al., 1974) to about one-half and lead to a doubling of plasma levels with concomitant increased clinical effect (Brooks et al., 1974).

According to Holt and Hawkins (1965), the symptomatic relief obtained using indomethacin in patients suffering from rheumatoid arthritis follows the plasma-level pattern. Clear relationships between plasma levels and CNS side

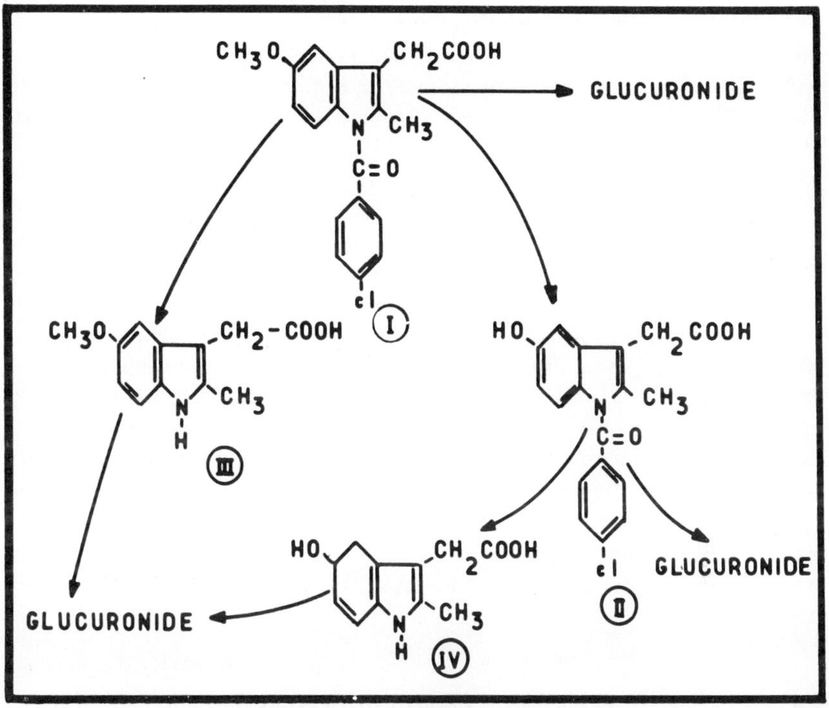

Fig. 3: Metabolism of indomethacin; (I) indomethacin; (II) desmethyl indomethacin; (III) deschlorobenzoyl indomethacin; (IV) desmethyl deschloro benzoyl indomethacin.

effects such as headache, disturbed equilibrium, feelings of unreality, dizziness and vertigo have been reported by Rothermich (1966) and by Caruso (1971). These authors stated that worsening of side effects was evident for plasma levels over 10 μg/ml. Kunze et al. (1974), on the other hand, could not confirm a similar relationship. Other commonly reported side effects which are not related to plasma levels include nausea, epigastric buring, diarrhea, skin rashes and ulcers. Two cases of glomerulonephritis, apparently correlated to indomethacin use, have also been recently described (Marsh et al., 1971).

Newborns, Infants and Children

Very limited data are available on indomethacin disposition in the pediatric patient; however, scanty as the information is, it suggests that considerable differences may be present in newborns and children. Traeger et al. (1973) recently observed that indomethacin crosses the placenta relatively quickly so that an equilibrium between maternal and umbilical cord plasma is achieved within 4-5 h. At peak time in the mother, concentrations in the cord plasma are about 50% of the maternal levels. Newborns who receive the drug transplacentally dispose of it at a very low rate, with an apparent plasma half-life of 15 h or more. This reduced disposition rate appears to be due mainly to the immaturity of kidney function. On the contrary, in children of 7-11 years of age, the renal excretion of indomethacin and its metabolites appears to be significantly faster than in adults, with about 40% of the dose excreted within 12 h (Kunze et al., 1974). Infants and children appear to be more susceptible to indomethacin side effects (Calabro and Marchesano, 1968; Chapman, 1966; Medical Letters, 1968). Toxic hepatitis, without evidence of infection, accompanied by ulcerative lesions of the g.i. tract has been described in a 12-year-old boy by Kelsey and Sharyi (1967). In addition, indomethacin may interfere with resistance to infections or active latent infections. Taking the existing clinical and pharmacological evidence under consideration, the *AMA Drug Evaluations* 1973 at present suggests that the use of indomethacin is contraindicated in pregnant women, nursing mothers, and infants and children under 14 years of age. Conditions under which it might be safely be used in these patients have not as yet been established.

PYRAZOLONE DERIVATIVES

Pyrazolone derivatives, introduced as analgesics and antipyretics in 1897, at present are seldom used in the United States because of their recognized ability to induce agranulocytosis and other blood dyscrasias. Among aminopyrine, dypirone and antipyrine, there is little difference in the pharmacologic and toxic effect. Despite their very limited use in the USA, Canada, Great Britain and Scandinavia, in countries of South America, Africa, Asia and southern Europe pyrazolone derivatives are still widely employed for analgesic and antipyretic therapy, given either alone or in fixed combination with phenacetin, acetaminophen, salicylates, etc. Since there are really no special advantages offered by these drugs to warrant the serious risk of possible fatal reactions, their use, especially in children, should be banned.

The kinetic data available on these compounds are mainly derived from studies in which aminopyrine or antipyrine were used, in volunteers or in patients, principally as a "tool" or "marker" to evaluate drug metabolism in several different conditions. It is, however, rather surprising to note that, even at present, there are investigations carried out with antipyrine or aminopyrine because "they may be taken as an index of drug metabolizing enzyme activity, for the complete absorption, the negligible binding to plasma protein and the

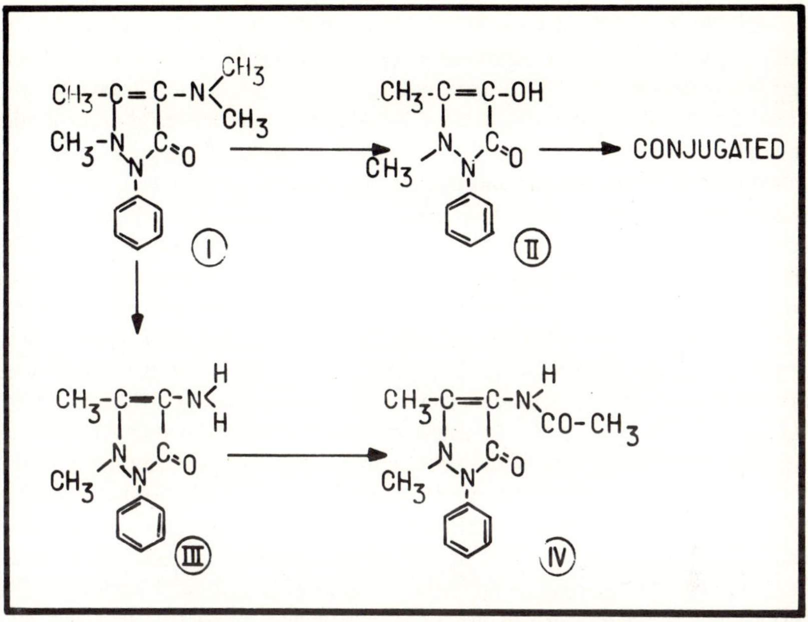

Fig. 4: Metabolism of aminopyrine; (I) aminopyrine; (II) 4-hydroxy antipyrine; (III) 4-amino antipyrine; (IV) N-acetyl-4-amino antipyrine.

virtual complete excretion in 48-72 hours of metabolites products." The utilization of these drugs as investigatory agents persists despite the fact that numerous reports clearly indicate that single-administration studies are not indicative or predictive for chronic treatment with several drugs and even though recent reports on antipyrine indicate that the drug is of no value at all in obtaining information on other drugs' metabolism (Smith and Rawlins, 1974; May et al., 1974; Davis et al., 1974).

Aminopyrine is promptly absorbed by the gastrointestinal tract, and peak plasma levels are attained within 2 h; it is about 15-20% bound to plasma proteins and distributes uniformly throughout the total body water (Brodie and Axelrod, 1950; Chen et al., 1962; Jori et al., 1972). The compound is rapidly metabolized through demethylation to 4-amino-antipyrine, which is further acetylated (Fig. 4) to N-acetyl-4-amino-antipyrine. A minor fraction may be converted to 4-hydroxyantipyrine (Brodie and Axelrod, 1950). About 50% of the dose is excreted in the 24 h urine and 75-80% within 72 h (Brodie and Axelrod, 1950). Unchanged aminopyrine accounts for 2-4% of the dose; 10% is present as 4-amino-antipyrine and about 65% as N-acetyl-4-amino-antipyrine. Pre-treatment with phenylbutazone may stimulate aminopyrine metabolism and lead to increased formation of 4-aminopyrine (Chen et al., 1962). In a one-day-old infant Reinicke et al. (1970) were able to observe a plasma decay value of aminopyrine concentrations corresponding to an apparent plasma half-life of about 40 h. This value was reduced to 13 h after 8 days of life. Certainly, the data are indicative of reduced aminopyrine catabolism in the neonate.

Antipyrine is also rapidly and completely absorbed in volunteers, with peak plasma levels reached in 1-2 h (Brodie and Axelrod, 1950b). In patients, however, the peak may be delayed to as much as 6 h (Huffman et al., 1974). The binding to plasma proteins is minimal, and the compound distributes to various organs in proportion to their water content, for these reasons, antipyrine has been used for the measurement of total body water (Soberman et al., 1949; Brodie and Axelrod, 1950b). Its reported apparent volume of distribution varies from 0.36 to 0.75 L/kg (Lindgren et al., 1974; Elfstrom and Lindgren, 1974; Flanagan and Richens, 1974; Adreasen and Vesell, 1975). The antipyrine rate of disappearance from plasma is slower than that of aminopyrine, and the reported plasma half-lives in adults vary from 6 to 30 h, with a mean value of about 10-12 h (Brodie and Axelrod, 1950b; Vesell and Page, 1968b; Breckenridge and Orme, 1971; Vesell et al., 1971; Davies and Thorgeirsson, 1971; O'Malley et al., 1971; Prescott et al., 1973; Breckenridge et al., 1973; Smith and Rawlins, 1974; Petruch et al., 1974; Davis et al., 1974; Huffman et al., 1974; Flanagan and Richens, 1974; Andreasen et al., 1974). In the elderly, the T½ may be significantly higher, with a mean value of 17 h (O'Malley et al., 1971).

The rate of antipyrine plasma disappearance was found to be increased by concomitant or previous administration of several other drugs, including phenobarbital (Vesell et al., 1971), glutethimide, amobarbital, methaqualone and phenhydramine (Ballinger et al., 1972), and diphenylhydantoin (Petruch et al., 1974); the same effect occurred after exposure to chlorinated hydrocarbon (Kolmodin-Hedman et al., 1969) and with chronic antipyrine administration (Davis et al., 1974). The compound is, in fact, a potent metabolic inducer (Breckenridge and Orme, 1971). Instead, reduction of the antipyrine disappearance rate was observed with administration of phenylbutazone (Davies and Thorgheirsson, 1971), oral contraceptive steroids (O'Malley et al., 1972), nortriptyline and allopurinol (Vesell et al., 1971), disulfuram (Vesell et al., 1971b) and tetrahydrocannabinol (Vesell and Passananti, 1973).

Reduced metabolism in the course of obstructive jaundice has been reported by Branch et al. (1973), but Elfstrom and Lindgren (1974) failed to confirm this finding. No significant differences between normal subjects and cirrhotic patients were observed by Andreasen and Vesell (1975), at variance with a previous report of Andreasen et al. (1974) in which a marked reduction of antipyrine clearance was described in patients with liver disease. A variation in apparent half-life in the presence of hyper- and hypothyroid conditions has been recently reported by Eichelbaum et al. (1974) for antipyrine, and by Brunck et

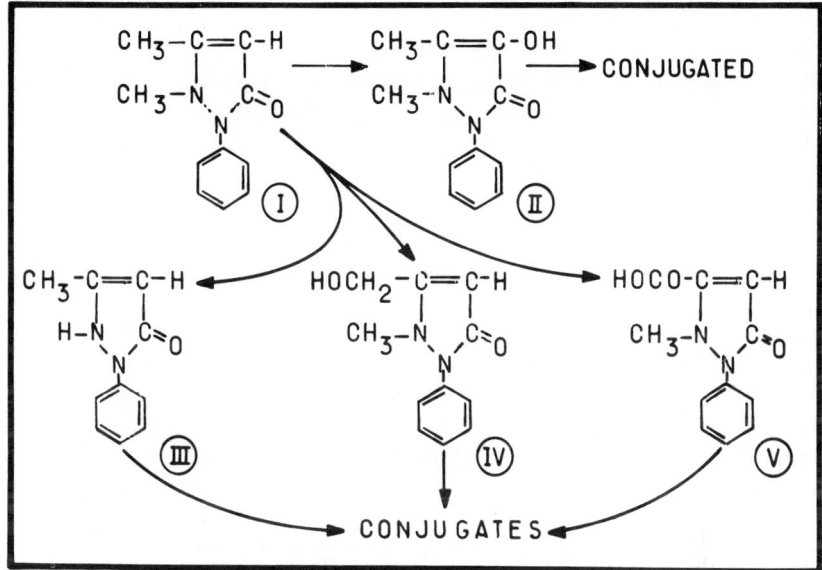

Fig. 5: Metabolism of antipyrine; (I) antipyrine; (II) 4-hydroxy antipyrine; (III) N-desmethyl antipyrine; (IV) 3-hydroxy methyl antipyrine; (V) 3-carboxy antipyrine.

al. (1974) for dipyrone. Although both papers suggest modification of metabolic rates, the bearing of variation in distribution volume, which were considerable, has been apparently underestimated and values of total body clearances were not reported. Antipyrine is about 70-80% hydroxylated to form 4-hydroxy-antipyrine, which is further conjugated with glucuronic acid (Brodie and Axelrod, 1950b). Other identified metabolites include 3-hydroxymethyl-antipyrine, 3-carbosy-antipyrine and N-desmethyl-antipyrine (Yoshimura et al., 1968; Baty and Evans, 1973; Lindgren et al., 1974) (Fig. 5).

Within 50 h, about 80% of the dose may be recovered in urine as 4OH-antipyrine, while unchanged antipyrine accounts for about 5% and minor metabolites for less than 10% of the dose (Huffman et al., 1974). In a recent study, Alvares et al. (1975) observed that, in children from 1-8 years of age, the apparent plasma half-life of antipyrine had a mean value of 6.6 ± 0.4 h, suggesting that children of that age metabolize the drug at almost twice the rate of adults. These authors suggest that the increased plasma disappearance is mainly the result of an increased metabolism which, in turn, is due to the greater liver-to-body weight ratio in children than in adults. However, difference in total body water might contribute to the observed differences.

In conclusion, the data available on the kinetics of pyrazolone derivatives,

292 DRUG DISPOSITION DURING DEVELOPMENT

although very detailed and complete, do not add any new information to the general knowledge on drug disposition in various age groups or in pathological conditions; furthermore, the data do not even help in defining situations where these compounds themselves might be used more appropriately and safely. The same effort spent on those drugs which are equally therapeutic, without danger of toxicity under normal conditions, might lead to useful advances in analgesic and/or antipyretic treatment.

ACETANILID, PHENACETIN AND ACETAMINOPHEN

Adults

In man, acetanilid and phenacetin are almost completely converted to acetaminophen very shortly after their absorption (Greenberg and Lester, 1946; Brodie and Axelrod, 1948b, 1949; Prescott et al., 1970), and for this reason the three drugs will be discussed together. *Acetanilid* and *phenacetin* administered orally, at doses ranging from 10 to 30 mg/kg, are rapidly absorbed with peak plasma levels attained within 1-2 h (Greenberg and Lester, 1946; Lester and Greenberg, 1947; Brodie and Axelrod, 1948b; Prescott et al., 1968, 1970; Prescott, 1969; Thomas et al., 1972; Cunningham et al., 1974). Several factors, such as rate of gastric emptying, size of particles, pharmaceutical formulations and concomitant administration of other drugs may induce significant variations in the gastrointestinal absorption rate. The relative bioavailability of phenacetin may range from 50 to 75%, with peak plasma levels varying from 0.5 to 25 μg/ml, after a single oral administration (Prescott et al., 1970; Prescott and Nimmo, 1971; Thomas et al., 1972; Chiou, 1974). When given rectally, phenacetin is very poorly absorbed (Hauser and Pfleger, 1965).

At variance with acetanilid, which is virtually completely converted into acetaminophen, *phenacetin* may give rise to other minor metabolites, and these have been considered, in several instances, as responsible for the toxic effects of the drug (Fig. 6). The "minor metabolites" include p-phenetidine, 2-hydroxyphenetidine, 2-hydroxyphenacetine and a hypothetical N-hydroxyphenacetin (Brodie and Axelrod, 1949; Buch et al., 1966, 1967; Klutch et al., 1966; Prescott et al., 1968; Dubach and Raaflaub, 1969; Prescott, 1969). According to Thomas et al. (1972), the formation of 2-hydroxyphenetidine may be increased from 1.9 to 3.4% of the dose by concomitant administration of aspirin, caffeine and codeine. In addition, the formation of 2-hydroxyphenetidine may be markedly enhanced at high doses of phenacetin (Raaflaub and Dubach, 1969).

Both acetanilid and phenacetin plasma levels decay very quickly, with an apparent half-life of about 60-70 and 35-104 min, respectively (Lester and Greenberg, 1947; Prescott et al., 1968; Prescott, 1969, 1974). Following administration of the usual doses of either acetanilid or phenacetin, under

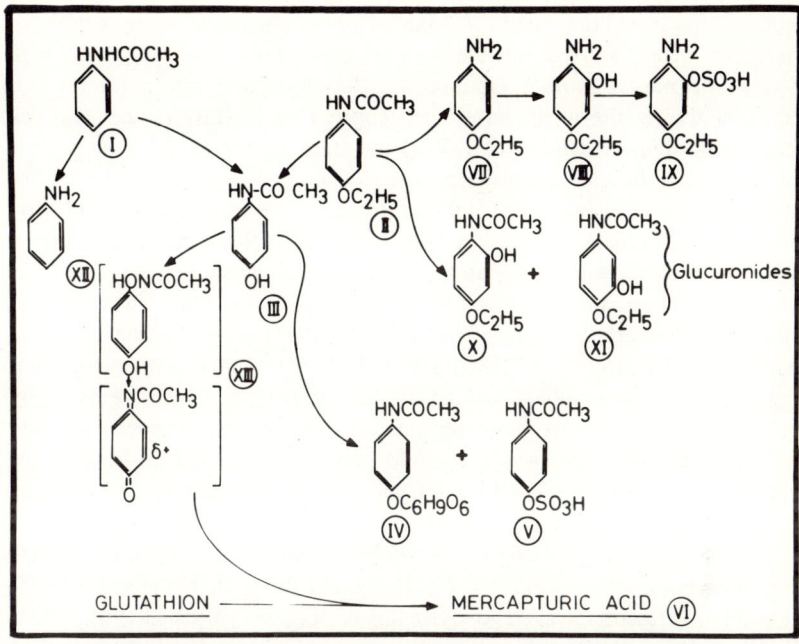

Fig. 6: Metabolism of phenacetin and acetaminophen; (I) acetanilide;
(II) phenacetin; (III) acetaminophen; (IV) acetaminophen glucuronide;
(V) acetaminophen sulfate; (VI) mercapturic acid; (VII) p-phenetidin;
(VIII) 2-hydroxyphenetidin; (IX) 2-hydroxy phenetidin sulfate
(X) 2-hydroxyphenacetin; (XI) 3-hydroxyphenacetin; (XII) aniline;
(XIII) postulated toxic intermediates.

normal conditions, peak plasma levels of acetaminophen (N-acetyl-p-aminophenol) are attained within 2-4 h, with plasma concentrations ranging from 5 to 25 µg/ml. When administered as such, acetaminophen reaches maximal plasma concentrations at 30-120 min, with levels which may vary from 5 to 37 µg/ml for doses of 500-1,800 mg (Brodie and Axelrod, 1948a; Gwilt et al., 1963; Cummings et al., 1967; Prescott et al., 1968, 1969; Albert et al., 1974; Hedges et al., 1974; Heading et al., 1973). The absorption rate and the relative bioavailability of *acetaminophen* can be significantly modified by the concomitant administration of propantheline or methoclopramide (Nimmo et al., 1973; Prescott, 1974). Ingestion of activated charcoal within 1 h of the acetaminophen intake may reduce the bioavailability by 65-70% (Levy et al., 1972). A significant relationship between gastric emptying half-time and both the maximum plasma acetaminophen concentrations and the time taken to reach the peak has been reported by Heading et al. (1973). Jaffe et al. (1971) reported no effect of food on the total amount of drug absorbed, while significant differences were observed on the rate of absorption, especially with high carbohydrate meals. Diurnal variations in the absorption rate, with reduced absorption during the night, have been reported by McGilveray and Mattock (1972). According to Farid et al. (1972) and Gazzard et al. (1973), acetaminophen is 25-50% bound to plasma proteins. From animal data, we can assume that the compound is evenly distributed throughout the various tissues and body fluids without evident localization (Davison et al., 1961). Acetaminophen is disposed of rapidly, with an apparent plasma half-life which may vary from 75 to 180 min (Nelson and Morioka, 1963; Cummings et al., 1967; Prescott et al., 1968, 1970; Prescott, 1969; Levy and Regardh, 1971; Levy and Yamada, 1971; McGilveray and Mattock, 1971; Pantuck et al., 1972). In man, acetaminophen is mainly converted into sulfate and glucuronide derivatives which are promptly excreted in proportions of about 25 and 70% of the dose, respectively; only 1-4% is found as unchanged acetaminophen in urine, and 3-4% may be excreted as the mercapturic acid conjugate (Nelson and Marioka, 1963; Cummings et al., 1967; Prescott et al., 1968; Levy and Regardh, 1971; Heading et al., 1973; Albert et al., 1974; Hedges et al., 1974; Mitchell et al., 1974). About 50% of the dose is excreted in the first 6 h (Levy and Regardh, 1971) and 80-90% within 24 h (Prescott et al., 1968; Heading et al., 1973; Mitchell et al., 1974) (Fig. 6).

The rate of formation of acetaminophen sulfate may be reduced by concomitant administration of salicylamide, and the effect may be counteracted by cysteine, which seems to increase the excretion of the sulfate conjugate (Levy and Yamada, 1971). On the other hand, salicylic acid has no effect on the formation of the acetaminophen conjugates (Levy and Regardh, 1971). Axelrod et al. (1957) reported decreased acetaminophen glucuronide formation during unconjugated hyperbilirubinemia, but the finding could not be confirmed later by Arias et al. (1969). At therapeutic doses, adverse reactions to phenacetin and acetaminophen are rare. Prescott et al. (1970) observed that for the usual doses of phenacetin common side effects are minimal and are mainly represented by CNS disturbances (dizziness, sense of unreality, impaired ability to concentrate) which last 60-90 min. These effects seemed to be related to the absorption peak of phenacetin and were present when plasma concentrations were over 8-10 μg/ml. The more severe side effects, such as hemolytic anemia in individuals with deficiency of glucose-6-phosphate dehydrogenase or methemoglobinemia in heavy, chronic users of phenacetin, do not appear to be related to plasma levels of phenacetin or acetaminophen, but are probably due to the formation of toxic metabolites (Prescott et al., 1968; Gault et al., 1974; Mitchell et al., 1974).

In cases of severe poisoning, either by voluntary overdosage or by the continued, heavy consumption of high doses of phenacetin and/or acetaminophen, reported side effects include the following: nausea, vomiting, myocardial damage, bleeding diatheses, gastric erosion, duodenal ulcer, hypoalbuminemia, acute elevation of biochemical indices of liver damage, jaundice and transient hypoglycemia. The clinical picture may evolve toward coma and death. Necroscopy findings have consistently shown massive centrilobular necrosis, renal distal tubular necrosis and cerebral edema (McLean et al., 1968; Prescott et al., 1971; Clark et al., 1973; Farid et al., 1972; Mitchell et al., 1974). Acetaminophen plasma levels as high as 500 µg/ml have been reported within a few hours after massive ingestion (15-30 g), and, according to Prescott et al. (1971), plasma levels over 120 µg/ml at 12 h after drug intake are very often connected with severe liver and kidney lesions. According to the same authors, however, the best guide to the degree of hepatic injury is the plasma half-life of acetaminophen, which, in these cases, may be considerably prolonged (7-16 h). Hepatic necrosis is very likely to occur if plasma T½ is more than 4 h, and hepatic coma will occur if plasma T½ is more than 12 h (Prescott et al., 1971). The prolonged apparent plasma half-life of acetaminophen is probably due to impaired conjugation as a result of the hepatic lesion. Mitchell et al. (1974) maintain that the threshold dose for severe toxic effect is around 10-15 g. The same authors were able to identify a mercapturic acid of acetaminophen in human urine. This might indicate that acetaminophen is converted to an electrophilic reactant which may deplete hepatic glutathion and, by extensive arylation of hepatic macromolecules, induce cell death. On this basis, according to Mitchell et al. (1974), the administration of cysteamine, a glutation-like nucleophile, may be indicated as specific treatment for acetaminophen intoxication if given not later than 6-8 h after drug intake. Mepyramine, promethazine and hydrocortisone generally fail to protect the patient, but forced diuresis and hemodialysis may have a positive effect if started within a few hours after the overdosage. The use of charcoal hemoperfusion does not seem to be of any benefit to these patients (Gazzard et al., 1974).

Newborns, Infants and Children

Acetaminophen in the last 4-6 years has received increased use as an analgesic and antipyretic both in Europe and the United States, especially in pediatric practice, where its use has been facilitated by the fact that it can be formulated into a stable suspension easy to administer to children. When taken in ordinary doses, the compound is virtually free of adverse side effects in children (Tarlin et al., 1972; Goulding, 1973). In children who have ingested up to 7 g of acetaminophen, only minimal ill effects, apart from drowsiness, have been reported (Goulding, 1973). On the contrary, phenacetin should be avoided in children because of the possibility of methemoglobinemia and hemolytic anemia. Considering its widespread use, the kinetic data on acetaminophen during development are not very numerous; however, they do indicate that, with the exception of the newborn, no differences would seem to exist in the disposition of the drug in infants, children and adults (Vest and Streiff, 1959; Vest and Rossier, 1963; Levy et al., 1975).

In newborns, following administration of acetanilid, the rate of hydroxylation of acetanilid to acetaminophen and the subsequent conjugation with glucuronic acid are significantly slower than in older children and adults (Vest, 1958; Vest and Streiff, 1959). In newborns of 1 to 10 days of age, after acetanilid administration acetaminophen and its glucoronyl conjugate were found to reach peak plasma concentration at 3-6 h and 12-20 h, respectively. The metabolic processes may be even slower in premature newborns (Vest and Streiff, 1959). The 24 h urinary excretion of acetaminophen (free and conjugate) accounts for only 15-25% of the dose, while in older children it is in the range of 75-80%. The percentage of conjugated acetaminophen excreted in urine increases steadily within the first 6 weeks after birth, with values near to the adult levels after 3 months (Vest, 1958; Careddu et al., 1961; Mereu et al., 1962; Vest and Rossier, 1963). In a more recent study, Levy et al. (1975), administering 12 mg/kg of acetaminophen to 2- to 3-day-old full-term infants confirmed the previous data of Vest by showing that the rate constant for the formation of acetaminophen glucuronide is smaller in newborns than in older children and adults. The impaired glucuronidation was not without an effect on the apparent plasma half-life, which was found to range from 2.2 to 5 h with a mean value of 3.5 ± 0.8 h. Longer half-life values, 8-22 h, in the newborns were reported by Windorfer (1972). This limited ability to conjugate acetaminophen with glucuronic acid appears, however, to be partially compensated for by a well-developed capability for sulfate conjugation. Acetaminophen sulfate was, in fact, found to have a formation rate constant higher than that in adults.

In the study of Levy et al. (1975), the total recovery from 48 h urine collections was of the order of 52-79%, about 20% less than the corresponding values in children and adults. The urinary excretion rate for unmetabolized acetaminophen was about one-half the magnitude of the adult value, which is in agreement with the known reduced kidney function in the neonate (see Chapter 5). No relationship could be observed between the rate constants for acetaminophen glucuronide or acetaminophen sulfate formation and bilirubin concentrations of D glucaric acid urinary excretion. The same authors, on the basis of urinary data, conclude that acetaminophen absorption is considerably slower in the neonate. This may be partially due to the prolonged gastric emptying in the first days of life (Weber and Cohen, 1975).

In infants with congenital nonobstructive, nonhemolytic jaundice, unconjugated hyperbilirubinemia does not seem to have any effect on the formation of acetaminophen glucuronides (Gorodischer et al., 1970; Levy and Ertel, 1971), while in the same situation the formation of salicylic and salicylamide glucuronide may be deficient.

CONCLUSIONS

As shown above, important differences, clearly linked to the developmental stage, are evident in the disposition rate of most of the compounds considered. Such differences are not without effect on the therapeutic outcome, especially in view of the high potential toxicity of this class of drugs. As for other drugs, monitoring of plasma levels in the course of chronic treatment of pediatric patients should help greatly to diminish the risk of toxic reactions. Several data on the disposition of new inflammatory agents have appeared in the last two years (Rubin et al., 1972a,b; Kaiser and Vangiessen, 1974; Hellenberg et al., 1974; Proctor et al., 1974; Runkel et al., 1974; Selley et al., 1975; Segre, 1975). The data are, however, still very preliminary, and no information at all is available for pediatric patients. Considering the high potential toxicity of most of the older drugs, information on the disposition of these compounds in children, and on the possible relationship between plasma levels and therapeutic effects, is urgently needed.

REFERENCES

Acute salicylate poisoning (1972): *British Medical Journal, 1:* 263-264.
Albert, K.S., Sedman, A.J. and Wagner, J.G. (1974a): Pharmacokinetics of orally administered acetaminophen in man. *Journal of Pharmacokinetics and Biopharmaceutics, 2:* 381-393.
Albert, K.S., Sedman, A.J., Wilkinson, P., Stoll, R.G., Murray, W.J. and Wagner, J.G. (1974b): Bioavailability studies of acetaminophen and nitrofurantoin. *Journal of Clinical Pharmacology, 14:* 264-270.
Ali, M.A. and Routh, J.I. (1969): The protein binding of acetylsalicylic acid and salicylic acid. *Clinical Chemistry, 15:* 1027-1038.
Alvares, A.P., Kapelner, S., Sassa, S. and Kappas, A. (1975): Drug metabolism in normal children, lead-poisoned children, and normal adults. *Clinical Pharmacology and Therapeutics, 17:* 179-183.
American Medical Association (1973): *AMA Drug Evaluations,* 2nd ed., Chapter 22, American Medical Association, Chicago.
American Medical Association (1973): *AMA Drug Evaluations,* 2nd ed., Chapter 26, American Medical Association, Chicago.
American Pharmaceutical Association (1973): *Evaluations of Drug Interactions,* 1st ed., American Pharmaceutical Association, Washington.
Andreasen, P.B., Ranek, L., Statland, B.E. and Tygstrup, N. (1974): Clearance of anti-pyrine-dependence of quantitative liver function. *European Journal of Clinical Investigation, 4:* 129-134.
Andreasen, P.B. and Vesell, E.S. (1975): Comparison of plasma levels of antipyrine, tolbutamide, and warfarin after oral and intravenous administration. *Clinical Pharmacology and Therapeutics, 16:* 1059-1065.
Anton, A.H. (1973): Increasing activity of sulfonamides with displacing agents: a review.

Annals of the New York Academy of Sciences, 226: 273-292.
Arias, I.M., Gartner, L.M., Cohen, M., Benezzer, J. and Levi, A.J. (1969): Chronic non-hemolytic unconjugated hyperbilirubinemia with glucuronyl transferase deficiency. *American Journal of Medicine, 47:* 395-409.
Axelrod, J., Schmid, R. and Hammaker, L. (1957): A biochemical lesion in congenital, non-obstructive, non-haemolytic jaundice. *Nature, 180:* 1426-1427.
Baldoni, A. (1915): Sull'eliminazione dell'acido salicilurico e dell'acido salicilico in seguito a somministrazione di acido salicilico, salicilato di sodio e diplasal. *Archivio di Farmacologia Sperimentale, 18:* 151-158.
Ballinger, B., Browning, M., O'Malley, K. and Stevenson, I.H. (1972): Drug-metabolizing capacity in states of drug dependence and withdrawal. *British Journal of Pharmacology, 45:* 638-643.
Barcelo', P. and Serra Peralba, A. (1964): Experimentacion clinica con la oxifenilbutazona (Tanderil) administrada por via rectal. *Anales de Medicina, 50:* 382-392.
Baty, J.D. and Evans, D.A.P. (1973): Norphenazone, a new metabolite of phenazone in human urine. *Journal of Pharmacy and Pharmacology, 25:* 83-84.
Bedford, C., Cummings, A.J. and Martin, B.K. (1965): A kinetic study of the elimination of salicylate in man. *British Journal of Pharmacology, 24:* 418-431.
Behrman, R.E. and Battaglia, F.C. (1967): Protein binding of human fetal and maternal plasmas to salicylate. *Journal of Applied Physiology, 22:* 125-130.
Bernstein, S.H. and Allerhand, J. (1964): Abnormalities of serum proteins as criteria for the diagnosis of acute rheumatic fever. *American Journal of Medical Sciences, 247:* 431-437.
Bleyer, W.A., Au, W.Y.W., Lange, W.A., Sr. and Raisz, L.G. (1970): Studies on the detection of adverse drug reactions in the newborn. I. Fetal exposure to maternal medication. *Journal of the American Medical Association, 213:* 2046-2048.
Bleyer, W.A. and Breckenridge, R.T. (1970): Studies on the detection of adverse drug reactions in the newborn. II. The effects of prenatal aspirin on newborn hemostasis. *Journal of the American Medical Association, 213:* 2049-2053.
Bluesteon, R., Kippen, I. and Klinengurg, J.R. (1969): Effect of drugs on mote binding to plasma proteins. *British Medical Journal, 4:* 590-593.
Boda, D., Pinter, S., Kovacs, L., Szepesy, G., Szollosi, J. and Maraz, A. (1971): Appearance of salicylate in the circulation of the newborn after administering the drug to the mother in the first minute of the placental stage. *Annals of Clinical Research, 3:* 150-152.
Branch, R.A., Herbert, C.M. and Read, A.E. (1973): Determinants of serum antipyrine half-life in patients with liver disease. *Gut, 14:* 569-573.
Breckenridge, A., Burke, C.W., Davies, D.S. and Orme, M. (1973): Immediate decrease by hydrocortisone of the plasma half-life of antipyrine. *British Journal of Pharmacology, 47:* 434-436.
Breckenridge, A. and Orme, M. (1971): Clinical implications of enzyme induction. *Annals of the New York Academy of Sciences, 179:* 421-431.
Brem, J., Pereli, E.M., Gopalan, S.K. and Miller, T.B. (1973): Salicylism, hyperventilation, and the central nervous system. *Journal of Pediatrics, 83:* 264-266.
Brodie, B.B. and Axelrod, J. (1948a): The estimation of acetanilide and its metabolic products, aniline, N-acetyl p-aminophenol, and p-amino-phenol (free and total conjugated) in biological fluids and tissues. *Journal of Pharmacology and Experimental Therapeutics, 94:* 22-28.
Brodie, B.B. and Axelrod, J. (1948b): The fate of acetanilide in man. *Journal of Pharmacology and Experimental Therapeutics, 94:* 29-38.
Brodie, B.B. and Axelrod, J. (1949): The fate of acetophenetidin (phenacetin) in man and methods for the estimation of acetophenetidin and its metabolites in biological material. *Journal of Pharmacology and Experimental Therapeutics, 97:* 58-67.

Brodie, B.B. and Axelrod, J. (1950a): The fate of aminopyrine (Pyramidon) in man and methods for the estimation of aminopyrine and its metabolites in biological material. *Journal of Pharmacology and Experimental Therapeutics, 99:* 171-184.

Brodie, B.B. and Axelrod, J. (1950b): The fate of antipyrine in man. *Journal of Pharmacology and Experimental Therapeutics, 98:* 97-104.

Brodie, B.B., Lowman, E., Burns, J.J., Lee, P.R., Chemkin, T., Goldman, A., Weiner, M. and Steele, J.M. (1954): Observations on the antirheumatic and physiologic effects of phenylbutazone (Butazolidin) and some comparisons with cortisone. *American Journal of Medicine, 16:* 181-190.

Brooks, P.M., Bell, M.A., Sturrock, R.D., Famaey, J.P. and Dick, W.C. (1974): The clinical significance of indomethacin-probenecid interaction. *British Journal of Clinical Pharmacology, 1:* 287-290.

Brown, S.S., Cameron, J.C. and Matthew, H. (1967): Plasma salicylate levels in acute poisoning in adults. *British Medical Journal, 2:* 738-739.

Bruck, E., Fearnley, M.E., Meanock, I. and Patley, H. (1954): Phenylbutazone therapy. Relation between the toxic and therapeutic effects and the blood level. *Lancet, I:* 225-227.

Brunck, S.F., Combs, S.P., Miller, J.D., Delle, M. and Wilson, W.R. (1974): Effects of hypothyroidism and hyperthyroidism on dipyrone metabolism in man. *Journal of Clinical Pharmacology, 14:* 271-279.

Buch, H., Gerhards, W., Karachristianidis, G., Pfleger, K. and Rummel, W. (1967): Hemmung der durch phenacetin und p-phenetidin verursachten Mathamoglobin-bildung durch Barbiturate. *Biochemical Pharmacology, 16:* 1575-1583.

Buch, H., Hauser, H., Pfleger, K. and Rudiger, W. (1966): Uber die Ausscheidung eines noch nicht beschriebenen phenacetinmetaboliten beim Menschen und bei der Ratte. *Archiv fur Experimentelle Pathologie und Pharmakologie, 253:* 25.

Buchanan, N. and Rabinowitz, L. (1974): Infantile salicylism. A reappraisal. *Journal of Pediatrics, 84:* 391-395.

Burns, J.J., Rose, R.K., Chenkin, T., Goldman, A., Schulert, A. and Brodie, B.B. (1953): Physiological disposition of butazolidine in man and method for its estimation in biological material. *Journal of Pharmacology and Experimental Therapeutics, 109:* 346-357.

Burns, J.J., Rose, R.K., Goodwin, S., Reichenthal, J., Horning, E.C. and Brodie, B.B. (1955): The metabolic fate of phenylbutazone (butazolidin) in man. *Journal of Pharmacology and Experimental Therapeutics, 113:* 481-489.

Burns, J.J., Yu, T.F., Dayton, P.G., Gutman, A.B. and Brodie, B.B. (1960): Biochemical pharmacological considerations of phenylbutazone and its analogues. *Annals of the New York Academy of Sciences, 86:* 253-262.

Calabro, J.J. and Marchesano, J.M. (1968): The early natural history of juvenile rheumathoid arthritis. A 10-year follow-up study of 100 cases. *Medical Clinics of North America, 52:* 567-591.

Careddu, P., Mereu, T. and Apollonio, T. (1961): Eliminazione urinaria di N-acetil-p-aminofenolo dopo carico con acetanilide nel neonato. *Bollettino Societa Italiana Biologia Sperimentale, 37:* 359-362.

Caruso, I. (1971): Verteilung von Indometacin in Blut und Synovialflussigkeit chronischer polyarthritiker. *Arzneimittel-Forschung, 21:* 1824-1826.

Casteels-Van Daele, M., Jaeken, J., Eggermont, E., de Gaetano, G. and Vermijlen, J. (1972): More on the effects of antenatally administered aspirin on aggregation of platelets of neonates. *Journal of Pediatrics, 80:* 685-686.

Champion, G.D., Paulus, H.E., Mongan, E., Okun, R., Pearson, C.M. and Sarkissian, E. (1972): The effect of aspirin on serum indomethacin. *Clinical Pharmacology and Therapeutics, 13:* 239-244.

Chapman, R.A. (1966): Suspected adverse reactions to indomethacin. *Canadian Medical Association Journal, 95:* 1156.
Chen, W., Vrindten, P.A., Dayton, P.G. and Burns, J.J. (1962): Accelerated aminopyrine metabolism in human subjects pretreated with phenylbutazone. *Life Sciences, 1:* 35-42.
Chiou, W.L. (1974): Dose- and dosage form-dependent pharmacokinetics of phenacetin and its metabolite in man. *Journal of Clinical Pharmacology, 14:* 418-425.
Chiou, W.L., and Onyemelukwe, I. (1974): Disintegration, dissolution and oral absorption in humans of five commercial buffered aspirin dosage forms. *Journal of Clinical Pharmacology, 14:* 597-603.
Clark, R., Thompson, R.P.H., Borirakchanyavat, V., Widdop, B., Davidson, A.R., Goulding, R. and Williams, R. (1973): Hepatic damage and death from overdose of paracetamol. *Lancet, I:* 66-69.
Cluff, L.E. and Petrie, J.C. (1974): *Clinical Effects of Interaction Between Drugs.* Elsevier, Amsterdam.
Cohen, S.N. and Armstrong, M.F. (1974): *Drug Interactions: A Handbook for Clinical Use,* Williams and Wilkins, Baltimore.
Coldwell, B.B., Solomonraj, G., Boyd, E.M., Jante, J. and Morrison, A.B. (1969): The effect of dosage form and route of administration on the absorption and excretion of acetylsalicylic acid in man. *Clinical Toxicology, 2:* 111-127.
Collins, E. and Turner, G. (1973): Salicylates and pregnancy. *Lancet, 2:* 1494.
Consolo, S., Morselli, P.L., Zaccala, M. and Garattini, S. (1970): Delayed absorption of phenylbutazone caused by desmethylimipramine in humans. *European Journal of Pharmacology, 10:* 239-242.
Corby, D.G. and Schulman, I. (1971): The effects of antenatal drug administration on aggregation of platelets of newborn infants. *Journal of Pediatrics, 79:* 307-313.
Craig, J.O., Ferguson, I.C. and Syme, J. (1966): Infants, toddlers and aspirin. *British Medical Journal, 1:* 757-761.
Crawford, J.S. and Hodi, H.W.Y. (1968): Binding of salicylic acid and sulphanilamide in serum from pregnant patients, cord blood and subjects taking oral contraceptives. *British Journal of Anaesthesiology, 40:* 825-833.
Cummings, A.J., King, M.L. and Martin, B.K. (1967): A kinetic study of drug elimination: the excretion of paracetamol and its metabolites in man. *British Journal of Pharmacology, 29:* 150-157.
Cunningham, J.L., Bullen, M.F. and Price Evans, D.A. (1974): The pharmacokinetics of acetanilide and of diphenylhydantoin sodium. *European Journal of Clinical Pharmacology, 7:* 461-466.
Currie, J.P. (1952): Treatment of rheumatoid arthritis with butazolidine. *Lancet, 2:* 15-16.
Davies, D.S. and Thorgeirsson, S.S. (1971): Mechanism of hepatic drug oxidation and its relationship to individual differences in rates of oxidation in man. *Annals of the New York Academy of Sciences, 179:* 411-420.
Davis, M., Simmons, C.J., Dordoni, B. and Williams, R. (1974): Urinary D-glucaric acid excretion and plasma antipyrine kinetics during enzyme induction. *British Journal of Clinical Pharmacology, 1:* 253-257.
Davison, C. (1971): Salicylate metabolism in man. *Annals of the New York Academy of Sciences, 179:* 249-268.
Davison, C., Guy, J.L., Levitt, M. and Smith, P.K. (1961): The distribution of certain non-narcotic analgetic agents in the CNS of several species. *Journal of Pharmacology and Experimental Therapeutics, 134:* 176-183.
Davison, C. and Mandel, H.G. (1971): Nonnarcotic analgesics and antipyretics. I. Salicylates. In: *Drill's Pharmacology in Medicine,* edited by J.R. Di Palma, pp. 379-403, McGraw-Hill, New York.

Davison, C. and Smith, P.K. (1961): The binding of salicylic acid and related substances to purified proteins. *Journal of Pharmacology and Experimental Therapeutics, 133:* 161-170.

Davison, C. and Strautz, R.L. (1961): The effect on the distribution and excretion of salicylate by drugs displacing that compound from plasma binding sites. *Pharmacologist, 3:* 81.

Dayton, P.G., Israili, Z.H. and Perel, J.M. (1973): Influence of binding on drug metabolism and distribution. *Annals of the New York Academy of Sciences, 226:* 172-194.

de Gaetano, G., Donati, M.B. and Garattini, S. (1975): Drugs affecting platelet function tests–their effects on haemostasis and surgical bleeding. *Thrombosis Diathesis Haemorrhagica,* in press.

Done, A.K. (1960): Salicylate intoxication. Significance of measurements of salicylate in blood in cases of acute ingestion. *Pediatrics, 26:* 800-807.

Done, A.K. (1974): Salicylate, pharmacokinetics, and the pediatrician. *Pediatrics, 54:* 670-672.

Dubach, U.S. and Raàflaub, J. (1969): Neue aspekte zur frage der Nephrotoxizitat von Phenacetin. *Experientia, 25:* 956-958.

Duggan, D.E., Hogans, A.F., Kwan, K.C. and McMahon, F.G. (1972): The metabolism of indomethacin in man. *Journal of Pharmacology and Experimental Therapeutics, 181:* 563-575.

Earle, R., Jr. (1961): Congenital salicylate intoxication. Report of a case. *Medical Intelligence, 265:* 1003-1004.

Ebadi, M.S. and Kugel, R.B. (1970): Alteration in metabolism of acetylsalicylic acid in children with Down's syndrome. Decreased plasma binding and formation of alicyluric acid. *Pediatrics Research, 4:* 187-193.

Editorial (1974): Aspirin-induced hepatic injury. *Annals of Internal Medicine, 80:* 103-105.

Eichelbaum, M., Bodem, G., Gugler, R., Schneider-Deters, C. and Dengler, H.J. (1974): Influence of thyroid status on plasma half-life of antipyrine in man. *New England Journal of Medicine, 290:* 1040-1042.

Elfstrom, J. and Lindgren, S. (1974): Disappearance of phenazone from plasma in patients with obstructive jaundice. *European Journal of Clinical Pharmacology, 7:* 467-471.

Elliott, H.C. (1966): Urinary excretion kinetics of salicyluric acid. *Proceedings of the Society for Experimental Biology and Medicine, 121:* 861-864.

Farid, N.R., Glynn, J.P. and Kerr, D.N.S. (1972): Haemodialysis in paracetamol self-poisoning. *Lancet, 2:* 396-398.

Flanagan, R.J. and Richens, A. (1974): The influence of elevated plasma hydrocortisone concentrations on antipyrine metabolism in man. *British Journal of Clinical Pharmacology, 1:* 409-412.

Ganshorn, A. and Kurz, H. (1968): Unterschiede zwischen der Proteinbindung Neugeborener und Erwachsener und ihre Bedeutung fur die pharmakologische Wirkung. *Naunyn-Schmiedebergs Archiv fur Pharmakologie und Experimentelle Pathologie, 260:* 117-118.

Garnham, J.C., Raymond, K., Shotton, E. and Turner, P. (1975): The effect of buffered aspirin on plasma indomethacin. *European Journal of Clinical Pharmacology, 8:* 107-113.

Garrettson, L.K., Procknal, J.A. and Levy, G. (1975): Fetal acquisition and neonatal elimination of a large amount of salicylate. *Clinical Pharmacology and Therapeutics, 17:* 98-103.

Gault, M.H., Shahidi, N.T. and Barber, V.E. (1974): Methemoglobin formation in analgesic nephropathy. *Clinical Pharmacology and Therapeutics, 15:* 521-527.

Gazzard, B.G., Ford-Hutchinson, A., Williams, R. and Smith, M.J. (1973): The binding of paracetamol to the plasma proteins of man and pig. *Journal of Pharmacy and Pharmacology, 25:* 964-967.

Gazzard, B.G., Wilson, R.A., Weston, M.J., Thompson, R.P.H. and Williams, R. (1974): Charcoal haemoperfusion for paracetamol overdose. *British Journal of Clinical Pharmacology, 1:* 271-275.

Giacoia, G.P., Levy, G., Catz, C.S., Procknal, J.A., Mauri, N. and Garrettson, L.K. (1975): Pharmacokinetics of salicylate in nursing mothers and their breast fed infants, in press.

Gibson, T., Zaphiropoulos, G., Grove, J., Widdop, B. and Berry, D. (1975): Kinetics of salicylate metabolism. *British Journal of Clinical Pharmacology, 2:* 233-238.

Gladtke, E. (1968): Pharmacokinetic studies on phenylbutazone in children. *Il Farmaco* (ed. sci.), *23:* 897-906.

Gorodischer, R., Levy, G., Krasner, J. and Yaffe, S.J. (1970): Congenital nonobstructive, nonhemolytic jaundice. *New England Journal of Medicine, 282:* 375-377.

Goulding, R. (1973): Acetaminophen poisoning. *Pediatrics, 52:* 883-884.

Greenberg, L.A. and Lester, D. (1946): The metabolic fate of acetanilid and other aniline derivatives. I. *Journal of Pharmacology and Experimental Therapeutics, 88:* 87-98.

Gwilt, J.R., Robertson, A., Goldman, L. and Blanchard, A.W. (1963): The absorption characteristics of paracetamol tablets in man. *Journal of Pharmacy and Pharmacology, 15:* 445-453.

Hauser, H. and Pfleger, K. (1965): Untersuchung über orale und rectale Resorption von phenacetin und N-acetyl-p-Aminophenol. *Archiv für Experimentelle Pathologie und Pharmakologie, 251:* 108-109.

Heading, R.C., Nimmo, J., Prescott, L.F. and Tothill, P. (1973): The dependence of paracetamol absorption on the rate of gastric emptying. *British Journal of Pharmacology, 47:* 415-421.

Helleberg, L., Rubin, A., Wolen, R.L., Rodda, B.E., Ridolfo, A.S., and Gruber, C.M., Jr. (1974): A pharmacokinetic interaction in man between phenobarbitone and fenoprofen, a new anti-inflammatory agent. *British Journal of Clinical Pharmacology, 1:* 371-374.

Herrmann, B. (1959): Uber den Stoffwechsel des Butazolidin. *Medicina Experimentalis, 1:* 170-178.

Hill, J.B. (1973): Salicylate intoxication. *New England Journal of Medicine, 288:* 1110-1113.

Hill, J.B. (1970): The effect of altering blood pH on rat tissue and plasma salicylate concentrations. *Federation Proceedings, 29:* 434 proc.

Hedges, A., Kaye, C.M., Maclay, W.P. and Turner, P. (1974): A comparison of the absorption of effervescent preparations of paracetamol and penicillin V (phenoxymethylpenicillin) with solid dose forms of these drugs. *Journal of Clinical Pharmacology, 14:* 363-368.

Hill, R., Horning, M. and Horning, E.C. (1972): Pattern of drug ingestion in gravid females. *Pediatrics Research, 6:* 410-416.

Hollister, L. and Levy, G. (1965): Some aspects of salicylate distribution and metabolism in man. *Journal of Pharmaceutical Sciences, 54:* 1126-1129.

Holt, L.P.J. and Hawkins, C.F. (1965): Indomethacin: studies of absorption and of the use of indomethacin suppositories. *British Medical Journal, 1:* 1354-1356.

Hucker, H.B., Zacchei, A.G., Cox, S.V., Brodie, D.A. and Cantwell, N.H.R. (1966): Studies on the absorption, distribution and excretion of indomethacin in various species. *Journal of Pharmacology and Experimental Therapeutics, 153:* 237-249.

Huffman, D.H., Shoeman, D.W. and Azarnoff, D.L. (1974): Correlation of the plasma elimination of antipyrine and the appearance of 4-hydroxyantipyrine in the urine. *Biochemical Pharmacology, 23:* 197-201.

Huguley, C.M., Jr. (1964): Agranulocytosis induced by Dipyrone, a hazardous antipyretic and analgesic. *Journal of the American Medical Association, 189:* 938-941.

Hunziker, H. (1956): *Zeitschrift für Rheumaforschung, 15:* 219-229 (cited by Rechenberg, 1962).

Hvidberg, E.F., Andreasen, P.B. and Ranek, L. (1974): Plasma half-life of phenylbutazone in patients with impaired liver function. *Clinical Pharmacology and Therapeutics, 15:* 171-177.

Hvidberg, E., Lausen, H.H., and Jansen, J.A. (1972): Indomethacin: plasma concentrations and protein binding in man. *European Journal of Clinical Pharmacology, 4:* 119-124.

Indomethacin (indocid.) (1968): *Medical Letters, 10:* 37-38.

Jaffe, J.M., Colaizzi, J.L. and Barry, H., III (1971): Effects of dietary components on GI absorption of acetaminophen tablets in man. *Journal of Pharmaceutical Sciences, 60:* 1646-1650.

Jakob, R. (1968): Klinisch-chemische untersuchungen mit Oxyphenbutazon. *Zentralblatt für Phlebologie, 2:* 162-175.

Jori, A., Di Salle, E. and Quadri, A. (1972): Rate of aminopyrine disappearance from plasma of young and aged humans. *Pharmacology, 8:* 273-279.

Kaiser, D.G. and Vangiessen, G.J. (1974): GLC determination of ibuprofen /(±)-2-(p-iso-butylphenyl) propionic acid/in plasma. *Journal of Pharmaceutical Sciences, 63:* 219-221.

Kelsey, W.M. and Sharyi, M. (1967): Fatal hepatitis probably due to indomethacin. *Journal of the American Medical Association, 199:* 586-587.

Kerckhoffs, H.P.M. and Huizinga, T. (1967): A comparative investigation about the absorption of drugs after oral, rectal and parenteral administration. *Pharmaceutisch Weekblad, 102:* 1183-1200.

Klutch, A., Harfenish, M. and Conney, A.N. (1966): Hydroxyacetophenetidine, a new metabolite of acetophenetidine. *Journal of Medicinal Chemistry, 9:* 63-66.

Kolmodin, B., Azarnoff, D.L. and Sjoqvist, F. (1969): Effect of environmental factors on drug metabolism: decreased plasma half-life of antipyrine in workers exposed to chlorinated hydrocarbon insecticides. *Clinical Pharmacology and Therapeutics, 10:* 638-642.

Kramer, E. and Routh, J.I. (1973): The binding of salicylic acid and acetylsalicylic acid to human serum albumin. *Clinical Biochemistry, 6:* 98-105.

Krasner, J., Giacoia, G.P. and Yaffe, S.J. (1973): Drug-protein binding in the newborn infant. *Annals of the New York Academy of Sciences, 226:* 101-114.

Krasner, J. and Yaffe, S.J. (1975): Drug-protein binding in the neonate. In: *Basic and Therapeutic Aspects of Perinatal Pharmacology,* edited by P.L. Morselli, S. Garattini and F. Sereni, pp. 357-366, Raven Press, New York.

Kucera, J.L. and Bullock, F.J. (1969): The binding of salicylate to plasma protein from several animal species. *Journal of Pharmacy and Pharmacology, 21:* 293-296.

Kunin, C.M. (1964): Enhancement of antimicrobial activity of penicillins and other antibiotics in human serum by competitive serum binding inhibitors. *Proceedings of the Society for Experimental Biology and Medicine, 117:* 69-73.

Kunze, M., Stein, G., Kunze, E. and Traeger, A. (1974): Zur Pharmakokinetik von Indomethazin in Abhägigkeit vom Lebeusalter, bei Patienten mit Gallenwegsverschluss, Nierenfunktionslin-schränkung und Unverträglichkeitserscheinungen. *Deutsche Gesundheitswesen, 29:* 351-353.

Lamont-Havers, R. and Wagner, B.M. (1968): *Proceedings, Conference of Effects of Chronic Salicylate Administration,* New York, 1966, U.S. Govt. Printing Office, Washington.

Larsen, P.R. (1972): Salicylate-induced increases in free triiodothyronine in human serum. *Journal of Clinical Investigation, 51:* 1125-1134.

Leonards, J.R. (1963): The influence of solubility on the rate of gastrointestinal absorption of aspirin. *Clinical Pharmacology and Therapeutics, 4:* 476-479.
Lester, D. and Greenberg, L.A. (1947): The metabolic fate of acetanilid and other aniline derivatives. II. *Journal of Pharmacology and Experimental Therapeutics, 90:* 68-75.
Levi, A.J., Sherlock, S. and Walker, D. (1968): Phenylbutazone and isoniazid metabolism in patients with liver disease in relation to previous drug therapy. *Lancet I:* 1275-1279.
Levy, G. (1965a): Salicylurate formation—demonstration of Michaelis-Menten kinetics in man. *Journal of Pharmaceutical Sciences, 54:* 496.
Levy, G. (1965b): Pharmacokinetics of salicylate elimination in man. *Journal of Pharmaceutical Sciences, 54:* 959-967.
Levy, G. (1975): Salicylate pharmacokinetics in the human neonate. In: *Basic and Therapeutic Aspects of Perinatal Pharmacology,* edited by P.L. Morselli, S. Garattini and F. Sereni, pp. 319-330, Raven Press, New York.
Levy, G., Amsel, L.P. and Elliott, H.C. (1969a): Kinetics of salicyluric acid elimination in man. *Journal of Pharmaceutical Sciences, 58:* 827-829.
Levy, G. and Ertel, I.J. (1971): Effect of bilirubin on drug conjugations in children. *Pediatrics, 47:* 811-817.
Levy, G. and Garrettson, L.K. (1974): Kinetics of salicylate elimination by newborn infants of mothers who ingested aspirin before delivery. *Pediatrics, 53:* 201-210.
Levy, G., Gumtow, R.N. and Rutowski, J.M. (1961): The effect of dosage form upon the gastrointestinal absorption rate of salicylates. *Canadian Medical Association Journal, 85:* 414-419.
Levy, G. and Gwilt, P.R. (1972): Activated charcoal for acute acetaminophen intoxication. *Journal of the American Medical Association, 219:* 621.
Levy, G. and Hollister, L.E. (1964): Inter- and intrasubject variations in drug absorption kinetics. *Journal of Pharmaceutical Sciences, 53:* 1446-1452.
Levy, G., Khanna, N.N., Soda, D.M., Tsuzuki, O. and Stern, L. (1975): Pharmacokinetics of acetaminophen in the human neonate: formation of acetaminophen glucuronide and sulfate in relation to plasma bilirubin concentration and D-glucaric acid excretion. *Pediatrics, 55:* 818-825.
Levy, G. and Leonards, J.R. (1966): Absorption, metabolism and excretion of salicylates. In: *The Salicylates: A Critical Bibliographic Review,* edited by M.J.H. Smith and P.K. Smith, pp. 5-48, Interscience, New York.
Levy, G. and Leonards, J.R. (1971): Urine pH and salicylate therapy. *Journal of the American Medical Association, 217:* 81.
Levy, G. and Procknal, J.A. (1968): Drug biotransformation interactions in man. I. Mutual inhibition in glucuronide formation of salicylic acid and salicylamide in man. *Journal of Pharmaceutical Sciences, 57:* 1330-1335.
Levy, G. and Regardh, C-G. (1971): Drug biotransformation interactions in man. V. Acetaminophen and salicylic acid. *Journal of Pharmaceutical Sciences, 60:* 608-611.
Levy, G. and Tsuchiya, T. (1972b): Effect of activated charcoal on aspirin absorption in man. I. *Clinical Pharmacology and Therapeutics, 13:* 317-322.
Levy, G., Tsuchiya, T. and Amsel, L.P. (1972): Limited capacity for salicyl phenolic glucuronide formation and its effect on the kinetics of salicylate elimination in man. *Clinical Pharmacology and Therapeutics, 13:* 258-268.
Levy, G., Vogel, A.W. and Amsel, L.P. (1969b): Capacity-limited salicylurate formation during prolonged administration of aspirin to healthy human subjects. *Journal of Pharmaceutical Sciences, 58:* 503-504.
Levy, G. and Yaffe, S.J. (1968): The study of salicylate pharmacokinetics in intoxicated infants and children. *Clinical Toxicology, 1:* 409-424.
Levy, G. and Yaffe, S.J. (1974): Relationship between dose and apparent volume of distribution of salicylate in children. *Pediatrics, 54:* 713-717.

Levy, G. and Yamada, H. (1971): Drug biotransformations interactions in man. II: Acetaminophen and salicylamide. *Journal of Pharmaceutical Sciences, 60:* 215-221.
Lewis, R.B. and Schulman, J.D. (1973): Influence of acetylsalicylic acid, an inhibitor of prostaglandin synthesis, on the duration of human gestation and labour. *Lancet, 2:* 1159-1161.
Lindgren, S., Collste, P., Norlander, B. and Sjöqvist, F. (1974): Gas chromatographic assessment of the reproducibility of phenazone plasma half-life in young healthy volunteers. *European Journal of Clinical Pharmacology, 7:* 381-385.
MacLean, D., Peters, T.J., Brown, R.A.G., McCathie, M., Baines, G.F. and Robertson, P.G.C. (1968): Treatment of acute paracetamol poisoning. *Lancet, 2:* 849-852.
Macpherson, C.R., Milne, M.D. and Evans, B.M. (1955): The excretion of salicylate. *British Journal of Pharmacology, 10:* 484-489.
Manso, C., Taranta, A. and Nydick, J. (1956): Effect of aspirin administration on serum glutamic oxaloacetic and glutamic pyrinic transaminases in children. *Proceedings of the Society for Experimental Biology and Medicine, 93:* 84-86.
Marsh, F.P., Almeyda, J.R. and Levy, I.S. (1971): Non-thrombocytopenic purpura and acute glomerulonephritis after indomethacin therapy. *Annals of the Rheumatic Diseases, 30:* 501-505.
May, B., Helmstaedt, D., Büstgens, L. and McLean, A. (1974): The relation between cytochrone P-450 in liver biopsies and drug metabolism in patients with liver disease and in morphine addiction. *Clinical Sciences, 46:* 11P.
McGilveray, I.J. and Mattok, G.L. (1972): Some factors affecting the absorption of paracetamol. *Journal of Pharmacy and Pharmacology, 24:* 615-619.
Menguy, R., Desbaillets, L., Masters, Y.F. and Okaba, S. (1972): Evidence for a sex-linked difference in aspirin metabolism. *Nature, 239:* 102-103.
Mereu, T., Apollonio, T., Sereni-Piceni, L., Careddu, P. (1962): Excretion of N-acetyl-p-aminophenol in the newborn. *Lancet, 1:* 1300.
Miller, R.L. and Melmon, K.L. (1972): Inflammatory disorders. In: *Clinical Pharmacology*, edited by H.F. Morrelli and K.L. Melmon, pp. 382-417, Macmillan, New York.
Mitchell, J.R., Thorgeirsson, S.S., Potter, W.Z., Jollow, D.J. and Keiser, H. (1974): Acetaminophen-induced hepatic injury: protective role of glutathione in man and rationale for therapy. *Clinical Pharmacology and Therapeutics, 16:* 676-684.
Morselli, P.L., Garattini, S. and Cohen, S.N. (eds.) (1974): *Drug Interactions*, Raven Press, New York.
Nelson, E. and Morioka, T. (1963): Kinetics of the metabolism of acetaminophen by humans. *Journal of Pharmaceutical Sciences, 52:* 864-868.
Nimmo, J., Heading, R.C., Tothill, P. and Prescott, L.F. (1973): Pharmacological modification of gastric emptying: effects of propantheline and metoclopromide on paracetamol absorption. *British Medical Journal, 1:* 587-589.
Nora, J.J., Nora, A.H., Sommerville, R.J., Hill, R.M. and McNamara, D.G. (1963): Maternal exposure to potential teratogens. *Journal of the American Medical Association, 202:* 1065-1069.
Nöschel, H., Bonow, A., Möller, R., Estel, Ch., and Müller, B. (1972): Plazentapassage von Natriumsalizylat. *Zentralblatt für Gynekologie, 94:* 437-442.
Nowak, M.M., Brundhofer, B. and Gibaldi, M. (1974): Rectal absorption from aspirin suppositories in children and adults. *Pediatrics, 54:* 23-26.
Ober, K.-F. (1974): Mechanism of interaction of tolbutamide and phenylbutazone in diabetic patients. *European Journal of Clinical Pharmacology, 7:* 291-294.
Odell, G.B. (1973): Influence of binding on the toxicity of bilirubin. *Annals of the New York Academy of Sciences, 226:* 225-237.
Øie, S. and Levy, G. (1975): Effect of certain drugs and drug metabolites on bilirubin binding in albumin solution and in plasma of newborns and adults, in press.

O'Malley, K., Crooks, J., Duke, E. and Stevenson, I.H. (1971): Effect of age and sex on human drug metabolism. *British Medical Journal, 3:* 607-609.
O'Malley, K., Stevenson, I.H. and Crooks, J. (1972): Impairment of human drug metabolism by oral contraceptive steroids. *Clinical Pharmacology and Therapeutics, 13:* 552-557.
Oppenheimer, J.H. (1973): Interaction of drugs with thyroid hormone binding sites. *Annals of the New York Academy of Sciences, 226:* 333-340.
O'Reilly, R.A. (1973): The binding of sodium warfarin to plasma albumin and its displacement by phenylbutazone. *Annals of the New York Academy of Sciences, 226:* 293-308.
Palmer, L., Bertilsson, L., Alvan, G., Orme, M., Sjöqvist, F. and Holmstedt, B. (1974): Indomethacin: quantitative determination in plasma by mass fragmentography including pilot pharmacokinetics in man. In: *Prostaglandin Synthetase Inhibitors,* edited by H.J. Robinson and J.R. Vane, pp. 91-97, Raven Press, New York.
Palmisano, P.A. and Cassady, G. (1969): Salicylate exposure in the perinate. *Journal of the American Medical Association, 209:* 556-558.
Pantuck, E.J., Kuntzman, R. and Conney, A.N. (1972): Decreased concentration of phenacetin in plasma of cigarette smokers. *Science, 175:* 1248-1250.
Paulus, H.E., Siegel, M., Mongan, E., Okun, R. and Calabro, J.J. (1971): Variations of serum concentrations and half-life of salicylate in patients with rheumatoid arthritis. *Arthritis and Rheumatism, 14:* 527-532.
Petruch, F., Schuppel, R.V.A. and Steinhilber, G. (1974): Effect of diphenylhydantoin on hepatic drug hydroxylation. *European Journal of Clinical Pharmacology, 7:* 281-285.
Pierce, A.W., Jr. (1974): Salicylate poisoning. *Pediatrics, 54:* 342-347.
Pinckard, R.N., Hawkins, D. and Farr, R.S. (1973): The influence of acetylsalicylic acid on the binding of acetrizoate to human albumin. *Annals of the New York Academy of Sciences, 226:* 341-354.
Pinedo, H.M., van de Putte, L.B.A. and Loeliger, E.A. (1973): Salicylate-induced consumption coagulopathy. *Annals of the Rheumatic Diseases, 32:* 66-68.
Prescott, L.F. (1969): The metabolism of phenacetin in patients with renal disease. *Clinical Pharmacology and Therapeutics, 10:* 383-394.
Prescott, L.F. (1974): Drug absorption interactions—gastric emptying. In: *Drug Interactions,* edited by P.L. Morselli, S. Garattini and S.N. Cohen, pp. 11-20, Raven Press, New York.
Prescott, L.F., Adjepon-Yamoah, K.K. and Roberts, E. (1973): Rapid gas liquid chromatographic estimation of antipyrine in plasma. *Journal of Pharmacy and Pharmacology, 25:* 205-207.
Prescott, L.F. and Nimmo, J. (1971): Generic inequivalence–clinical observations. *Acta Pharmacologica et Toxicologica, 29,* suppl. 3, 288-303.
Prescott, L.F., Sansur, M., Levin, W. and Conney, A.H. (1968): The comparative metabolism of phenacetin and N-acetyl-p-aminophenol in man, with particular reference to effects on the kidney. *Clinical Pharmacology and Therapeutics, 9:* 605-614.
Prescott, L.F., Steel, R.F. and Ferrier, W.R. (1970): The effects of particle size on the absorption of phenacetin in man. *Clinical Pharmacology and Therapeutics, 11:* 496-504.
Prescott, L.F., Wright, N., Roscoe, P. and Brown, S.S. (1971): Plasma-paracetamol half-life and hepatic necrosis in patients with paracetamol overdosage. *Lancet, 1:* 519-522.
Proctor, J.D., Evans, E.F., Campos, V., Velandia, J., Pollack, D., Wingfield, W.L. and Wasserman, A.J. (1974): Tolerance to pirprofen and preliminary efficacy trial in rheumatoid arthritis. *Clinical Pharmacology and Therapeutics, 16:* 69-76.
Raaflaub, J. and Dubach, U.C. (1969): Dose-dependent change in the pattern of phenacetin metabolism in man and its possible significance in analgesic nephropathy. *Klinische Wochenschrift, 47:* 1286-1287.

Rechenberg, H.K. (1962): *Phenylbutazone—Butazolidin*, Edwards Arnold, London.
Rechenberg, H.K. and Herrmann, B. (1961): Untersuchungen über die Resorption des Antiphlogisticums G 27202 (Tanderil). *Schweizer Medizinische Wochenschrift, 91:* 403-405.
Reimold, E.W., Worthen, H.G. and Phillip Reilly, T. (1973): Salicylate poisoning. Comparison of acetazolamide administration and alkaline diuresis in the treatment of experimental salicylate intoxication in puppiies. *American Journal of Diseases of Children, 125:* 668-674.
Reinicke, C., Rogner, G., Frenzel, J., Maak, B. and Klinger, W. (1970): Die Wirkung von Phenylbutazon und Phenobarbital auf die Amidopyrin-Elimination, die Bilirubin-Gesamtkonzentration im Serum und einige Blutgerinnungsfaktoren bei neugeborenen Kindern. *Pharmacologia Clinica, 2:* 167-172.
Reynolds, R.C. and Cluff, L.E. (1960): Interaction of serum and sodium salicylate: changes during acute infection and the influence on pharmacological activity. *Bulletin of Johns Hopkins Hospital, 107:* 278-290.
Rich, R.R. and Johnson, J.S. (1973): Salicylate hepatotoxicity in patients with juvenile rheumatoid arthritis. *Arthritis and Rheumatism, 16:* 1-9.
Rothermich, N.O. (1966): An extended study of indomethacin. I. Clinical pharmacology. *Journal of the American Medical Association, 195:* 531-536.
Rothermich, N.O. (1971): The fate of rectally administered radioactive indomethacin in human subjects: a preliminary report. *Clinical Pharmacology and Therapeutics, 12:* 300-301.
Rowland, M. and Riegelman, S. (1968): Pharmacokinetics of acetylsalicylic acid and salicylic acid after intravenous administration in man. *Journal of Pharmaceutical Science, 57:* 1313-1319.
Rowland, M., Riegelman, S., Harris, P.A. and Sholkoff, S.D. (1972): Absorption kinetics of aspirin in man following oral administration of an aqueous solution. *Journal of Pharmaceutical Sciences, 61:* 379-385.
Rowland, M., Riegelman, S., Harris, P.A., Sholkoff, S.D. and Eyring, E.J. (1967): Kinetics of acetylsalicylic acid disposition in man. *Nature, 215:* 413-414.
Rubin, A., Rodda, B.E., Warrick, P., Ridolfo, A. and Gruber, C.M. (1972a): Physiological disposition of fenoprofen in man. II. *Journal of Pharmaceutical Sciences, 61:* 739-745.
Rubin, A., Warrick, P., Walen, R.L., Chernish, S.M., Ridolfo, A. and Gruber, C.M. (1972b): Physiological disposition of fenoprofen in man. III. *Journal of Pharmacology and Experimental Therapeutics, 183:* 449-457.
Rubin, A., Rodda, B.E., Warrick, P., Gruber, C.M., Jr. and Ridolfo, A.S. (1973): Interactions of aspirin with nonsteroidal antiinflammatory drugs in man. *Arthritis and Rheumatism, 16:* 635-645.
Runkel, R., Forchielli, E., Sevelius, H., Chaplin, M. and Segre, E. (1974): Nonlinear plasma level response to high doses of naproxen. *Clinical Pharmacology and Therapeutics, 15:* 261-266.
Russell, A.S., Sturge, R.A. and Smith, M.A. (1971); Serum transaminases during salicylate therapy. *British Medical Journal, 2:* 428-429.
Schachter, D. and Manis, J.G. (1958): Salicylate and salicyl-conjugates: fluorimetric estimation, biosynthesis and renal excretion in man. *Journal of Clinical Investigation, 37:* 800-807.
Seaman, W.E., Ishak, K.G. and Plotz, P.H. (1974): Aspirin-induced hepatotoxicity in patients with systemic Lupus Erythematosus. *Annals of Internal Medicine, 80:* 1-8.
Segar, W.E. (1969): The critically ill child: salicylate intoxication. *Pediatrics, 44:* 440-444.
Segre, E.J. (1975): Naproxen metabolism in man. *Journal of Clinical Pharmacology, 15:* 316-323.

Selley, M.L., Glass, J., Triggs, E.J. and Thomas, J. (1975): Pharmacokinetic studies of tometin in man. *Clinical Pharmacology and Therapeutics, 17:* 599-605.

Sholkoff, S.D., Eyring, E.J., Rowland, M. and Riegelman, S. (1967): Plasma and synovial fluid concentrations of acetylsalicylic acid in patients with rheumatoid arthritis. *Arthritis and Rheumatism, 10:* 348-351.

Sir, S. (1964): Bekämpfung und Verhütung postoperativer Entzüdungs-erscheinungen mit einem neuen Antphlogisticum (Tanderil). *Zeitschrift für Laryngologie-Rhinologie-Otologie und ihre Grenzgebiete, 43:* 639-646.

Siurala, M., Mustala, O. and Jussila, J. (1969): Absorption of acetylsalicylic acid by a normal and an atrophic gastric mucosa. *Scandinavian Journal of Gastroenterology, 4:* 269-273.

Skeith, M.D., Simkin, P.A. and Healey, L.A. (1967): The renal excretion of indomethacin and its inhibition by probenecid. *Clinical Pharmacology and Therapeutics, 9:* 89-93.

Smith, P.K., Gleason, H.L., Stoll, C.G. and Ogorzalek, S. (1946): Studies on the pharmacology of salicylates. *Journal of Pharmacology and Experimental Therapeutics, 87:* 237-255.

Smith, S.E. and Rawlins, M.D. (1974): Prediction of drug oxidation rates in man: lack of correlation with serum gamma-glutamyl transpeptidase and urinary excretion of D-glucaric acid and 6-hydroxycortisol. *European Journal of Clinical Pharmacology, 7:* 71-75.

Soberman, R., Brodie, B.B., Levy, B.B., Axelrod, J., Hollander, V. and Steele, J.M. (1949): The use of antipyrine in the measurement of total body water in man. *Journal of Biological Chemistry, 179:* 31-42.

Solomon, H.M., Schrogie, J.J. and Williams, D. (1968): The displacement of phenylbutazone-^{14}C and warfarin-^{14}C from human albumin by various drugs and fatty acids. *Biochemical Pharmacology, 17:* 143-151.

Soren, A. (1975): Kinetics of salicylates in blood and joint fluids. *Journal of Clinical Pharmacology, 15:* 173-177.

Spector, R., Korkin, D.T. and Lorenzo, A.V. (1972): A rapid method for the determination of salicylate binding by the use of ultrafilters. *Journal of Pharmacy and Pharmacology, 24:* 786-789.

Tarlin, L., Landrigan, P., Rabineau, R., Mass, F. and Alpert, J.J. (1972): A comparison of the antipyretic effect of acetaminophen and aspirin. *American Journal of Diseases of Children, 124:* 880-882.

Thomas, B.H., Coldwell, B.B., Zeitz, W. and Solomonraj, G. (1972): Effect of aspirin, caffeine, and codeine on the metabolism of phenacetin and acetaminophen. *Clinical Pharmacology and Therapeutics, 13:* 906-910.

Traeger, A., Noschel, H. and Zaumseil, J. (1973): Zur pharmakokinetik von Indomethazin bei Schwangeren, Kreissenden und deren Neugeborenen. *Zentralblatt Für Gynäekologie, 95:* 635-641.

Traeger, A., Stein, G., Kunze, M. and Zausmeil, J. (1972): Zur Pharmakokinetik von Indomethazin bei nierengschädigten Patienten. *International Journal of Clinical Pharmacology, 63:* 237-242.

Tsuchiya, T. and Levy, G. (1972): Biotransformation of salicylic acid to its acyl and phenolic glucuronides in man. *Journal of Pharmaceutical Sciences, 61:* 800-801.

Van Petten, G.R., Feng, H., Withey, R.J. and Letton, H.F. (1971): The physiologic availability of solid dosage forms of phenylbutazone. I. *Journal of Clinical Pharmacology, 11:* 177-186.

Vesell, E.S. and Page, J.G. (1968a): Genetic control of drug levels in man: phenylbutazone. *Science, 159:* 1479-1480.

Vesell, E.S. and Page, J.G. (1968b): Genetic control of drug levels in man: antipyrine. *Science, 161:* 72-73.
Vesell, E.S. and Passananti, G.T. (1973): Inhibition of drug metabolism in man. *Drug Metabolism and Disposition, 1:* 402-410.
Vesell, E.S., Passananti, G.T., Greene, F.E. and Page, J.G. (1971a): Genetic control of drug levels and of the induction of drug-metabolizing enzymes in man: individual variability in the extent of allopurinol and nortriptyline inhibition of drug metabolism. *Annals of the New York Academy of Sciences, 179:* 752-773.
Vesell, E.S., Passananti, G.T. and Lee, C.H. (1971b): Impairment of drug metabolism by disulfiram in man. *Clinical Pharmacology and Therapeutics, 12:* 785-792.
Vest, M.F. (1958): Insufficient glucuronide formation in the newborn and its relationship to the pathogenesis of Icterus neonatorum. *Archives of Disease in Childhood, 33:* 473-476.
Vest, M.F. and Rossier, R. (1963): Detoxification in the newborn: the ability of the newborn infant to form conjugates with glucuronic acid, glycine, acetate and glutathione. *Annals of the New York Academy of Sciences, 111:* 183-197.
Vest, M.F. and Streiff, R.R. (1959): Studies on glucuronide formation in newborn infants and older childrenn. *A.M.A. Journal of Diseases of Children, 98:* 688-693.
Von Lehmann, B., Wan, S.H., Riegelman, S. and Becker, C. (1973): Renal contribution to overall metabolism of drugs. IV. Biotransformation of salicylic acid to salicyluric acid in man. *Journal of Pharmaceutical Sciences, 62:* 1483-1486.
Weber, W.W. and Cohen, S.N. (1975): Aging effects and drugs in man. In: *Concepts in Biochemical Pharmacology,* V. 28, 3, edited by J.R. Gillette and J.R. Mitchell, pp. 213-233, Springer-Verlag, Berlin.
Whittaker, J.C. and Price Evans, D.A. (1970): Genetic control of phenylbutazone metabolism in man. *British Medical Journal, 4:* 323-328.
Wiegand, R.G. and Sanders, P.G. (1964): Calculation of kinetic constants from blood levels of drugs. *Journal of Pharmacology and Experimental Therapeutics, 146:* 271-275.
Willis, A.L. (1974): An enzymatic mechanism for the antithrombotic and antihemostatic actions of aspirin. *Science, 183:* 325-3277.
Windorfer, A. (1972): Steigerung der geucuronidierings rate in der neugeborenenperiode durch therapeutische Phenobarbitaldosen. *Zeitschrift für Kinderheilkunde, 113:* 33-41.
Windorder, A. Jr., Kuenzer, W. and Urbanek, R. (1974): The influence of age on the activity of acetylsalicylic acid-esterase and protein salicylate binding. *European Journal of Clinical Pharmacology, 7:* 227-231.
Wunderls, Ch. (1956): Die Proteinbindung von 3,5-dioxo-1,2-diphenyl-4-n-butyl-pyrazolidin und werteren Pharmaka. *Arzneimittel-Forschung, 6:* 731-734.
Wurster, D.E. and Kramer, S.F. (1961): Investigation of some factors influencing percutaneous absorption. *Journal of Pharmaceutical Sciences, 50:* 288-293.
Yaffe, S.J., Levy, G., Matsuzawa, T. and Boliah, T. (1966): Enhancement of glucuronide-conjugating capacity in a hyperbilirubinemic, infant due to apparent enzyme induction by phenobarbital. *New England Journal of Medicine, 275:* 1461-1466.
Yoshimura, H., Shimeno, H. and Tsukamoto, H. (1968): Metabolism of drugs. LIX. A new metabolite of antipyrine. *Biochemical Pharmacology, 17:* 1511-1516.
Yu, T.F., Burns, J.J., Paton, B.C., Gutman, A.B. and Brodie, B.B. (1958): Phenylbutazone metabolites: antirheumatic, sodium-retaining and uricosuric effects in man. *Journal of Pharmacology and Experimental Therapeutics, 123:* 63-69.

11

Antiepileptic Drugs

PAOLO LUCIO MORSELLI

Antiepileptic drugs comprise the class of compounds in which, probably more than in any other, monitoring of plasma levels and knowledge of pharmacokinetic behavior of each single agent have proven to be very useful for a more rational, correct and safer therapeutic approach. Clear relationships between drug plasma levels and effects have been in fact observed for most of the compounds, and in several instances therapeutic and toxic thresholds could also be defined (Woodbury et al., 1972; Eadie and Tyrer, 1974; Livingston, 1972; Penry and Dale, 1975). Moreover, antiepileptics comprise the class of drugs for which very extensive information exists on drug kinetic parameters in the various age groups. From the available data, the importance of the age factor on drug disposition is clearly emerging. The drugs considered in this chapter are diphenylhydantoin, phenobarbital, primidone, ethosuximide, carbamazepine, clonazepam and di-N-propylacetate.

Diazepam, although widely used in the treatment of epilepsy, is not included in this chapter, but will be discussed in detail in Chapter 15, among psychotropic drugs.

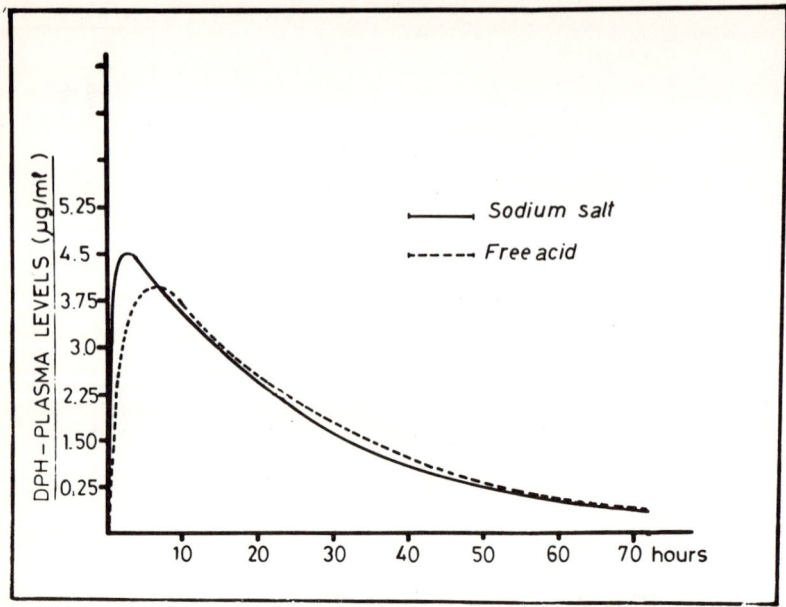

Fig. 1: Mean plasma levels of diphenylhydantoin (DPH) in four healthy volunteers following an oral intake of 200 mg of diphenylhydantoin administered in tablets as sodium salt (continuous line) or free acid (dotted line) form.

DIPHENYLHYDANTOIN

Adults

In adults, the absorption of diphenylhydantoin from the gastrointestinal tract is nearly complete, the main absorption site being the duodenum. The sodium salt is absorbed more rapidly than the free acid form (Fig. 1). Peak levels are frequently reached between 4 and 8 h after a single oral intake, but considerable interindividual differences may be observed in the course of chronic treatment (Woodbury and Swinyard, 1972; Glazko and Chang, 1972; Wilder et al., 1972). Administering loading doses of 500–600 mg, the peak may occur as late as 48–96 h (Wilder et al., 1973a). Intramuscular administration leads to slower and less effective absorption due to the fact that DPH injected into muscular tissue precipitates into the crystalline form, which is then very slowly released from the tissue site. Twice as much drug has to be given intramuscularly in order to achieve the same plasma levels as obtained by oral administration (Dam and Olesen, 1966; Wallis et al., 1968; Serrano et al., 1973; Wilder et al., 1974). Following absorption, the drug equilibrates quite rapidly with the various tissues. DPH is also distributed in all extracellular fluids (CSF, saliva, bile, gastrointestinal fluid) as the free form. The possibility of an enterohepatic recycling of the drug may be hypothized in man on the basis of recent results of Albert et al. (1974). In adult subjects with normal renal and liver functions, DPH is bound to plasma proteins for about 89–93%, while in uremic patients with compromised renal function the binding may be as low as 75% (Triedman et al., 1960; Lunde et al., 1970, 1972; Reidenberg et al., 1971; Bochner et al., 1973; Odar-Cederlöf and Borgå, 1974; Albert et al., 1974). The reduced binding in uremia is probably due both to the lowered protein concentration and to a qualitative change in the drug-binding proteins (Reidenberg et al., 1971; Shoeman et al., 1973). Compounds such as salicylic acid, sulfafurazol and phenylbutazone may exert a significant displacing effect on DPH-binding (Lunde et al., 1970). The binding to plasma proteins appears to involve several sites, and, according to Lightfoot and Christian (1966), DPH is bound to albumin and to two α-globulins, identified as those to which thyroxine is also bound.

The DPH brain concentrations usually range from 0.75 to 1.52 times the concentration of total drug in plasma (Sherwin et al., 1973a; Vajda et al., 1974), while CSF concentrations correspond to the DPH free fraction in plasma water (Lund et al., 1972).

A direct relationship between free drug in plasma water and concentration in red blood cells has also been reported (Borondy et al., 1973; Hansotia and Keran, 1974; Wilkinson and Kurata, 1974). The apparent volume of distribution in adults has been calculated to be about 1.6–2.5 L/kg by Woodbury and Swinyard (1972), while more recently Odar-Cederlöf and Borgå (1974) reported an apparent volume of distribution of 0.60–0.67 L/kg in subjects with normal kidney function and a value of 1.0–1.8 L/kg in uremic patients with altered renal function. A reduced binding to plasma proteins, as well as expansion of the extracellular water, is the probable reason underlying the observed phenomenon.

The biological transformation pathways of diphenylhydantoin are reported in Fig. 2. The most important catabolic step in man is the parahydroxylation of one of the phenol rings which leads to the formation of 5-(p-hydroxyphenyl)-5-phenylhydrantoin (HPPH) (Butler, 1957; Mayert, 1960; Chang and Glazko, 1972).

The HPPH is readily conjugated with glucuronic acid, and the conjugated derivatives is cleared rapidly from the blood in subjects with normal kidney function, however, it may accumulate in cases of renal impairment (Letteri et al., 1971). HPPH is practically devoid of toxic and anticonvulsant effects. The presence of 5-meta HPPH has also been described in human urine, but in man its amount seems to be negligible (Atkinson et al., 1970). Other metabolites include

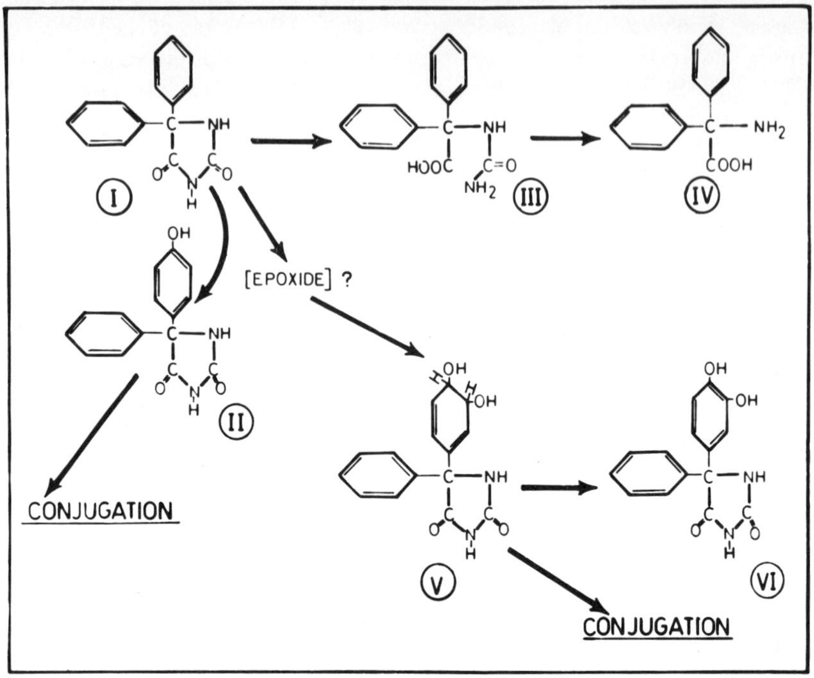

Fig. 2: Metabolism of diphenylhydantoin in man. I. Diphenyhydantoin (DPH); II. 5-(p-hydroxyphenyl)-5-phenylhydantoin (5-HPPH); III. Di-phenylhydantoic acid; IV. Aminodiphenylacetic acid; V. 5-(3,4-dihydroxy-1,5-cycloexadien-1-yl)-5-phenylhydantoin; VI. t-(3,4-dihydroxyphenyl)-5-phenylhydantoin.

the dihydrodiol and the 5-(3,4 dihydroxyphenyl)-5-phenylhydantoin.

The dihydrodiol (V) results from the oxidation on an aromatic double bound in one of the phenyl rings (Horning et al., 1971; Chang et al., 1970). The possibility of the formation of an epoxide intermediate has been suggested, but no conclusive evidence to support this is available at present. The 3,4-dihydroxy derivative (VI) is formed by the oxidation of the nonaromatic diol (Borgå et al., 1972). The binding of pHPPH to plasma protein is about 63-65% (Glazko and Chang, 1972).

The apparent plasma half-life may vary from 7 to 40 h, with an average of 20-22 h, while after i.v. administration the half-life may range from 10 to 18 h (Arnold and Gerber, 1970; Glazko et al., 1969; Letteri et al., 1971; Odar-Cederlöf and Borgå, 1974). The disappearance of the drug, however, is not always a simple monoexponential process, and apparently does not follow first-order kinetics (Arnold and Gerber, 1970; Letteri et al., 1971; Gerber et al., 1972; Bochner et al., 1972; Atkinson and Shaw, 1973; Richens, 1974). The nonexponential decline of DPH is explained by the fact that, at higher plasma levels, the biotransformation mechanism to the major metabolites approaches saturation. The decline of plasma DPH can, in fact, be described in terms of the Michaelis-Menten equation. From this it derives that disproportionately great increases in plasma DPH levels may be observed with small increases in dosages, in the course of chronic treatment (Fig. 3). It appears that there are important, and wide, individual variations in the levels at which the rate-limiting drug metabolizing enzymes become saturated. The level of saturation probably results from the net sum of different phenomena such as saturation, autoinduction, product inhibition, genetic factors and presence of other drugs.

The fraction of unchanged DPH in urine accounts for less than 5% of the administered dose, and a similar amount may be found in the feces. The drug is mainly excreted in the urine as pHPPH glucuronide, in a ranges of 33-48% of administered dose in 24 h, and 75% in 5 days (Glazko et al., 1969). For the reason explained above (the saturation of rate-limiting enzyme metabolic reactions), the amount excreted as HPPH is inversely related to the administered dose. Recent studies (Bochner et al., 1973) on renal handling of DPH and HPPH indicate that the renal clearance of DPH (3-23 ml/min) is very low, suggesting a net resorption in the kidney, while HPPH has a clearance of 76 to 420 ml/min, which exceeds the insulin clearance. This suggests that a net secretion of HPPH occurs in the nephron. The clearance of both compounds (DPH and HPPH) appears to be flow-dependent. For this reason it is possible that renal handling of DPH and HPPH involves passive resorption for both the compounds, as well as secretion in the case of HPPH. It is, in fact, known that a moderate water diuresis tends to increase the renal clearance of compounds subject to passive resorption in the renal tubule.

The dihydrodiol and the 3,4-dihydroxy derivatives are probably excreted by active tubular secretion, as are most organic anions and cations.

Alkalinization of urine may enhance the urinary excretion of unchanged DPH. Hypoxia may lead to diminished binding to plasma proteins with increased transfer of free drug in tissues such as brain.

Several interactions between DPH and other drugs have been described in the last 10 years, and detailed information on this topic can be found in recent reviews (Hartshorn, 1972; Kutt, 1972b, 1974; Buchanan and Sholiton, 1972). In adults, the therapeutic range is considered to be between 8 and 25 μg/ml (Schiller and Buchthal, 1958; Buchthal et al., 1960, Buchthal and Lennox-Buchthal, 1958; Kutt, 1972a, Stensrud and Palmer, 1964) Toxic signs such as horizontal nystagmus, ataxia, gait incoordination, disarthria and intention tremor are very frequent with a plasma level of 30 μg/ml or more (Kutt et al., 1964a,b,c; Kutt, 1972a). It must be remembered that seizures may occur as evidence of DPH in-

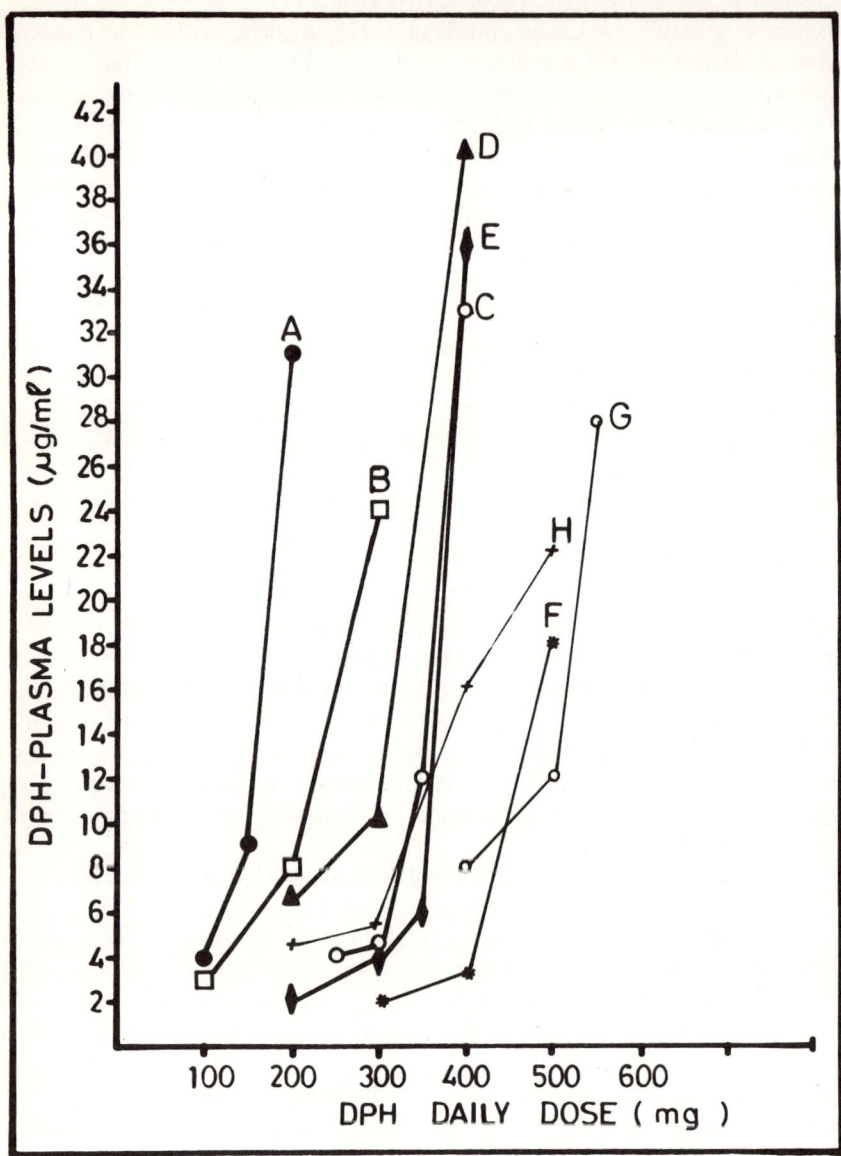

Fig. 3: Effect of dosage increment on diphenylhydantoin plasma levels during chronic treatment in eight epileptic patients. The behavior of plasma levels is indicative of saturation kinetics.

Table 1. Diphenylhydantoin Plasma Protein-Binding in Newborns and Adults

Normal Newborn	Hyperbilirubinemic Newborn	Adult	References
25.7 ±1.5	–	14.2 ±0.6	Ganshorn and Kurz, 1968
16	20.4	10.6	Ernhebo et al., 1971
10.6 ±1.4	15.5 ±0.7	7-4 ±0.7	Rane et al., 1971

Data are expressed as % of free fraction (unbound DPH).

toxication (Lascelles et al., 1970; Levy and Fenichel, 1964). Conditions such as hypoalbuminemia and liver diseases may increase the risk of toxicity (Kutt et al, 1964b; BCDSP., 1973). Hematological complications secondary to DPH therapy are not considered to be dose-related (Glaser, 1972) and are frequently attributed to idiosyncrasy on an immunological basis. However, Reynolds (1972) found a significative negative correlation between folate and DPH levels both in serum and in CSF. Furthermore, a dose-dependent blood discrasia has been recently described by Parker and Gumnit (1974).

Newborns

The date available on diphenylhydantoin in newborns are mainly derived from observations carried out on neonates who received the drug transplacentally. The few observations in which the drug was administered, either orally or intramuscularly, to newborns tend to indicate that the drug absorption is relatively slow and incomplete. Jalling et al. (1970) reported that after intramuscular administration the DPH plasma levels, 4 and 8 h after drug administration (9.3 mg/kg) in a 3-day newborn, were lower than the levels observed before the injection. A similar trend was observed in a 22-day-old newborn after oral administration of 10.4 mg/kg.

Several data (Table 1) indicate that the binding to plasma protein is significantly reduced in the neonate and even more in cases of hyperbilirubinemia (Ganshorn and Kurz, 1968; Ehrnebo et al., 1971; Rane et al., 1971). By equilibrium dialysis, Ehrnebo et al. (1971) found that in the normal neonate the free DPH fraction was about 16%, while in hyperbilirubinemic neonates the free fraction was about 20%. In adults, the corresponding value was 10-11%. By untrafiltration Rane et al. (1971) found a free fraction mean value of 10.6 ± 1.4 in normal neonates, of 15.5 ± 0.7 in hyperbilirubinemic neonates, of 7.4 ± 0.7 in adults. In the same study, an inverse relationship between the plasma albumin concentration and the percentage of unbound DPH, as well as a significant correlation between free DPH and the total bilirubin concentration, were observed. A higher red blood cell/plasma ratio (0.84 against a value of 0.38 in adults) has been recently reported by Borondy et al. (1973) in normal newborns. The low albumin concentration and the increased bilirubin are not the only cause of the reduced binding in newborns; other factors, such as acidosis and hypoxia, could play a role in contributing to lower binding. According to Rane (1974), the apparent volume of distribution of DPH in the newborn is twice the adult value, but the data need to be confirmed.

The elimination rate of transplacentally transferred DPH in the neonates appears in most cases to be characterized by two distinct phases: a first phase that seems to follow zero-order kinetics and may last for 24 to 56 h, and a second phase apparently following first-order kinetics (Mirkin, 1971; Rane et al., 1974). The shift from zero-order to first-order seems to take place for concentrations ranging from 10 to 20 μg/ml (Fig. 2). This biphasic pattern of elimination could be attributed to a dose-dependent rate of elimination due to saturation of the hydroxylase system responsible for metabolism of the drug, but could also be attributed to the elimination after 2-3 days of endogenous substrates capable of competitively inhibiting the DPH metabolism at microsomal levels (Feuer and Liscio, 1969; Kardish and Feuer, 1972; Wilson, 1970; Sereni et al., 1973; see also Chapter 4). Whatever the explanation, further studies are needed to clarify contradictions in the available data. Mirkin has reported an average apparent plasma half-life of 60 h, while Rane et al. reported an apparent half-life, during the first-order phase, of 6 to 34 h (mean: 17.5 h).

According to Horning et al. (1971), Rane et al. (1974) and Reynolds and Mirkin (1973), the newborns of mothers who received DPH or other anticonvulsant agents during pregnancy have the capacity to hydroxylate diphenylhydantoin to pHPPH and to conjugate the resulting pHPPH. The dihydrodiol, also, has been found in the urine of newborns who received the drug either transplacentally or by direct administration (Horning et al., 1971). Whether these data, which are in apparent disagreement with findings on other drugs (see page 55), are due to the peculiarity of the DPH moiety, or may be explained by induction of drug-metabolizing enzymes during fetal life, has not yet been clarified. Recent data by Hoppel et al. (1975), who found that measurable levels of conjugated and unconjugated HPPH are already present at birth, tend to suggest that at least part of the metabolites found in newborn urines are of maternal origin. Further support for this hypothesis is given by the observation of Reynolds and Mirkin (1973), who reported that the percentage of urinary unconjugated HPPH to conjugated HPPH increased as the newborn infant matured. This suggests that the high output of conjugate HPPH during the first 2 to 3 days of life is due to the presence of conjugated compounds of maternal origin. On the whole, the data available indicate that, in newborns who received the drug transplacentally, the elimination rate of DPH may be either very slow or close to adult values. Various factors, such as modification of microsomal enzyme activities either toward induction or inhibition, modification of plasma protein-binding concomitant to rises in bilirubin concentrations (possibly contributing to the fast drop of plasma levels on days 4 and 5), and/or elimination of endogenous substances received from the mother, probably underlie the observed phenomenon and do not allow a clear definition of the problem.

Infants

The data available on DPH plasma levels and kinetics in infants are extremely scarce and refer to four cases ranging from 36 to 78 days of age. In all four cases, the plasma levels following repeated DPH administration, either by oral or intramuscular route, were extremely low when compared to the administered dose (Jalling et al., 1970). Whether this can be attributed to poor absorption or to decreased binding, which would thus facilitate increased tissue uptake and metabolism, or to enhanced catabolism because of enzyme induction, as seen with other compounds, cannot be concluded on the basis of the available data. However, it may be of interest to underline the fact that one of the four cases, a premature infant of 34 days, whose mother received anticonvulsivant treatment throughout the pregnancy, had plasma levels of 1-2 μ/ml with an oral dose of 9.4 mg/kg.

Children

Orally administered diphenylhydantoin is efficiently absorbed in children, with peak plasma levels attained 2 to 6 h after the dose. A poor oral absorption was reported by Borofsky et al. (1973) in an 18-month-old child, where 18 mg/kg had to be given in order to reach therapeutic levels. From the data of Weiss et al. (1969), capsules containing the sodium form or suspensions containing free acid lead to more or less similar levels in the course of chronic treatment. According to Buchanan et al. (1969b), a single oral dose of 10 mg/kg gives peak plasma levels of 8 to 12 μg/ml, while in the course or repeated phenobarbital administration DPH peak plasma levels following the same oral dose are reduced from 3 to 7 μg/ml. Despite the fact that the authors invoke an increased metabolic rate, due to PB, to explain the observed phenomenon, the data seem to point to an interaction at the absorption level.

As reported for adults and newborns, DPH administered by intramuscular route is absorbed very slowly and inefficiently. In a recent study, Wilensky and Lowden (1973) were unable to reach the therapeutic range, despite very high i.m. doses of DPH; the levels rose 3 to 4 times when the dose was switched to the oral route. The reducted absorption during the i.m. administration period was documented not only by very low plasma levels but also by a very low urinary excretion of HPPH (10-20% of the administered dose).

No data are available on DPH plasma protein-binding in children. The existing few data on the CSF content of DPH in epileptic children on chronic DPH treatment suggest that, at ages of 4 to 7 years, the binding of DPH to plasma proteins is of the same order as that observed in adults (89-90%) (Borofsky et al., 1973).

Several papers indicate that the individual variability and the wide scattering of the plasma level-dose relationship during chronic treatment are more pronounced in children than in adults (Svensmark and Buchthal, 1964; Diamond and Buchanan, 1971; Buchanan and Allen, 1971; Garrettson and Dayton, 1970; Borofsky et al., 1972; Buchanan et al., 1973b). Even if no clear kinetic data are available, there seems to be a general agreement on the fact that younger children (below 20-25 kg of body weight, 1 to 6 years of age) require higher doses of DPH than older children and adults in order to obtain plasma levels in the therapeutic range (Buchthal and Svensmark, 1971; Melchior et al., 1971; Gauchel et al., 1973; Dawson and Jamieson, 1971, Sherwin et al., 1974). The higher drug requirements may be due, as for other drugs (see Chapters 8, 14), to an increased drug clearance that is sustained by an increased metabolic rate. Buchanan and Allen (1971) found that in about 50% of the children receiving DPH alone the serum level-dose ratio was 1 or less. More recent observations of Borofsky et al. (1972) clearly indicate that in children from birth to 4 years of age there is a definite tendency to unusually low levels with levels/dose ratios less than 1. Extending these data, Berlet (1975) demonstrated that, assigning the ratios of serum level per drug dose to the most frequently represented age groups of 4 to 8, 8 to 12, and 12 to 16 years, the ratios of serum levels to drug doses rise significantly as the children grow older. This phenomenon reflects a decrease in the overall elimination of DPH and appears to be a continuous phenomenon from infancy to adolescence. Similar data with different age groups (1-6, 6-11 and 11-16) were also reported by Nolte and Brugmann (1975), who showed that in order to reach plasma levels of about 10 μg/ml, the younger children required about twice as much DPH as the older group.

If knowledge of these age differences is the basis for a correct therapeutic approach, it is also very true that, because of wide individual differences, both in therapeutic response and metabolism, a common therapeutic level is not to be expected; monitoring of plasma levels is always necessary. In children, the apparent plasma T½ of DPH may vary from less than 12 h to 35 h or more (Borofsky et al., 1973; Berlet, 1975) and the mean urinary excretion of HPPH from 59 to 88%. This mean value of 59-88% in 24 h is higher than that reported for adults and suggests an increased metabolic rate in the pediatric patients. In cases of rapid metabolism, the HPPH excretion may be as high as 91% of administered DPH (Borofsky et al., 1973), and in cases with unusually high serum DPH levels the HPPH excretion may be as low as 40-27% of the administered dose. In the three cases of acute intoxication in young children (2 to 4 years) following a massive accidental ingestion of DPH, the recorded apparent T½ was 66, 62 and 46 h with a DPH/HPPH ratio in urine of about 9%, the usual ratio being less than 2% (Wilder et al., 1973a). These data suggest a limited capacity of liver enzymes. The daily fluctuations in plasma DPH levels appear to be minimal (12-17%) if the drug is given t.i.d., but they may reach higher values (40-50%) if the drug is given only once or twice daily (Berlet, 1975, Buchthal and Svensmark, 1971). Minimal fluctuations following a single daily dose are, on the contrary, reported by Buchanan et al. (1973b) in a limited number of children. The whole body of data clearly indicates that in prescribing DPH to children, two distinct and very important factors must be considered: the age of the patient and the dose.

The findings of Borofsky et al. (1973) and of Nolte and Brugmann (1975) demonstrate that in children, like adults, DPH follows Michaelis-Menten kinetics. This means that small increases in dosages may result in unexpected and unusually high plasma DPH concentrations. According to Borofsky et al. (1973), with doses lower than 5 mg/kg the serum level/dose ratio is usually around 1, but with doses from 5 to 8 mg/kg this ratio may rise to 2 or 3 and may be even higher for bigger dosages. Similar data are reported by Garrettson and Dayton (1970) and by Nolte and Brugmann (1975). The individual variability is probably linked to individual differences (due to both genetic and environmental factors) in the saturation point of parahydroxylating enzymes, as has been well documented in adults. Regarding the possible influence of PB on DPH, and vice versa, there is a considerable amount of data which indicate that PB may enhance the metabolism of DPH, and that DPH may competitively inhibit the PB hydroxylation (Morselli et al., 1971b). This phenomenon is not an absolute one and depends on the preexisting levels of enzymatic activity, as well as on the relative concentrations of the two drugs (Garrettson and Dayton, 1971; Morselli et al., 1971b; Buchthal and Svensmark, 1971);

The therapeutic level in children is generally considered to range between 7 to 20 μg/ml, and a clear relationship between serum levels and seizure control in individual cases (Fig. 4) has been reported recently by Borofsky et al. (1973) and Morselli (1974). Patients not responding to DPH plasma levels of 20-25 μg/ml should be considered refractory to DPH, and the drug should not be administered.

With regard to the chronic toxic side effects, there seems to be general agreement on the following two facts: there is not sufficient reliability in the clinical signs of intoxication, especially in younger children, and common side effects

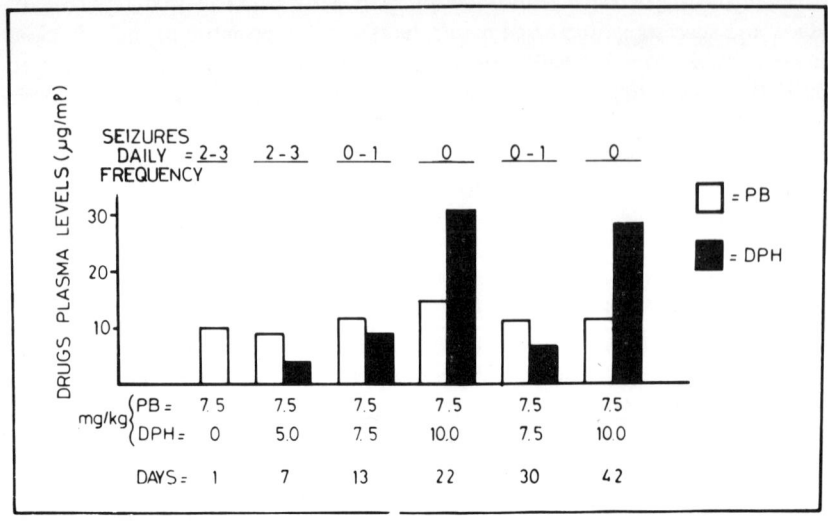

Fig. 4: Relationships between diphenylhydantoin plasma levels and clinical effects in an epileptic child (8 years old). On day 23, ataxia was evident and conditioned a dose reduction with subsequent drop in plasma levels of DPH and reappearance of crisis. By returning to 10 mg/Kg day, full control of attacks was achieved although a certain degree of ataxia could not be avoided.

are frequently absent even for concentrations of 30-40 µg/ml (Patel and Crichton, 1968; Weiss et al., 1969, Melchior, 1971, Buchanan and Allen, 1971; Nolte and Brügmann, 1975; Berlet, 1975). When present, the most common signs of toxicity are vomiting, gingivitis, hypertrophy, somnolence and ataxia, while nystagmus apparently is not frequent in children. According to Buchanan and Allen, more than 50% of their patients with DPH levels over 20 µg/ml were free of any clinical symptoms of toxicity. On the other hand, as in adults, an increase in seizure frequency may be observed with plasma levels over the toxic threshold (Patel and Crichton, 1968). Once more, this stresses the fact that in children excessive DPH plasma or serum concentration cannot always be detected by clinical signs, and that monitoring of plasma levels may have an important role in therapeutic management. In cases of acute intoxication, impaired levels of consciousness may be associated with behavior instability or stimulation (Holcomb et al., 1972; Wilder et al., 1973a). Episodes of opistontonus have been described with plasma DPH levels over 100 µg/ml (Tenckhoff et al., 1968). The level of consciousness and the neurological picture appears to improve as the plasma DPH levels descend below 40-35 µg/ml (Tenckhoff et al., 1968; Holcomb et al.,

1972; Wilder et al., 1973a). Besides neurological signs of toxicity, hyperglycemia and hypoinsulinemia may be present in course of an acute intoxication (Glaser, 1972; Holcomb et al., 1972). The possible psychiatric implication linked to a folate deficiency induced by DPH or PB have been extensively reviewed by Reynolds (1972). Hypersensitivity reactions, skin rashes and depression of the hematopoietic system appear to have in children more or less the same incidence as in adults (Glaser, 1972; Reynolds, 1972). Hypocalcemia with radiologic evidence of rickets or decreased bone density is, on the contrary, a toxic side effect which may be of greater relevance in a developing organism, and whose significant incidence has been clearly documented by several reports in the last years (Kruse, 1968; Richens and Rowe, 1970; Hunter et al., 1971; Borgstedt et al., 1972; De Luca et al., 1972; Lifshitz and Maclaren, 1973; Hahn et al., 1975). The probable increased catabolism of vitamin D induced by DPH and PB is supposed to play a major role in the pathogenesis of the disorder. The incidence of hypocalcemia associated with bone disorders may vary from 4 to 30%, according to the various authors; however, low serum calcium and phosphorus with elevated alkaline phosphates are a quite common finding in epileptic children treated with DPH and/or PB. In a recent study, a significant decrease in serum calcium, serum 25-hydroxycalciferol, and a significant reduction in bone mass, was a constant finding in 32 children treated with either DPH alone or in combination with PB (Hahn et al., 1975). According to Lifshitz and Maclaren (1973), vitamin D-dependent rickets associated with long-term anticonvulsant medication may occur in a significant percentage of the population after one year of treatment. These studies suggest that vitamin D supplementation should be given to children who need long-term anticonvulsant drug therapy.

PHENOBARBITAL

Adults

Phenobarbital administered by the oral route to adult epileptic patients, at daily dosages of 2-3 mg/kg, is almost completely absorbed (80-90%), with a peak plasma level between 4 to 18 h after the drug intake (Maynert, 1972a; Butler et al., 1954; Lous, 1954a; Svensmark and Buchthal, 1963a). The rate of absorption from the gastrointestinal tract is variable and depends on various factors, such as the preparation, the rate of gastric emptying and the presence of food or other drugs. The sodium salt form is absorbed more rapidly than the free acid (Sjogren et al., 1965).

During chronic treatment, it is assumed that phenobarbital is more or less evenly distributed throughout the various organs and extracellular fluids, while with acute parenteral (i.v.) administration it distributes more rapidly to the

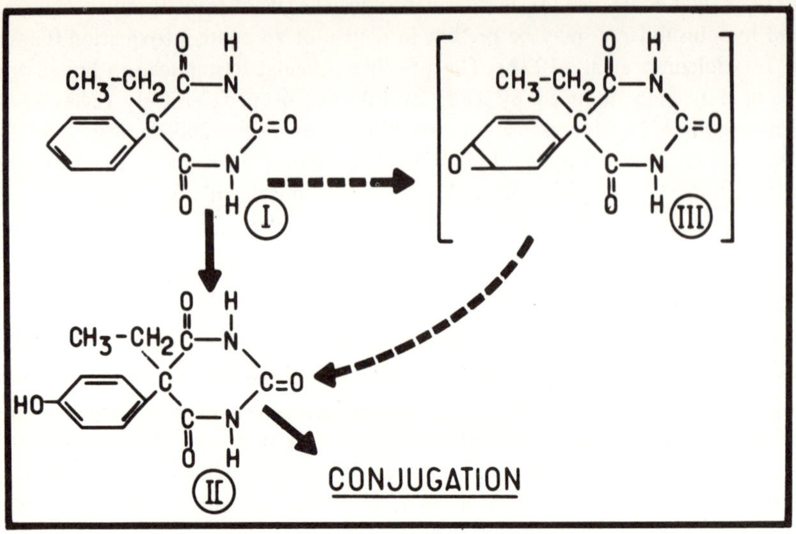

Fig. 5: Metabolism of phenobarbital in man. I. Phenobarbital; II. 5-Ethyl-5(4-hydroxyphenyl)barbituric acid; III. Hypothyzed epoxide.

high blood flow organs (Maynert, 1972a). Moreover, it enters the brain relatively slowly; therefore, immediate efficacy cannot be expected in the case of status epilepticus. With chronic PB treatment, the brain/plasma ratios of the drug are about 0.59-0.91 (Ploman and Persson; 1957, Sherwin et al., 1973; Vajda et al., 1974).

Under normal conditions, the apparent volume of distribution of PB is 0.60-0.75 L/kg. and the drug is about 46-48% bound to plasma proteins (Lous, 1954b, Waddel and Butler, 1957). Due to its pKa value of 7.2, the drug is extremely sensitive to pH variations in the plasma, with an increased transfer from plasma to the tissues every time the blood pH decreases (acidosis) and the reverse during increased blood pH (alkalosis) (Waddel and Butler, 1957; Maynert, 1972a).

The apparent plasma half-life is prolonged and may range from 60 to 140 h (Butler et al., 1954; Lous, 1954a; Morselli et al., 1971b; Maynert, 1972b).

About 55 to 75% of the dose of phenobarbital is metabolized very slowly in the liver, and another 20-35% is excreted unchanged in the urine (Butler, 1956; Maynert, 1972a,b). The main metabolic pathway of PB in man is via parahydroxylation of the phenyl ring (Fig. 5) (Butler, 1956). The resulting p-hydroxyphenobarbital is then partially (50-54%) excreted as such and partially (46-49%)

as the glucuronide derivative after conjugation with clucuronic acid (Butler, 1956; Algeri and McBay, 1956; Maynert, 1972b). Dihydrodiols have not been reported in the biotransformation of phenobarbital in man; also, the formation of an oxirane derivative as the initial step of the oxidation of the aromatic ring has been hypothyzed (Horning et al., 1973; Maynert, 1972b). The p-hydroxyphenobarbital is practically devoid of any anticonvulsant activity and, due to its higher polarity, is not reabsorbed at the tubular level, thus it is rapidly excreted. On the contrary, phenobarbital is probably reabsorbed at the tubular level, since its renal clearance is about 4-5 mg/min at normal urinary pH and urine flow-dependent. A rise in urinary pH may condition a significant increase in the renal clearance of the drug, which may reach values of 29 ml/min (Waddel and Butler, 1957). The toxicity of phenobarbital may be increased in patients with renal disease (Maynert, 1972a), and unusually high plasma levels, if referred to the dose, have also been described in obesity and liver disease (Svensmark and Buchthal, 1963a; Kutt et al., 1964b). Phenobarbital may interact with several drugs and its toxicity may increase in cases of metabolic inhibition (Cucinell, 1972; Hartshorn, 1972) or in cases of low urinary pH (e.g., instances of elevated ingestion of vitamin C).

In adults, the therapeutic range is generally considered to be between 16 and 30 µg/ml (Buchthal and Lennox-Buchthal, 1972b). Toxic symptoms such as drowsiness, sedation, nystagmus on lateral gaze, ataxia and dysarthria may occur frequently at plasma concentrations over 40 µg/ml and present at levels over 80 µg/ml (Lous, 1954c; Sunshine, 1957; Buchthal and Svensmark, 1959, 1960; Plaa and Hine, 1960; Booker, 1972a; Browning and Maynert, 1972). As in the case of DPH, a high level of PB may increase frequency of seizures. Blood discarsia (macrocitosis and megaloblastic anemia) and musculoskeletal and coagulation disorders may also be occasionally observed in the course of chronic treatment (Browning and Maynert, 1972; Richens and Rowe, 1970; Kirboe and Plum, 1966; Klipstein, 1964; Chanarin et al., 1958; De Vries, 1965). According to Hutt et al. (1968), at levels appropriate for the control of seizures, mental performance may not be optimal.

Newborns

A considerable amount of data on phenobarbital pharmacokinetics in newborns has become available in recent years, mainly through the studies of Boréus' group. In the newborn, phenobarbital is absorbed promptly if administered by the intramuscular route. Maximal levels are generally attained within 2 to 4 h, followed by a plateau, and in some cases the absorption peak may be delayed to as much as 8 h. The peak levels expressed in µg/ml are on the order of 1.3 times the dose (mg/kg) (Boréus et al., 1975; Jalling, 1976). After oral administration, the peak concentrations are lower in relation to the dose, and the time of maximal concentrations may range from 4 to 14 h (Boréus et al., 1975; Jalling, 1976). These data indicate that in newborns 1 to 15 days of age the absorption following oral administration is less reliable and predictable than that following intramuscular injection. The plasma protein-binding is significantly reduced in newborns compared to that in adults. The "free fraction" oscillates from 57 to 64% of the total drug in the plasma, and in hyperbilirubinemia it may be as high as 72% (Ganshorn and Kurz, 1968; Ehrnebo et al., 1971).

Jalling (1976) has shown that during chronic treatment phenobarbital is present in the CSF at concentrations ranging from 48 to 83% of those in the plasma. It is of interest to note that the higher value was observed in a case with documented alteration of the blood-brain barrier and that the lower values (0.48-0.58) were observed in 2 newborns, 14 and 21 days of age. The fact that no phenobarbital was found in the CSF, despite plasma levels of 3 and 4 μg/ml, in two cases where lumbar puncture was performed within 40 min of oral administration, may be taken as an example of the slow entry of PB into the brain. The apparent volume of distribution in the neonate is somewhat larger than in infants or adults and may vary between 0.59 to 1.54 l/kg (Boréus et al., 1975; Jalling, 1976).

The apparent plasma disappearance rate of PB, administered either directly to the newborn or prenatally through the mother, appears to be significantly lower than that observed in infants or in adults. Prenatally administered, the apparent plasma half-life may vary from 75 to 577 h (Melchior et al., 1967; Jalling et al., 1973), and the data point to a significant (P <0.001) inverse correlation between the newborn apparent plasma half-life and the time exposure to the drug. In other words, a long period of prenatal treatment seems to be associated with a plasma disappearance rate similar to, or shorter than, that in adults, whereas a short period of medication is associated with a very long plasma half-life (Jalling et al., 1973; Boréus et al., 1975). Induction of the newborn liver microsomal enzymes taking place during intrauterine life is the probable explanation of this phenomenon.

In most cases, the phenobarbital plasma disappearance rate follows first-order kinetics, but, as described for diphenylhydantoin (p. 318), a biphasic plasma disappearance curve may also be observed. Jalling et al. (1973) and Boréus et al. (1975) described 3 newborns in whom a change from a slow to a fast disappearance rate was observed between the 5th and 7th day of life. As stated before, several factors may condition such a phenomenon. Product inhibition, sudden variation in diuresis or displacement from binding to plasma proteins due to increased levels of bilirubin (which reaches its maximal concentrations after 3-4 days in full-term newborns and 5-7 days in prematures) seem the most likely reasons, but the phenomenon might also be due to the disappearance of endogenous competitive inhibitors.

After direct administration to the newborn, the apparent plasma half-life may range from 69 to 165 h (mean: 97 h), according to Wallin et al. (1974), and from 59 to 182 (mean: 109 h) according to Jalling (1976); yet premature newborns all show slower rates of disposition. This emphasizes the importance of careful age characterization when pharmacokinetic data in the newborn period are interpreted. The same authors also demonstrated that a prophylactic phenobarbital administration of 5 mg/kg in the first 4 h, followed by the daily administration of the same dose, is inadequate to reach PB levels effective against hyperbilirubinemia. Under such conditions, effective PB levels are generally reached only after 4-5 days. According to Wallin et al. (1974), the PB administration should be carried out in such a way that "the effect on bilirubin concentration is manifest as early as possible and well before the maximal levels of bilirubin are attained." The authors quote favorably the report of Zacka and Frenzel (1971), who noted a significant reduction of bilirubin levels administering PB intramuscularly at 10 mg/kg, twice a day, during the first 2 days of life.

In the treatment of neonatal convulsions, PB should be administered not in repeated small doses, which result in a slow approach to a steady-state level, but in a relatively large first dose, aimed at quickly attaining a therapeutic PB concentration in the CNS.

The newborn is capable of metabolizing phenobarbital, even if at a lower rate than infants and children. Horning et al. (1973) reported that newborns could hydroxylate PB but that no traces of conjugated derivatives could be detected. On the contrary, according to Boréus et al. (1975), both the p-hydroxyphenobarbital and its conjugated derivative are present, even if in traces, in newborn urine within 4-8 h after the drug intake. The portion of unchanged PB excreted in the urine appears to be directly related to the diuresis, while the maximum excretion of conjugated p-OH is reached after 5-6 days. It is interesting that, in the case reported by Boréus, during the first 24-48 hours of life the unchanged PB represented about 70% of the urinary output of the drug, while it was only 40-35% on the 5th-6th day of life. According to Jalling (1976), in the first 2 weeks of life day-to-day variations may be present in the rate of disappearance of PB from the plasma, and in some cases this phenomenon may be accompanied by an alteration in renal function. The effective phenobarbital levels in newborns range between 12 and 20 $\mu g/ml$, and sedation may be evident with plasma levels of 41 $\mu g/ml$ (Jalling, 1976).

Infants

In infants, phenobarbital is well absorbed after both intramuscular and oral administration; peak plasma levels are generally attained after 2-4 h, and no significant differences are evident between intramuscular and oral administration (Jalling, 1976; Boreus et al., 1975). Following a single dose, the peak concentration expressed as $\mu g/ml$ is generally equal to 1.6 times the dose expressed in

Table 2. Phenobarbital Apparent Plasma Half-Life and Apparent Volume of Distribution During Development

	Newborns	Infants	Children	Adults
Apparent plasma half-life (h)	*234 ±43 (6)a 199 ±20 (9)a 186 ±56 (10)b 107 ±10 (10)c 110 ±11 (13)d	68 ±6 (18)e 51 ±8 (4)f 47 ±8 (15)g	38 ±10 (5)h 36 ±64 (2)f	132 ±18 (5)h 64 ±141 l,m,n
Apparent volume of distribution (L/Kg)	0.59-1.54	0.46-1.31	0.50-0.55	0.50-0.60

The reported values have been calculated from the available literature data:
(a) Jalling et al., 1973; (b) Melchior et al., 1967; (c) Wallin et al., 1974; (d) Jalling, 1975a;
(e) Jalling, 1975b; (f) Garrettson and Dayton, 1970; (g) Heinz and Kampffmeyer, 1971;
(h) Morselli et al., 1971; (l) Lous, 1954; (m) Butler et al., 1964; (n) Maynert, 1972a.
*Premature newborns. Number of patients in brackets.

mg/kg. No data are available on protein-binding; however, the CSF/plasma concnetration ratios observed by Jalling in 6 infants (3 to 16 months of age) suggest that plasma protein-binding of phenobarbital is close to adult values. The observed ratios varied from 0.44 to 0.57, with a mean value of 0.51, and the equilibrium between plasma and CSF was attained within 4 h. The apparent volume of distribution for infants of 1 to 3 months of age may vary from 0.41 to 1.31 L/kg, with a mean value of 0.69 ± 0.16 according to Heinze and Kampffmeyer (1971). A similar value has recently been reported by Jalling (1975b), who, in infants of 6 to 18 months of age, described an apparent volume of distribution of 0.63 ± 0.09 L/kg, with individual values ranging from 0.47 ± 0.76 L/Kg.

The plasma disappearance rate of phenobarbital is generally faster in infants than in newborns or adults (Table 2). Heinze and Kampffmeyer (1971) reported apparent plasma half-lives ranging from 21 to 68 h (mean: 47 ± 8 h) in infants of 1 to 3 months of age, and Wilson and Wilkinson (1973) reported an apparent plasma half-life of 39 h in a 6-month-old girl. Similarly, Garrettson and Dayton (1970), in 4 infants from 10 to 18 months of age, described an apparent plasma half-life for phenobarbital of 38-78 h (mean 51 ± 8 h). More recently, in a larger study, Jalling (1976) demonstrated that in 15 infants (11-19 months) the apparent phenobarbital half-life varied from 37 to 133 h, with a mean value of

69 h. In this group of patients, only 1 had plasma half-lives over 100 h, and in 9 of the 15 the T½ was below 60 h. The same author has also reported an unexpected relationship between the PB dose and the plasma half-life; the higher the dose, the shorter the half-life. No explanations for such a phenomenon are available, but similar data have recently been described with digoxin (Morselli et al., 1975).

In infants, a biexponential decay of the phenobarbital plasma concentration curve may also be observed in selected cases (Wilson and Wilkinson, 1973; Jalling, 1976). No data are available on urinary excretion of phenobarbital and its metabolites in infancy. The therapeutic level in this age group is supposed to be above 15 μg/ml (Faero et al., 1972).

Our knowledge on adverse phenobarbital effects in infancy is very poor; in fact, the evaluation of common phenobarbital side effects may be very difficult in the acutely ill infant. Respiratory depression seems to be rare, even at very high plasma levels (80-100 μg/ml) (Wilson and Wilkinson, 1973; Buchthal and Svensmark, 1971). Recently, we observed a marked improvement in the psychomotor performance in a series of 8 cases (12-18 months of age) with a lowering of the PB levels from 45-50 to 20-15 μg/ml. These factors, the difficulty in accurate objective evaluation of PB side effects and the fact that high levels may impair the psychomotor development stress both the need and the value of continuous monitoring of plasma levels during therapy with phenobarbital in infancy.

Children

In children, phenobarbital is absorbed quite rapidly either orally or after intramuscular administration. In both situations, after a single dose of about 3-5 mg/kg, peak plasma levels are attained between 2 and 4 h (Fig. 6). However, in cases of combined treatment with other anticonvulsant drugs, or in cases using higher doses, the absorption peak following oral intake may be delayed up to 8-12 h. Even if no data are available on protein-binding, it is generally assumed that this parameter is in the adult range, and the same applies to the apparent volume of distribution.

It is generally agreed that children dispose of phenobarbital at a faster rate than do adults (Plaa and Hine, 1960; Svensmark and Buchthal, 1964; Buchthal and Svensmark, 1971). In children from 5 to 10 years of age, we found that the apparent plasma half-life varied from 21 to 78 h (mean value: 38 ± 10). In four cases, the disappearance curve followed first-order kinetics (21,25,30 and 38 h) while in the fifth case there were zero-order kinetics (Morselli et al., 1971). The reasons for such behavior are not obvious but do not seem related to the initial phenobarbital levels. Apparent plasma half-lives of 37 and 64 h have been re-

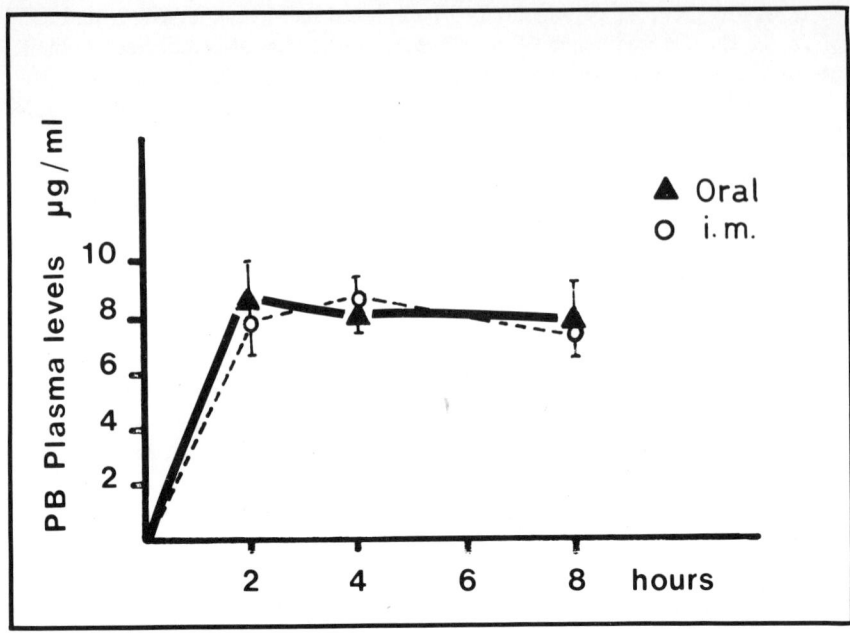

Fig. 6: Phenobarbital plasma levels in five epileptic children (3 to 5 years of age) following an administration of 5 mg/Kg by oral and intramuscular route.

ported by Garrettson and Dayton (1970) in two children of 2 and 4 years, respectively.

A point which emerges quite clearly from the data in the literature is that significant differences in the rate of phenobarbital disposition linked to the individual's maturational stage may be present within the pediatric age group. Svensmark and Buchthal, by grouping patients according to body weight and age, could show significant differences in the level/dose relationship, with values of 4.8 ± 0.2 for the 10-20 kg group (1-6 year) and 6.9 ± 0.3 for the 30-48 kg group (10-14 years). The adult value in their study was 9.9 ± 0.4. A level/dose ratio of 4 to 7 is reported by Buchanan et al. (1969b) in 4 children of 5 to 7.5 years of age. According to our observations, more or less similar results were obtained with children receiving phenobarbital alone (Fig. 7), while the differences between age groups appear to be smaller in cases of combined therapy. However, a wide scattering of data was present in each group considered; therefore, even if useful for determining the initial dose, those ratios do not permit a precise prediction of the dosage required by the individual patient. The PB plasma levels are usually unpredictable during combined therapy.

The practical implication of these data is not only that children require a

ANTIEPILEPTICS

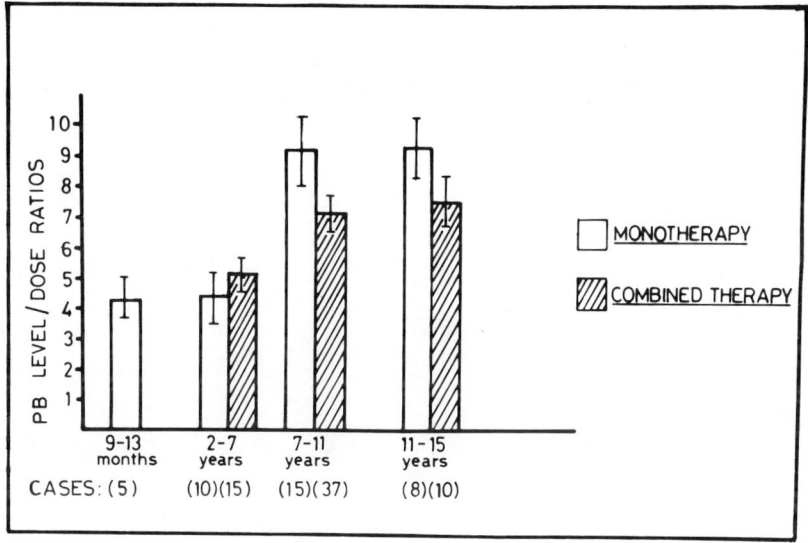

Fig. 7: Effect of age and associated treatment on phenobarbital level/dose ratios in course of chornic treatment.

higher dose to maintain therapeutic levels, but also that the compound should be administered 2 or 3 times daily to avoid large serum fluctuations. The therapeutic level is considered to be between 15 and 30 µg/ml (Buchthal and Svensmark, 1960; Melchior, 1965; Buchthal and Svensmark, 1971; Morselli et al., 1971). Regarding side effects, there is general agreement that children may tolerate exceptionally high levels of phenobarbital without evident toxic effects, and levels as high as 80 µg/ml are compatible with a clear sensorium (Solow and Green, 1972; Wilson and Wilkinson, 1973; Buchthal and Svensmark, 1971; Rizzo et al., 1976). In the case of vitamin D-dependent hypocalcemia, it seems that what has been described for DPH holds true for PB also. A decline in scholastic performance may be observed after a few months of PB therapy, and according to Eadie and Tyrer (1974) personality changes and insidious blunting of intellectual function may occur in the course of chronic phenobarbital therapy.

PRIMIDONE

Adults

Following a single oral dose of 500 mg, peak primidone plasma levels of 5-10 µg/ml are attained between 0.5 and 9 h with an average of 3 h, while in the

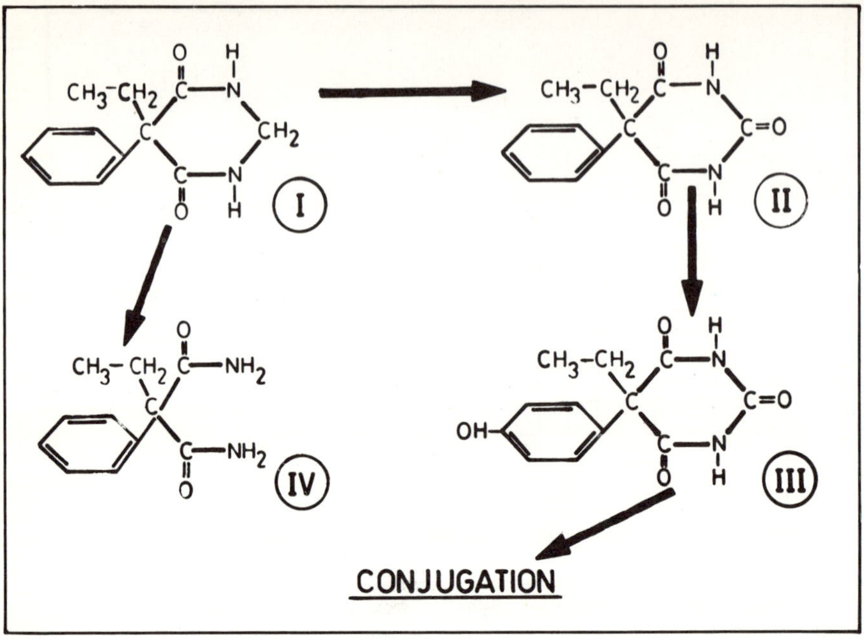

Fig. 8: Metabolism of primidone in man. I. Primidone; II. Phenobarbital-(5-ethyl-5-phenyl)barbituric acid; III. 5-ethyl-5(p-hydroxyphenyl)barbituric acid; IV. Phenylethylmalonamide.

course of chronic treatment peak plasma levels tend to occur later (Booker et al., 1970; Gallagher and Baumel, 1972a). The compound is not bound to plasma proteins, and the CSF/plasma ratios are close to unity in agreement with the binding data (Reynolds et al., 1971; Gallagher and Baumel, 1972a). The apparent plasma half-life may vary from 3.3 to 12.5 h (Booker et al., 1970; Gallagher and Baumel, 1972; Baumel et al., 1972). In man, primidone is quickly metabolized to phenylethylmalonamide (PEMA) and more slowly to phenobarbital (Fig. 8). PEMA is, in fact, measurable 1-2 h after primidone dosing and reaches a peak plasma level after 7-8 h (Gallagher and Baumel, 1971; Baumel et al., 1972; Gallagher et al., 1972). Like primidone, PEMA is not bound to plasma proteins and is present in CSF at concentrations similar to those in the plasma (Baumel et al., 1972), and its apparent plasma half-life may vary from 29 to 36 h. Phenobarbital is measurable only 24-48 h after initiating a repeated primidone treatment. There are no data on the urinary excretion of primidone and PEMA in man. In the case of chronic treatment, PEMA levels appear to be relatively stable and on the same order, or less, than those of phenobarbital (Baumel et al., 1972; Gallagher and Baumel, 1972b). Since PEMA has been proven in animals to possess anticonvulsant activity independent from that of pehnobarbital, it may also contribute to the therapeutic effect (Gallagher et al., 1970; Baumel et al., 1972; Gallagher and Baumel, 1972c). However, no clear data in man are available at this time. From the study of Gallagher et al. (1973), the early toxicity of primidone (nystagmus, drowsiness and nausea) is clearly produced by the drug itself and not by its metabolites. Phenobarbital, moreover, may induce tolerance to the toxic effects of primidone. There are no clear data on the therapeutic levels of primidone and PEMA. Levels of primidone over 10-15 µg/ml may be associated with sedation, vertigo, nausea, nystagmus, ataxia and lethargy (Booker, 1972b; Gallagher et al., 1973). Immunological reactions, hematological disorders, probably due to folic acid deficiency and osteomalacia, may also be present. Whether they are solely related to primidone or PEMA or PB is as yet unknown (Booker, 1972b). According to Cereghino et al. (1973), carbamazepine may lead to a rise in plasma primidone levels

Newborns

Primidone per se crosses the placenta and may be present in the urine of newborns during the first 24-30 h (Martinez and Snyder, 1973). No appreciable formation of phenobarbital from primidone could be detected in newborns for the first 48 h. The data are in agreement with the adult data, which indicate that formation of phenobarbital from primidone is not detectable until 24-48 h. No other kinetic data are as yet available on primidone levels in infancy or childhood.

ETHOSUXIMIDE

Adults

In adults, ethosuximide seems to be promptly and efficiently absorbed following oral administration. Blood levels, after an oral dose of 500-1,000 mg, reach peak levels of 15-24 µg/ml within 1 to 4 h (Hansen and Feldberg, 1964; Chang et al., 1972b; Buchanan et al., 1973a). The peak is generally followed by a plateau for 12-20 h and steady-state levels are reached (depending on the dose) between 5 and 9 days. Once the steady state is reached and constant intake is maintained, there are very minimal daily fluctuation (11-20%) of the plasma level (Hansen and Feldberg, 1964; Chang et al., 1972b; Buchanan et al., 1973a; Sherwin, 1973; Sherwin and Robb, 1972; Sherwin et al., 1973b). No significant degree of protein-binding occurs for ethosuximide, and a CSF/plasma ratio of

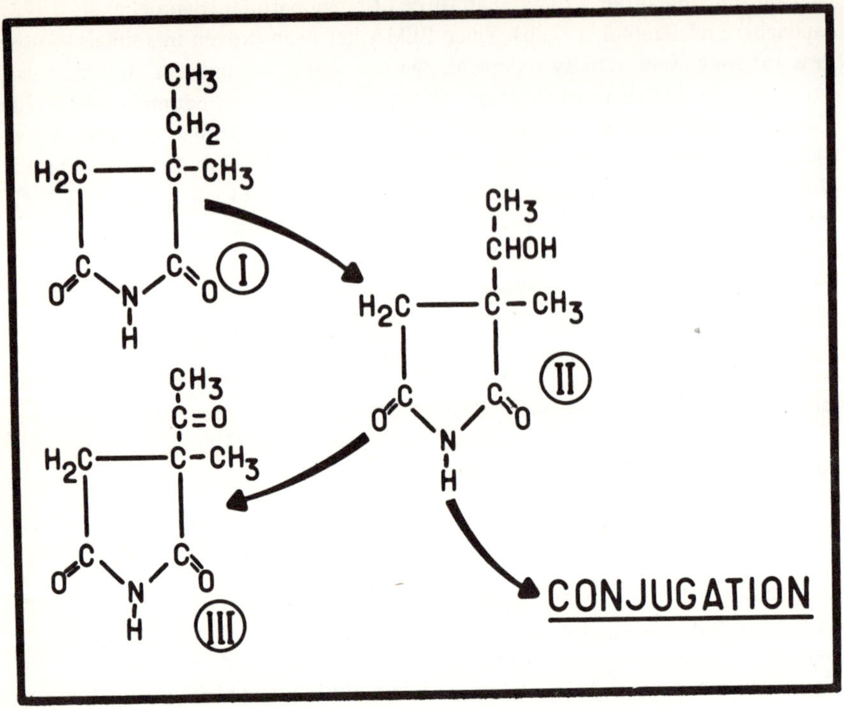

Fig. 9: Metabolism of ethosuximide in man. I. Ethosuximide; II. 2(1-hydroxyethyl)-2methylsuccinimide; III. 2-acetyl-2-methylsuccinimide.

1.01 ± 0.15 has been reported by Sherwin et al. (1972). The apparent volume of distribution of the drug is about 0.61 L/kg, according to Buchanan et al. (1973a). The apparent plasma half-life in man may vary from 55 to 66 h following a single dose (Dill et al., 1965; Chang et al., 1972b; Sherwin et al., 1972) On the basis of this finding, both a single daily treatment schedule (Buchanan et al., 1973a) and one using medication twice daily (Sherwin, 1973) have been proposed.

The compound is rather extensively metabolized since only 12 to 24% of the administered dose can be recovered as such in the urine (Chang et al., 1972b; Buchanan et al., 1973). As reported in Fig. 9, so far two major metabolites have been identified in the urine of patients and volunteers; these are the 2-(1-hydroxyethyl)-2-methylsuccinimide (which is further conjugated with glucuronic acid and is present in urine representing 40% of the administered dose) and the 2-acetyl-2-methylsuccinimide (Chang et al., 1972a). The presence of 2-(2-hydroxyethyl)-2-methylsuccinimide has also been reported (Hill et al., 1973). The urinary clearance of ethosuximide is very low (1.9 ml/min (Buchanan et al., 1973a), and, since the drug is not bound to plasma protein at any significant extent, the data are indicative of a significant resorption at tubular level.

The therapeutic level of ethosuximide is generally considered to range between 40 and 80 µg/ml (Penry et al., 1972; Sherwin and Robb, 1972; Sherwin et al., 1973b). Side effects appear to be dose-related and usually manifest upon initiating the therapy and when the dose is increased. The most common toxic signs include gastric disturbances, fatigue, lethargy, headache and dizziness. Skin and the hematopoietic system may also be target organs (Buchanan, 1972).

Psychotic episodes following ethosuximide therapy have been described by Roger et al. (1968), in adolescent and young adults. Even if side effects appear to be dose-dependent in some cases, plasma levels as high as 170 µg/ml have been described without toxic effects (Buchanan, 1972; Sherwin and Robb, 1972).

Newborns, Infants and Children

Only one report is available on ethosuximide in newborns (Hill et al., 1973). The data refer to transplacentally administered ETS, and in this case analysis carried out on the mother's and neonate's urine by means of MS-GC showed the presence of the same compounds which were identified as 2-(1-hydroxyethyl)2-methylsuccinimide and 2-(2-hydroxyethyl)-2-methylsuccinimide. No quantitative estimate was performed and no traces of ethosuximide were identified in the newborn early urine. Whether the compounds found in newborn urine were of maternal origin or not cannot be concluded on the basis of the available data.

In children, ethosuximide is rapidly absorbed, both as capsule and as syrup. Wechselberg and Hübel (1967) described a peak level of about 20 µg/ml 1-2 h after an oral dose of 250 mg. Peak levels between 1 and 7 h are reported by Buchanan et al. (1969a) and Haerer et al. (1970) after a 500 mg dose administered as syrup or as capsule. The syrup absorption is faster, but the forms are equivalent. As in adults, peak levels are followed by a plateau which lasts about 12 h. In the course of repeated treatment, minimal fluctuations (10-20%) are present in plasma levels. The calculated volume of distribution in children from 6 to 8 years of age is 0.69 L/kg, very close to the adult value (Buchanan et al., 1969a). It appears evident from the various reports that children require relatively higher dosages of ethosuximide to achieve levels comparable to adult levels.

Some of the data available in the literature have been calculated in term of level-dose ratios (Table 3). It is demonstrated that, within each group, younger children have a lower ratio. In several studies, the plasma levels appear to be statistically correlated with the dose (Solow and Green, 1971; Sherwin and Robb, 1972; Penry et al., 1972). However, notwithstanding the positive statisti-

Table 3. Influence of Age on Ethosuximide Level-Dose Ratios According to Literature Data

Age Groups (yrs)	Level-Dose Ratios	No. of Patients	Reference
4-9	1.6 ± 0.2	7	Harer et al., 1970
12-25	2.3 ± 0.2	14	
8-11	1.4 ± 0.4	3	Solow and Green, 1971
13-25	3.5 ± 0.5	9	
5-8	2.8 ± 0.4	8	Penry et al., 1972
9-14	3.3 ± 0.3	10	
3-7	0.7 ± 0.1	3	Baruzzi et al., 1975
8-15	2.1 ± 0.2	10	
16-40	2.5 ± 0.2	7	

cal correlation, the wide variability in plasma levels, present among patients receiving similar doses, makes the dose an "unreliable predictor" of plasma levels for the individual child (Penry et al., 1972).

The possibility that the lower level-dose ratio observed for younger children may be due to an increased metabolic clearance is supported by the shorter half-life values observed in children in respect to adults. Buchanan et al. (1969a) found that the apparent plasma half-life in children of 6 to 8 years of age varied from 24 to 41 h, with a mean value of about 30 h. Sherwin et al. (1972) described apparent plasma half-lives of 30 h in a 3-year old child and of 24 h in a 10-year old boy.

According to Penry et al. (1972), maximal clinical control is achieved in children when plasma ethosuximide levels range from 40 to 80 µg/ml. In their study, these authors reported that "no patients with plasma levels below 41 µg/ml" were completely controlled, while in those patients who had control greater than 95% the mean plasma level was 66.8% µg/ml, with a range of 41 to 89 µg/ml. Similar data are reported by Sherwin (1973).

CARBAMAZEPINE

Adults

In adult healthy volunteers, the gastrointestinal absorption of carbamazepine is rather slow. Single doses of 4 to 6.6 mg/kg lead to peak plasma levels of 2-4

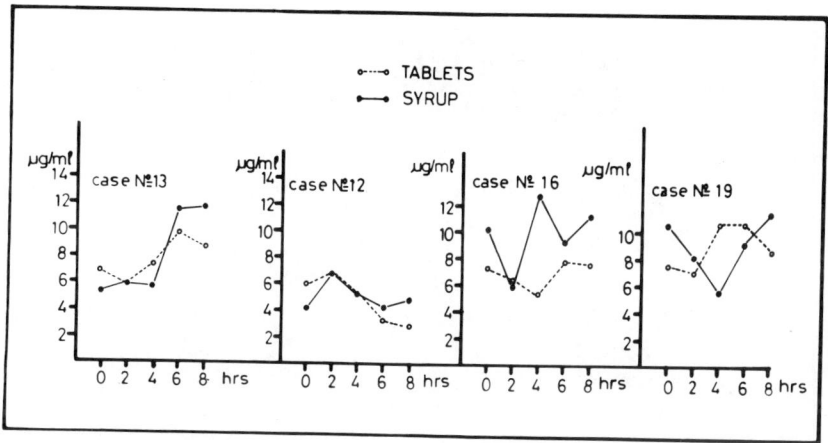

Fig. 10: Carbamazepine plasma level absorption curve in the course of chronic treatment after oral administration of 200 mg given in both tablet and syrup form in four epileptic patients.

µg/ml within 6-18 h (Morselli et al., 1971a, 1972, 1975b; Palmer et al., 1973; Faigle and Feldmann, 1975; Strandjord and Johannessen, 1975). During chronic treatment, there is a trend toward a more rapid absorption, with peak plasma levels attained between 2.5 and 6 h (Meinardi, 1972; Cereghino et al., 1973; Troupin et al., 1974; Morselli, 1975; Strandjord and Johannessen, 1975). However, recent data indicate that in the course of repeated dosing the absorption curves of carbamazepine (Fig. 10) are erratic and practically unpredictable (Morselli et al., 1975b). A direct effect of carbamazepine on gastric motility has been hypothized, but no precise data are available. No differences in plasma levels could be observed administering CBZ chronically as tablets and as suspension preparation (Morselli et al., 1975b).

At therapeutic concentrations, carbamazepine is about 75% bound to plasma proteins; the association constant for the albumin-carbamazepine complex is rather low; and proteins other than albumin are also implicated in the binding (Di Salle et al., 1974). Other antiepileptic drugs commonly used in association with carbamazepine (DPH, PB, dipropyl acetate, ethosuximide and benzodiazepines) do not have any significant displacing effect on carbamazepine *in vitro* (Morselli et al., 1975a; Rawlins et al., 1975). CSF concentration may vary from 17 to 31% of respective plasma levels, with a mean value of 23% (Johannessen and Strandjord, 1972, 1973; Meinardi, 1972; Morselli et al., 1975a), while brain-to-plasma ratios range from 1 to 2 (Morselli et al., 1975a; Morselli et al., 1976b). The apparent volume of distribution, calculated from oral data and assuming complete bioavailability, is 0.82-1.86 l/kg (Palmer et al., 1973; Morselli

338 DRUG DISPOSITION DURING DEVELOPMENT

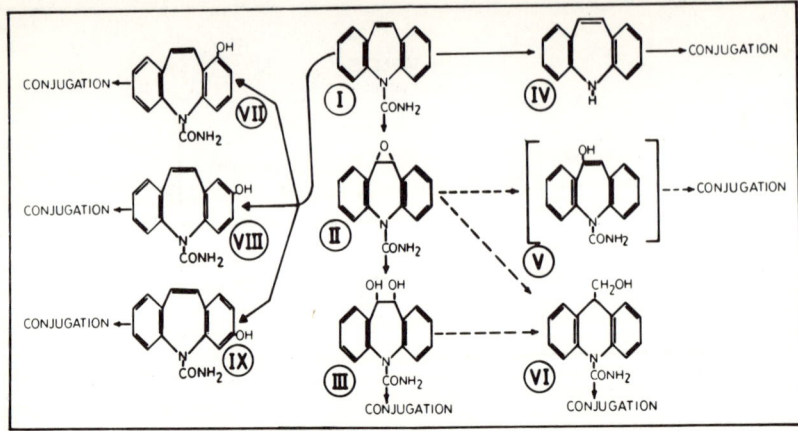

Fig. 11: Metabolism of carbamazepine in man. I. Carbamazepine;
II. Carbamazepine-10,11-epoxide; III. 10,11-dihydroxy-10,11-dihydrocarbamazepine; IV. Iminostilbene; V. 10-hydroxy-10,11-dihydrocarbamazepine; VI. 9-hydroxymethyl-10-carbamoylacridin; VII. 1-hydroxycarbamazepine; VIII. 2-hydroxycarbamazepine; IX. 3-hydroxycarbamazepine.

et al., 1975a; Rawlins et al., 1975). While after a single dose the apparent plasma half-life of carbamazepine is 26-25 h, in epileptic patients dosed chronically the disappearance rate is significantly faster, with values of 10-17 h (Troupin et al., 1974; Morselli et al., 1975a, 1976a). These observations suggest that, as was found in experimental animals (Morselli et al., 1972; Farghali Hassan et al., 1976), an induction of liver microsomal enzymes may take place during repeated treatment with carbamazepine (Morselli, 1975). The possibility that carbamazepine could be an inducer was first hypothized by Hansen et al. (1971).

In man, carbamazepine is extensively metabolized (Fig. 11), and the major degradation products so far identified are represented by the carbamazepine-10, 11-oxide (Baker et al., 1973; Goenechea and Hecke-Seibicke, 1972). A second minor distinct pathway for the biotransformation of carbamazepine, catalyzed by hepatic oxygenases, involving hydroxylation of the aromatic rings and subsequent conjugation with glucuronic acid, has very recently been described by Faigle et al. (1975).

Among the identified metabolites, the carbamazepine-10, 11-oxide has shown an anticonvulsant activity in mice and rats close to the range of the parent compound (Frigerio and Morselli, 1975). Whether this is true also for man is not

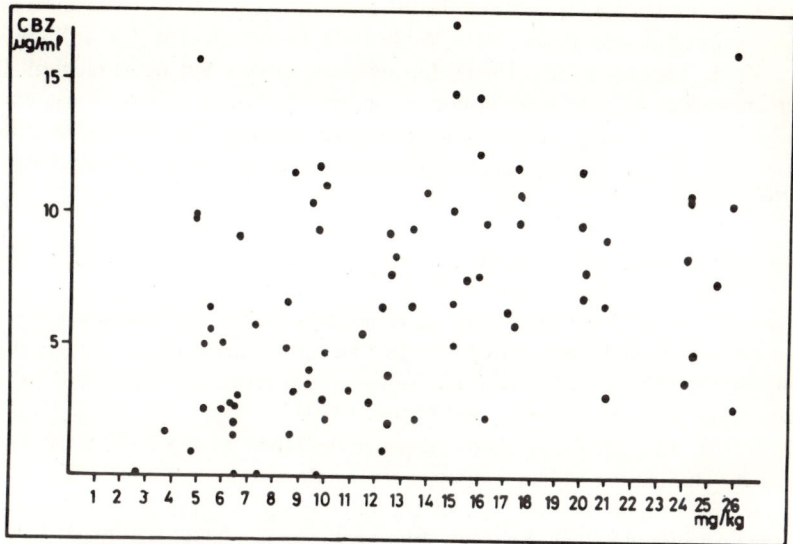

Fig. 12: Relationships between carbamazepine steady-state plasma levels and daily doses (mg/Kg) in epileptic patients following chronic treatment with the drug.

known. The epoxide is about 50% bound to plasma proteins, and its apparent plasma half-life is 8-14 h (Di Salle et al., 1974; Morselli et al., 1975a). Carbamazepine is excreted as such for only 1% of the dose, while the identified metabolites account for about 30% of the administered amount, the main portion being represented by the glycol (Morselli, 1975). Plasma levels during chronic treatment are quite variable and may range from 0.5 to 25 μg/ml (Cereghino et al., 1973; Rodin et al., 1974; Troupin et al., 1974; Morselli et al., 1975b, 1976a; Monaco et al., 1976; Strandjord and Johannessen, 1975). There is no apparent relationship between the daily dose and plasma levels at steady state (Fig. 12)

During chronic treatment, carbamazepine-10, 11-oxide is constantly present at levels of 0.5-4.5 μg/ml. The epoxide plasma levels are not related to carbamazepine concentrations by a constant ratio, but they may range from 15 to 50% of the carbamazepine levels (Christiansen and Dam, 1975; Morselli et al., 1975a). Although there does not seem to be general agreement on the therapeutic and toxic thresholds, recent data tend to suggest that the therapeutic level of carbamazepine may be between 5 and 12 μg/ml (Morselli et al., 1975a; Monaco et al., 1976), while concentrations of over 15-20 μg/ml are clearly associated with toxic side effects. The most frequent side effects encountered with carbamazepine are nausea, drowsiness, disturbances in vision, ataxia, restlessness and nystagmus (Kutt and Penry, 1974; Wink, 1973; Cereghino et al., 1974; Rodin et al., 1974; Troupin et al., 1974). Idiosyncratic effects and hematological disturbances such as bone marrow depression may occasionally be observed, while more frequent findings appear to be a transient leukopenia and a modest reduction in platelets (Cereghino et al., 1974; Monaco et al., 1976; Livingston et al., 1967; Killian, 1969; Crill, 1973).

Newborns, Infants and Children

There are only two reports on carbamazepine plasma levels in newborns. In the cases described, carbamazepine was transferred in utero from the mother, who received the drug for treatment of epilepsy together with other anticonvulsant drugs such as phenytoin and phenobarbital (Hoppel et al., 1975; Rane et at., 1975). The calculated plasma apparent half-lives were 8.2, 10.5, 10.8 and 27.7 h. The plasma apparent disappearance rate seemed to follow a first-order kinetic. The reported values are of the same order as those observed in adult epileptic patients following chronic treatment. The possibility that the fetal drug metabolizing enzymes were induced in utero by continuous treatment with carbamazepine and diphenylhydantoin is very likely. These data are consistent with the possibility of intrauterine induction of liver drug-metabolizing enzymes (Morselli et al., 1974). No kinetic data have been described in infants. The data available on carbamazepine plasma levels in children refer to levels observed in the course of combined treatment in patients of 6 to 15 years of age (Morselli et al., 1975a,b,c). For doses varying from 5.4 to 33.3 mg/kg, the plasma concentrations were found to range from 0.5 to 1.4 μg/ml, with no apparent relationship between the daily doses and the plasma levels. The carbamazepine-10, 11-oxide was constantly present. A wide scattering, comparable to that described in adults, was observed in the plasma level-dose ratios. The majority of the children, however, showed plasma level/dose ratios of 0.22-0.67 (mean: 0.36) while in adults the mean ratio was 0.78, with values oscillating from 0.5 to 1.44 (Fig. 13). These observations suggest that also for carbamazepine a faster disposition rate may be present in children. As for other anticonvulsants, the incidence of side effects seems to be lower in children (Gamstorp, 1966; Lerman and Kivity-Ephraim, 1974; Scheffner and Schiefer, 1972).

CLONAZEPAM

Clonazepam has very recently been introduced as a new tool for treatment of seizures. Kinetic data on this molecule are still very few and can be summarized rather briefly. In adult volunteers, clonazepam, administered as a

ANTIEPILEPTICS 341

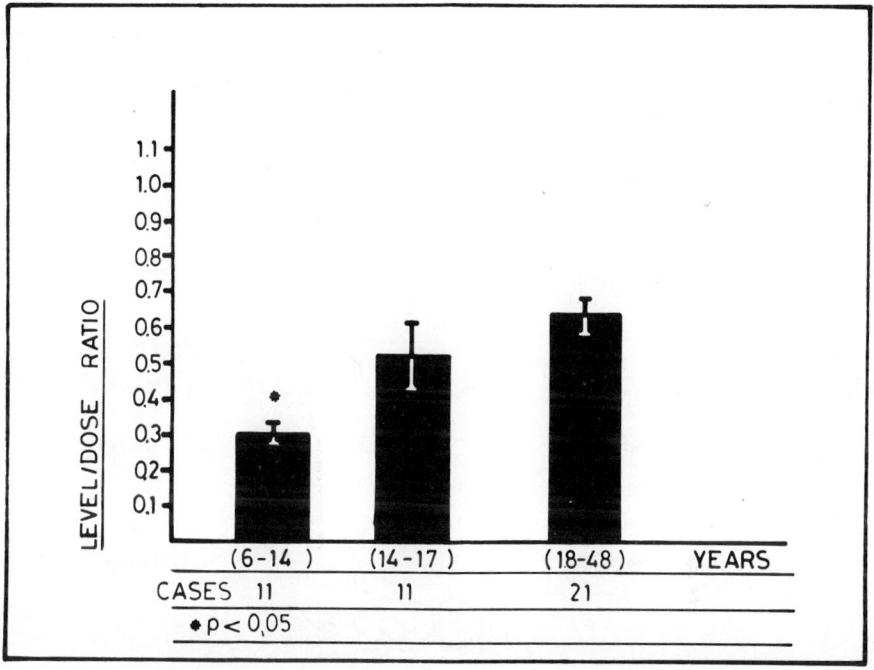

Fig. 13: Effect of age on carbamazepine level/dose ratios in epileptic patients treated chronically with the drug.

single oral dose, is virtually completely absorbed (Eschenof, 1973). Peak plasma levels are attained, in most instances, between 1 and 3 h and may be followed by a plateau for the subsequent 4-6 h (Eschenhof, 1973; Naestoft et al., 1973; Kaplan et al., 1974). Peak plasma levels as late as 8 h have been described in a few cases (De Silva et al., 1974; Kaplan et al., 1974). For doses ranging from 0.02 to 0.003 mg/kg, peak levels are between 6 and 15 ng/ml. In the course of chronic treatment with dosages of 0.1-0.3 mg/kg/daily, plasma levels may range from 20 to 85 ng/ml (Naestoft et al., 1973; Huang et al., 1974; Dreifuss et al., 1975; Hvidberg, 1975; Sjo et al., 1975). The apparent volume of distribution is between 2 and 3 L/kg, according to Kaplan et al. (1974), Van der Kleijn (1975) and Hvidberg and Sjö (1975). The apparent plasma half-life may vary from 19 to 40 h, but the clonazepam disappearance rate seems to be accelerated by a concomitant treatment with phenobarbital and diphenylhydantoin (Hvidberg and Sjö, 1975; Van der Kleijn, 1975).

About 1-4% of the dose is excreted intact and the rest is extensively metabolized (Fig. 14). The two major metabolites identified in humans are the 7-amino

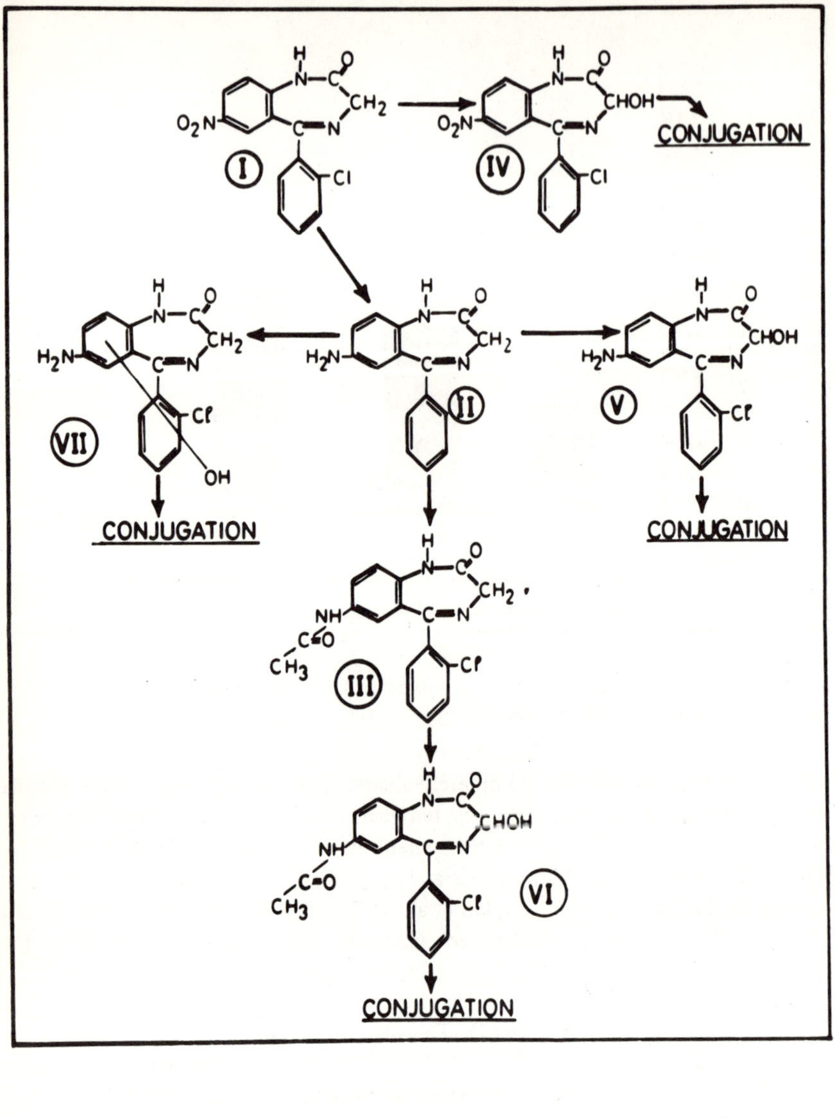

Fig. 14: Metabolism of clonazepam in man. I. Clonazepam; II. 7-aminoclonazepam; III. 7-acetamidoclonazepam; IV. 3-hydroxyclonazepam; V. 7 amino-3-hydroxyclonazepam; VI. 7 acetamido-3-hydroxyclonazepam; VII. 7-phenolaminoclonazepam.

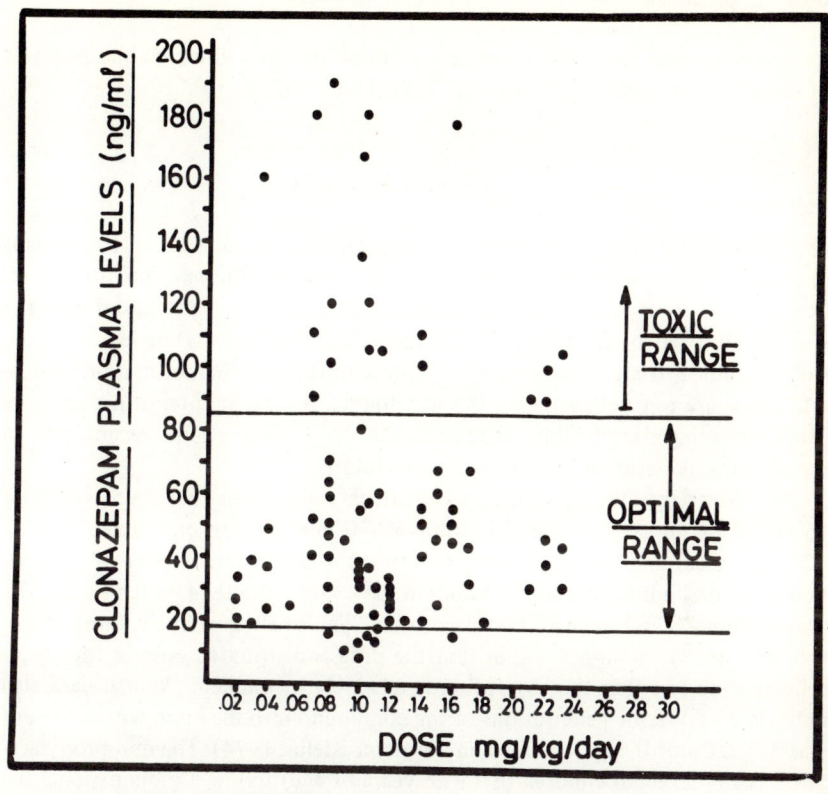

Fig. 15: Relationships between clonazepam steady-state plasma levels and daily doses (mg/Kg) in epileptic patients following chronic treatment with the drug in association with other anticonvulsant drugs.

clonazepam and the 7-acetamido clonazepam, which are excreted both as free and as conjugated compounds, and account for about 25-30% of the administered dose (Eschenhof, 1973; Sjö et al., 1975).

In adults, as well as in children, a direct relationship between plasma levels and dose has been described by Penry (1974), Huang et al. (1974), Hvidberg and Sjö (1975) and Sjö et al. (1975). However, in a recent study in children receiving clonazepam in association with other anticonvulsant drugs, we were unable to confirm such a finding (Fig. 15) (Gerna and Morselli, 1976; Baruzzi et al., 1977).

The clonazepam therapeutic and toxic thresholds are not yet well defined. According to Penry (1974) and Dreyfuss et al. (1975), the best therapeutic results are attained with plasma concentrations ranging from 25 to 70 ng/ml. Our experience tends to confirm such an assumption. Dysphoria may be present with levels over 60 ng/ml (Sjö et al., 1975). Higher levels of clonazepam, or of its metabolites, may be associated with severe ataxia and worsening of the clinical picture (Baruzzi et al., 1977). In the case of therapy discontinuation, withdrawal symptoms appear to be more frequent in those patients with high plasma levels of metabolites (Hvidberg and Sjo, 1975; Sjo et al., 1975).

DI-N-PROPYLACETATE

Di-n-propylacetate is a drug which has been introduced as an anticonvulsant in several European countries since 1967-68. However, the real activity and efficacy of the compound in man is still discussed, and it is not yet sure if the drug is active by itself or via an eventual unidentified metabolite. Double-blind, controlled, clinical trials documenting a real anticonvulsant effect of di-n-propylacetate alone are not yet available. Despite doubts, it may be interesting, since its use is spreading considerably, at least in Europe, to report some recent data on the pharmacokinetics of the compound in children.

Di-n-propylacetate is supposed to be quickly absorbed. Peak levels of about 15 to 60 μg/ml can be observed within 60-90 min after an oral intake of 300-400 mg. According to Schobben et al. (1975), the apparent volume of distribution after oral administration in children may vary from 0.14 to 0.41 l/kg. The drug is about 85% bound to plasma protein. The small apparent volume of distribution tends to suggest either that the drug is distributed only in the extracellular water, or that the absorption is relatively incomplete. Animal data also indicate a very poor penetrations of the compound into the brain with a "brain/plasma" ratio of 0.30 (Schobben and Van der Kleijn, 1974). The di-n-propylacetate plasma levels in children (3 to 12 years of age) follow a monoexponential decay, with an apparent plasma half-life of 8-11 h (Schobben et al., 1975). In the course of chronic treatment, plasma levels fluctuate considerably during the dosing intervals (Meinardi and Bongers, 1975; Schobben et al., 1975), and no evident relationships can be observed between plasma levels and the daily drug intake (Fig. 16). Di-n-propylacetate is excreted as such in the urine in very limited amounts (6-7%) (Schobben et al., 1975), and this points toward an extensive metabolic degradation of the compound, although no metabolites have as yet been identified in man and theoretically another way of elimination (fecal) could play an important role.

While Schobben et al. (1975) were unable to demonstrate any evident relationship between age and drug clearance, in a recent series of observations on adults and children we found a clear effect of age, as shown in Fig. 17. The drug is well tolerated even in high dosages (Mises and Plantade, 1967; Bergamini et al., 1970; Kerfriden et al., 1970; Mairlot, 1970; Matthes and Schmutterer, 1971). The most current side effects appear to be gastric complaints (nausea, vomiting) which can be reduced or abolished by the use of enteric tablets (Sonne et al., 1975). According to Schobben et al. (1975), therapeutic concentrations range

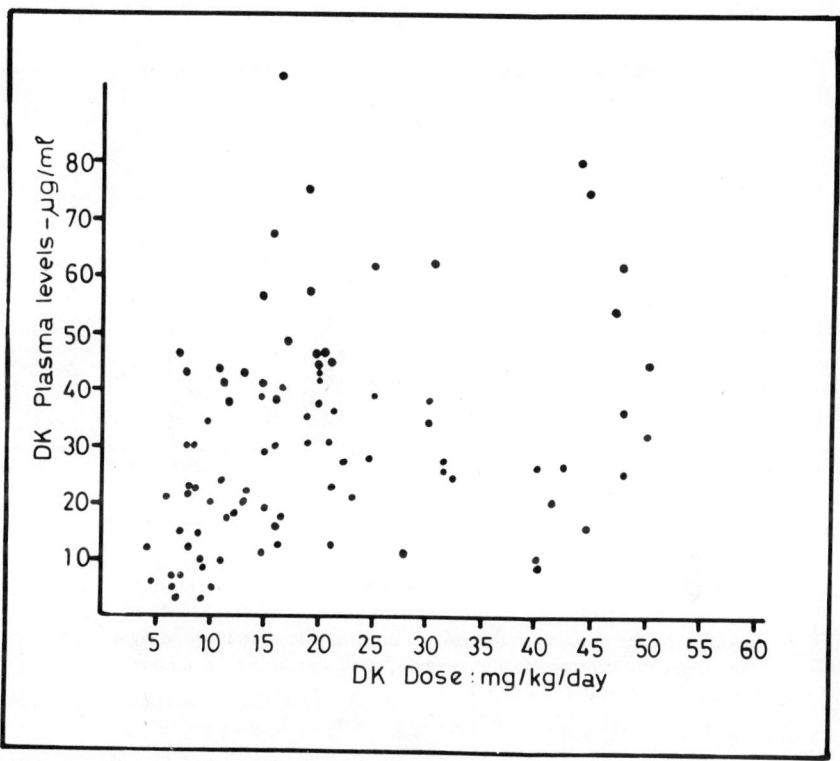

Fig. 16: Relationships between di-n-propylacetate (DK) plasma levels and daily doses (mg/kg) in epileptic patients following chronic treatment with the drug in association with other anticonvulsant drugs.

from 50 to 100 µg/ml, but the data are very preliminary and further observations are needed.

The onset of "therapeutic effect" is usually observed only after several days. This behavior has been attributed to the possible elevation of an inhibitory neurotransmitter in the brain, or to the low accumulation of an eventual unidentified metabolite. A third possibility is that di-n-propylacetate could exert an inhibitory effect on the clearance of other antiepileptic drugs given in association. A consistent rise in phenobarbital plasma levels, following the introduction of di-n-propylacetate in the therapeutic regimen, has in fact been reported by Schobben et al. (1975).

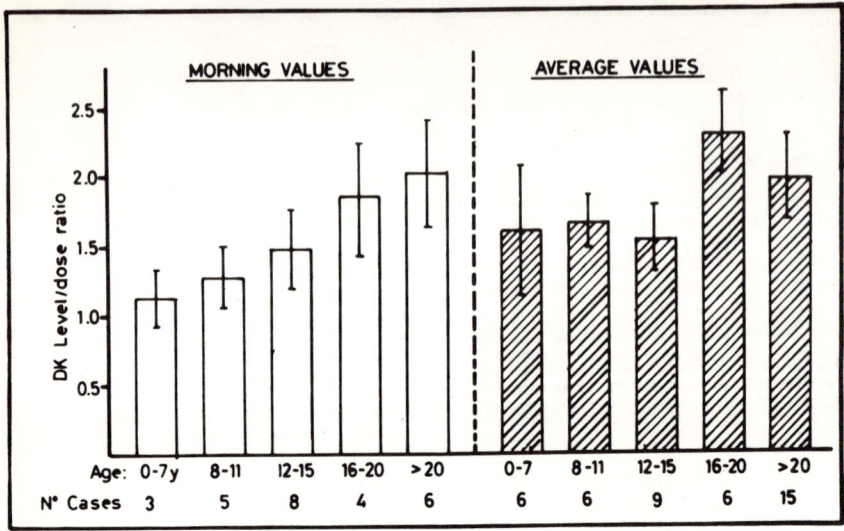

Fig. 17: Effect of age on di-n-propylacetate (DK) level/dose ratios in epileptic patients treated chronically with the drug. A clear age effect is evident on the morning values (before the drug administration), but not on values derived from data obtained by sampling during the absorptive and early postabsorptive phase.

CONCLUSIONS

At present, the disposition of anticonvulsants drugs in man appears reasonably well-described in adults; for most of the compounds, valuable and significant data are also available for newborns, infants and children. Clear relationships exist between plasma drug concentrations and therapeutic and/or toxic side effects. From the reported data, the age factor, or, better, the development factor, emerges as a very important variable which should not be neglected in programming a rational therapeutic schedule with this class of drugs. Another point to be underlined is the fact that this therapeutic class of drugs is represented by compounds with very different physicochemical properties that have in common a similar metabolic pathway, and this factor indeed seems to be the common denominator in sustaining age differences.

Absorption, in fact, may be fast or relatively slow and erratic, binding to plasma proteins may be extensive or nil, the apparent volume of distribution may range from 0.4 to 3 L/kg; all drugs, however, undergo considerable metabolic breakdown through the liver mixed-oxygenase-enzymatic microsomal system to give rise to hydroxylated products which are further conjugated and excreted. This step appears to be the most important one in determining differences in clearances, which in infants and children are clearly faster than in adults, while apparent volume of distribution does not seem to be significantly different in the various age groups.

For newborns, previous exposure (in utero) to inducing agents can be a very important determinant of the metabolic rate in the neonate. This, too, is a factor which should always be taken into account when administering drugs to newborns.

Other points which up to the present have scarcely been considered deserve a more systematic approach. The possible influence of sexual maturation on the metabolism of anticonvulsant drugs has as yet received very little attention. Both the loss of control in epileptic adolescents, as well as the appearance of toxic signs in the course of chronic constant therapy in coincidence with puberty, could be linked to hormone interference with drug metabolism or to the modification of body mass subsequent to sexual maturation. The answer to these questions probably could only be determined through long-term monitoring of plasma levels.

Another fact that clearly emerges from the available data is the great individual variability of the plasma level/dose ratios, variability which makes it impossible to predict the plasma concentrations reached in the individual patient with a certain dose. This factor necessitates the long-term monitoring of plasma levels in epileptic patients in order to assure regular achievement of plasma levels within the therapeutic range. The necessity for constant monitoring of drug plasma levels in infants and children is also supported by the difficulty in identifying the presence of toxic effects such as sedation or alteration of psychomotor activity, effects which may have a strongly negative imprint on the developing child. (Morselli 1976a)

REFERENCES

Albert, K.S., Sakmar, E., Hallmark, M.R., Weidler, D.J. and Wagner, J.G. (1974): Bioavailability of diphenylhydantoin. *Clinical Pharmacology and Therapeutics, 16:* 727-735.

Algeri, E.J. and McBay, A.J. (1956): Metabolites of phenobarbital in human urine. *Science, 123:* 183-184.

Arnold, K. and Gerber, N. (1970): The rate of decline of diphenylhydantoin in human plasma. *Clinical Pharmacology and Therapeutics, 11:* 121-134.

Atkinson, A.J., Jr., MacGee, J., Strong, J., Garteiz, D. and Gaffney, T.E. (1970): Identification of 5-meta-hydroxyphenyl-5-phenylhydantoin as a metabolite of diphenylhydantoin. *Biochemical Pharmacology, 19:* 2483-2491.

Atkinson, A.J. and Shaw, J.M. (1973): Pharmacokinetic study of a patient with diphenylhydantoin toxicity. *Clinical Pharmacology and Therapeutics, 14:* 521-528.

Baker, K.M., Csetenyi, J., Frigerio, A., Morselli, P.L., Parravicini, F. and Pifferi, G. (1973): 10,11-dihydro-10,11-dihydroxy-5H-dibenz[b,f]azepine-5-carboxamide, a metabolite of carbamazepine isolated from human and rat urine. *Journal of Medicinal Chemistry, 16:* 703-705.
Baruzzi, A., Bossi, L., Castelli, D., Gerna, M., Righetti, A., Morselli, P.L. (1975): Alcune considerazioni sulla farmacocinetica dei farmaci anti-convulsivanti in eta evolutiva. *Rivista Gaslini 7:* 125-130.
Baruzzi, A., Gerna, M., Altamura, A.C., Avanzini, G., Langer, R., Zagnoni, P., Morselli, P.L. (1977): Clonazepam plasma levels in epileptic patients - in preparation.
Baumel, I.P., Gallagher, B.B. and Mattson, R.H. (1972): Phenylethylmalonamide (PEMA). An important metabolite of primidone. *Archives of Neurology, 27:* 34-41.
Bergamini, L., Mutani, R., Furlan, P.M. and Riccio, A. (1970): Le Dêpakine dans le traitement de l'epilepsie essentielle ou idiopathique. *Archives Suisses de Neurologie, Neurochirurgie et de Psychiatrie, 106:* 1-7.
Berlet, H. (1975): Serum levels of diphenylhydantoin in children. In: *Pharmacology of Anti-Epileptic Drugs,* edited by H. Schneider, et al. Springer-Verlag, pp. 63-69.
Bochner, F., Hooper, W.D., Sutherland, J.M., Eadie, M.J. and Tyrer, J.H. (1973): The renal handling of diphenylhydantoin and 5-(p-hydroxyphenyl)-5-phenylhydantoin. *Clinical Pharmacology and Therapeutics, 14:* 791-796.
Bochner, F., Hooper, W.D., Tyrer, J.H. and Eadie, M.J. (1972): Effect of dosage increments on blood phenytoin concentrations. *Journal of Neurology, Neurosurgery and Psychiatry, 35:* 873-876.
Booker, H.E., (1972a): Phenobarbital, mephobarbital and metharbital. Relation of plasma levels to clinical control. In: *Antiepileptic Drugs,* edited by D.M. Woodbury, J.K. Penry and R.P. Schmidt, pp. 329-334, Raven Press, New York.
Booker, H.E. (1972b): Primidone. Toxicity. In: *Antiepileptic Drugs,* edited by D.M. Woodbury, J.K. Penry and R.P. Schmidt, pp. 377-383, Raven Press, New York.
Booker, H.E., Hosokowa, K., Burdette, R.D. and Darcey, B. (1970): A clinical study of serum primidone levels. *Epilepsia* (Amsterdam), *11:* 395-402.
Boreus, L.O., Jalling, B. and Kallberg, N. (1975): Clinical pharmacology of phenobarbital in the neonatal period. In: *Basic and Therapeutic Aspects of Perinatal Pharmacology,* edited by P.L. Morselli, S. Garattini and F. Sereni, Raven Press, New York, in press.
Borgå, O., Garle, M. and Gutova, M. (1972): Identification of 5 (3,4-dihydroxyphenyl)-5-phenylhydantoin as a metabolite of 5,5-diphenylhydantoin (henytoin) in rats and man. *Pharmacology, 7:* 129-137.
Borgstedt, A.D., Bryson, M.F., Young, L.W. and Forbes, G.B. (1972): Long-term administration of antiepileptic drugs and the development of rickets. *Journal of Pediatrics, 81:* 9-15.
Borofsky, L.G., Louis, S. and Kutt, H. (1973): Diphenylhydantoin in children (pharmacology and efficacy). *Neurology, 23:* 967-972.
Borofsky, L.G., Louis S., Kutt, H. and Roginsky, M. (1972): Diphenylhydantoin: efficacy, toxicity and dose-serum level relationships in children. *Journal of Pediatrics, 81:* 995-1002.
Borondy, P., Dill, W.A., Chang, T., Buchanan, R.A. and Glazko, A.J. (1973): Effect of protein binding on the distribution of 5,5-diphenylhydantoin between plasma and red cells. *Annals of the New York Academy of Sciences, 226:* 82-87.
Boston Collaborative Drug Surveillance Program (BCDSP)(1973): Diphenylhydantoin side effects and serum albumin levels. *Clinical Pharmacology and Therapeutics, 14:* 529-532.
Browning, R.A. and Maynert, E.W. (1972): Phenobarbital, mephobarbital and metharbital.

ANTIEPILEPTICS 349

Toxicity. In: *Antiepileptic Drugs*, edited by D.M. Woodbury, J.K. Penry and R.P. Schmidt, pp. 345-351, Raven Press, New York.

Buchanan, R.A. (1972): Ethosuximide, Toxicity. In: *Antiepileptic Drugs*, edited by D.M. Woodbury, J.K. Penry and R.P. Schmidt, pp. 449-454, Raven Press, New York.

Buchanan, R.A. and Allen, R.J. (1971): Diphenylhydantoin (Dilantin R) and phenobarbital blood levels in epileptic children. *Neurology, 21:* 866-871.

Buchanan, R.A., Fernandez, L. and Kinkel, A.W. (1969a): Absorption and elimination of ethosuximide in children. *Journal of Clinical Pharmacology and New Drugs, 9:* 393-398.

Buchanan, R.A., Heffelfinger, J.C. and Weiss, C.F. (1969b): The effect of phenobarbital on diphenylhydantoin metabolism in children. *Pediatrics, 43:* 114-116.

Buchanan, R.A., Kinkel, A.W. and Smith, T.C. (1973a): The absorption and excretion of ethosuximide. *International Journal of Clinical Pharmacology and New Drugs, 7:* 213-218.

Buchanan, R.A. and Sholiton, L.J. (1972): Diphenylhydantoin. Interactions with other drugs in man. In: *Antiepileptic Drugs*, edited by D.M. Woodbury, J.K. Penry and R.P. Schmidt, pp. 181-191, Raven Press, New York.

Buchanan, R.A., Turner, J.L., Moyer, C.E. and Heffelfinger, J.C. (1973b): Single daily dose of diphenylhydantoin in children. *Journal of Pediatrics, 83:* 479-483.

Buchthal, F. and Lennox-Buchthal, M.A. (1972a): Diphenylhydantoin. Relation of anticonvulsant effect to concentration in serum. In: *Antiepileptic Drugs*, edited by D.M. Woodbury, J.K. Penry and R.P. Schmidt, pp. 193-209, Raven Press, New York.

Buchthal, F. and Lennox-Buchthal, M.A. (1972b): Phenobarbital. Relation of serum concentration to control of seizures. In: *Antiepileptic Drugs*, edited by D.M. Woodbury, J.K. Penry and R.P. Schmidt, pp. 335-343, Raven Press, New York.

Buchthal, F. and Svensmark, O. (1959/1960): Aspects of the pharmacology of phenytoin (Dilantin R) and phenobarbital relevent to their dosage in the treatment of epilepsy. *Epilepsia* (Amsterdam), *1:* 373-384.

Buchthal, F. and Svensmark, O. (1971): Serum concentrations of diphenylhydantoin (Phenytoin) and phenobarbital and their relation to therapeutic and toxic effects. *Psychiatria, Neurologia, Neurochirurgia, 74:* 117-136.

Buchthal, F., Svensmark, O. and Schiller, P.J. (1960): Clinical and electroencephalographic correlations with serum levels of diphenylhydantoin. *Archives of Neurology, 2:* 624-630.

Butler, T.C. (1956); The metabolic hydroxylation of phenobarbital. *Journal of Pharmacology and Experimental Therapeutics, 116:* 326-336.

Butler, T.C. (1957): The metabolic conversion of 5,5-diphenyl hydantoin to 5-(p-hydroxyphenyl) 5-phenyl hydantoin. *Journal of Pharmacology and Experimental Therapeutics, 119:* 1-11.

Butler, T.C. Mahaffee, C. and Waddell, W.J. (1954): Phenobarbital: studies of elimination, accumulation, tolerance, and dosage schedules. *Journal of Pharmacology and Experimental Therapeutics, 111:* 425-435.

Cereghino, J.J., Brock, J.T., Van Meter, J.C., Penry, J.K., Smith, L.D. and White, B.G. (1974): Carbamazepine for epilepsy. A controlled prospective evaluation. *Neurology, 24:* 401-410.

Cereghino, J.J., Van Meter, J.C., Brock, J.T. Penry, J.K., Smith, L.D. and White, B.G. (1973): Preliminary observations of serum carbamazepine concentration in epileptic patients. *Neurology, 23:* 357-366.

Chanarin, I., Mollin, D.L. and Anderson, B.B. (1958): Folic acid deficiency and the megaloblastic anaemias. *Proceedings of the Royal Society of Medicine, 51:* 757.

Chang, T., Burkett, A.R. and Glazko, A.J. (1972a): Ethosuximide. Biotransformation.

In: *Antiepileptic Drugs,* edited by D.M. Woodbury, J.K. Penry and R.P. Schmidt, pp. 425-429, Raven Press, New York.
Chang, T., Dill, W.A. and Glazko, A.J. (1972b): Ethosuximide. Absorption, distribution, and excretion. In: *Antiepileptic Drugs,* edited by D.M. Woodbury, J.K. Penry and R.P. Schmidt, pp. 417-423, Raven Press, New York.
Chang, T. and Glazko, A.J. (1972): Diphenylhydantoin. Biotransformation. In: *Antiepileptic Drugs,* edited by B.M. Woodbury, J.K. Penry and R.P. Schmidt, pp. 149-162, Raven Press, New York.
Chang, T., Savory, A. and Glazko, A.J. (1970): A new metabolite of 5,5-diphenylhydantoin (Dilantin R). *Biochemical and Biphysical Research Communications, 38:* 444-449.
Christiansen, J. and Dam, M. (1975): Drug interaction in epileptic patients. In: *Clinical Pharmacology of Antiepileptic Drugs,* edited by H. Schneider, et al., Springer-Verlag, Berlin, pp. 197-200.
Crill, W.E. (1973): Carbamazepine. *Annals of Internal Medicine, 79:* 844-847.
Csetenyi, J., Baker, K.M., Frigerio, A. and Morselli, P.L. (1973): Iminostilbene–a metabolite of carbamazepine isolated from rat urine. *Journal of Pharmacy and Pharmacology, 25:* 340-341.
Cucinell, S.A. (1972): Phenobarbital. Interactions with other drugs. In: *Antiepileptic Drugs,* edited by D.M. Woodbury, J.K. Penry and R.P. Schmidt, pp. 319-327, Raven Press, New York.
Dam, M. and Olesen, V. (1966): Intramuscular administration of phenytoin. *Neurology, 16:* 288-292.
Dawson, K.P. and Jamieson, A. (1971): Value of blood phenytoin estimation in management of childhood epilepsy. *Archives of Disease in Childhood, 46:* 386-388.
De Luca, K., Masotti, R.E. and Partington, M.W. (1972): Altered calcium metabolism due to anticonvulsant drugs. *Developmental Medicine and Child Neurology, 14:* 318-321.
de Silva, J.A.F., Puglisi, C.V. and Munno, N. (1974): Determination of clonazepam and flunitrazepam in blood and urine by electron-capture GLC. *Journal of Pharmaceutical Sciences, 63:* 520-527.
De Vries, S.I. (1965): Haematological aspects during treatment with anticonvulsant drugs. *Epilepsia* (Amsterdam), *6:* 1-15.
Diamond, W.D. and Buchanan, R.A. (1970): A clinical study of the effect of phenobarbital on diphenylhydantoin plasma levels. *Journal of Clinical Pharmacology and New Drugs, 10:* 306-311.
Dill, W.A., Peterson, L., Chang, T. and Glazko, A.J. (1965): Phsiologic disposition of α-methyl-α-ethyl succinimide (Ethosuximide)–zarontin in animals and man. *American Chemical Abstracts,* 19th Meeting, Detroit, p. 30N.
Di Salle, E., Pacifici, G.M. and Morselli, P.L. (1974): Studies on plasma protein binding of carbamazepine. *Pharmacological Research Communications, 6:* 193-202.
Dreifuss, F.E., Penry, J.K., Rose, S.W., Kupferberg, H.J., Dyken, P. and Sato, S. (1975): Serum clonazepam concentrations in children with absence seizures. *Neurology, 25:* 255-258.
Eadie, M.J. and Tyrer, J.H. (eds.) (1974): *Anticonvulsant Therapy. Pharmacological Basis and Practice,* p. 87, Churchill Livingstone, Edinburgh.
Ehrnebo, M., Agurell, S., Jalling, B. and Boréus, L.O. (1971): Age differences in drug binding by plasma proteins: studies on human foetuses, neonates and adults. *European Journal of Clinical Pharmacology, 3:* 189-193.
Eschenhof, E. (1973): Untersuchungen über das Schicksal des Antikonvulsivums Clonazepam im Organismus der Ratte, des Hundes und des Menschen. *Arzneimittel-Forschung, 23:* 390-400.

Faero, O., Kastrup, K.W., Lykkegaard Nielsen, E., Melchoir, J.C. and Thorn, I. (1972): Successful prophylaxis of febrile convulsions with phenobarbital. *Epilepsia* (Amsterdam), *13:* 279-285.
Faigle, J.W., Brechbühler, S. and Feldmann, K.F. (1975): The biotransformation of carbamazepine. In: *International Symposium on Epileptic Seizure, Behaviour, Pain*, St. Moritz, January, edited by W. Birkmayer, Springer-Verlag, Berlin, in press.
Faigle, J.W. and Feldmann, K.F. (1975): Pharmacokinetic data of carbamazepine and its major metabolites in man. In: *Clinical Pharmacology of Antiepileptic Drugs*, edited by H. Schneider, Springer-Verlag, Berlin, in press.
Farghali-Hassan, Assael, B.M., Gerna, M., Garattini, S. and Morselli, P.L. (1976): Carbamazepine pharmacokinetics in young, adult and pregnant rats. Relationships to the pharmacologic effect. *Archives Internationales de Pharmacolynamie et de Therapie 219:* 197-211.
Feuer, G. and Liscio, A. (1969): Origin of delayed development of drug metabolism in the newborn rat. *Nature* (London), *223:* 68-70.
Frigerio, A., Fanelli, R., Biandrate, P., Passerini, G., Morselli, P.L. and Garattini, S. (1972): Mass spectrometric characterization of carbamazepine-10,11-eposide, a carbamazepine metabolite isolated from human urine. *Journal of Pharmaceutical Sciences, 61:* 1144-1147.
Frigerio, A., Morselli, P.L. (1975): Carbamazepine Biotransformation. In: *Advances in Neurology*, Vol. 11, pp. 295-308 - Raven Press, New York.
Gallagher, B.B. and Baumel, I.P. (1971): Diphenylhydantoin, phenobarbital, and primidone: serum concentrations, distribution and toxicity in a large population of epileptic patients. *Neurology, 21:* 394-395.
Gallagher, B.B. and Baumel, I.P. (1972a): Primidone. Absorption, distribution, and excretion. In: *Antiepileptic Drugs*, edited by D.M. Woodbury, J.K. Penry and R.P. Schmidt, pp. 357-359, Raven Press, New York.
Gallagher, B.B. and Baumel, I.P. (1972b): Primidone. Biotransformation. In: *Antiepileptic Drugs*, edited by D.M. Woodbury, J.K. Penry and R.P. Schmidt, pp. 361-366, Raven Press, New York.
Gallagher, B.B. and Baumel, I.P. (1972c): Primidone. Interactions with other drugs. In: *Antiepileptic Drugs*, edited by D.M. Woodbury, J.K. Penry and R.P. Schmidt, pp. 367-371, Raven Press, New York.
Gallagher, B.B., Baumel, I.P. and Mattson, R.H. (1972): Metabolic disposition of primidone and its metabolites in epileptic subjects after single and repeated administration. *Neurology, 22:* 1186-1192.
Gallagher, B.B., Baumel, I.P., Mattson, R.H. and Woodbury, S.G. (1973): Primidone, diphenylhydantoin and phenobarbital. Aspects of acute and chronic toxicity. *Neurology, 23:* 145-149.
Gallagher, B.B., Smith, D.B. and Mattson, R.H. (1970): The relationship of the anticonvulsant properties of primidone to phenobarbital. *Epilepsia* (Amsterdam), *11:* 293-301.
Gamstorp, I. (1966): A clinical trial of tegretol in children with severe epilepsy. *Developmental Medicine and Child Neurology, 8:* 296-300.
Ganshorn, A. and Kurz, H. (1968): Unterschiede zwischen der Proteinbindung Neugeborener und Erwachsener und ihre Bedeutung für die pharmakologische Wirkung. *Naunyn-Schmiedeberg's Archiv für Pharmakologie und Experimentelle Pathologie, 260:* 117-118.
Garrettson, L.K. and Dayton, P.G. (1970): Disappearance of phenobarbital and diphenylhydantoin from serum of children. *Clinical Pharmacology and Therapeutics, 11:* 674-679.
Gauchel, F.D., Lehr, H.J., Gauchel, G. and von Harnack, G.A. (1973): Diphenylhydantoin

bei Kindem. Klinische-pharmakologische Untersuchungen. *Deutsche Medizinische Wochenschrift, 98:* 1391-1396.

Gerna, M., Morselli, P.L. (1976): A simple and sensitive gas-chromatographic method for the determination of clonazepam in human plasma. *J. Chromatography, 116:* 445-450.

Gerber, N., Lynn, R. and Oates, J. (1972): Acute intoxication with 5,5-diphenylhydantoin (Dilantin R) associated with impairment of biotransformation. Plasma levels and urinary metabolites, and studies in healthy volunteers. *Annals of Internal Medicine, 77:* 765-771.

Glaser, G.H. (1972): Diphenylhydantoin. Toxicity. In: *Antiepileptic Drugs,* edited by D.M. Woodbury, J.K. Penry and R.P. Schmidt, pp. 219-226, Raven Press, New York.

Glazko, A.J. and Chang, T. (1972): Diphenylhydantoin. Absorption, distribution, and excretion. In: *Antiepileptic Drugs,* edited by D.M. Woodbury, J.K. Penry and R.P. Schmidt, pp. 127-136, Raven Press, New York.

Glazko, A.J., Chang, T. Baukema, J., Dill, W.A., Goulet, J.R. and Buchanan, R.A. (1969): Metabolic disposition of diphenylhydantoin in normal human subjects following intravenous administration. *Clinical Pharmacology and Therapeutics, 10:* 298-504.

Goenechea, S. and Hecke-Seibicke, E. (1972): Beitrag zum Stoffwechsel von Carbamazepine. *Zeitschrift für Klinische Chemie und Klinische Biochemie, 10:* 112-113.

Haerer, A.F., Buchanan, R.A. and Wiygul, F.M. (1970): Ethosuximide blood levels in epileptics. *Journal of Clinical Pharmacology and New Drugs, 10:* 370-374.

Hahn, T.J., Hendin, B.A., Scharp, C.R., Boisseau, V.C. and Haddad, J.G. (1975): Serum 25-hydroxycalciferol levels and bone mass in children on chronic anticonvulsant therapy. *New England Journal of Medicine, 292:* 550-554.

Hansen, J.M., Sierboek-Neilsen, K. and Skovsted, L. (1971): Carbamazepine induced acceleration of diphenylhydantoin and Warfarin metabolism in man. *Clinical Pharmacology and Therapeutics, 12:* 539-543.

Hansen, S.E. and Feldberg, L. (1964): Absorption and elimination of Zarontin. *Danish Medical Bulletin, 11:* 54-55.

Hansotia, P. and Keran, E. (1974): Diphenylhydantoin binding by red blood cells of normal subject. *Neurology, 24:* 575-578.

Hartshorn, E.A. (1972): Drug interactions. Central nervous system drugs: anticonvulsants, *Drug Intelligence and Clinical Pharmacy, 6:* 130-137.

Heinze, E. and Kampffmeyer, H.G. (1971): Biological half-life of phenobarbital in human babies. *Klinische Wochenschrift, 49.* 1146-1147.

Hill, R.M., Horning, M. and Horning, E. (1973): Identification of transplacentally acquired anticonvulsant agents in the neonate. In: *Methods of Analysis of Anti-Epileptic Drugs,* edited by J.W.A. Meijer, H. Meinardi, C. Gardner-Thorpe and E. Van der Kleijn, pp. 143-147, Excerpta Medica, Amsterdam.

Holcomb, R., Lynn, R., Harvey, B., Jr., Sweetman, B.J. and Gerber, N. (1972): Intoxication with 5,5-diphenylhydantoin (Dilantin). Clinical features, blood levels, urinary metabolites and metabolic changes in a child. *Journal of Pediatrics, 80:* 627-632.

Hoppel, C., Rane, A. and Sjöqvist, F. (1975): Kinetics of phenytoin and carbamazepine in the newborn. In: *Basic and Therapeutic Aspects of the Perinatal Pharmacology,* edited by P.L. Morselli, S. Garattini and F. Sereni, Raven Press, New York, in press.

Horning, M.G., Stratton, C., Nowlin, J., Wilson, A., Horning, E.C. and Hill, R.M. (1973): Placental transfer of drugs. In: *Fetal Pharmacology,* edited by L. Boréus, pp. 355-372, Raven Press, New York.

Horning, M.G., Stratton, C., Wilson, A., Horning, E.C. and Hill, R.M. (1971): Detection of 5-3,4-dihydroxy-1,5-cyclohexadien-1-yl)-5-phenylhydantoin as a major metabolite of 5,5-diphenylhydantoin (Dilantin) in the newborn human. *Analytical Letters, 4:* 537-545.

Huang, C.Y., McLeod, J.C., Sampson, D. and Hensely, W.J. (1974): Clonazepam in the treatment of epilepsy, *Medical Journal of Australia, 2:* 5-8.

Hunter, J., Maxwell, J.D., Stewart, D.-A., Parson, V. and Williams, R. (1971): Altered calcium metabolism in epileptic children on anticonvulsants. *British Medical Journal. 4:* 202-204.

Hutt, S.J., Jackson, P.M., Belsham, A. and Higgins, G. (1968): Perceptual-motor behaviour in relation to blood phenobarbitone level: a preliminary report. *Developmental Medicine and Child Neurology, 10:* 626-632.

Hvidberg, E.F. and Sjö, O. (1975): Clinical pharmacokinetic experiences with clonazepan. In: *Clinical Pharmacology of Antiepileptic Drugs,* edited by H. Schneider et al., Springer-Verlag, Berlin, pp. 242-246.

Jalling, B. (1976): Plasma concentrations of phenobarbital in the treatment of convulsions in newborns. *Acta Paediatrica Scandinavica,* in press.

Jalling, B. (1976): Plasma and cerebrospinal fluid concentrations of phenobarbital in infants given single doses. *Developmental Medicine in Child Neurology, 16:* 781-783.

Jalling, B., Boréus, L.O., Kållberg, N. and Agurell, S. (1973): Disappearance from the new born of circulating prenatally administered phenobarbital. *European Journal of Clinical Pharmacology, 6:* 234-238.

Jalling, B. Boréus, L.O., Rane, A. and Sjöqvist, F. (1970): Plasma concentrations of diphenylhydantoin in young infants. *Pharmacologia Clinica, 2:* 200-202.

Johannessen, S.I. and Strandjord, R.E. (1972): The concentration of carbamazepine (Tegretol R) in serum and in cerebrospinal fluid in patients with epilepsy. *Acta Neurologica Scandinavica, 48,* suppl. 51: 445-446.

Johannessen, S.I. and Standjord, R.E. (1973): Concentration of carbamazepine (Tegretol R) in serum and in cerebrospinal fluid in patients with epilepsy. *Epilepsia, 14:* 373-379.

Kaplan, S.A., Alexander, K., Jack, M.L., Puglisi, C.V., de Silva, J.A.F., Lee, T.L. and Weinfeld, R.E. (1974): Pharmacokinetic profiles of clonazepam in dog and humans and of fluritrazepam in dog. *Journal of Pharmaceutical Sciences, 63:* 527-532.

Kardish, R. and Feuer, R. (1972): Relationship between maternal progesterones and the delayed drug metabolism in the neonate. *Biology of the Neonate, 20:* 58-67.

Kerfriden, P., Kerfriden, M. and Albe-Fessard, D. (1970): L'Expérience de Toul-ar-c'Hoat le depakine dans le traitement des enfants épileptiques. Observations longitudinales de 74 enfants. *Presse Medicale, 73:* 1943-1944.

Killian, J.M. (1969): Tegretol in trigeminal neuralgia with special reference to hematopoietic side effects. *Headache, 9:* 58-63.

Kiørboe, E. and Plum, C.M. (1966): Megaloblastic anaemia developing during treatment of epilepsy. *Acta Medica Scandinavica, 179,* suppl. 445: 349-357.

Klipstein, F.A. (1964): Subnormal serum folate and macrocytosis associated with anticonvulsant drug therapy. *Blood, 23:* 68-86.

Kruse, R. (1968): Osteopathien bei antiepileptischer Langzeittherapie (Vorläufige Mitteilung). *Monatsschrift für Kinderheikunde, 116:* 378-381.

Kutt, H. (1972a): Diphenylhydantoin. Relation of plasma levels to clinical control. In: *Antiepileptic Drugs,* edited by D.M. Woodbury, J.K. Penry and R.P. Schmidt, pp. 211-218, Raven Press, New York.

Kutt, H. (1972b): Diphenylhydantoin. Interactions with other drugs in man. In: *Antiepileptic Drugs,* edited by D.M. Woodbury, J.K. Penry and R.P. Schmidt, pp. 169-180, Raven Press, New York.

Kutt, H. (1974): Interactions with antiepileptic drugs involving multiple mechanisms. In: *Drug Interactions,* edited by P.L. Morselli, S. Garattini and S.N. Cohen, pp. 211-222, Raven Press, New York.

Kutt, H., Winters, W., Kokenge, R. and McDowell, F. (1964a): Diphenylhydantoin meta-

bolism, blood levels and toxicity. *Archives of Neurology, 11:* 642-648.
Kutt, H., Winters, W., Scherman, R. and McDowell, F. (1964b): Diphenylhydantoin and phenobarbital toxicity. The role of liver disease. *Archives of Neurology, 11:* 649-656.
Kutt, H., Wolk, M., Scherman, R. and McDowell, F. (1964c): Insufficient parahydroxylation as a cause of diphenylhydantoin toxicity. *Neurology, 14:* 542-548.
Lascelles, P.T., Kocen, R.S. and Reynolds, E.H. (1970): The distribution of plasma phenytoin levels in epileptic patients. *Journal of Neurology, Neurosurgery and Psychiatry, 33:* 501-505.
Lerman, P. and Kivity-Ephraim, S. (1974): Carbamazepine sole anticonvulsant for focal epilepsy of childhood, *Epilepsia, 15:* 229-234.
Letteri, J.M., Mellk, H., Louis, S., Kutt, H., Durante, P. and Glazko, A. (1971): Diphenylhydantoin metabolism in uremia. *New England Journal of Medicine, 285:* 648-652.
Levy, L.L. and Fenichel, G.M. (1964): Diphenylhydantoin activated seizures. *Neurology, 15:* 716-722.
Lifshitz, F. and Maclaren, N.K. (1973): Vitamin D-dependent rickets in institutionalized, mentally retarded children receiving long-term anticonvulsant therapy. I. A survey of 288 patients. *Journal of Pediatrics, 83:* 612-620.
Lightfoot, R.W., Jr. and Cristian, C.-L. (1966): Serum protein binding of thyroxin and diphenylhydantoin. *Journal of Clinical Endocrinology and Metabolism, 26:* 305-308.
Livingston, S. (1972): *Comprehensive Management of Epilepsy in Infancy, Childhood and Adolescence,* C.C. Thomas, Springfield.
Livingston, S., Villamater, C., Sakata, Y. and Pauli, L.L. (1967): Use of carbamazepine in epilepsy. *Journal of the American Medical Association, 200:* 204-208.
Lous, P. (1954a): Plasma levels and urinary excretion of three barbituric acids after oral administration to man. *Acta Pharmacologica et Toxicologica, 10:* 147-165.
Lous, P. (1954b): Blood serum and cerebrospinal fluid levels and renal clearance of phenemal in treated epileptics. *Acta Pharmacologica et Toxicologica, 10:* 166-177.
Lous, P. (1954c): Barbituric acid concentration in serum from patients with severe actue poisoning. *Acta Pharmacologica et Toxicologica, 10:* 261-280.
Lund, L., Berlin, A. and Lunde, P.K.M. (1972): Plasma protein binding of diphenylhydantoin in patients with epilepsy. Agreement between the unbound fraction in plasma and the concentration in the cerebrospinal fluid. *Clinical and Pharmacology and Therapeutics, 13:* 196-200.
Lunde, P.K.M., Rane, A., Yaffe, S.J., Lund, L. and Sjöqvist, F. (1970): Plasma protein binding of diphenylhydantoin in man. Interaction with other drugs and the effect of temperature and plasma dilution. *Clinical Pharmacology and Therapeutics, 11:* 846-855.
Mairlot, F. (1970): Observations cliniques sur l'effet de l'acide dipropylacetique dans les manifestations epileptiques et caracterielles. *Revue de Neuropsychiatrie Infantile, 18:* 269-278.
Martinez, G. and Snyder, R.D. (1973): Transplacental passage of primidone. *Neurology, 23:* 381-383.
Matthes, A. and Schmutterer, J. (1971): 3Klinische Erfahrungen mit einem neunen Antiepileptikum: dipropylessig säue. *Deutsche Medizinische Wochenschrift, 96:* 63-66.
Maynert, E.W. (1960): The metabolic fate of diphenylhydantoin in the dog, rat, and man. *Journal of Pharmacology and Experimental Therapeutics, 130:* 275-284.
Maynert, E.W. (1972a): Phenobarbital, mephobarbital, and metharbital. Absorption, distribution and excretion. In: *Antiepileptic Drugs,* edited by D.M. Woodbury, J.K. Penry and R.P. Schmidt, pp. 303-310, Raven Press, New York.
Maynert, E.W. (1972b): Phenobarbital, mephobarbital and metharbital. Biotransformation.

In: *Antiepileptic Drugs*, edited by D.M. Woodbury, J.K. Penry and R.P. Schmidt, pp. 311-317, Raven Press, New York.
Medlinsky, H.-L. (1974): Rickets associated with anticonvulsant medication. *Pediatrics*, *53:* 91-95.
Meinardi, H. (1972): Other antiepileptic drugs. Carbamazepine. In: *Antiepileptic Drugs*, edited by D.M. Woodbury, J.K. Penry and R.P. Schmidt, pp. 487-496, Raven Press, New York.
Meinardi, H. and Bongers, E. (1975): Analytical data related to the use of dipropylacetic acid in the treatment of epilepsy. In: *Clinical Pharmacology of Antiepileptic Drugs*, edited by H. Schneider, et al., Springer-Verlag, Berlin, pp. 235-240.
Melchior, J.C. (1965): The clinical use of serum determinations of phenytoin and phenobarbital in children. *Developmental Medicine and Child Neurology, 7:* 387-391.
Melchior, J.C., Buchthal, F. and Lennox-Buchthal, M. (1971): The ineffectiveness of diphenylhydantoin in preventing febrile convulsions in the age of greatest risk, under three years. *Epilepsia* (Amsterdam), *12:* 55-62.
Melchior, J.C., Svensmark, O. and Trolle, D. (1967): Placental transfer of phenobarbitone in epileptic women, and elimination in newborns. *Lancet, 2:* 860-861.
Mirkin, B.L. (1971): Diphenylhydantoin: placental transport, fetal localization, neonatal metabolism, and possible teratogenic effects. *Journal of Pediatrics, 78:* 329-337.
Misès, R. and Plantade, A. (1967): Étude éxperimentale d'un nouvel antiépiloptique: le Dépakène. *Proceedings, Congrés de Psychiatrie et de Neurologie*, Dijon, July 4-9, pp. 964-966.
Monaco, F., Riccio, A., Gerna, M. and Morselli, P.L. et al., (1976): Further observations on carbamazepine plasma levels in epileptic patients. Relationship with therapeutic and side effects. *Neurology, 26:* 936-943.
Morselli, P.L. (1974): Significato ed importanza della misura e del controllo delle concentrazioni plasmatiche dei farmaci nella terapia dell'epilessia. *Prospettive in Pediatria, n. 12:* 523-541.
Morselli, P.L. (1975): Carbamazepine: absorption, distribution and excretion. In: *Complex Partial Seizures and Their Treatment—Advances in Neurology*, Vol. 11, edited by D.D. Daly and J.K. Penry, Raven Press, New York, pp. 279-283.
Morselli, P.L. (1976a): Pediatric Clinical Pharmacology—Routine monitoring or clinical trials? In: *Clinical Pharmacy and Clinical Pharmacology*, edited by Gouveia, Tognoni and Van der Kleijn. North-Holland Biomedical Press, pp. 279-289.
Morselli, P.L. Assael, B., Gomeni, R., Mandelli, M., Marini, A., Reali, E. Visconti di Massimo, U. and Sereni, F. (1975d): Digoxin pharmacokinetic during human development. In: *Basic and Therapeutic Aspects of Perinatal Pharmacology*, edited by P.L. Morselli, S. Garattini and F. Sereni, pp. 367-392, Raven Press, New York.
Morselli, P.L., Biandrate, P., Frigerio, A. and Garattini, S. (1972): Pharmacokinetics of carbamazepine in rats and humans. *European Journal of Clinical Investigation, 2:* 297.
Morselli, P.L., Biandrate, P., Frigerio, A., Gerna, M. and Tognoni, G. (1973): Gas chromatographic determination of carbamazepine and carbamazepine-10,11-epoxide in human body fluids. In: *Methods of Analysis of Antiepileptic Drugs*, edited by J.W.A. Meijer, H. Meinardi, C. Gardner-Thorpe and E. van der Kleijn, pp. 169-175, Excerpta Medica, Amsterdam.
Morselli, P.L. and Frigerio, A. (1975): Metabolism and pharmacokinetics of carbamazepine. *Drug Metabolism Reviews, 4:* 97-113.
Morselli, P.L., Garattini, S. and Cohen, S. (eds.) (1974): *Drug Interactions*, Raven Press, New York.

Morselli, P.L., Baruzzi, A., Bossi, L., Gerna, M., Porta, M. (1976b): Carbamazepine and carbamazepine-10,11-epoxide concentrations in human brain. In: *British Journal of Clinical Pharmacology*, in press.

Morselli, P.L., Bossi, L., Gerna, M. (1976): Pharmacokinetic studies with carbamazepine in epileptic patients. In: *Epileptic Seizures, Behavior, Pain*, edited by W. Birkmayer, Hans Huber Publ., Vienna, pp. 141-150.

Morselli, P.L., Gerna, M., de Maio, D., Zanda, G., Viani, F. and Garattini, S. (1975a): Pharmacokinetic studies on carbamazepine in volunteers and in epileptic patients. In: *Clinical Pharmacology of Antiepileptic Drugs*, edited by H. Schneider, et al., Springer-Verlag, Berlin, pp. 166-180.

Morselli, P.L., Gerna, M. and Garattini, S. (1971a): Carbamazepine plasma and tissue levels in the rat. *Biochemical Pharmacology, 20:* 2043-2047.

Morselli, P.L., Monaco, F., Gerna, M., Recchia, M. and Riccio, A. (1975b): Bioavailability of two different carbamazepine preparations in course of chronic administration to epileptic patients. *Epilepsia* (Amsterdam), *16:* 759-764.

Morselli, P.L., Rizzo, M. and Garattini, S. (1971b): Interaction between phenobarbital and diphenylhydantoin in animals and in epileptic patients. *Annals of the New York Academy of Sciences, 179:* 88-107.

Naestoft, J., Lund, M., Larsen, N.-E. and Hvidberg, E. (1973): Assay and pharmacokinetics of clonazepam in humans. *Acta Neurologica Scandinavica, 49,* suppl. 53: 103-108.

Nolte, R. and Brügmann, G. (1975): Problems in controlled anticonvulsive treatment with phenytoin in children. I. In: *Clinical Pharmacology of Antiepileptic Drugs*, edited by H. Schneider, et al., Springer-Verlag, Berlin, pp. 70-78.

Odar-Cederlöf, I. and Borgå, O. (1974): Kinetics of diphenylhydantoin in uraemic patients: consequences of decreased plasma protein binding. *European Journal of Clinical Pharmacology, 7:* 31-37.

Palmér, L., Bertilsson, L., Collste, P. and Rawlins, M. (1973): Quantitative determination of carbamazepine in plasma by mass fragmentography. *Clinical Pharmacology and Therapeutics, 14:* 827-832.

Parker, W.A. and Gumnit, R.J. (1974): Diphenylhydantoin toxicity: dose-dependent blood dyscrasia. *Neurology, 24:* 1178-1180.

Patel, H. and Crichton, J.U. (1968): The neurologic hazards of diphenylhydantoin in childhood. *Journal of Pediatrics, 73:* 676-684.

Penry, J.K. (1974): Usefulness of serum antiepileptic drug levels in the treatment of epilepsy. In: *Drug Interactions*, edited by P.L. Morselli, S. Garattini and S.N. Cohen, pp. 299-308, Raven Press, New York.

Penry, J.K. (1975): *Complex Partial Seizures and Their Treatment. Advances in Neurology*, V. 11, Raven Press, New York.

Penry, J.K., Porter, R.J. and Dreifuss, F.E. (1972): Ethosuximide. Relation of plasma levels to clinical control. In: *Antiepileptic Drugs*, edited by D.M. Woodbury, J.K. Penry and R.P. Schmidt, pp. 431-441, Raven Press, New York.

Plaa, G.L. and Hine, C.H. (1960): Hydantoin and barbiturate blood levels observed in epileptics. *Archives Internationales de Pharmacodynamie et de Thérapie, 128:* 375-382.

Ploman, L. and Persson, B.H. (1957): On transfer of barbiturates to human foetus and their accumulation in some of its vital organs. *Journal of Obstetrics and Gynaecology of the British Commonwealth, 64:* 706.

Rane, A. (1974): Urinary excretion of diphenylhydantoin metabolites in newborn infants. *Journal of Pediatrics, 85:* 543-545.

Rane, A., Bertilsson, L. and Palmér, L. (1975): Disposition of placentally transferred carbamazepine (Tegretol) in the newborn. *European Journal of Clinical Pharmacology, 8:* 283-284.

Rane, A., Garle, M., Borgå, O. Sjöqvist, F. (1974): Plasma disappearance of transplacentally transferred diphenylhydantoin in the newborn studied by mass fragmentography. *Clinical Pharmacology and Therapeutics, 15:* 39-45.

Rane, A., Lunde, P.K.M., Jalling, B., Yaffe, S.J. and Sjöqvist, F. (1971): Plasma protein binding of diphenylhydantoin in normal and hyperbilirubinemic infants. *Journal of Pediatrics, 78:* 877-882.

Rawlins, M.D., Collste, P., Bertilsson, L. and Palmér, L. (1975): Distribution and elimination kinetics of carbamazepine in man. *European Journal of Clinical Pharmacology, 8:* 91-96.

Reidenberg, M.M., Odar-Cederlöf, I., Von Bahr, C., Borgå, O. and Sjöqvist, F. (1971): Protein binding of diphenylhydantoin and desmethylimipramine in plasma from patients with poor renal function. *New England Journal of Medicine, 285:* 264-267.

Reynolds, E.H. (1972): Diphenylhydantoin. Hematologic aspects of toxicity. In: *Antiepileptic Drugs*, edited by D.M. Woodbury, J.K. Penry and R.P. Schmidt, pp. 247-262, Raven Press, New York.

Reynolds, E.H., Mattson, R.H. and Gallagher, B.B. (1971): Relationships between serum and cerebrospinal fluid anticonvulsant drug and folic acid concentrations in epileptic patients. *Neurology, 21:* 394.

Reynolds, J.W. and Mirkin, B.L. (1973): Urinary corticosteroid and diphenylhydantoin metabolite patterns in neonates exposed to anticonvulsant drugs in utero. *Clinical Pharmacology and Therapeutics, 14:* 891-897.

Richens, A. (1974): Drug estimation in the treatment of epilepsy. *Proceedings of the Royal Society of Medicine, 67:* 1227-1229.

Richens, A. and Rowe, D.J. (1970): Disturbance of calcium metabolism by anticonvulsant drugs. *British Medical Journal, 4:* 73-76.

Righetti, A., Baruzzi, A., Bossi, L., Gerna, M., Canger, R., Viani, F. and Morselli, P.L. (1976): Factors influencing ethosuximide plasma levels in epileptic patients. In preparation.

Rizzo, M., Breschi, F., Bossi, L., Avanzini, G. and Morselli, P.L. (1976): Plasma levels of phenobarbital and diphenylhydantoin in epileptic children. In preparation.

Rodin, E.A., Rim, C.S. and Rennick, P.M. (1974): The effects of carbamazepine on patients with psychomotor epilepsy: results of a double-blind study. *Epilepsia* (Amsterdam, *15:* 547-561.

Roger, J., Grangeon, H., Gueyj, J. and Lob, H. (1968): Incidences psychiatriques et psychologiques du traitement par l'éthosuccimide chez les épileptiques. *Encephale, 57:* 704-438.

Scheffner, D. and Schiefer, I.S. (1972): The treatment of epileptic children with carbamazepine. *Epilepsia* (Amsterdam), *13:* 819-828.

Schiller, P.J. and Buchthal, F. (1958): Diphenylhydantoin and phenobarbital in serum in patients with epilepsy. *Danish Medical Bulletin, 5:* 161-163.

Schobben, F. and van der Kleijn, E. (1974): Pharmacokinetics of distribution and elimination of sodium di-n-propylacetate in mouse and dog. *Pharmaceutisch Weekblad, 109:* 33-42.

Schobben, F., van der Kleijn, E. and Gabreels, F.J.M. (1975): Pharmacokinetics of di-n-propylacetate in epileptic patients. *European Journal of Clinical Pharmacology, 8:* 97-105.

Sereni, F., Mandelli, M., Principi, N., Tognoni, G., Pardi, G. and Morselli, P.L. (1973): Induction of drug metabolizing enzyme activities in the human fetus and in the newborn infant. *Enzyme, 15:* 318-329.
Serrano, E.E., Roye, D.B., Hammer, R.H. and Wilder, B.J. (1973): Plasma diphenylhydantoin values after oral and intramuscular administration of diphenylhydantoin. *Neurology, 23:* 311-317.
Sherwin, A.L. (1973): Does monitoring of anti-epileptic drugs lead to improved seizure control? Ethosuximide levels in absence attacks. In: *Methods of Analysis of Anti-Epileptic Drugs,* edited by J.W.A. Meijer, H. Meinardi, C. Gardner-Thorpe and E. van der Kleijn, pp. 1-5, Excerpta Medica, Amsterdam.
Sherwin, A.L. Eisen, A.A. and Sokolowski, C.D. (1973a): Anticonvulsant drugs in human epileptogenic brain. Correlation of phenobarbital and diphenylhydantoin levels with plasma. *Archives of Neurology, 29:* 73-77.
Sherwin, A.L., Loynd, J.S., Bock, G.W. and Sokolowski, C.D. (1974): Effects of age, sex, obesity and pregnancy on Plasma diphenylhydantoin levels. *Epilepsia* (Amsterdam), *15:* 507-521.
Sherwin, A.L., and Robb, J.P. (1972): Ethosuximide. Relation of plasma levels to clinical control. In: *Antiepileptic Drugs,* edited by D.M. Woodbury, J.K. Penry and R.P. Schmidt, pp. 443-448, Raven Press, New York.
Sherwin, A.L., Robb, J.P. and Lechter, M. (1973b): Improved control of epilepsy by monitoring plasma ethosuximide. *Archives of Neurology, 28:* 178-181.
Shoeman, D.W., Benjamin, D.M. and Azarnoff, D.L. (1973): The alteration of plasma proteins in uremia as reflected in the ability to bind diphenylhydantoin. *Annals of the New York Academy of Sciences, 226:* 127-130.
Sjö, O., Hvidberg, E.F., Naestoft, J. and Lund, M. (1975): Pharmacokinetics and side-effects of clonazepam and its 7-amino-metabolite in man. *European Journal of Clinical Pharmacology, 8:* 249-254.
Sjögren, J., Solvell, L. and Karlsson, I. (1965): Studies on the absorption rate of barbiturates in man. *Acta Medica Scandinavica, 178:* 553-559.
Solow, E.B. and Green, J.B. (1971): The determination of ethosuximide in serum by gas chromatography. Preliminary results of clinical application. *Clinica Chimica Acta, 33:* 87-90.
Solow, E.B. and Green, J.B. (1972): The simultaneous determination of multiple anti convulsant drug levels by gas-liquid chormatography. *Neurology, 22:* 540-550.
Sonnen, A.E.H., Blom, G.F. and Meijer, J.W.A. (1975): Enteric coated depakine. In: *Clinical Pharmacology of Antiepileptic Drugs,* edited by H. Schneider, et al., Springer-Verlag, Berlin, pp. 229-236.
Stensrud, P.A. and Palmer, H. (1964): Serum phenytoin determination in epileptics, *Epelepsia* (Amsterdam), *5:* 364370.
Strandjord, R.E. and Johannessen, S.I. (1975): A preliminary study of serum carbamazepine levels in healthy subjects and in patients with epilepsy. In: *Clinical Pharmacology of Antiepileptic Drugs,* edited by H. Schneider, et al., Springer-Verlag, Berlin, pp. 181-188.
Sunshine, I. (1957): Chemical evidence of tolerance to phenobarbital. *Journal of Laboratory and Clinical Medicine, 50:* 127-133.
Svensmark, O. and Buchthal, F. (1963a): Accumulation of phenobarbital in man. *Epilepsia* (Amsterdam), *4:* 199-206.
Svensmark, O. and Buchthal, F. (1963b): Dosage of phenytoin and phenobarbital in children. *Danish Medical Bulletin, 10:* 234-235.
Svensmark, O. and Buchthal, F. (1964): Diphenylhydantoin and phenobarbital. Serum levels in children. *American Journal Diseases of Children, 108:* 82-87.

Tenckhoff, H., Sherrard, D.J., Hickman, R.O. and Ladda, R.L. (1968): Acute diphenylhydantoin intoxication. *American Journal Diseases of Children, 116:* 422-425.
Triedman, H.M., Fishman, R.A. and Yahr, M.D. (1960): Determination of plasma and cerebrospinal fluid levels of Dilantin in the human. *Transactions of the American Neurological Association, 85:* 166-170.
Troupin, A.S., Green, J.R. and Levy, R.H. (1974): Carbamazepine as an anticonvulsant: a pilot study. *Neurology, 24:* 863-869.
Vajda, F., Williams, F.M., Davidson, S., Falconer, M.A. and Breckenridge, A. (1974): Human brain, cerebrospinal fluid, and plasma concentrations of diphenylhydantoin and phenobarbital. *Clinical Pharmacology and Therapeutics, 15:* 597-603.
van der Kleijn, E. (1975): Personal communication.
Waddel, W.J. and Butler, T.C. (1957): The distribution and excretion of phenobarbital. *Journal of Clinical Investigation, 36:* 1217-1226.
Wallin, A., Jalling, B. and Boréus, L.O. (1974): Plasma concentrations of phenobarbital in the neonate during prophylaxis for neonatal hyperbilirubinemia. *Journal of Pediatrics, 85:* 392-397.
Wallis, W., Kutt, H. and McDowell, F. (1968): Intravenous diphenylhydantoin in treatment of acute repetitive seizures. *Neurology, 18:* 513-525.
Wechselberg, K. and Hübel, G. (1967): Zur Resorption und Verteilung von Methyl-Alt hyl-suxcinimid (MAS) im Serum und Liquor bei Kindern. *Zeitschrift für Kinderheilkunde, 100:* 10-19.
Weiss, C.F., Heffelfinger, J.C. and Buchanan, R.A. (1969): Serial Dilantin levels in mentally retarded children. *American Journal of Mental Deficiency, 73:* 826-830.
Wilder, B.J., Buchanan, R.A. and Serrano, E.E. (1973a): Correlation of acute diphenylhydantoin intoxication with plasma levels and metabolite excretion. *Neurology, 23:* 1329-1332.
Wilder, B.J., Serrano, E.E. and Ramsay, R.E. (1973b): Plasma diphenylhydantoin levels after loading and maintenance doses. *Clinical Pharmacology and Therapeutics, 14:* 797-801.
Wilder, B.J., Serrano, E.E., Ramsey, E. and Buchanan, R.A. (1974): A method for shifting from oral to intramuscular diphenylhydantoin administration. *Clinical Pharmacology and Therapeutics, 16:* 507-513.
Wilder, B.J., Streiff, R.R. and Hammer, R.H. (1972): Diphenylhydantoin. Absorption, distribution, and excretion: clinical studies. In: *Antiepileptic Drugs*, edited by D.M Woodbury, J.K. Penry and R.P. Schmidt, pp. 137-148, Raven Press, New York
Wilensky, A.J. and Lowden, J.A. (1973): Inadequate serum levels after intramuscular administration of diphenylhydantoin. *Neurology, 23:* 318-324.
Wilkinson, G.R. and Kurata, D. (1974): The uptake of diphenylhydantoin by the human erythrocyte and its application to the estimation of plasma binding. In: *Drug Interactions*, edited by P.L. Morselli, S. Garattini and S.N. Cohen, pp. 289-297, Raven Press, New York.
Wilson, J.T. (1970): Alteration of normal development of drug metabolism by injection of growth hormone. *Nature* (London) *225:* 861-863.
Wilson, J.T. and Wilkinson, G.R. (1973): Chronic and severe phenobarbital intoxication in a child treated with primidone and diphenylhydantoin. *Journal of Pediatrics, 83:* 484-489.
Wink, C.A.S. (1972): *Tegretol in Epilepsy.* Report of an international clinical symposium held in London, Nicholls, Manchester.
Woodbury, D.M., Penry, J.K. and Schmidt, R.P. (eds.) (1972): *Antiepileptic Drugs*, Raven Press, New York.

Woodbury, D.M. and Swinyard, E.A. (1972): Diphenylhydantoin, Absorption, distribution, and excretion. In: *Antiepileptic Drugs,* edited by D.M. Woodbury, J.K. Penry and R.P. Schmidt, pp. 113-123, Raven Press, New York.

Zwacka, G. and Grenzel, J. (1971): Untersuchungen zur Beinflussung der Hyperbilirubinamie unreifer Neugeborener durch Kurzzeit-induktion mit Phenobarbital. *Paediatrie und Paedologie, 6:* 102.

12

Hypnotics

LAURA BOSSI AND PAOLO LUCIO MORSELLI

Hypnotics (barbiturates and non-barbiturates) are widely used for the symptomatic relief of insomnia. Their effectiveness has generally been determined by clinical evaluation, while only in recent years has information become available on their kinetics in humans. These drugs are usually administered chronically, hence, knowledge of their metabolism and disposition is of considerable importance, since a distinct limitation of the duration of action is needed.

Many commonly used hypnotics have a half-life which exceeds the duration of a night's sleep, giving rise to unpleasant "hangover" effects and to accumulation in the course of chronic therapy, a highly undesirable event. Furthermore, some compounds with a short half-life, such as flurazepam, have active metabolites which are slowly cleared from the organism and contribute substantially to the drug's action. For others, the accumulation is counteracted to a certain degree by the development of autoinduction phenomena which determine a shortening of the half-life. Often this also results in interactions with other drugs. It must be underlined that accumulation does not necessarily imply a persistence of the CNS depression, since tolerance may develop.

In this chapter, we have included some compounds which may actually be excluded from clinical practice in the United States but which are nevertheless widely prescribed in children in many other countries. To the best of our knowledge, very few data are available on pharmacokinetics of hypnotics at pediatric age. We feel that such information is needed, even if the use of hypnotics in pediatrics is questionable for ethical reasons.

CHLORAL HYDRATE

Adults

Chloral hydrate is one of the oldest known hypnotic agents. Although its popularity has greatly diminished since the introduction of barbiturates and benzodiazepines in the treatment of insomnia, it is still a widely used hypnotic (Hartmann and Cravens, 1973), particularly in children and in elderly patients (Maynert, 1971; Ferguson Anderson, 1973). It has also been recommended for the treatment of infantile febrile convulsions (Martindale, 1972), and for preoperative sedation (Root, 1962; Ilingworth, 1968). Small doses produce sedation (0.5 g), larger doses facilitate sleep (1-2 g), overdosage leads to anesthesia or coma (4-20 g). Chloral hydrate is very rapidly reduced to trichloroethanol, which is responsible for the pharmacological effect of the drug (Butler, 1948; Marshall and Owens, 1954). This reaction occurs in the liver and other tissues, as well as erythrocytes (Butler, 1949; Sellers et al., 1972a), and is catalyzed by the enzyme alcohol dehydrogenase (Friedman and Cooper, 1960). Alcohol may severely enhance the central depressant action of chloral hydrate (Adams, 1940; Kaplan et al., 1969; Sellers et al., 1972b). In man, this interaction results in higher trichloroethanol levels and, also, in higher blood alcohol concentrations (Sellers, 1972a). A small amount of trichloroethanol is excreted unchanged in the urine; the rest is conjugated to an inactive glucuronide before excretion (Marshall and Owens, 1954). Apart from reduction, chloral hydrate can be oxidized to trichloroacetic acid (Butler, 1948; Marshall and Owens, 1954; Cooper and Friedman, 1958), which is excreted unchanged in the urine (Paykoc and Powell, 1954). The metabolic fate of chloral hydrate is summarized in Fig. 1. Few quantitative studies on the pharmacokinetics of chloral hydrate have been available up to now. The early investigations by Marshall and Owens (1954) and by Owens and Marshall (1955) are very accurate metabolic studies, but are not useful in the determination of pharmacokinetic parameters. Sellers et al. (1972a), in a more recent study on the interaction of chloral hydrate and alcohol, determined an average half-life for trichloroethanol of 8.2 h. The pharmacokinetics of chloral hydrate and its metabolites have recently been reviewed by Breimer (1974), who developed a sensitive method for the simultaneous determination of chloral hydrate and its metabolites in biological fluids with which he determined their kinetics after both oral and rectal administration.

Unaltered chloral hydrate does not reach the blood circulation in measurable amounts; the CNS depressant activity after oral and rectal administration may therefore be entirely attributed to trichloroethanol. Peak levels of 7.6 $\mu g/ml$ (range: 5.2 to 11.2) of trichloroethanol are attained 20-60 min after an oral dose of 15 mg/kg; the trichloroethanol glucuronide reaches its maximum value of 6.7 $\mu g/ml$ (range: 2.7 to 10.7) in about the same time as does free trichloroe-

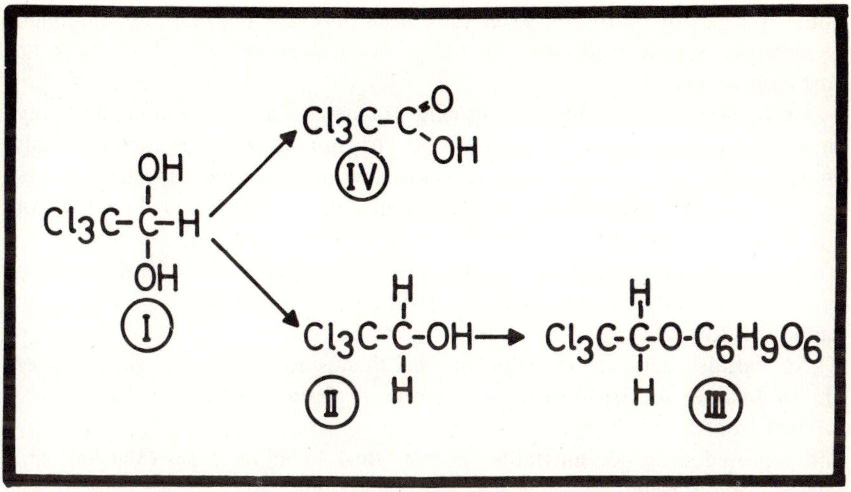

Fig. 1: Metabolism of chloralhydrate in man. I. Chloralhydrate; II. Trichloroethanol; III. Trichloroacetic acid glucuronide; IV. Trichloroacetic acid.

thanol. The concentrations of the two compounds then decay in a biphasic manner, the average half-lives of the beta-phase being about 8.0 h (range: 6.5 to 9.5 h) for trichloroethanol and about 6.7 h for the glucuronide (range: 6.8 to 8.0 h), respectively (Breimer, 1974). After rectal administration, absorption appears to be slower, but the apparent plasma half-lives of trichloroethanol are in the same range as those after oral administration.

A third important metabolite is trichloroacetic acid; this compound is rapidly formed after a single oral dose, considerable blood levels being reached in about 1 h. The plasma levels of trichloroacetic acid then increase slowly up to 12 h. Probably, the initial rapid formation of this acid occurs during the first passage of chloral hydrate through the liver as a result of oxidation by aldehyde dehydrogenase or, possibly, by the mixed-function oxygenase system, while the lower increase in trichloroacetic acid is most likely due to the oxidation of trichloroethanol. The half-life of trichloroacetic acid is very long: about 100 h (Breimer, 1974). These data agree with the earlier finding of Paykoc and Powell (1954), who found a T½ of 80-100 h after an i.v. infusion of the sodium salt in 6 human volunteers.

The compound is highly bound to plasma proteins, 84-94% for concentrations of 30-100 μg/ml plasma (Sellers and Koch-Weser, 1971), and, because of this characteristic, interactions with other drugs such as warfarin should be considered (Sellers and Koch-Weser, 1971). During repetitive administration of chloral hydrate, considerable accumulation of trichloroacetic acid takes place; concentrations of up to 100 µg/ml have been observed. Because this compound is a strong organic acid, the possibility of its eventual toxicity needs to be further investigated.

Unchanged chloral hydrate is usually not detectable in the urine, and only small quantities (2.6 to 7.7 mg) of free trichloroethanol are excreted. This finding could be consistent with the existence of significant tubular reabsorption. The urinary excretion of the glucuronide accounts for about 11 to 24% of the dose, whereas within 2 days up to 50% of the dose may be excreted as trichloroacetic acid. At present, there are no data available on the fecal excretion of chloral hydrate in man, and the possibility of other ways of elimination cannot be excluded.

No definite data are available on the therapeutic and toxic threshold of chloral hydrate and trichloroethanol; however, plasma levels of trichloroethanol ranging from 5 to 20 µg/ml were observed by several authors following single and repeated drug administration in the usual hypnotic doses (Marshall and Owens, 1954; Owens and Marshall, 1955; Sellers et al., 1972a,b; Breimer, 1974). The central depressant action of chloral hydrate or, more accurately, of trichloroethanol, resembles that of alcohol, the barbiturates and the gaseous anesthetics, and overdosage (4-20 g) causes anesthesia and coma.

Like many hypnotics, chronic chloral hydrate usage can result in habituation, tolerance and addiction; the abstinence syndrome resembles delirium tremens. Because of the drug's irritant properties, chloral hydrate addicts often manifest gastric symptoms. The drug may give rise to idiosyncratic cutaneous reactions (Christianson and Perry, 1956), although their incidence is very low. High concentrations of chloral hydrate inhibit cholinesterase and exert eserine-like actions (Dybing and Dybing, 1955; Brown, 1962), but trichloroethanol does not have this property.

Newborns, Infants and Children

There are little existing data on chloral hydrate kinetics in children or newborns, the one exception being a report by Rezza (1956), who, in children of 4-8 years, determined an apparent plasma half-life of 10 min after an i.v. administration. This lack of information on chloral hydrate metabolism and kinetics is somewhat surprising since the drug is used in pregnancy, it can cross the placenta, together with its metabolites, and, in addition, both trichloroethanol and trichloroacetic acid have been detected in human milk (Maynert, 1971; Lacey, 1971). Furthermore, as stated before, the drug is commonly used in pediatrics (Illingworth, 1968; Maynert, 1971; Martindale, 1972; Ferguson and Anderson, 1973). To the best of our knowledge, there has been only one report on chloral hydrate poisoning in the pediatric age group (Lansky, 1974).

GLUTETHIMIDE

Adults

The absorption rate of glutethimide is variable, peak levels ranging from 2.9 to 7.1 µg/ml and occurring at any time from 1 to 6 h after oral administration of sedative doses (500 mg) of the drug (Curry et al., 1971). Ambre and Fisher (1972) found plasma concentrations ranging from 6.2 to 6.8 µg/ml about 2 h after the administration of 1,000 mg dose in 3 healthy subjects. Parker et al. (1970) reported peak concentrations of 6.3 to 12.2 µg/ml after hypnotic doses of 2,000 mg. Erratic absorption has been reported in overdosed patients (Curry, 1971).

In the therapeutic concentration ranges, an average of 54.2% of the drug is bound to plasma proteins (range: 47.3 to 59.3%) (Curry et al., 1971). In normal volunteers given hypnotic doses of glutethimide, Curry et al. (1971) observed a biphasic decay of plasma concentrations, a rapid phase with an apparent plasma half-life of 3.85 h (range: 2.7-4.3) and a slow phase, which lasted from the 4th-8th hour to the 24th hour, with a mean apparent plasma half-life of 11.6 h (range: 5.1-22 h). These data agree with previous reports on healthy volunteers that described plasma half-lives of about 10 h in subjects given glutethimide in single doses ranging from 250 to 750 mg (Bütikofer et al., 1962).

In most reports on intoxicated patients, the plasma half-life of glutethimide are similar to the ones reported in normal subjects after sedative doses (Goldbaum et al., 1960; Curry et al., 1971; Hansen et al., 1975), with values of 10 to 11 h. Maher (1970) described in intoxicated patients serum apparent half-lives ranging from 10 to 175 h, together with a positive linear relationship between the initial serum levels and the half-life values. This finding could be explained by a rate-limited enzymatic degradation of glutethimide. Observations carried out on 3 renal patients without evidence of hepatic failure showed no correlation between urine flow and the serum half-life of glutethimide. Half-lives varying from 17 to 43 h were observed in anuric and chronic renal failure patients (Maher, 1970).

Glutethimide is mainly metab olized through hydroxylation by the microsomal enzyme system (Fig. 2) and rapidly excreted via the urine as 4-hydroxy-glutethimide glucuronide and alpha-phenyl-alpha-hydroxyethyl glutarimide, which account for about 90% of the dose. Less than 2% of the dose is excreted unmetabolized in the urine (Bütikofer et al., 1962; Curry et al., 1971). Mallein et al. (1960) found in the urine of humans given glutethimide traces of two other metabolites, alpha-phenylglutarimide, and alpha-phenyl-alpha-ethylglutaconimide, which are known to account for about 6% of the administered dose in dogs (Keberle et al., 1962). Bütikofer et al. (1962) were not able to confirm this finding. Early studies claimed that the enterohepatic circulation played a significant role in glutethimide toxicity on the basis of

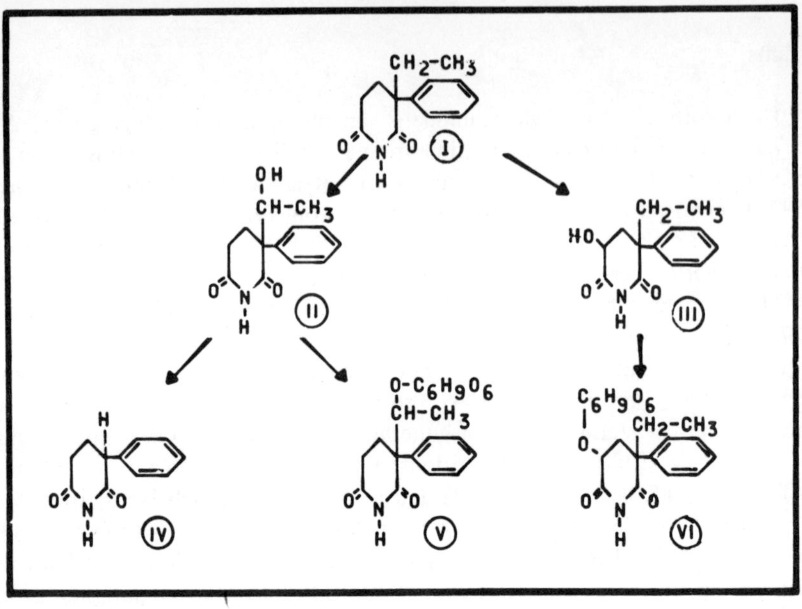

Fig. 2: Metabolism of glutethimide in man. I. glutethimide (α-phenyl-α-ethylglutharimide); II. αphenyl-α(1-hydroxyethylglutharimide); III. 4-hydroxyglutethimide (4-hydroxy-2-ethyl-2-phenylglutharimide; IV. αphenylglutharimide; V. αphenyl-α(1-hydroxy)ethylglutharimide glucuronide; VI. α-phenyl-α-ethylglutaconimide.

animal studies with labeled glutethimide (Bernhard et al., 1957); further studies by the same authors, however, demonstrated that 97–98% of the radioactivity found in the bile was associated with inactive metabolites (Keberle et al., 1962). More recently, Charytan et al. (1970) showed that in 5 patients with T-tube biliary drainage who had received 500 mg of glutethimide per os (with a mean 4 h serum level of 2.1 µg/ml) only 0.13% of the dose could be recovered in the bile. No data are available on 4-hydroxyglutethimide biliary excretion in man.

In intoxicated patients, accumulation of 4-hydroxyglutethimide takes place in plasma and tissues (Ambre and Fischer, 1972, 1974; Hansen and Fischer, 1974; Hansen et al., 1975). This fact is of considerable clinical interest, because 4-hydroxyglutethimide is pharmacologically active, and could play an important role in glutethimide poisoning.

In patients taking hypnotic doses of glutethimide, peak plasma levels from 5 to 7 µg/ml have been reported (Bütikofer et al., 1962; Curry et al., 1971; Ambre and Fischer, 1972). In cases of glutethimide overdose, plasma levels as high as 110 µg/ml have been found (Chazan and Cohen, 1969; Maher and Schreiner, 1969). There seems to be general agreement on the fact that the relationship between plasma levels and the severity of intoxication is very poor (Chazan and Cohen, 1969; Wright and Roscoe, 1970; Rosenbaum et al., 1971; Chazan and Garella, 1971). Gold et al. (1973), in patients in coma caused by glutethimide, found CSF concentrations which were from 10 to 82% ((mean: 35 ± 5) of those in the plasma (which ranged from 9 to 31 µg/ml). The serum levels at the time of arousal varied from 4 toto 18 µg/ml, with corresponding CSF values of 1.5 to 5.8 µg/ml. The poor relationship between the clinical picture and the plasma or CSF glutethimide levels in all likelihood can be explained by the presence of a significant accumulation of the active metabolite 4-hydroxyglutethimide in plasma and tissues (Ambre and Fischer, 1972, 1974; Hansen and Fischer, 1974; Hansen et al., 1975). Plasma levels of 16.8-22.7 µg/ml were observed in 3 cases of nonfatal intoxication, while brain levels of 6-44 µg/ml were found in human post-mortem samples (Hansen and Fischer, 1974). Probably a relationship exists to a certain degree between severity of intoxication and plasma levels if one considers the total level of both compounds, as may be suggested considering the two fatal cases recently reported by Hansen and Fischer (1974).

The most frequently occurring side effect of glutethimide is a generalized rash, which usually disappears within 2 or 3 days after withdrawal of the drug. On the other hand, nausea, residual sedation, paradoxical excitement, blurred vision, acute hypersensitivity reactions, acute intermittent porphyria, thrombocytopenic purpura, aplastic anemia, urticaria, exfoliative dermatitis and leukopenia have all been reported, but rarely occur (AMA, 1973). Greenwood et al. (1973) reported a case of osteomalacia associated with long-term glutethimide administration. There was evidence of hepatic enzyme induction, and the plasma half-life of ^{3}H-vitamin D_3 was decreased. These changes were reversed by suspending the drug. Long-term use of "larger than usual" therapeutic doses may result in psychic and physical dependence (Sharpless, 1970). The clinical picture usually is that of a toxic psychosis, with mydriasis and dryness of the mouth. Withdrawal of the drug under these conditions may provoke hallucinations or convulsions. There are some reports on the development of neurological abnormalities in cases of glutethimide (Lingl, 1966; Nover, 1967; Haas and Marasigan, 1968). Overdosage (20-30 times the usual dose) has caused prolonged coma with cyclic variations in depth, associated with more marked hypotension and a lesser degree of respiratory depression than in barbiturate poisoning (McBay and Katsas, 1957). Areflexia or intermittent spasticity of the extremities and fever (less frequently, hypothermy) are often observed (Myess and Stockard, 1975). Peritomeal dialysis or hemodialysis has not proven to be more effective in treating overdosage than intensive supportive therapy (Wright and Roscoe, 1970; Chazan and Cohen, 1969).

Newborns, Infants and Children

No data are available on glutethimide disposition in newborns and infants. It is known that the drug readily crosses the placenta; similar meternal and neonatal plasma concentrations were found by Curry et al. (1971) in newborns of mothers taking glutethimide chronically during the last days of pregnancy. The drug is also excreted in mother's milk but at very low concentrations (<0.3 µg/ml) (Curry et al., 1971); therefore, it seems unlikely that important amounts of glutethimide are transferred from nursing mothers to breast-fed infants. Certainly, it is important to remember that newborns of mothers dependent on glutethimide may also show an abstinence syndrome (Maynert, 1971).

METHAQUALONE

Methaqualone appears to be well absorbed from the gastrointestinal tract both in healthy volunteers and in patients. After a single oral dose of 170-150 mg, peak concentrations of 1.1-2.7 µg/ml are usually attained with 1-2 h, while concentrations of 1.8-5.2 µg/ml have been described following a 300 mg dose (Berry, 1969; Morris et al., 1972; Alvan et al., 1973; Clifford et al., 1974; Nayak et al., 1974). The preparation in salt form is better absorbed than the free base (Goenechea et al., 1973). In a study on the relative bioavailability of different tablet and capsule dosage forms, using both C^{14}-labeled and unlabeled drug, Smith et al. (1973) observed higher plasma levels and earlier urinary excretion of administered radioactivity with the loose-filled capsule form.

Presence of diphenhydramine hydrochloride in the pharmaceutical preparation does not seem to alter the methaqualone absorption pattern (Williams et al., 1974). No differences in the area-under-the-curve seem to occur after single or repeated administration (Nayak et al., 1974) and between fasted and unfasted subjects (Smyth et al., 1973; Nayak et al., 1974). Methaqualone has a high tissue affinity, and in animal studies it appears to be widely distributed in most tissues (Cohen et al., 1962; Akagi et al., 1963; Smart and Brown, 1970); the apparent volume of distribution in humans may range from 5.4 to 7.7 L/kg (Alvan et al., 1974).

Under normal conditions, methaqualone is extensively bound to plasma proteins (Smart and Brown, 1970). At concentrations within the therapeutic range (1.2-4 µg/ml), a fractional binding to plasma proteins of 80-81.5% has been reported by Alvan et al. (1974), whereas for plasma levels of 40 µg/ml (toxic concentrations) the binding is about 70% (Smyth et al., 1973). Methaqualone is largely excluded from red blood cells; in fact, only 20% of the amount present in blood has been found to be bound to erythrocytes (Berry, 1969; Mitchard and Williams, 1972; Williams et al., 1974).

While a previous report by Morris et al. (1972) gave an average apparent plasma half-life of 2.6 h, recent reports utilizing more specific and sensitive analytical methods (GLC-MS) describe a biexponential decay of the plasma concentrations and a longer half-life. The fast component of the plasma apparent half-life may range from 0.9 to 5 h, while the slow component (β-phase) may vary from 16 to 41.5 h (Alvan et al., 1973; Clifford et al., 1974; Nayak et al., 1974). The multiple-dose kinetics of methaqualone have recently been studied by Alvan et al. (1974). As suggested by the drug's long half-life, steady-state plasma levels were reached in about 10 days. For daily doses of 1 mg/kg, steady-state plasma levels ranged from 0.2 to 0.5 µg/ml, while the dosages of 300 mg/day steady-state plasma levels of 1.2 to 1.7 µg were reported (Nayak et al., 1974). The apparent plasma half-life of methaqualone with multiple dosing was considerably shorter than after a single dose, thus suggesting induced metabolism (Alvan et al., 1974).

Methaqualone is extensively metabolized, the major route of degradation in man involving hydroxylation of the 2 and 2' methyl groups and of the tolyl and quinazoline rings (Fig. 3). Subsequent O-methylation and glucuronide-derivative formation occurs prior to excretion (Agaki et al., 1963; Preuss et al., 1966a,b; Nowak et al., 1966; Preuss and Hassler, 1970; Bonnichsen et al., 1972; Brown and Goenechea, 1973). At the present time, no data are available on the possible activity of these methaqualone metabolites in man.

The primary routes of drug excretion are renal and biliary, with some enterohepatic recirculation of the metabolites (Brown and Goenechea, 1973; Smyth et al., 1973; Nayak et al., 1974). Very little of the unchanged drug is excreted in the urine, either after therapeutic doses or following overdosage (Heyndricks and de Leenheer, 1969; Geldmacher-Mallinckrodt and Mang, 1970; Allen et al., 1970; Goudie and Burnett, 1971). Studies with C^{14}-labeled methaqualone have shown that in man about 50 to 70% of the dose is excreted in the urine as the metabolites over a 72 h period (Smyth et al., 1973). In the same study, the fecal recovery of C^{14}, representing unchanged drug and metabolites, accounted for 1 to 4% of the dose over a 96 h collection period. At high doses, methaqualone may be a consistent inducer of liver microsomal enzymes (Ballinger et al., 1972; Zarolinsky et al., 1972). A 2-3 fold increase in D-glucaric acid excretion has been reported by Nayak et al., (1974) following an 8-28 day administration.

According to the various reports, therapeutic plasma levels may range from 0.9 to 2.2 µg/ml (Brown and Smart, 1969; Berry, 1969; Morris et al., 1972; Goenechea et al., 1973; Bailey and Jatlow, 1973), while levels over 5-10 µg/ml are often associated with severe toxic, and even fatal, complications. Mild methaqualone overdosage leads to a picture of central nervous system depression,

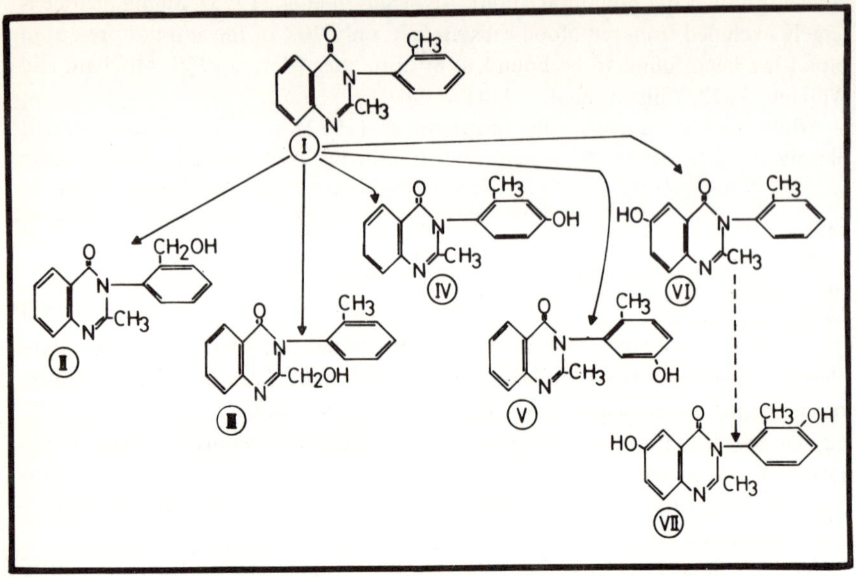

Fig. 3: Metabolism of methaqualone in man. I. methaqualone-(2-methyl-3-o-tolyl-4(3H)-quinazolinone; II. 2-methyl-3-(3-hydroxymethylphenyl)-4(3H)-quinazolinone; III. 2-hydroxymethyl-3-o-tolyl-4(3H)-quinazolinone; IV. 2-methyl-3(4-hydroxy-2-methylphenyl)-3H)-quinazolinone; V. 2-methyl-3(5-hydroxy-2-methylphenyl)-4(3H)-quinazolinone; VI. 2-methyl-3(o-tolyl)-6-hydroxy-4(3H)-quinazolinone; VII. 6-hydroxy-2-methyl-3(3' hydroxy-2'methylphenyl)-4(3H)-quinazolinone.

associated with dizziness, mild ataxia and visual distortion (Matthew et al., 1972; Alvan et al., 1974). In cases of severe poisoning, pyramidal signs, hypertonicity, increased limb reflexes and myoclonia are frequently present (Matthew et al., 1972; Abboud et al., 1974). It is worth noting that, as opposed to barbiturate poisoning, marked respiratory depression is rare (Johnstone et al., 1971; Matthew et al., 1972). With therapeutic doses, minor gastric distress, nausea, headaches and skin rashes, as well as excitation and chronic neuropathy, have been reported (Geldmacher-Mallinckrodt and Lautenbach, 1963; Matthew et al., 1968; Malmlund et al., 1972; Finke and Spiegelberg, 1973; Editorial, 1973).

No data are presently available on the kinetics of methaqualone in infancy, childhood and adolescence. Being metabolized through hepatic oxidative systems, it is likely that methaqualone shows an age-dependent metabolic rate; however, more specific information is both important and necessary since it is known that the drug crosses the placenta and that physical tolerance may result from its long-term use. Furthermore, in many countries among young people methaqualone has become a drug that is widely abused (de Alarcon, 1969).

BARBITURATES

Adults

Amobarbital is readily absorbed from the gastrointestinal tract. After a single dose of 200 mg, peak levels of 2.4–2.7 µg/ml are attained within 2 h (Sjögren et al., 1965); comparable absorption will result following i.m. administration (Krauer et al., 1973). Amobarbital is distributed rather uniformly throughout the body; changes in body pH may alter its distribution but not so strikingly as with phenobarbital (Garrett et al., 1974). The apparent Vd ranges from 0.9 to 1.2 L/kg (Balasubramaniam et al., 1970a,b; Mawer et al., 1970). In normal adult subjects, 58–61% binding to plasma proteins has been reported (Mawer et al., 1972; Ehrnebo and Odar-Cederlof, 1975). The plasma protein-binding of amobarbital does appear to increase with pH (Goldbaum and Smith, 1954; Branstad et al., 1972); however, this change should be negligible within the range of physiological variations and over the pH range in alkalotic and acidotic conditions. In chronic liver disease, the binding may be significantly decreased (31%) in those patients with low albumin concentration (3.5 g/100 ml). The main metabolite of amobarbital, hydroxyamobarbital, does not show any significant binding to plasma proteins (Grove and Toseland, 1971).

The amobarbital disappearance curve in plasma appears to fit a two-compartment open model with a biexponential decay. The alpha-phase has an apparent T½ of 0.5–0.6 h, while the apparent plasma half-life for the beta-phase may vary from 16 to 24 h (Balasubramaniam et al., 1970a,b; Grove and Toseland, 1971; Mawer et al., 1972). The disappearance rate of amobarbital is dose-dependent, according to Balasubramaniam et al. (1970b), although such data have recently been criticized by Garrett et al. (1974). Mawer et al. (1972) have described a prolonged amobarbital apparent plasma half-life (beta-phase = 39.4 ± 6.6 h; control group: 21.1 ± 1.23 h) in patients with chronic liver disease, concomitant with a reduced excretion of hydroxyamobarbital. It might be of interest to note that a prolonged half-life was observed only in those cases with hypoalbuminemia and that the longest half-lives (about 49 h) were found in two patients with portocaval anastomosis (Mawer et al., 1970).

Amobarbital is metabolized primarily by oxidation to its 3-hydroxymetabolite, 5-ethyl-5(3-hydroxyisoamyl) barbituric acid (Fig. 4) (Maynert, 1965), which has been reported to have some hypnotic activity in mice (Irrgang, 1965). The urinary excretion of this polar derivative accounts (at therapeutic doses) for about half of the dose over a period of 120 h (Maynert, 1965; Kamm and Van Loon, 1966). A greater urine output (diuretically augmented or increased by

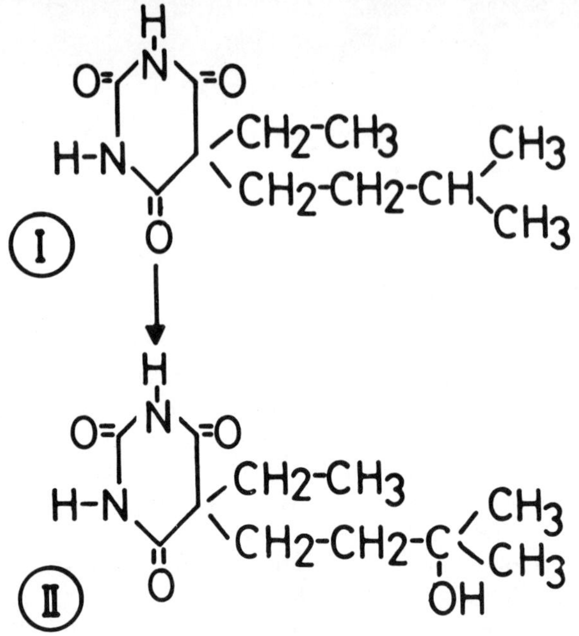

Fig. 4: Metabolism of amobarbital. I. amobarbital; II. 3-hydroxyamobarbital.

extra fluid intake) is accompanied by a greater excretion of hydroxyamobarbital (Grove and Toseland, 1971), lending some support to the application of forced diuresis in amobarbital overdosage (Mawer and Lee, 1968). Essentially no unchanged amobarbital is excreted via the urine, even after an overdose (Maynert, 1965; Kamm and Van Loon, 1966; Mawer and Lee, 1968; Balasubramaniam et al., 1970b). Although Kamm and Van Loon (1966) and Maynert (1965) did not detect any glucuronide that was susceptible to beta-glucuronide hydrolysis in the urine of amobarbital-treated patients, non-glucuronide conjugates may be present. In fact, Balasubramaniam and his group (1970a) showed that some individuals do excrete hydroxyamobarbital partly as a conjugate which is readily hydrolyzed in acid but not by beta-glucuronidase. The remainder of the dose may be eliminated as undetected conjugates of hydroxyamobarbital in feces or urine, or as further oxidation products not yet identified. In elderly subjects, the rate of hydroxylation of amobarbital is significantly lower than that in young adults;

this is indicated by a significantly reduced excretion of the 3-hydroxyderivative and by significantly higher plasma levels of the unchanged drug after a single dose (Grove et al., 1974). In a study of the kinetics of hydroxyamobarbital, Grove and Toseland (1971) observed that the compound is rapidly excreted, with 57% of the dose eliminated in the first 8 h and 91% in the first 24 h. Plotting these data on a sigma-minus function, the rapid elimination is emphasized, with a T½ of 5.7 h. The rate of elimination of this metabolite is thus much faster than its rate of formation. This explains the negligible accumulation of hydroxyamobarbital in the blood of patients taking amobarbital.

No definite data exist on the therapeutic and toxic thresholds for amobarbital in the course of chronic treatment. From the available information, it does appear, however, that plasma levels between 1 and 11 µg/ml are associated with clinically positive effects (Balasubramaniam, 1970a; Grove et al., 1974; Tansella et al., 1975).

Pentobarbital is well absorbed from the gastrointestinal tract. After oral administration of 200 mg of pentobarbital in various dosage forms, peak levels of 1.5 to 4.5 µg/ml are reached after 0.5 to 2 h, the sodium salts being absorbed more rapidly than the free acid form, and solutions or suspensions better than capsules or tablets (Sjögren et al., 1965; Ehrnebo et al., 1972). In a more recent study, an absorption half-life of 13 min was observed; the time lag until absorption began was about 30 min from the moment of tablet intake. The bioavailability of the drug was high (94%), and this was in agreement with the calculated bioavailability of completely absorbed oral pentobarbital by application of i.v. clearance concepts (Ehrnebo, 1974). The presence of food significantly reduces the apparent absorption rate constant, but the amount absorbed is not altered (Smith et al., 1973). The same authors showed that the absorption of a second 50 mg dose, given 1.5 h after the first dose, in non-fasting subjects, was not altered and that a rapid increase in plasma levels occurred after this administration. This finding has considerable importance in clinical practice: for example, if a patient takes a dose of barbiturates shortly after a meal and is not sedated in about one hour, he may be tempted to take an additional dose just as the first one is being absorbed; the result would be a rapid rise in barbiturate serum level and a significant danger of exaggerated response (Smith et al., 1973).

Until recently, the lack of sensitive methods for the determination of pentobarbital in biological fluids did not allow the pharmacokinetics of the drug to be studied at therapeutic doses. In an early work, Brodie et al. (1953) reported that 45% of the pentobarbital present in plasma was bound to plasma proteins, at drug plasma levels of 10 to 20 µg/ml. These authors also determined the plasma levels of the drug after i.v. injection of high doses (750–1,000 mg) to 6 volunteers, but no kinetic parameters were evaluated. From these data, Riegelman et al. (1968), applying a two-compartment model, calculated values of 62 L for the central compartment and 130 L for the Vdss, with a plasma half-life of 41 h. A similar value (T½ = 35 ± 6.1h) was reported by Misra et al. (1971) in four

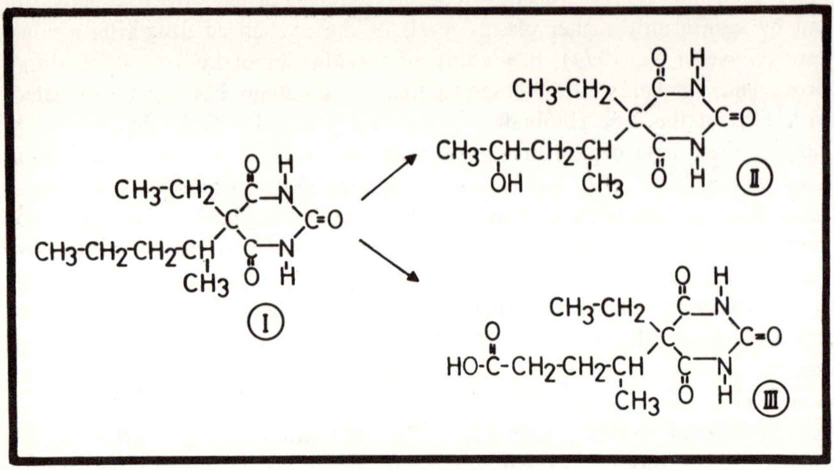

374 DRUG DISPOSITION DURING DEVELOPMENT

Fig. 5: Metabolism of pentobarbital. I. Pentobarbital; II. 5-ethyl-5(3-hydroxy-1-methylbutyl)barbituric acid; III. 5-ethyl-5(1-methylbutyric acid)barbituric acid.

healthy subjects given 6 mg/kg of pentobarbital orally. More recently, Ehrnebo (1974), using a sensitive and specific GLC method, was able to study pentobarbital kinetics in 7 volunteers after oral and i.v. administration of a therapeutic dose (100 mg). Using a two-compartment open model, the apparent volume of distribution was calculated to be about 0.99 L/kg, suggesting uniform distribution of the drug in all body fluids and tissues. The plasma half-life of the beta-phase following i.v. administration was found to be about 22 h, with similar values for the plasma half-life after oral administration. These data differ slightly from those reported by Smith et al. (1973), who found, after i.v. administration of 50 mg of pentobarbital, a mean plasma half-life value of about 50 h. Differences in the experimental technique, as well as more complex pharmacokinetic factors, could account for these discrepant values; therefore, in order to obtain more detailed knowledge of pentobarbital pharmacokinetics, further investigations are required.

Pentobarbital, like many other barbiturates, is metabolized primarily by the hepatic microsomal enzyme system through oxidation of the penultimate carbon of the methyl-butyl side chain (Brodie et al., 1953) (Fig. 5). The oxidation produces a diastereo-isomeric pair of 3-hydroxymetabolites, pentobarbital being a racemic mixture of the R (+) and S (−) compounds (Brodie et al., 1953; Maynert, 1965). Less than 1% of the drug is excreted unchanged in the urine (Brodie et al., 1953) and studies with ^{15}N-labeled drug have shown that isomeric alcohols are excreted during about 4 to 5 days, the dextrorotatory alcohol accounting for 7 to 8%, and the levorotatory, for 40 to 43% of the excreted isotope (Maynert, 1965); the remainder of the isotope in the urine (about 35% of the dose) was not identified; urinary urea and ammonia contained only very small amounts of radioactivity. Glucuronide derivatives of the alcohols, or metabolites containing a carboxyl group, might account for the remainder of the dose (Bush and Sanders, 1967). A carboxyl acid derivative has, indeed, been isolated from the urine of subjects taking pentobarbital (Algeri and McBay, 1953; Titus and Weiss, 1955; Frey et al., 1959). Data are accumulating on the diastereoisomeric metabolites, indicating the existence of steric effects on drug metabolism and disposition (Maynert and Dawson, 1952; Goldstein and Aronow, 1960; Maynert, 1965; Dickert et al., 1966; Kunzmann et al., 1967; Büch et al., 1969; Palmer et al., 1969, 1970; Christensen and Lee, 1973; Christensen et al., 1973; Mark et al., 1973; Freudenthal and Carroll, 1974); however, the clinical relevance of this information has not as yet been clarified.

Hexobarbital [5(1,2-cyclohesenyl)-1,5-dimethyl barbituric acid] has been widely used as an anesthetic and for hypnotic therapy. A very accurate study of its pharmacokinetic properties has recently been performed by Breimer (1974), to whom we refer for more detailed information. In adults, hexobarbital is rather rapidly absorbed from the gastrointestinal tract, peak levels of 4.3 to 6.1 μg/ml being attained to 1 to 3 h after oral administration of 400 to 600 mg of the drug in different formulations (Sjögren et al., 1965; Breimer and Van Rossum, 1973; Breimer, 1974). Sodium salts are absorbed more rapidly than the free acid (Sjögren et al., 1965; Breimer, 1974). When the drug is administered rectally (600 mg), the absorption is not yet complete after 4 h, and the levels then remain constant (about 2 μg/ml) for several hours.

The bioavailability relative to oral administration is 40-60%. Administering doses of only 100 mg, the relative bioavailability approached unity, indicating that the absorption is related to the dosage (Breimer, 1974).

No data are available, to our knowledge, on hexobarbital *in vivo* protein-binding in man. Binding to 3% serum albumin, investigated by equilibrium dialysis at pH 7.4 at 37° C, indicated a binding of 20 to 18%. No significant differences were noted for the two hexobarbital diastereoisomers, indicating that there is no stereospecificity in the interaction of the drug with albumin (Breimer, 1974). The apparent volume of distribution is relatively constant, ranging from 0.98 to 1.23 L/kg. The V of the central compartment is two- or threefold smaller than the apparent Vd, indicating extensive tissue distribution of the drug (Breimer, 1974; Breimer et al., 1975).

The first observations on hexobarbital elimination kinetics were made by Brodie (1952), who administered high doses (3 g) of hexobarbital to a volunteer, following the plasma concentrations for 24 h. He observed a slow rate of decline, probably because of the large dose. More recent studies by Breimer, applying a two-compartment open model, indicate that hexobarbital is eliminated following first-order kinetics, with a mean plasma half-life of 4.4 h (range: 2.6 to 7 h)

(Breimer and Van Rossum, 1973; Breimer, 1974; Breimer et al., 1975). The same authors followed the plasma elimination kinetics of the two diastereoisomers (a racemic mixture of (+) and (−) hexobarbital) and observed for (+) hexobarbital an apparent plasma half-life of 4.6 h (range: 3.5 to 6), while (−) hexobarbital was eliminated significantly faster, with a half-life of only 1.4 h. The half-life ratio between the two isomers is 3.2. Since hardly any unchanged drug is excreted with the urine and feces, and there is no reason to assume a different Vd, the differences in half-life are likely to be due to different metabolic rates. Probably a significant first-pass effect occurs for (−) hexobarbital (Breimer, 1974). Theoretically, a first-order elimination curve is not expected to occur for racemic hexobarbital, since two different elimination rate constants of the enantiomers underlie this process; however, the (−) isomer is eliminated during the first few hours, in which absorption still takes place, so that its contribution to the pure elimination phase of the racemic mixture should be negligible. With respect to the hypnotic activity of the two diastereoisomers in man, Breimer and Van Rossum (1973), report that human volunteers experienced a clear hypnotic effect after oral administration of 400 mg of (+) hexobarbital, whereas after (−) hexobarbital hardly any effect was noted. This is probably due to a difference in potency between the 2 enantiomers, but it could also be explained on the basis of the different elimination rates of the compounds. While there is much information on the metabolic fate of the hexobarbital in various animal species (see the extensive review by Bush and Weller, 1970), the data in humans are scarce. There are reports on urinary metabolites of hexobarbital, indicating that hexobarbital undergoes oxidation and demethylation, and is excreted as 3-ketohexobarbital, norhexobarbital and ketonorhexobarbital (Raventos, 1954; Frey et al., 1959; Mark, 1963; Bush and Weller, 1973). Breimer (1974) studied the renal excretion of hexobarbital and its 3-ketometabolite and found that the unchanged drug accounted for less than 0.5% of the dose, while 3-ketohexobarbital accounted for 29 to 63% of the dose, therefore appearing to be an important metabolite, at least in quantitative terms, since it does not seem to possess hypnotic properties (Bush et al., 1953). In a further study, Breimer et al. (1975) examined the urinary excretion of the two compounds after administration of the (+) and (−) isomers. Hexobarbital appears to be metabolized to 3-ketohexobarbital to a significantly greater extent than is (+) hexobarbital. The urinary half-life of 3-ketohexobarbital in this study varied between 3 and 5 h. In patients with liver disease, the elimination half-life was found to be prolonged in most cases: patients with hepatitis showed half-lives ranging from 4.28 to 15.2 h (mean: 7.9 h), while patients with cirrhosis had T½ values from 4.3 to 38.0 h (mean: 13.9). The metabolic clearance constants were significantly reduced, indicating a decreased metabolic capacity of the liver. The mean excretion of 3-ketohexobarbital was also diminished. The average apparent Vd was enlarged in some patients with cirrhosis. This fact was supposed to be in relation to the accumulation of ascitic fluid (Breimer, 1974).

HYPNOTICS

Secobarbital has been widely used as a hypnotic and as an anesthetic; in pediatrics, it has been recommended for premedication (Root, 1971). Secobarbital is rapidly absorbed from the gastrointestinal tract. In adults, after oral administration of about 200 mg of secobarbital sodium, Sjögren et al. (1965) observed peak plasma levels of 2.0 to 4.9 μg/ml after 0.5-2 h. If given in solution, peak plasma levels may be attained within 30 min. After oral administration of 3.3 mg/kg of the acid form, Clifford et al. (1974) noticed peak levels (determined on whole blood) of 1.83 to 2.14 μg/ml after 2 to 4 h. Secobarbital is slowly cleared from blood, its half-life ranging from 28 to 30 h in different studies, for doses ranging from 200 to 600 mg (Fazekas et al., 1956; Parker et al., 1970; Clifford et al., 1974). Secobarbital is almost completely metabolized before excretion. In man, the main process seems to be oxidation of the two side chains, giving rise to hydroxyderivatives (Mark, 1963; Bush and Sanders, 1967). The three major urinary metabolites are secodiol (5-2,3-dihydroxypropyl-5-1-methylbutyl barbituric acid), and two diastereoisomeric forms of hydroxysecobarbital. Together, these compounds account for about 50% of the administered 2 g dose in the first 2 days (Waddel, 1965). About 5% of the unchanged drug is eliminated with the urine in the first 2 days. Furthermore, a dealkylated derivative, 5-(1-methylbutyl barbituric acid) has been isolated in the urine (Cochin and Daly, 1963; Waddell, 1965). By forced saline diuresis, the urinary excretion of secobarbital can be significantly increased (Rice et al., 1972).

The most common side effects of barbiturates are drowsiness, lethargy and residual sedation ("hangover"). Idiosyncratic reactions (skin rashes, angioedema, etc.) and gastrointestinal distress are occasionally encountered. Particularly in children and in elderly patients, paradoxical restlessness can occur. Barbiturates may aggravate the symptoms of acute intermittent porphyria, which therefore constitutes a contraindication for the use of this class of compounds. Prolonged use of barbiturates may cause tolerance and psychic and physical dependence (Fraser et al., 1958; Katz, 1972). The symptoms of chronic intoxication include disorientation, ataxia and euphoria resembling acute alcohol intoxication. The withdrawal syndrome is usually more severe than the opiate withdrawal syndrome, being characterized by generalized convulsions, delirium and, sometimes, coma and death.

Newborns, Infants and Children

Amobarbital, as with the other barbiturates, readily crosses the placental barrier and becomes widely distributed in the fetal tissue (Ploman and Persson, 1957). Krauer et al. (1973) studied the elimination kinetics of amobarbital in mothers at term and in their newborn infants after administration of a single dose of 200 mg of sodium amobarbital i.m. 0.7-3.5 h before delivery. Similar drug concentrations (ranging from 0.5 to 2.8 μg/ml) were found in both the cord and the maternal plasma immediately after delivery. From the decreasing drug concentration values, first-order kinetics were observed in both the mothers and the newborns. The plasma half-life in the mothers was 11 to 17 h (mean values: 15.83 ± 1.71 h). These values are similar to those found in non-pregnant women and adult men (Balasubramaniam et al., 1970a; Grove and Toseland, 1971; Mawer et al., 1972). In the newborn infants, the mean plasma half-life for amobarbital varied from 17 to 59 h (mean: 38.9 ± 4.8 h), that is 2.5 times as long as in the mothers. The plasma concentrations of hydroxyamobarbital increased during the first 12 to 24 h after delivery in 2 of the mothers and 2 of the neonates, decreasing thereafter. In one newborn, a constant slow increase of plasma hydroxyamobarbital, present in traces at birth, was evident for up to 67 h. None of the mothers or newborns in this study showed toxic signs, and a good Apgar score was obtained in all the infants.

The slow elimination rate seen in the newborn is probably due to the limited capacity of his liver mocrosomes to hydroxylate the drug. Product inhibition caused by accumulation of hydroxyamobarbital as a result of the reduced filtration rate present in newborns was not considered likely by the authors, since it occurs only at very high concentrations of the metabolite. It is also unlikely that the additional drug intake through breast-feeding plays any role in determining the slow elimination of amobarbital in the babies, since the amobarbital concentration in the colostrum of one mother was found to be only about two-thirds of that in the plasma, and a newborn baby ingests only a few ml of colostrum at each feeding during the first days of life.

No other data are available, to the best of our knowledge, on the pharmacokinetics in pediatric age of the barbituric compounds reviewed in this chapter. More information would be useful, since it is known, as already said, that barbiturates freely cross the placental barrier (Ploman and Persson, 1957; Persson, 1960; Villa, 1965; Carrier et al., 1969; Boulos et al., 1971; Editorial, 1972; Bleyer and Marshall, 1972; Desmond et al., 1972) and distribute rapidly in the fetus, undergoing preferential storage in the midbrain, where they reach levels higher than in the circulating blood (Ploman and Persson, 1957). The ingestion of high doses of barbiturates in pregnancy (in addicted mothers or for therapeutic reasons) may determine congenital addiction and a consequent neonatal withdrawal syndrome characterized by restlessness, neurological distress such as convulsions, hypertonus, hyperreflexia, tremor, etc., and autonomic and gastrointestinal disturbances (Desmond et al., 1972; Bleyer and Marshall, 1972; Editorial, 1972).

BENZODIAZEPINES

Flurazepam is considered to be one of the safest and most effective hypnotic agents (Greenblatt and Shader, 1974c; Greenblatt and Miller, 1974). Its pharmacological properties have been outlined in the classical study by Randall et al. (1969), and have been recently reviewed by Greenblatt et al. (1975). Flurazepam appears to be, together with N-desmethyldiazepam, the only known hypnotic conserving its efficacy during long-term administration (Kales et al., 1973; Kales and Sharf, 1973; Greenblatt and Shader, 1974a,b,c; Tansella et al., 1975). It is also said to have a less marked potential to depress dreaming than the other hypnotics (Frost et al., 1973; Dement et al., 1972), but the significance of this difference is still be to assessed (Greenblatt and Shader, 1974c). Guidelines for the choice and clinical use of hypnotics have been presented in recent works (Lasagna, 1972; Greenblatt et al., 1974; Kales and Kales, 1974; Greenblatt and Miller, 1974). Flurazepam seems to be rapidly absorbed from the gastrointestinal tract, peak blood concentrations of 10-20 ng/ml being observed about 1 h after administration of large single doses (90 mg) of the drug (De Silva and Strojny, 1971). The blood levels of the unchanged drug then fall under the sensitivity limit of the analytical method employed, probably because of both tissue distribution and rapid biotransformation. The metabolism of flurazepam is outlined in Fig. 6. It prpceeds by progressive dealkylation of the 1-diethylaminoethyl side chain, followed by oxidation of the amino group to an alcohol. An aldehydic intermediate is postulated (Schwartz et al., 1968; Schwartz and Postma, 1970; Schwartz, 1973). The main metabolites detectable in plasma are the hydroxyethyl (V) and N-1 unsubstituted analog (IV), which reach peak concentrations about 4 times greater than the parent compound about 1 h after dosing (De Silva and Strojny, 1971). According to the same authors, the apparent plasma half-life of the hydroxyethyl metabolite is about 2 h. The N-1 unsubstituted metabolite is eliminated much slower, with an apparent plasma half-life of 47 to 100 h (Kaplan et al., 1973). During chronic treatment with therapeutic doses (30 mg/day) of flurazepam, plasma levels are generally below 2 ng/ml. The hydroxyethylmetabolite is seen only in the early hours, samples, while the N-1 unsubstituted metabolite (IV) accumulates in plasma, reaching steady-state plasma levels 5 to 6 times as high as the plasma levels present 24 h after the first administration. Since this compound has shown in animal studies a pharmacological activity similar to the parent drug, it may contribute to therapeutic and toxic effects of flurazepam (Kaplan et al., 1973). With the exception of metabolite (IV), the other known metabolites of flurazepam are rapidly excreted with the urine and feces. After an oral dose of 28 mg ^{14}C-labeled flurazepam, about 81% of the radioactivity was recovered in the urine and 8-9% in the feces in 18 days (after 3 days the excretion was essentially completed). Glucuronide and sulfate conjugates of the hydroxyethyl analog of flurazepam (V) accounted for 27 to 31% of the urinary radioactivity. Small amounts of the free N-1 unsubstituted analog and of the conjugated N-1 unsubstituted, 3-hydroxy analog (VII) were also present (Schwartz and Postma, 1970). Investigations using a spectrophotofluorimetric method (De Silva and Strojny, 1971) give slightly different results: in 48 h, 51 to 56% of a 90 mg oral dose is eliminated with the urine, the glucuronide and sulfate conjugates of the

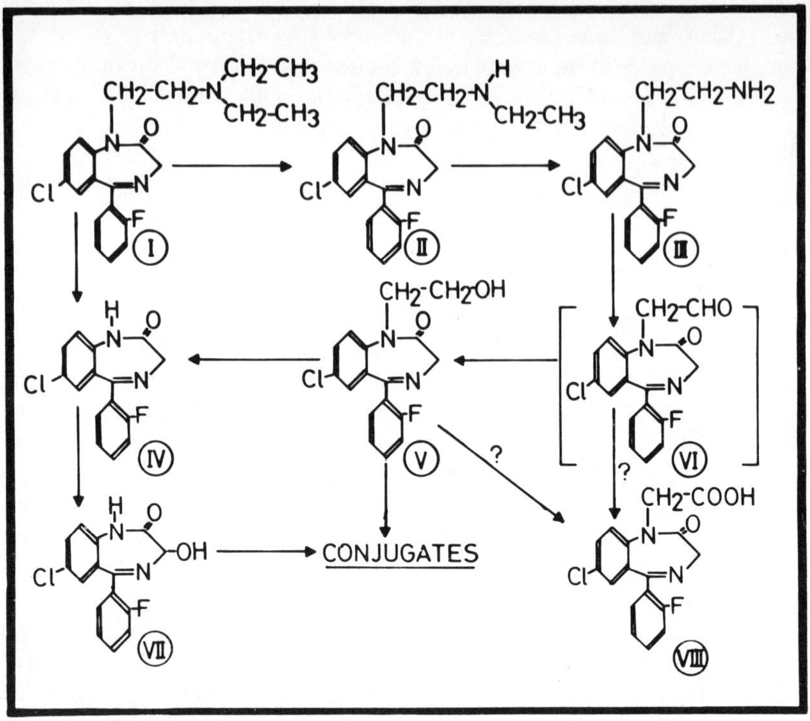

Fig. 6: Metabolism of flurazepam. I. Flurazepam; II. Ethylaminoethyl analog; III. Aminoethyl analog; IV. N-1 unsubstituted analog; V. Hydroxyethyl analog; VI. (Postulated) aldehyde; VII. Carboxymethyl analog; VIII. Acetic acid analog.

hydroxyethyl metabolite accounting for 91 to 92% of the urinary metabolites. No data are available (to our knowledge) on the plasma protein-binding characteristics of flurazepam and its derivatives. Circular dichroism studies (Muller and Wollert, 1973) suggest that flurazepam is less protein-bound than the other benzodiazepines, probably because of the 2 halogen groups and the large N-1 alkyl substitution. The most common side effect of flurazepam is morning drowsiness ("hangover") (Bond and Lader, 1972; Greenblatt et al., 1975). Other subjective side effects are headache, dry mouth, psychomotor depression (Sambrooks et al., 1972; Greenblatt et al., 1975). The side effects seem to occur only slightly more frequently with flurazepam than with placebos (Greenblatt et al., 1975). Flurazepam can determine habituation and tolerance, but this seems to be a rare event (Greenblatt et al., 1975). Swanson et al. (1973) reviewed 225 cases of patients hospitalized because of prescription drug abuse; only in one case was flurazepam implicated. One case of swelling of the tongue following flurazepam use has been

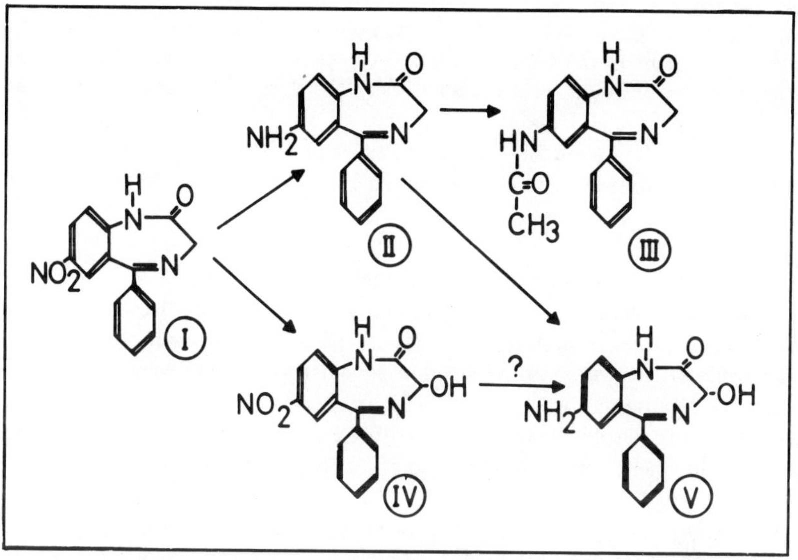

Fig. 7: Metabolism of nitrazepam. I. Nitrazepam; II. 7-amino analog; III. 7-acetamido analog; IV. hydroxylated analog; V. hydroxylated 7-amino analog.

reported by Rapp (1971), possibly on an idiosyncratic base. No data are available on flurazepam disposition in the pediatric age group.

Nitrazepam is another benzodiazepine marketed as a hypnotic in several countries, while in others it is known mostly for its activity in myoclonic epilepsy.

The pharmacokinetics of the compound have been nicely described by Rieder and Wendt (1973). Nitrazepam is variably absorbed following oral administration, its bioavailability ranging from 53 to 94% of the dose. After an oral dose of 10 mg, peak levels of 68 to 108 ng may be attained within 2 h. The compound is about 86-97% bound to plasma proteins and the apparent volume of distribution may range from 1.5 to 2.5 L/kg. After single oral or intravenous administration, the plasma concentrations decay biexponentially with an apparent plasma half-life of the terminal phase of 17-30 h. For daily doses of 5 mg, steady-state plasma levels of 40 to 50 ng have been reported by Rieder and Wendt (1973) in healthy subjects. In patients, we could observe a higher variability, with plasma concentrations ranging from 30 to 150 ng/ml. No differences in the apparent plasma half-life could be noticed after repeated treatment with nitrazepam (Rieder and Wendt, 1973). The compound is extensively metabolized, the 7-acetamide derivative being the major metabolite

(Fig. 7). The 7-amino and the hydroxy metabolites appear to be less important. The drug is mainly excreted via the kidney, 65–71% of the dose appearing in the urine and 14–20% in the feces over a 5–6 day period. Only traces of unchanged nitrazepam can be found in urine and feces. The drug and its metabolites cross the placenta easily, and plasma concentrations similar to those present in the mother are rapidly attained in the fetus. Three to 4 h after oral administration of 10 mg to the mother, plasma levels of 10 to 39 ng/ml were observed in the newborns (Rieder and Wendt, 1973).

Nitrazepam has also been detected in milk, but in very small quantities. No other data are available for children and infants.

Nitrazepam possesses a definite hypnotic activity; however, the availability of other benzodiazepines and the capacity of nitrazepam to induce several disturbing side effects (more pronounced in the elderly) such as severe "hangover," confusion, disorientation, ataxia, disarthria, nightmares and vivid dreams (Greenblatt and Shader, 1974c) have reduced its use as a hypnotic in several countries. Furthermore, habituation to the compound may occur (Greenblatt and Shader, 1974c).

N-desmethyldiazepam has recently been marketed as a hypnotic in Europe. Its activity on sleep resembles that of flurazepam, in the sense that it appears not to modify the REM stage and conserves its activity during long-term administration (Tansella et al., 1975; Tognoni et al., 1975). Its pharmacokinetic profile will be described together with diazepam in Chapter 14.

CONCLUSIONS

From the data reported, it emerges clearly that, despite the old and wide use of sedative-hypnotic agents, our knowledge on the disposition of these compounds in pediatric patients is very poor. The problem of wider knowledge on this topic is not a secondary one since hypnotics either old or new are probably one of the classes of drugs most used in all ages. Surprisingly, the recommended dosages for barbiturates in children (AMA Drug Evaluation, 1973) are more or less the same for the various compounds despite differences in their kinetic profiles in adults. For other drugs, the information is "inadequate" to establish dosage. The result is that no rationale may exist behind the choice that the pediatrician or the general practitioner, or, as often happens, the parents, have to make when they decide to administer a hypnotic to an infant or child.

REFERENCES

Adams, L.V. (1940): The toxicity of chloral alcoholate. *Journal of Pharmacology and Experimental Therapeutics, 69*: 273-274.

Akagi, M., Oketani, Y., Takada, M. and Suga, T. (1963): Studies on metabolism of 2-methyl-3-o-tolyl-4 (3H)-quinazolinone. II. *Chemical Pharmaceutical Bulletin, 11:* 321.
Algeri, E.I. and McBay, A.J. (1953): The identification of pentobarbital by paper chromatography in a medicolegal death. *New England Journal of Medicine, 248:* 423-424.
Allen, J.T., Fry, D. and Marks, V. (1970): Urine spot-test for methaqualone. *Lancet, 1:* 951-952.
Alvan, G., Ericsson, O., Levander, S. and Lindgren, J.-E. (1974): Plasma concentrations and effects of methaqualone after single and multiple oral doses in man. *European Journal of Clinical Pharmacology, 7:* 449-454.
Alvan, G., Lindgren, J.-E., Bogentoft, C. and Ericsson, O. (1973): Plasma kinetics of methaqualone in man after single oral doses. *European Journal of Clinical Pharmacology, 6:* 187-190.
Ambre, J.J. and Fischer, L.J. (1972): Glutethimide intoxication: plasma levels of glutethimide and a metabolite in humans, dogs and rats. *Research Communications in Chemical Pathology and Pharmacology, 4:* 307-326.
Ambre, J.J. and Fischer, L.J. (1974): Identification and activity of the hydroxy metabolite that accumulates in the plasma of humans intoxicated with glutethimide. *Drug Metabolism Disposition, 2:* 151-158.
American Medical Association (1973): *AMA Drug Evaluation*, 2nd ed., Ch. 27, AMA, Chicago.
Bailey, D.N. and Jatlow, P.I. (1973): Methaqualone overdose: analytical methodology, and the significance of serum drug concentrations. *Clinical Chemistry, 19:* 615-620.
Balasubramaniam, K., Lucas, S.B., Mawer, G.E. and Simons, P.J. (1970a): The kinetics of amylobarbitone metabolism in healthy men and women. *British Journal of Pharmacology, 39:* 564-572.
Balasubramaniam, K., Mawer, G.E. and Simons, P.J. (1970b): The influence of dose on the distribution and elimination of amylobarbitone in healthy subjects. *British Journal of Pharmacology, 40:* 578P-579P.
Ballinger, B., Browning, M., O'Malley, K. and Stevenson, I.H. (1972): Drug-metabolizing capacity in states of drug dependence and withdrawal. *British Journal of Clinical Pharmacology, 45:* 638-643.
Bernhard, K., Just, M. and Vuilleumier, J.P. (1957): Zur Bestimmung des zeitlichen Ablaufes in der Leber stattfindender Detoxikationen durch Analyse der Galle. *Helvetica Physiologica Acta, 15:* 177-183.
Berry, D.J. (1969): Gas chromatographic determination of methaqualone, 2-methyl-3-o-tolyl-4 (3H)-quinazolinone, at therapeutic levels in human plasma. *Journal of Chromatography, 42:* 39-44.
Bleyer, W.A. and Marshall, R.E. (1972): Barbiturate withdrawal syndrome in a passively addicted infant. *Journal of the American Medical Association, 221:* 185-186.
Bond, A.J. and Lader, M.H. (1972): Residual effects of a new benzodiazepine: flurazepam. *British Journal of Pharmacology, 44:* 343P-344P.
Bonnichsen, R., Fri, C.-G., Negoita, C. and Ryhage, R. (1972): Identification of methaqualone metabolites from urine extract by gas chromatography-mass spectrometry. *Clinica Chimica Acta, 40:* 309-318.
Boulos, B.M., Davis, L.E., Larks, S.D., Larks, G.G., Sirtori, C.R. and Almond, C.H. (1971): Placental transfer of drugs. IV. *Archives Internationales de Pharmacodynamie et Therapie, 194:* 403-414.
Brånstad, J.O., Meressar, V. and Agren, A. (1972): Complex formation between macromolecules and drugs. VII. *Acta Pharmaceutica Suecica, 9:* 129-134.
Breimer, D.D. (1974): *Pharmacokinetics of Hypnotic Drugs.* Drukkerij-Uitgevenj Brakkenstein, Nijmegen.

Breimer, D.D., Honhoff, C., Zilly, W., Richter, E. and Van Rossum, J.M. (1975): Pharmacokinetics of hexobarbital in man after intravenous infusion. *Journal of Pharmacokinetics and Biopharmaceutics, 3:* 1-11.

Breimer, D.D. and Van Rossum, J.M. (1973): Pharmacokinetics of (+),(−)- and (±)-hexobarbitone in man after oral administration. *Journal of Pharmacy and Pharmacology, 25:* 762-764.

Brodie, B.B. (1952): Physiological disposition and chemical fate of thiobarbiturates in the body. *Federation Proceedings, 11:* 632-639.

Brodie, B.B., Burns, J.J., Mark, L.C., Lief, P.A., Bernstein, E. and Papper, E.M. (1953): The fate of pentobarbital in man and dog and a method for its estimation in biological material. *Journal of Pharmacology and Experimental Therapeutics, 109:* 26-34.

Brown, D.A. (1962): An eserine-like action of chloral hydrate. *British Journal of Pharmacology, 19:* 111-119.

Brown, S.S. and Goenechea, S. (1973): Methaqualone: metabolic kinetic and clinical pharmacologic observations. *Clinical Pharmacology and Therapeutics, 14:* 314-324.

Brown, S.S. and Smart, G.A. (1969): Fluorimetric assay of methaqualone in plasma by reduction to 1,2,3,4-tetrahydro-2-methyl-4-oxo-3-o-tolylquinazoline. *Journal of Pharmacy and Pharmacology, 21:* 466-468.

Buch, H., Grund, W., Buzello, W. and Rummel, W. (1969): Narkotische Wirksamkeit und Gewebsvesteilung der optischen Antipoden des Pentobarbitals bei der Ratte. *Biochemical Pharmacology, 18:* 1005-1009.

Bush, M.T., Butler, T.C. and Dickison, H.L. (1953): The metabolic fate of 5-(1-cyclohexen-1-yl)-1,5-dimethyl-barbituric acid (hexobarbital Evipal) and of 5-(1-cyclohexen-1-yl)-5-methylbarbituric acid (Norevipal). *Journal of Pharmacology and Experimental Therapeutics, 108:* 104-111.

Bush, M.T. and Sanders, E. (1967): Metabolic fate of drugs: barbiturates and closely related compounds. *Annual Review of Pharmacology, 7:* 57-76.

Bush, M.T. and Weller, L. (1973): Metabolic fate of hexobarbital (Hb). *Drug Metabolism Reviews, 1:* 249-290.

Bütikofer, E., Cottier, P., Imhof, P., Keberle, H., Riess, W. and Schmid, K. (1962): Uber die Eliminierungsgeschwindigkeit von Glutethimid (Doriden R) und die Natur der Ausscheidungsprodukte beim Messchen. *Arkiv für Experimentelle Pathologie und Pharmakologie, 244:* 97-108.

Butler, T.C. (1948): The metabolic fate of chloral hydrate. *Journal of Pharmacology and Experimental Therapeutics, 92:* 49-58.

Butler, T.C. (1949): Reduction and oxidation of chloral hydrate by isolated tissue in vitro. *Journal of Pharmacology and Experimental Therapeutics, 95:* 360-362.

Carrier, G., Hume, A.S., Douglas, B.H. and Wiser, W.L. (1969): Disposition of barbiturates in maternal blood, fetal blood, and amniotic fluid. *American Journal of Obstetrics and Gynecology, 105:* 1069-1071.

Charytan, C. (1970): The enterohepatic circulation in glutethimide intoxication. *Clinical Pharmacology and Therapeutics, 11:* 816-820.

Chazan, J.A. and Cohen, J.J. (1969): Clinical spectrum of glutethimide intoxication. *Journal of the American Medical Association, 208:* 837-839.

Chazan, J.A. and Garella, S. (1971): Glutethimide intoxication: a prospective study of 70 patients treated conservatively without hemodialysis. *Archives of Internal Medicine, 128:* 215-219.

Christensen, H.D., Barnett, L. and Carroll, F.I. (1973): Biological activity of pentobarbital metabolites. *Journal of Pharmaceutical Sciences, 62:* 1722-1723.

Christensen, H.D. and Lee, I.S. (1973): Anesthetic potency and acute toxicity of optically

active disubstituted barbituric acids. *Toxicology and Applied Pharmacology, 26:* 295-503.
Christianson, H.B. and Perry, H.O. (1956): Reactions to chloral hydrate. *A.M.A. Archives of Dermatology, 74:* 232-240.
Clifford, J.M., Cookson, J.H. and Wickham, P.E. (1974): Absorption and clearance of secobarbital, heptabarbital, methaqualone, and ethinamate. *Clinical Pharmacology and Therapeutics, 16:* 376-389.
Cochin, J. and Daly, J.W. (1963): The use of thin layer chromatography for the analysis of drugs. II. *Journal of Pharmacology and Experimental Therapeutics, 139:* 154-159.
Cohen, Y., du Picard, Y.F. and Boissier, J.R. (1962): Étude de la distribution chez la souris d'un hypnotique marqué au carbone 14, la methyl-2, orthotolyl-3, quinazolone-4. *Archives Internationales de Pharmacodynamie et Thérapie, 137:* 271-282.
Cooper, J.R. and Friedman, P.J. (1958): The enzymic oxidation of chloral hydrate to trichloroacetic acid. *Biochemical Pharmacology, 1:* 76-81.
Curry, S.H., Riddall, D., Gordon, J.S., Simpson, P., Binns, T.B., Rondel, R.K. and McMartin, C. (1971): Disposition of glutethimide in man. *Clinical Pharmacology and Therapeutics, 12:* 849-857.
De Alarcon, R. (1969): Mandrax and methaqualone. *British Medical Journal, 1:* 319.
Dement, W.C., Zarcone, V.P., Hoddes, E., Smythe, H. and Carskadon, M. (1973): Sleep laboratory and clinical studies with flurazepam. In: *The Benzodiazepines,* edited by S. Garattini, E. Mussini and L.O. Randall, pp. 599-612, Raven Press, New York.
De Silva, J.A.F. and Strojny, N. (1971): Determination of flurazepam and its major biotransformation products in blood and urine by spectrophotofluorimetry and spectrophotometry. *Journal of Pharmaceutical Sciences, 60:* 1303-1314.
Desmond, N.M., Schwanecke, R.P., Wilson, G.S., Yasunaga, S. and Burgdorff, I. (1972): Maternal barbiturate utilization and neonatal withdrawal symptomatology. *Journal of Pediatrics, 80:* 190-197.
Dickert, Y.J., Shea, P.J. and McCarty, L.P. (1966): The synthesis and pharmacological activity of 5-ethyl-5-(3-hydroxy-1-methylbutyl) barbituric acid. *Journal of Medicinal Chemistry, 9:* 249-253.
Dybing, F. and Dybing, O. (1955): Anticholinesterase and anticurare effects of chloral hydrate and trichloroethanol. *Acta Pharmacologica et Toxicologica, 11:* 398-404.
Editorial (1972): Neonatal behaviour and maternal barbiturates. *British Medical Journal, 4:* 63-64.
Editorial (1973): Does methaqualone cause neuropathy? *British Medical Journal, 3:* 307.
Ehrnebo, M. (1974): Pharmacokinetics and distribution properties of pentobarbital in humans following oral and intravenous administration. *Journal of Pharmaceutical Sciences, 63:* 1114-1118.
Ehrnebo, M., Agurell, S. and Boréus, L.O. (1972): Gas chromatographic determination of therapeutic levels of amobarbital and pentobarbital in plasma. *European Journal of Clinical Pharmacology, 4:* 191-195.
Ehrnebo, M. and Odar-Cederlof, I. (1975): Binding of amobarbital, pentobarbital and diphenylhydantoin to blood cells and plasma proteins in healthy volunteers and uraemic patients. *European Journal of Clinical Pharmacology, 8:* 445-453.
Fazekas, J.F., Goldbaum, L.R., Koppanyi, T. and Shea, I.G. (1956): Study on the effect of overdoses of pentylenetetrazol and barbiturate combinations in human volunteers. *American Journal of Medical Sciences, 231:* 531-537.
Ferguson Anderson, W. (1973): *Prescriber's Journal, 13:* 109.
Finke, J. and Spiegelberg, V. (1973): Polyneuropathie nach Methaqualon. *Nervenarzt, 44:* 104-106.

Fraser, H.F., Wikler, A., Essig, C.F. and Isbell, H. (1958): Degree of physical dependence induced by secobarbital or phenobarbital. *Journal of the American Medical Association, 166:* 126-130.

Freudenthal, R.I. and Carroll, F.I. (1974): Metabolism of certain commonly used barbiturates. *Drug Metabolism Reviews, 2:* 265-278.

Frey, H.H., Sudendey, F. and Krause, D. (1959): Vergleichende Untersuchungen uber Stoffwechsel, Ausscheidung und Nachweis von Schlafmitteln aus der Barbitursaurereike. *Arzneimittel-Forschung, 9:* 294-297.

Friedman, P.J. and Cooper, J.R. (1960): The role of alcohol dehydrogenase in the metabolism of chloral hydrate. *Journal of Pharmacology and Experimental Therapeutics, 129:* 373-376.

Frost, J.D., Carrie, J.R.G., Borda, R.P. and Kellaway, P. (1973): The effects of Dalmane (flurazepam hydrochloride) on human EEG characteristics. *Electroencephalography and Clinical Neurophysiology, 34:* 171-175.

Garrett, E.R., Bres, J., Schnelle, K., and Rolf, L.L., Jr. (1974): Pharmacokinetics of saturably metabolized amobarbital. *Journal of Pharmacokinetics and Biopharmaceutics, 2:* 43-103.

Geldmacher-Mallinckrodt, M. and Lautenbach, L. (1963): Zum Nachweis der Revonalvergiftung. *Archiv für Toxikologie, 20:* 31.

Geldmacher-Mallinckrodt, M. and Mang, V. (1970): Rapid detection of metabolites of methaqualone and of the chlordiazepoxide group in urine. *Zeitschrift fur Klinische Chemie und Klinische Biochemie, 8:* 259-262.

Goenechea, S., Brown, S.S. and Ferguson, M.M. (1973): Gaschromatographische Bestimmung von Methaqualone in Kleinen Mengen Serum nach Einnaschme Therapeutischer Dosen. *Archiv für Toxikologie, 31:* 25-30.

Gold, M., Tassoni, E. and Etzl, M. (1973): Comparison of glutethimide concentration in the serum and cerebrospinal fluid of humans in drug overdose. *Clinical Chemistry, 19:* 1158-1161.

Goldbaum, L.R. and Smith, P.K. (1954): The interaction of barbiturates with serum albumin and its possible relation to their disposition and pharmacological actions. *Journal of Pharmacology and Experimental Therapeutics, 111:* 197-209.

Goldbaum, L.R., Williams, M.A. and Koppanyi, T. (1960): Determination of glutethimide in biological fluids. *Analytical Chemistry, 32:* 95.

Goldstein, A. and Aronow, L. (1960): The durations of action of thiopental and pentobarbital. *Journal of Pharmacology and Experimental Therapeutics, 128:* 1-6.

Goudie, J.H. and Burnett, D. (1971): A rapid method for the detection of methaqualone metabolites. *Clinica Chimica Acta, 35:* 133-135.

Greenblatt, D.J. and Miller, R.I. (1974): Rational use of psychotropic drugs. I. Hypnotics. *Hospital Pharmacy Forum, New England Medical Center Hospital, III,* 5, June.

Greenblatt, D.J. and Shader, R.I. (1974a): Drug therapy: benzodiazepines. 1. *New England Journal of Medicine, 291:* 1011-1015.

Greenblatt, D.J. and Shader, R.I. (1974b): Drug therapy: benzodiazepines. 2. *New England Journal of Medicine, 291:* 1239-1243.

Greenblatt, D.J. and Shader, R.I. (1974c): *Benzodiazepines in Clinical Practice*, Raven Press, New York.

Greenblatt, D.J., Shader, R.I. and Koch-Weser, J. (1975): Flurazepam hydrochloride. *Clinical Pharmacology and Therapeutics, 17:* 1-14.

Greenwood, R.H., Prunty, F.T.G. and Silver, J. (1973): Osteomalacia after prolonged glutethimide administration. *British Medical Journal, 1:* 643-645.

Grove, J., Irvine, R.E., Toseland, P.A. and Trounce, J.R. (1974): The effect of age on the

hydroxylation of amylobarbitone sodium in man. *British Journal of Clinical Pharmacology, 1:* 41-43.
Grove, J. and Toseland, P.A. (1971): The excretion of hydroxyamylobarbitone in man after oral administration of amylobarbitone and hydroxyamylobarbitone. *Journal of Pharmacy and Pharmacology, 23:* 936-940.
Haas, D.C. and Marasigan, A. (1968): Neurological effects of glutethimide. *Journal of Neurology, Neurosurgery and Psychiatry, 31:* 561-564.
Hansen, A.R. and Fischer, L.J. (1974): Gas-chromatographic simultaneous analysis for glutethimide and an active hydroxylated metabolite in tissues, plasma and urine. *Clinical Chemistry, 20:* 236-242.
Hansen, A.R., Kennedy, K.A., Ambre, J.J. and Fischer, L.J. (1975): Glutethimide poisoning. A metabolite contributes to morbidity and mortality. *New England Journal of Medicine, 292:* 250-252.
Hartmann, E. and Cravens, J. (1973): The effects of long term administration of psychotropic drugs on human sleep. IV. *Psychopharmacologia, 33:* 219-232.
Hetland, L.B. and Couri, D. (1974): Effects of ethanol on glutethimide absorption and distribution in relationship to a mechanism for toxicity enhancement. *Toxicology and Applied Pharmacology, 30:* 26-35.
Heyndrick, A. and de Leenheer, A. (1969): Clinical toxicology of the metabolites of methaqualone in man. *European Journal of Toxicology, 11:* 56-63.
Illingworth, S.L. (1968): *Prescriber's Journal, 8:* 64-71.
Irrgang, K. (1965): Zur Pharmakologie von 5-Aethyl-5-(3-hydroxyisoamyl)-barbitursäure einem Stoffwechselprodukt der 5-Aethyl-5-isoamyl-barbitursäure. *Arzneimittel-Forschung, 15:* 688-691.
Johnstone, R.E., Manitsas, G.T. and Smith, E.J. (1971): Apnea following methaqualone ingestion. *Ohio State Medical Journal, 67:* 1018-1020.
Kales, A., Kales, J.D., Leo, L.A., Bixler, E.O. (1973): Evaluation of the effectiveness of hypnotic drugs under conditions of prolonged use. Presented at the *Annual Meeting of the Radiation for the Psychophysiological Study of Sleep*, San Diego, California, May.
Kales, A. and Kales, J.D. (1974): Sleep disorders. Recent findings in the diagnosis and treatment of disturbed sleep. *New England Journal of Medicine, 290:* 487-499.
Kales, A. and Sharf, M.B. (1973): Sleep laboratory and clinical studies of benzodiazepines on sleep: flurazepam, diazepam, chlordiazepoxide, and RO 5-4200. In: *The Benzodiazepines*, edited by S. Garattini, E. Mussini and L.O. Randall, pp. 577-598, Raven Press, New York.
Kaplan, H.L., Jain, N.C., Forney, R.B. and Richards, A.B. (1969): Chloral hydrate-ethanol interactions in the mouse and dog. *Toxicology and Applied Pharmacology, 14:* 127-130.
Kaplan, S.A., de Silva, J.A.F., Jack, M.L., Alexander, K., Strothy, N., Weinfeld, R.E., Puglisi, C.V. and Weissman, L. (1973): Blood level profile in man following chronic oral administration of flurazepam hydrochloride. *Journal of Pharmaceutical Sciences, 62:* 1932-1935.
Kamm, J.J. and Van Loon, E.J. (1966): Amobarbital metabolism in man. *Clinical Chemistry, 12:* 789-796.
Katz, R.L. (1972): Sedatives and Tranquilizers. *New England Journal of Medicine, 286:* 757-758.
Keberle, H., Hoffmann, K. and Bernhard, K. (1962): The metabolism of glutethimide (Doriden). *Experientia, 18:* 105-111.
Krauer, B., Draffan, G.H., Williams, F.M., Clare, R.A., Dollery, C.T. and Hakins, D.F. (1973): Elimination kinetics of amobarbital in mothers and their newborn infants.

Clinical Pharmacology and Therapeutics, 14: 442-447.
Kuntzman, R., Ideda, M., Jacobson, M. and Conney, A.H. (1967): A sensitive method for the determination and isolation of pentobarbital-C14 metabolites and its application to *in vitro* studies of drug metabolism. *Journal of Pharmacology and Experimental Therapeutics, 157:* 220-230.
Lacey, J.H. (1971): Dichloralphenazone and breast milk. *British Medical Journal, 4:* 684.
Lansky, L.L. (1974): Unusual case of childhood chloral hydrate poisoning. *American Journal of Diseases of Children, 127:* 275-276.
Lasagna, L. (1972): Drug therapy: hypnotic drugs. *New England Journal of Medicine, 287:* 1182-1184.
Lingl, F.A. (1966): Irreversible effects of glutethimide addiction. *American Journal of Psychiatry, 123:* 349-351.
Maher, J.F. (1970): Determinants of serum half-life of glutethimide in intoxicated patients. *Journal of Pharmacology and Experimental Therapeutics, 174:* 450-455.
Maher, J.F., Schreiner, G.E. (1969): Current status of dialysis of poisons and drugs. *Transactions of the American Society of Artificial Internal Organs, 15:* 461-477.
Mallein, R., Treger, J., Vague, A. and Cottaz, G. (1960): Un cas d'intoxication par absorption massive (24.5 g) de glutethimide. *Bulletin Transaction Societé de Pharmacie, Lyon, 4:* 53-57.
Malmlund, H.O., Matell, G. and von Reis, G. (1972): Methaqualone poisoning. *Opuscula Medica, 17:* 216-223.
Mark, L.C. (1963): Metabolism of barbiturates in man. *Clinical Pharmacology and Therapeutics, 4:* 504-530.
Mark, L.C., Brand, L., Heiber, S., Smith, D. and Carroll, F.I. (1973): Pharmacological activity and biotransformation of R+ and S-barbiturate enantioners in mouse and man. *Federation Proceedings, 32,* abstr. 2638.
Marshall, E.K., Jr. and Owens, A.H., Jr. (1954): Absorption, excretion and metabolic fate of chloral hydrate and trichloroethanol. *Bulletin of Johns Hopkins Hospital, 95:* 1-18.
Martindale, (1972): *The Extra Pharmacopoeia,* 26th ed., p. 898, Pharmaceutical Press, London.
Matthew, H., Proudfoot, A.T., Brown, S.S. and Smith, A.C.A. (1968): Mandrax poisoning: conservative management of 116 patients. *British Medical Journal, 2:* 101.
Matthew, H., Roscoe, P. and Wright, N. (1972): Acute poisoning: a comparison of hypnotic drugs. *Practitioner, 208:* 254-258.
Mawer, G.E. and Lee, H.A. (1968): Value of forced diuresis in acute barbiturate poisoning. *British Medical Journal, 2:* 790-793.
Mawer, G.E., Miller, N.E. and Turnberg, L.A. (1972): Metabolism of amylobarbitone in patients with chronic liver disease. *British Journal of Pharmacology, 44:* 549-560.
Mawer, G.W., Miller, N.E. and Turnberg, L.A. (1970): Preliminary observations on the elimination of amylobarbitone by patients with chronic liver disease. *British Journal of Pharmacology, 40:* 579P-580P.
Maynert, E.W. (1965): The alcoholic metabolites of pentobarbital and amobarbital. *Journal of Pharmacology and Experimental Therapeutics, 150:* 118-121.
Maynert, E.W. (1971): Sedatives and hypnotics. I. Nonbarbiturates. In: *Drill's Pharmacology in Medicine,* edited by J.R. Di Palma, pp. 227-230, McGraw-Hill, New York.
Maynert, E.W. and Dawson, J.M. (1952): Ethyl (3-hydroxy-1-methylbutyl) barbituric acids as metabolites of pentobarbital. *Journal of Biological Chemistry, 195:* 389-395.
McBay, A.J. and Katsas, G.G. (1957): Glutethimide poisoning. *New England Journal of Medicine, 257:* 97-103.
Misra, P.S., Lefevre, A., Ishii, H., Rubin, E. and Lieber, C.S. (1971): Increase of ethanol,

meprobamate and pentobarbital metabolism after chronic ethanol administration in man and rats. *American Journal of Medicine, 51:* 346-356.

Mitchard, M. and Williams, M.E. (1972): An improved quantitative gas-liquid chromatographic assay for the estimation of methaqualone in biological fluids. *Journal of Chromatography, 72:* 29-34.

Morris, R.N., Gunderson, G.A., Babcock, S.W. and Zarolinski, J.F. (1972): Plasma levels and absorption of methaqualone after oral administration to man. *Clinical Pharmacology and Therapeutics, 13:* 719-723.

Muller, W. and Wollert, U. (1973): Interactions of benzodiazepines with human serum albumin. Circular dichroism studies. *Naunyn Schmiedebergs Archiv für Pharmakologie, 278:* 301-312.

Myers, R.R. and Stockard, J.J. 1975): Neurologic and electroencephalographic correlates in glutethimide intoxication. *Clinical Pharmacology and Therapeutics, 17:* 212-220.

Nayak, R.K., Smyth, R.D., Chamberlain, J.H., Polk, A., De Long, A.F., Herczeg, T., Chemburkar, P.B., Joslin, R.S., and Reavey-Cantwell, N.H. (1974): Methaqualone pharmacokinetics after single- and multiple-dose administration in man. *Journal of Pharmacokinetics and Biopharmaceutics, 2:* 107-121.

Nover, R. (1967): Persistent neuropathy following chronic use of glutethimide. *Clinical Pharmacology and Therapeutics, 8:* 283-285.

Owens, A.H., Jr. and Marshall, E.K., Jr. (1955): Further studies on the metabolic fate of chloral hydrate and trichloroethanol. *Bulletin of Johns Hopkins Hospital, 97:* 320-326.

Palmer, K.H., Fowler, M.S., Wall, M.E., Rhodes, L.S., Waddell, W.J. and Baggett, B. (1969): The metabolism of R (+) and RS- pentobarbital. *Journal of Pharmacology and Experimental Therapeutics, 170:* 355-363.

Palmer, K.H., Fowler, M.S. and Wall, M.E. (1970): Metabolism of optically active barbiturates. II. S(−) pentobarbital. *Journal of Pharmacology and Experimental Therapeutics, 175:* 38-41.

Parker, K.D., Elliott, H.W., Wright, J.A., Nomof, N. and Hine, C.H. (1970): Blood and urine concentrations of subjects receiving barbiturates, meprobamate, glutethimide or diphenylhydantoin. *Clinical Toxicology, 3:* 131-145.

Paycoc, Z.W. and Powell, J.F. (1954): The excretion of sodium trichloroacetate. *Journal of Pharmacology and Experimental Therapeutics, 85:* 289-295.

Persson, B.H. (1960): Studies on the accumulation of certain barbiturates in the brain of the human foetus. *Acta Obstetrica Gynecologica Scandinavica, 39:* 88-99.

Ploman, L. and Persson, B.G. (1957): On the transfer of barbiturates to the human foetus and their accumulation in some of its vital organ. *Journal of the Obstetrics and Gynecology of the British Empire, 64:* 706.

Preuss, Fr. R., Hassler, H.-M. and Köpf, R. (1966a): Zur Biotransformation des 2-Methyl-3-o-tolyl-4(3H)-chinazolinon (Methaqualon). I. *Arzneimittel-Forschung, 16:* 395-401.

Preuss, Fr. R., Hassler, H.-M. and Köpf, R. (1966b): Zur Biotransformation des 2-Methyl-3-o-tolyl-4(3H)-chinazolinon (Methaqualon). 2. *Arzneimittel-Forschung, 16:* 401-407.

Preuss, Fr. R. and Hassler, H.-M. (1970): Zur Biotransformation des 2-Methyl-3-o-tolyl-4(3H)-chinazolinon (Methaqualon). *Arzneimittel-Forschung, 20:* 1920-1922.

Randall, L.O., Schallek, W., Scheckel, C.L., Stefko, P.L., Banziger, R.F., Pool, W. and Moe, R.A. (1969): Pharmacological studies on flurazepam hydrochloride (RO-5-6901), a new psychotropic agent of the benzodiazepine class. *Archives Internationales de Pharmacodynamie, 178:* 216-241.

Rapp, M.S. (1971): Reaction to flurazepam. *Canadian Medical Association Journal, 105:* 1020-1021.

Raventos, J. (1954): The distribution in the body and metabolic fate of barbiturates. *Journal of Pharmacy and Pharmacology, 6:* 217-235.

Remmer, H., Siegert, M. and Neuhaus, G. (1963): Die Elimination von Glutethimid und von Langwirkenden Barbituraten nach toxisch und Therapeutisch Wirksamen Dosen. *Naunyn-Schmiedeberg's Archiv für Experimentelle Pathologie und Pharmacologie, 245:* 471-483.

Rezza, E. (1956): Richerche sul metabolismo del chloralio idrato nel bambino. *Minerva Pediatrics, 8:* 368.

Rich, A.J., Gruhn, S.W., Gibson, T.P., Delle, M. and Di Bona, G.F. (1972): Effect of saline infusion on the renal excretion of secobarbital, glutethimide, meprobamate, and chlordiazepoxide. *Journal of Laboratory and Clinical Medicine, 80:* 56-62.

Rieder, J. and Wendt, G. (1973): Pharmacokinetics and metabolism of the hypnotic nitrazepam. In: *The Benzodiazepines,* edited by S. Garattini, E. Mussini and L.O. Randall, pp. 99-127, Raven Press, New York.

Riegelman, S., Loo, J. and Rowland, M. (1968): Concept of a volume of distribution and possible errors in evaluation of this parameter. *Journal of Pharmaceutical Sciences, 57:* 129.

Root, B. (1962): Oral premedication of children with chloral hydrate and scopolamine. *Anesthesia and Analgesia, 41:* 194.

Root, B. and Loveland, J.P. (1971): A comparative evaluation of chlorprothixene and secobarbital for pediatric premedication. *Journal of Clinical Pharmacology, 11:* 56-68.

Rosenbaum, J., Kramer, M., Raja, R. and Boreyko, C. (1971): Resin hemoperfusion: a new treatment for acute drug intoxication. *New England Journal of Medicine, 284:* 874-877.

Sambrooks, J.E., MacCulloch, M.J., Birtles, C.J. and Smallmann, C. (1972): Assessment of the effects of flurazepam and nitrazepam on visual motor performance using an automated assessment technique. *Acta Psychiatrica Scandinavica, 48:* 443-454.

Schwartz, M.A., Vane, F.M. and Postma, E. (1968): Urinary metabolites of 7-chloro-1-(2-diathylaminoethyl)-5-(2-fluorophenyl)-1,3-dihydro-2H-1,4-benzodiazepin-2-one dihydrochloride. *Journal of Medicinal Chemistry, 11:* 770-774.

Schwartz, M.A. and Postma, E. (1970): Metabolism of flurazepam a benzodiazepine, in man and dog. *Journal of Pharmaceutical Sciences, 59:* 1800-1806.

Schwartz, M.A. (1973): Pathways of metabolism of the benzodiazepines. In: *The Benzodiazepines,* edited by S. Garattini, E. Mussini and L.O. Randall, pp. 53-74, Raven Press, New York.

Sellers, E.M. and Koch-Weser, J. (1971): Kinetics and clinical importance of displacement of warfarin from albumin by acidic drugs. *Annals of the New York Academy of Sciences, 179:* 213-225.

Sellers, E.M., Carr, G., Bernstein, J.G., Sellers, S. and Koch-Weser, J. (1972b): Interaction of chloral hydrate and ethanol in man. II. *Clinical Pharmacology and Therapeutics, 13:* 50-58.

Sellers, E.M., Lang, M., Koch-Weser, J., Le Blanc, E. and Kalant, H. (1972a): Interaction of chloral hydrate and ethanol in man. I. Metabolism. *Clinical Pharmacology and Therapeutics, 13:* 37-49.

Sharpless, S.K. (1970): Hypnotics and sedatives. In: *The Pharmacological Basis of Therapeutics,* 4th ed., Macmillan, New York.

Sjögren, J., Sölvell, L. and Karlsson, I. (1965): Studies on the absorption rate of barbiturates in man. *Acta Medica Scandinavica, 178:* 553-559.

Smart, G.A. and Brown, S.S. (1970): Preparative ultracentrifugation of small samples of plasma and the protein binding of methaqualone. *Analytical Biochemistry, 35:* 518-523.

Smith R.B., Dittert, L.W., Giften, W.O. and Doluisio, J.T. (1973): Pharmacokinetics of pentobarbital after intravenous and oral administration. *Journal of Pharmacokinetics and Biopharmaceutics, 1:* 5-15.

Smyth, R.D., Lee, J.K., Polk, A., Chemburkar, P.B. and Savacool, A.M. (1973): Bioavailability of methaqualone. *Journal of Clinical Pharmacology, 13:* 391-401.
Swanson, D.W., Weddige, R.L. and Morse, R.M. (1973): Abuse of prescription drugs. *Mayo Clinic Proceedings, 48:* 359-367.
Tansella, M., Siciliani, O., Burti, O., Schiavon, M., Zimmermann Tansella, Ch., Gerna, M., Tognoni, G. and Morselli, P.L. (1975): N-desmethyldiazepam and amylobarbitone sodium as hypnotics in anxious patients. Plasma levels, clinical efficacy and residual effects. *Psychopharmacologia, 41:* 81-85.
Titus, E. and Weiss, H. (1955): The use of biologically prepared radioactive indicators in metabolic studies metabolism of pentobarbital. *Journal of Biological Chemistry, 214:* 807-920.
Tognoni, G., Gomeni, R., De Maio, D., Alberti, G.G., Franciosi, P. and Scieghi, G. (1975): Pharmacokinetics of N-desmethyldiazepam in patients suffering from insomnia and treated with nortriptyline. *British Journal of Clinical Pharmacology, 2:* 227-232.
Villa, C.A. (1965): Placental drug transfer. *Annals of the New York Academy of Sciences, 123:* 237-245.
Waddell, W.J. (1965): The metabolic fate of 5-allyl-5-(1-methylbutyl) barbituric acid (Secobarbital). *Journal of Pharmacology and Experimental Therapeutics, 149:* 23-28.
Williams, M.E., Davis, S.S., Poxon, R., Kendall, M.J. and Mitchard, M. (1974): The influence of diphenhydramine on the absorption of methaqualone in man. *British Journal of Clinical Pharmacology, 1:* 259-264.
Wright, N. and Roscoe, P. (1970): Acute glutethimide poisoning. *Journal of the American Medical Association, 214:* 1704-1706.
Zarolinsky, J., Browne, R. and Possley, L. (1972): Effects of subacute administration of methaqualone and glutethimide on plasma levels of bishydroxycoumarin. *Archives Internationales de Pharmacodynamie et Thérapie, 195:* 185-191.

13

Cardiovascular Agents

PAOLO LUCIO MORSELLI AND GABRIO BIANCHETTI

Cardiovascular drugs are a very heterogeneous group of pharmacological agents which include compounds such as the cardioactive glycoside, used since 2,000 years ago, as well as compounds of very recent introduction such as the β-blockers and some antihypertensive compounds. In this chapter, we will take into consideration three classes of drugs, for which the available data permit a partial definition of the pharmacokinetic profile in various physiopathological conditions, at least in adults. The drugs considered are digitalis glycoside, antiarrhythmic agents and β-blockers.

DIGITALIS GLYCOSIDES

Digitalis glycosides have been used for more than 2,000 years in the treatment of cardiac disease. Despite their wide use, they are still poorly understood drugs. A large number of reports on digitalis glycoside levels in human biological fluids have appeared in the last few years, but nevertheless the risk of overdose or of underdigitalization is still very great. Their kinetics and the factors capable of modifying them are not yet completely clarified. In this section, we will describe the available data on digoxin and digitoxin dispositions, emphasizing both the differences due to age and the lack of some important information.

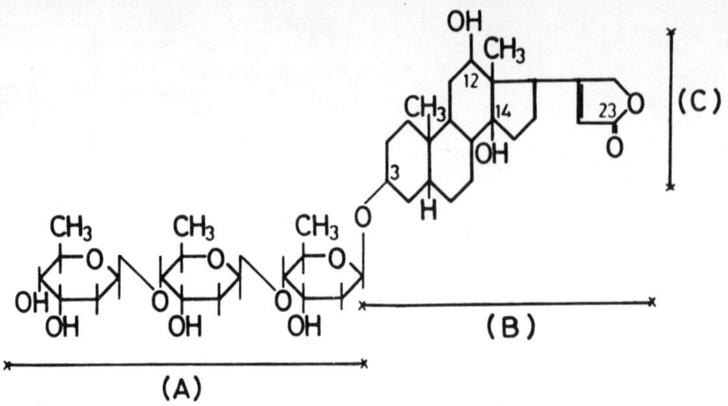

Fig. 1: Structural formula of digoxin; A = D. digitoxose; B = Digoxigenin; C = Lactone ring.

Digoxin

Adults. Digoxin is the pure crystalline glycoside obtained from "digitalis lanata." The structural formula given in Fig. 1 evidences a steroidic nucleus (digoxigenin), an exose chain (digitoxose) and a lactone ring in C_{17}. A hydroxy group in C_{12} confers a considerable polarity to the molecule. Digoxin is the most studied cardioactive glycoside, and numerous reviews have recently fully described its pharmacokinetic profile in adults in various pathological conditions as well as in volunteers (Soyka, 1972; Doherty and Kane, 1973; Smith and Haber, 1973; Doherty, 1973; Jusko, 1974; Marcus, 1975).

Administered by oral route, digoxin is mainly absorbed at the level of the small intestine, and its bioavailability may range from 70 to 100% if given in liquid form and from 35 to 60% if given as tablets (Doherty and Perkins, 1965; Huffman and Azarnoff, 1972; Dengler et al., 1973; Lindenbaum, 1973; Greenblatt et al., 1973; Steiness et al., 1973; Nyberg et al., 1974b; Huffman, 1975). The numerous papers appearing in the last few years on digoxin bioavailability have clearly documented important differences among the various preparations and showed that bioavailability and rate of absorption are strictly related to the rate of dissolution in the gut (Shaw et al., 1972; Lindenbaum, 1973; Steiness et al., 1973; Sanchez et al., 1973; Nyberg et al., 1974b; Fleckenstein et al., 1974a,b; Shaw and Carless, 1974; Butler and Lindenbaum, 1975; Lindenbaum, 1975; Jounela et al., 1975).

The gastrointestinal absorption of digoxin does not seem to be significantly affected by the presence of food (White et al., 1971; Greenblatt et al., 1974a), and in normal conditions, after a single oral dose of 0.25-0.75 mg, peak serum levels of 0.6-3.1 ng/ml are attained within 2-4 h (Huffmann and Azarnoff, 1972; Dengler et al., 1973; Steiness et al., 1973; Fraser et al., 1973; Greenblatt et al., 1973, 1974a; Nyberg et al., 1974b; Binnion, 1974; Fleckenstein et al., 1974a,b; Huffmann, 1975). Propantheline and metoclopramide may, on the contrary, significantly alter digoxin absorption (Manninen et al., 1973).

The bioavailability of digoxin given by intramuscular injection is about 80%, with serum peak concentration of 1.5-2.7 ng/ml, usually attained within 1-3 h after a dose of 0.25-0.75 mg (Doherty and Perkins, 1965; Soyka, 1972; Doherty, 1973; Steiness et al., 1974). It must be remembered that, as recently reported by Steiness et al. (1974), the intramuscular administration of digoxin may result in large areas of tissue necrosis at the injection site. The use of this route of administration appears questionable in view of these recent findings. Following an intravenous administration, digoxin serum levels decay biexponentially with a distribution phase which has an apparent half-life of 60-90 min (Doherty and Perkins, 1962; Dengler et al., 1973; Doherty, 1973; Doherty and Kane, 1973; Bertler et al., 1974; Greenblatt et al., 1974b; Nyberg et al., 1974a).

After oral absorption the distribution phase of digoxin may be rather long, and an equilibrium is usually reached only after 4-6 h. For this reason, a correct evaluation of steady-state concentrations may be obtained only if sampling is performed at least 6-8 h after drug intake.

Digoxin is bound to serum proteins for about 23-40% (Ohnhaus et al., 1972, 1974; Dengler et al., 1973; Wallace and Whiting, 1974; Kramer et al., 1974), and a linear relationship between serum and saliva digoxin concentrations has been recently reported (Jusko, 1974; Huffmann, 1975).

The apparent volume of distribution may range from 5.1-7.3 L/kg in subjects with normal kidneys to a value of 2.6-4.3 L/kg in patients with impaired renal function (Dengler et al., 1973; Reuning et al., 1973; Nyberg et al., 1974a; Jusko et al., 1974; Wagner, 1974a). A reduction in the volume of extracellular fluids and/or a decreased binding to quantitatively important tissues (such as skeletal muscle) probably underlies the reduced apparent volume of distribution in uremic patients (Jusko, 1974). Digoxin distributes to all tissues, higher concentrations usually being found in kidneys and heart; a heart/serum concentration ratio of 30 or higher may be observed in renal patients as well as in subjects with normal kidney function (Doherty et al., 1967a,b; Coltart et al., 1974; Karjalainen et al., 1974; Gullner et al., 1974; Jusko and Weintraub, 1974; Smith, 1975).

The apparent half-life of the serum terminal exponential decay may vary from 15 to 90 h in subjects with a creatinine clearance within normal values, and from 60 to 183 h in anephric patients or patients with renal insufficiency (Doherty and Perkins, 1965; Doherty et al., 1967a,b; Luchi and Gruber, 1968; Butler, 1970; Dettli et al., 1972; Huffmann and Azarnoff, 1972; Doherty, 1973; Brown and Abraham, 1973; Greenblatt et al., 1974c; Marcus, 1975). A recent study by

Finkelstein et al. (1975) indicates that extreme care should be taken when administering digoxin to patients undergoing regular dialytic treatment. Steady-state serum concentrations, on a maintenance dose of 0.125 mg 5 days a week are, in fact, achieved only after 21-35 days of treatment. In the presence of moderate hepatic diseases, the apparent digoxin serum half-life does not appear to be significantly altered (Marcus and Kapadia, 1964), while an increased serum disappearance rate (probably due to a decreased binding) has been observed in cases of acute hepatitis (Zilly et al., 1975). In cases of suicide attempts, an inverse relationship between serum concentrations and apparent serum half-life was observed by Smith and Willerson (1971). Similar data have been more recently reported by Bertler et al. (1973) and by Hobson and Zettner (1973). A decreased protein-binding at very high concentrations could be a possible explanation for the elevated clearances. More recently, Wagner (1974b) has proposed that the "shorter half-lives" were probably estimated during the absorption-distribution phase, which is very likely to be considerably prolonged after massive digoxin doses.

The reported cumulative (6 to 8 days) urinary excretion following an intravenous administration of digoxin, in subjects with a normal renal function, may vary from 29 to 90% of the administered dose, with an apparent urinary half-life of 1.4–2.7 days (Marcus et al., 1966; Doherty et al., 1970; Dengler et al., 1973; Bisset et al., 1973; Greenblatt et al., 1973). According to several reports, digoxin is mainly eliminated unchanged in urine, being subject to a very limited metabolic degradation (Doherty and Perkins, 1962; Doherty et al., 1970; Doherty, 1973; Jusko, 1974; Marcus, 1975) (Fig. 2). However, mechanisms other than renal excretion of the unchanged compound may play a significant part in the disposition of digoxin in man in several instances (Hernandez et al., 1963; Luchi and Gruber, 1968; Clark and Kalman, 1974b; Abshagen et al., 1974). A marked individual difference in the ability to metabolize digoxin was first reported by Hernandez et al. (1963). Subsequently, an increased conversion of digoxin to less active and/or inactive metabolites (Fig. 2) was observed by Luchi and Gruber (1968) in a patient requiring unusually high amounts of digoxin. In such a case, digoxin accounted for less than 50% of the extractable excreted material, while the remainder was represented by digoxigenin and dihydrodigoxigenin. More recently, Watson et al. (1973) described the identification of dihydrodigoxin as a metabolite of digoxin. This derivative may range from 7 to 40% of the methylene chloride extractable material in urine of patients on maintenance therapy, and it may also be present in plasma at concentrations of 0.18–0.36 ng/ml (Clark and Kalman, 1974a,b). It may be of interest to note that dihydrodigoxin has the same mobility of digoxin in many TLC systems.

Several reports indicating a linear relationship between creatinine clearance and digoxin renal clearance suggest that the drug is mainly excreted by glomerular filtration (Doherty and Perkins, 1965; Doherty et al., 1970; Doherty, 1973; Bisset et al., 1973; Falch, 1973; Jusko, 1974; Ohnhauss et al., 1974; Marcus,

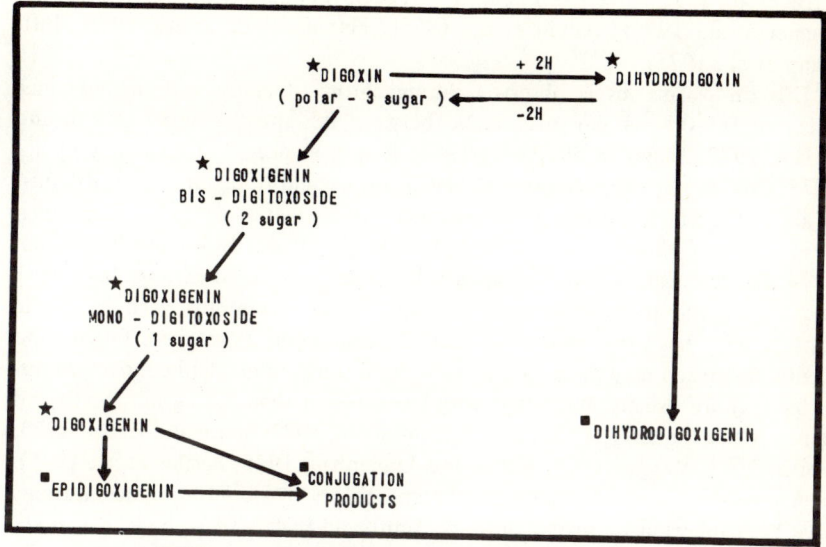

Fig. 2: Metabolic pathway of digoxin; * = Cardioactive; ■ = Cardioinactive.

1975). Steiness (1974) has recently presented evidence that digoxin may be subject to tubular secretion, a fact which could explain some of the unusually high digoxin clearances observed in some patients. Further evidence was given by the fact that spironolactone decreases the digoxin clearance, suggesting an inhibition of the tubular secretion of digoxin in the distal tubules. Reabsorption of digoxin in both proximal and distal tubules was observed by Doherty et al. (1969) in the dog. Marcus et al. (1964), Bisset et al. (1973) and Steiness (1974) could not confirm such data in man; however, Halkin et al. (1975b) presented data which suggest that, in man as well, digoxin may undergo passive tubular resorption in addition to filtration and secretion. These authors could in fact observe that, independent from creatinine clearance, urine flow rate and urea clearance are both related to digoxin renal clearance.

The possibility of using creatinine clearance values as a predictor of digoxin maintenance doses has been supported by several authors, and more recently a clear relationship has also been observed between BUN and digoxin clearance. However, these relationships, even if valid from a statistical point of view for groups of patients, do not allow a precise prediction of the dose for the single individual patient, and the measure of the serum concentration is still the best way to assess correct therapy. A better index of digoxin bioavailability and disposition may be obtained by evaluating the amount of drug excreted in 24 h together with the area-under-the-plasma-concentration curve (Jellife et al., 1970;

Shaw et al., 1972; Greenblatt et al., 1973; Peck et al., 1973; Bertler et al., 1974; Wagner et al., 1974a; Halkin et al., 1975b; Marcus, 1975; Smith, 1975; Huffmann et al., 1975).

Digoxin plasma levels observed during chronic therapy with maintenance doses of 0.1–0.5 mg/day may range between 0.5 and 8.2 ng/ml (Smith and Haber, 1970; Hayes et al., 1971, 1973; Rogers et al., 1972; O'Malley et al., 1973; Cree et al., 1973; Iisalo et al., 1973; Brown and Abraham, 1973; Ritzman et al., 1973; Sanchez et al., 1973; Falch, 1973; Sheiner et al., 1974; Karjalainen et al., 1974; Güllner et al., 1974; Nyberg et al., 1974b; Jusko and Weintraub, 1974; Bertler et al., 1974). Therapeutic levels are considered to range between 1 and 2.5 ng/ml in normokalemic patients. Toxic symptoms such as gastric disturbances, headache, anorexia, loss of visual acuity, weakness, fatigue and mental confusion as well as cardiac symptoms (arrhythmias and conduction disturbances) are usually associated with levels higher than 3.0 ng/ml (Smith and Haber, 1970; Doherty, 1973; Doherty and Kane, 1973; Smith and Haber, 1973; Smith, 1975; Marcus, 1975; Butler and Lindenbau, 1975; Bertler et al., 1975).

A considerable overlap between therapeutic and toxic serum concentrations have been reported by several authors (Smith and Haber, 1970; Fogelman et al., 1971; Beller et al., 1971; Christiansen et al., 1973; Doherty, 1973; Bertler et al., 1975). Despite this overlapping, the usefulness of monitoring serum digoxin levels is today not only generally accepted but considered an essential step for a more rational therapy.

Newborns, infants and children. Digoxin may easily cross the placenta, and concentrations similar to those present in serum of mothers have been found in cord serum (Rogers et al., 1972). The data of Rogers et al. (1972) showing that serum concentrations in the newborn, 12 h after delivery, were practically identical to the levels at birth, are indicative of a very low disposition of digoxin, if any, during the first hours of life.

Administered directly to newborns of 10–20 days of life, digoxin is efficiently absorbed if given by oral route in liquid form, while absorption is less and slower if digoxin is injected intramuscularly. In the latter case, peak plasma levels may be attained 6–10 h after dosing (Assael et al., 1973; Morselli, 1976). Given the incomplete and erratic absorption, and considering the recent report of Steiness et al. (1974) documenting the occurrence of tissue necrosis at the injection sites, the use of this parenteral route should be avoided as far as possible in newborns and infants.

The binding of digoxin to cord serum proteins is apparently lower but not significantly different from that observed in adults. According to Gorodischer et al. (1974), for serum concentrations of 2 ng/ml, the bound fraction in cord serum may vary from 14 to 26%.

Following an i.v. administration of 7–21 µg/kg to five newborns (four premature and one full-term newborn) of 3–9 days of age, an apparent volume of distribution of 5–10 L/kg has been described (Morselli et al., 1975). The data are in apparent agreement with the higher extracellular fluid volume in the newborn, with the lower binding and also with the report of Kim et al. (1974) describing, in five newborns of 10–24 days of age, myocardial and skeletal muscle concentrations higher than those found in children and adults. It must be remembered, however, that due to the different methods employed, to the different material analyzed (biopsy and autopsy) as well as to the different sampling times after the last dose, a comparison of the various data available on digoxin tissue concentrations is practically impossible.

The apparent plasma or serum disappearance rate of digoxin in newborns of 3 to 9 days of age may be extremely slow, and the drug total clearance seems to be closely related to the maturation state (Morselli, 1974, 1975). In five newborns, we could in fact observe an apparent plasma half-life ranging from 26 to 170 h, with corresponding values of body clearances of 3.9–0.54 ml/min/kg (Morselli et al., 1975). These values obtained after a single i.v. administration are of the same order of the values of relative clearances calculated on steady-state levels from the data available in the literature, which may range from 1.9 to 6.1 ml/min/kg (O'Malley et al., 1973; Cree et al., 1973; Iisalo et al., 1973; Larese and Mirkin, 1974; Wettrel et al., 1974). The very low clearances observed in newborns of 3 to 20 days of age are clearly related to the immaturity of the renal function (see Chapter 4).

In infants, digoxin is absorbed at a rate comparable to those observed in children and adults. Following an oral administration of 10–20 µg/kg, peak serum levels are generally attained within 60–180 min, with concentrations of 3 to 5 ng/ml (Hernandez et al., 1963, 1969; Krasula et al., 1972; Larese and Mirkin, 1974). According to Hernandez et al. (1969), after an intramuscular injection peak serum levels may be achieved within 15–30 min, while in a more recent report peak levels were observed after 2–4 h (Assael et al., 1973).

No data are available on plasma protein-binding in infants. The apparent volume of distribution may range from 10 to 28 L/kg, according to the published data (Morselli et al., 1975). As before, this data is in good agreement with the reports of Hernandez et al. (1969) and Gorodischer et al. (1976b), indicating that also in infants and tissue uptake and the tissue-binding of digoxin may be higher than in children and adults. The greater myocardium concentrations of digoxin found in infants raises the question whether the cardiac receptor in this age group is more resistant to the action of the drug. On the other hand, digoxin may be present at the receptor site at concentrations different from those present in the myocardium biophase. The relative differences in extra- and intracellular fluids may partially play a role in such a situation (Jusko, 1974).

In infants, digoxin is disposed of at a rate which is considerably faster than in children and adults. Apparent plasma half-lives of 18–27 h have been reported by Soyka (1972) and of 11–37 h by Morselli et al. (1975). Dungan et al. (1972), using H^3 digoxin, reported values of 18–26 h, while Hernandez et al. (1969) described an apparent serum half-life of 40 h. The dose may have a remarkable effect on digoxin apparent half-life, and higher doses seem to be disposed of at faster rates (Morselli et al., 1975).

The possibility of an increased metabolic breakdown of digoxin in infants has been postulated by our group, but convincing evidence for such an assumption is not yet available.

According to Dungan et al. (1972), the metabolism of digoxin in infants is of the same order of that in adults, with only 6% of the dose metabolized within 24 h. Major metabolites found in urine were digoxigenin bisdigitoxoside and digoxigenin. Yanagi et al. (1975) could not observe any significant difference in the urinary digoxin excretion in various age groups (from 2 months to 5 years).

At variance with these findings, very recent observations of Gorodischer et al. (1976a) clearly document that the renal clearances of digoxin relative to creatinine clearances may be considerably greater in infants than in adults. In agreement with the data of Steiness (1974) in adults, and at variance with the findings of Jalkin et al. (1974, 1975b), no relationship could be observed between digoxin clearance and urine flow.

The higher renal clearances described by Gorodischer et al. (1976a) are in good agreement with the increased total body clearances (8.5–13.5 ml/min/kg) reported by our group (Morselli et al., 1975), and with the fact that daily dosages of about 20 µg/kg or more are usually necessary to achieve therapeutic steady-state levels in infants. However, these new findings documenting a faster disposition rate in infants do not fully explain the higher requirement of digoxin in these age groups.

In fact, the serum concentrations at which the drug induces toxic effects appear to be higher in infants than in adults. According to Soyka et al. (1975), toxic signs become evident only at concentrations over 3.5 ng/ml, and Hayes et al. (1973) found no toxic effects in 65% of the cases with serum levels over 2 ng/ml, while clear symptoms of toxicity developed for concentrations over 4 ng/ml. At variance with these data, no relationship between digoxin levels and toxic effects could be found by Larese and Mirkin (1974).

In children, peak serum levels following an oral intake are usually attained within 60–120 min, and steady-state plasma levels of 0.7–3.5 ng/ml may be reached with maintenance doses of 9 to 15 µg/kg (Hayes et al., 1971, 1973; Cree et al., 1973; Iisalo et al., 1973; Krasula et al., 1974; Larese and Mirkin, 1974; Moss et al., 1975). Tissue distribution appears to be very similar to that observed in adults (Soyka et al., 1975). The apparent volume of distribution in children of 2–5 years of age is still considerably greater than in adults (Morselli et al., 1975). No data are available for older children.

Major metabolites identified in children's urine are digoxigenin and mono- and bis-digitoxosides (Soyka et al., 1975).

According to Hayes et al. (1971) and Krasula et al. (1972, 1974), the threshold value of toxic levels in children is around 2.9 ng/ml. Further data of Hayes et al. (1973) and of Iisalo et al. (1973) are in good agreement with this

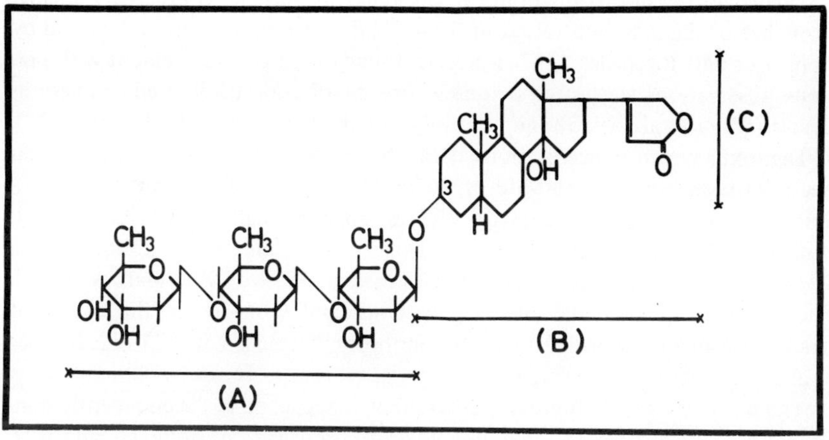

Fig. 3: Structural formula of digitoxin; A = D. digitoxose; B = Digitoxigenin; C = Lactone ring.

finding. These authors, in fact, noted that about 70% of the patients with serum levels over 2 ng/ml had toxic effects. In contrast with these data, no relationship could be observed between serum levels and effects by Larese and Mirkin (1974).

Digitoxin

At variance with digoxin, digitoxin is well and rapidly absorbed from the gastrointestinal tract, and its bioavailability is practically complete (90–100%). Such a difference is mainly due to the lack of the hydroxy group in C_{12} (Fig. 3), a fact which increases the lipid solubility of the molecule and facilitates its diffusion throughout membranes. After an oral dose of 0.25–1 mg, peak serum concentrations of 8–40 ng/ml may be achieved within 40–120 min, and a linear relationship between the dose expressed in mg/kg and the serum levels has been reported (Lukas, 1971; Rasmussen et al., 1972; Doherty, 1973; Vohringer and Rietbrock, 1974; Storstein, 1974a,b). At variance with digoxin, no differences in the amount absorbed nor in the absorption rate could be observed by Finkelstein et al. (1975) in dialyzed patients after a dose of 0.25 mg.

Digitoxin is bound to serum protein for 90 to 97%, with an association constant for albumin of 4.64×10^4 liter/mole (Lukas, 1971; Rasmussen et al., 1972; Storstein, 1974b). According to Kramer et al. (1974), in uremic patients the binding is reduced (88 ± 1.4%) and this is accompanied by a more rapid onset of action of the drug.

Digitoxin appears to distribute in an apparent volume considerably smaller than that of digoxin, and values of 0.5–0.7 L/kg have been recently reported by Vohringer and Rietbrock (1974). Such a finding is in good agreement with previous observations suggesting a nonselective distribution of digitoxin in various tissues (Okita et al., 1955) and relatively low tissue/serum ratios (Lukas, 1971).

Digitoxin serum concentrations decay biexponentially: a rapid distribution phase with an apparent half-life of 70 to 150 min is followed by a very prolonged terminal exponential phase with an apparent half-life of 102 to 220 h (Lukas, 1971; Rasmussen et al., 1972; Doherty and Kane, 1973; Ritzman et al., 1973; Vohringer and Rietbrock, 1974; Storstein, 1974a, 1975; Marcus, 1975). The terminal apparent half-life may be considerably shorter in the course of renal impairment, according to various authors (Rasmussen et al., 1972; Kramer et al., 1974; Storstein, 1974b).

The existence of an important enterohepatic recycling has been recently confirmed by Storstein (1975). Bile peak concentrations may be observed within 15 to 60 min after an i.v. administration of 0.6 mg, and after the distribution phase bile levels are constantly higher than those of serum. Concomitant administration of cholestiramine may significantly reduce the recycling of digitoxin, with a consequent drop in serum concentrations (Caldwell and Greenberger, 1971).

Digitoxin is metabolized in the body for about 60–80%, and a scheme of its metabolic degradation is presented in Fig. 4. The β-hydroxylation in C_{12} to yield digoxin does not appear to be an important metabolic route in man, and it may account for about 7.5–10% (Vohringer and Rietbrock, 1974). This pathway may, however, be increased by concomitant administration of "inducing" agents such as phenobarbital (Solomon and Abrams, 1972; Hutcheon, 1975).

Following a single administration, about 15–21% of the dose may be recovered in urine, and 13% in feces, over an 8-day collection period. The unchanged drug accounts for about 50% of the excreted material during the first 8 days, but over a period of 30 days it represents only 10–15% of the dose (Okita et al., 1955; Lukas, 1971; Doherty, 1973; Vohringer and Rietbrock, 1974; Storstein, 1974a). In the course of maintenance therapy, the percentage of the daily dose excreted as cardioactive substances may range from 20 to 70% (mean: 37.9 ± 18.7) in subjects with normal renal function and from 3 to 40% (mean: 13.6 ± 11.5) in subjects with renal impairment (Lukas, 1971; Storstein, 1974b; Finkelstein et al., 1975).

The reduced renal clearance of digitoxin and of its cardiactive metabolites in uremic patients and the faster serum disappearance suggest the presence of a compensatory mechanism such as an increased hepatic metabolism and/or an increased fecal excretion. From the available data (Storstein, 1974b), a modification of the apparent volume of distribution also seems very likely. A remarkable fluctuation of serum digitoxin levels has been recently observed by Finkelstein et al. (1975) in dialyzed patients on maintenance therapy.

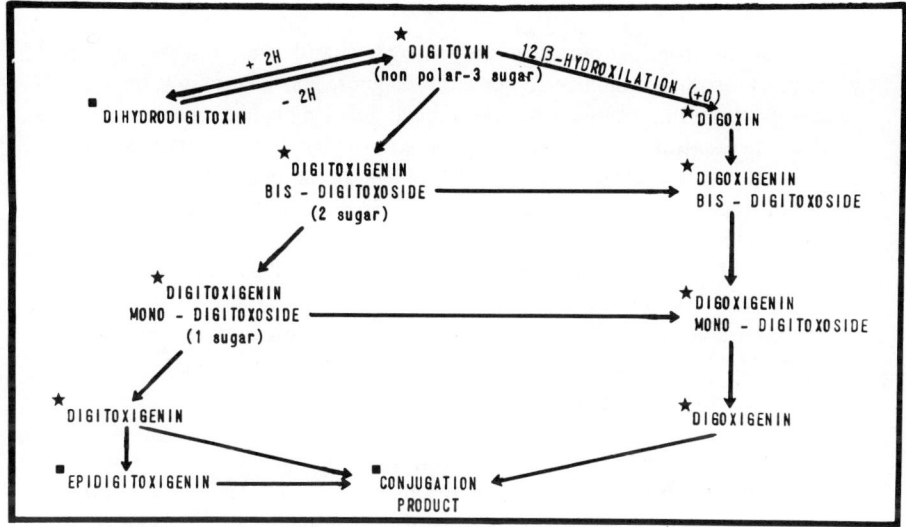

Fig. 4: Metabolic pathway of digitoxin; * = Cardioactive; ■ = Cardioinactive.

Renal excretion of digitoxin is dependent upon glomerular filtration and tubular resorption, but a net tubular secretion may also be present in cases of increased urine flow (Lukas, 1971). Digitoxin serum levels do correlate well with the inotropic action of the drug (Lukas, 1971), and the concentrations in the course of maintenance therapy range from 15 to 35 ng/ml (Beller et al., 1971; Rasmussen et al., 1972; Doherty, 1973; Doherty and Kane, 1973; Ritzman et al., 1973; Peters et al., 1974; Smith, 1975; Marcus, 1975).

In normokalemic patients, toxic effects at gastrointestinal levels are usually observed with serum concentrations higher than 40 ng/ml, while blurred vision, scotomata and xanthopsia are often associated with serum levels over 50 ng/ml. Cardiac toxicity is always evident for serum concentrations over 60 ng/ml (Lukas, 1971; Ritzman et al., 1973; Peters et al., 1974). Severe CNS disturbances were present in one case, reported by Lukas (1971), where serum concentrations were higher than 100 ng/ml.

Digitoxin and its metabolites can easily cross the placenta and be present in the fetus at concentrations higher than those present in the mother (Okita et al., 1956). No information is presently available on digitoxin disposition in pediatric age.

ANTIARRHYTHMIC AGENTS

One of the major advances in the management of heart diseases in recent years has been the possibility to correctly diagnose and successfully treat arrhythmias. Such an improvement has been made possible by a better understanding of their mechanism of action and by the knowledge of their pharmacokinetic profiles. However, despite the considerable body of data on antiarrhythmic agents in adults, very few or no data on their disposition in pediatric age are available. The drugs included in this section are quinidine, procainamide (as representative of the group depressing the normal electrophysiological properties) and lidocaine (as representative of the group facilitating conduction and reducing refractoriness). Propranolol will be treated with the β-blockers and diphenylhydantoin has already been described with the anticonvulsants.

Quinidine

Quinidine has been used as antiarrhythmic agent since 1918, and it may be considered the prototype of this class of drugs. Administered by oral route as quinidine sulfate, it is well absorbed and peak plasma levels of 4–9 µg/ml are usually attained with 1–2 h after a 400–600 mg dose; when sustained-release tablets are used, peak levels of 1.8–5.4 µg/ml are achieved within 4–8 h (Cramer et al., 1963; Cullhed et al., 1966; Lindseth-Ditlefsen and Bjerkelund, 1966; Lindseth-Ditlefsen and Löken, 1966; Mason et al., 1973; Aviado and Salem, 1975). According to Courthamel (1974), the bioavailability of quinidine may be greatly reduced in congestive heart failure.

Quinidine is bound to plasma proteins (mainly to albumin) for about 80–90% (Mason et al., 1973; Chien et al., 1974). A slight increase in the bound fraction may be observed in uremic patients, while a binding of 40 to 70% was reported for cirrhotic patients (Reidenberg and Affrime, 1974), and values ranging from 73 to 96% were described in cardiac patients by Kessler et al. (1974).

The apparent volume of distribution may range from 2.5 to 3 L/kg, according to Ronfeld and Chow (1975), while it may be reduced to 1.2–1.5 L/kg in patients with heart failure. Quinidine distributes rapidly to all tissues, with the exception of the brain, and concentrations four to ten times those in plasma may be achieved in heart muscle, kidney and skeletal muscle (Aviado and Salem, 1975).

In subjects with normal heart and kidney functions, the compound has a mean apparent half-life of 6–7 h, while in renal and cardiac patients a slight increase up to 8–11 h has been reported (Bellet et al., 1971; Crouthamel, 1974; Kessler et al., 1974; Ronfeld and Chow, 1975). Because of the individual variability in plasma half-lives, which in all the above-mentioned groups may range from 3 to 19 h, there are practically no differences in the apparent disappear-

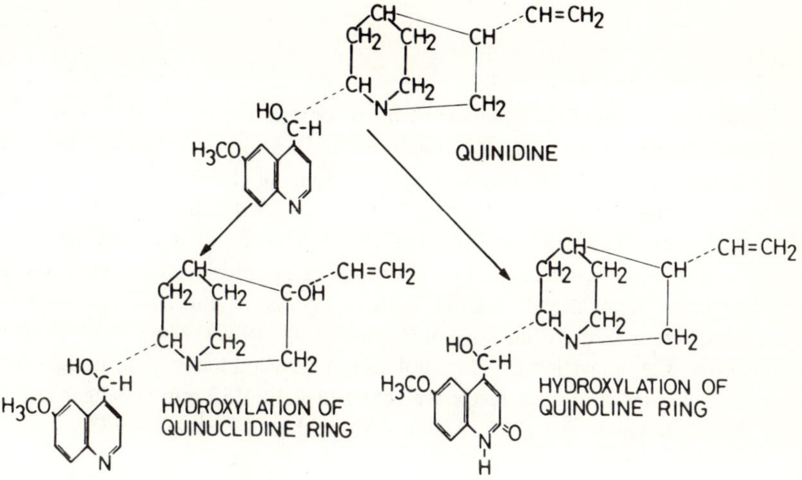

CARDIOVASCULAR DRUGS 405

Fig. 5: Structural formula of quinidine and its metabolic pathway.

ance rate of quinidine from plasma. Higher plasma concentrations observed in patients in some of the quoted studies are probably due (for the lack of specificity of the methods used) to the presence of metabolites.

Quinidine is partially metabolized to monohydroxyquinidine and dihydroxyquinidine, which are further conjugated in limited amounts (Hartel and Korhoner, 1968; Palmer et al., 1969; Carrol et al., 1974) (Fig. 5).

Quinidine may be present in urine for about 50% of the administered dose, and alkalinization of the urine may result in an increased serum level and occurrence of toxic effects (Palmer et al., 1969; Aviado and Salem, 1975). A reduced excretion of quinidine metabolites has been observed in cardiac and renal patients (Bellet et al., 1971; Aviado and Salem, 1975). It must be remembered that dihydroxyquinidine may already be present in tablets and capsules of quinidine sulfate in amounts ranging from 4 to 12% of the dose (Smith et al., 1973).

Therapeutic plasma levels range from 2 to 4 µg/ml with specific analytical methods (Henning and Nyberg, 1973) and from 4 to 7 µg/ml if less specific methods are used (Cullhed et al., 1966; Kessler et al., 1974).

Common toxic signs include anorexia, nausea, vomiting, diarrhea, headache, tinnitus, vertigo and blurred vision. More serious adverse effects, usually present for concentrations above 6–8 µg/ml, are represented by conduction blocks in sinoatrial and atrioventricular nodes, ventricular ectopic beats and ventricular tachycardia or fibrillation. Trombocitopenia is not a rare occurrence (Mason et al., 1973; Aviado and Salem, 1975).

Lidocaine

Lidocaine is usually administered by parenteral route, mostly intravenously by constant infusion. Adequate blood levels can also be reached by intramuscular administration. Peak plasma concentrations of 1.2–2.5 µg/ml are in fact achieved within 10–30 min after a 200 mg dose (Scott et al., 1968; Cohen et al., 1972; Adjepon-Yamoah and Prescott, 1973). The site of injection may significantly influence the absorption of lidocaine. A deltoid injection leads to higher plasma levels than lateral thigh or buttock injections, and peak concentrations are usually observed within 10 min (Cohen et al., 1972). When administered by oral route, the bioavailability does not seem to exceed the 35%, although the absorption is rapid and peak levels are achieved within 30 min (Eisinger and Hellier, 1968; Boyes et al., 1971; Adjepon-Yamoah and Prescott, 1973).

In normal subjects, lidocaine is bound to plasma protein for about 66% (Chow and Ronfeld, 1975), and it has an apparent volume of distribution of 1.6–1.7 L/kg (Rowland, 1974). The apparent volume of distribution may be increased up to 2.3 L/kg in patients with liver diseases, while it may be reduced to 0.8–1.0 L/kg in patients with congestive heart failure, and is practically unmodified in renal patients (Thomson et al., 1969, 1971, 1973; Rowland, 1974; Halkin et al., 1975a).

Lidocaine disappears from plasma according to a biexponential decay. Following an intravenous bolus of 50–100 mg, the distribution (alpha) phase has an apparent half-life of 6 to 9 min, while the apparent plasma half-life of the terminal exponential phase may range from 1.5 to 1.8 h (Rowland et al., 1971; Thomson et al., 1971, 1973; Rowland, 1974; Halkin et al., 1975a). The apparent plasma disappearance rate may be significantly prolonged in patients with liver diseases, while minor or no variations have been observed in renal and heart failure patients (Thomson et al., 1969, 1971, 1973; Rowland, 1974).

Lidocaine is extensively metabolized in the liver. Main metabolites so far identified are monoethylglycinexylidide (MEGX), glycinexylidide (GX) and 4-hydroxy-2,6-dimethylaniline (Beckett et al., 1966; Keenaghan and Boyes, 1972; Strong and Atkinson, 1972; Adjepon-Yamoah and Prescott, 1973; Halkin et al., 1975a) (Fig. 6).

Lidocaine as such may be present in the 24 h urine for about 2–3%, MEGX for 3–4% and GX for 2–3%, while 4-hydroxy-2,6-dimethylaniline represents about 70% of the administered dose (Keenaghan and Boyes, 1972). Plasma levels of the metabolites are about one-sixth to one-fifth of those of lidocaine. Monoethylglycinexylidide may play a role in the effects of lidocaine. After administration of the parent compound, MEGX reaches its peak within 1 h and has an apparent plasma half-life of 2.8 h, the apparent half-life of GX is con-

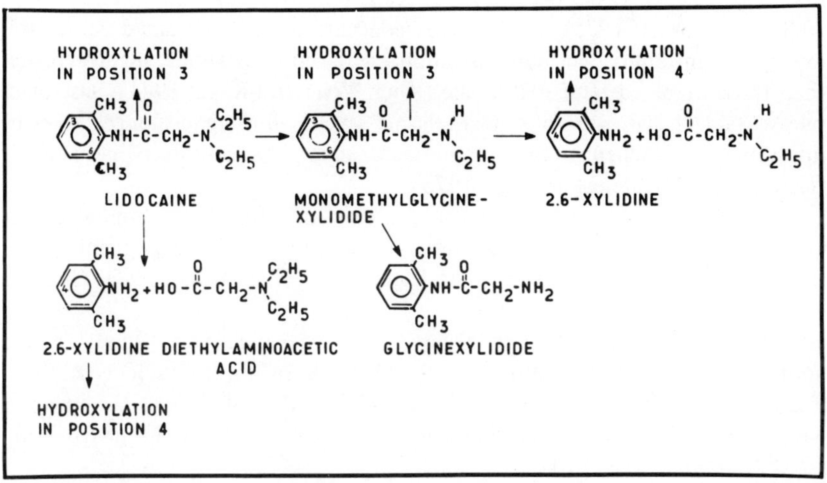

Fig. 6: Structural formula of lidocaine and its metabolic pathway.

siderably longer (~ 15 h) (Strong and Atkinson, 1972; Adjepon-Yamoah and Prescott, 1973; Halkin et al., 1975a).

Therapeutic plasma levels of lidocaine range from 2 to 5 μg/ml (Scott et al., 1968; Rowland, 1974; Zito and Reid, 1975). To maintain such a level, the usual procedure is to give an intravenous bolus of 1 mg/kg followed by a constant intravenous infusion of 40 μg/kg/min for the subsequent 2-3 h (Stenson et al., 1971; Rowland et al., 1971; Rowland, 1974; Zito and Reid, 1975).

Toxicity usually becomes evident with plasma levels over 5 μg/ml. The most common side effects are drowsiness, muscle twitching, paresthesias and, in some cases, convulsions. MEGX may also contribute to some of the adverse effects, and it must be kept in mind that unusually high levels of MEGX (up to one-third of those of lidocaine) have been observed in patients with congestive heart failure (Strong and Atkinson, 1972; Halkin et al., 1975a).

Procainamide

Procainamide is rapidly and quite well absorbed if administered by oral route, its rate of absorption depending mainly on the gastric transit time (Weliky and Neiss, 1975). According to the various authors, the bioavailability of procainamide by oral route may range from 70 to 95% (Koch-Weser and Klein, 1971; Dreyfuss et al., 1972; Fremstad et al., 1973; Weliky et al., 1975; Bigger, 1975). Peak levels of 4-6 μg/ml are usually observed within 60-90 min after an oral dose of 1 g (Koch-Weser, 1971; Karlsson, 1973; Fremstad et al., 1973; Weliky and Neiss, 1975). Peak plasma concentrations are attained earlier following an intramuscular administration, with concentrations slightly higher than those observed after oral intake (Koch-Weser and Klein, 1971). Sustained-release tablets give rise to similar plasma levels, allowing prolonged (6–8 h) intervals in dose schedule and a good maintenance of steady-state plasma levels (Karlsson, 1973; Fremstad et al., 1973).

Procainamide is bound to plasma proteins only for a very limited extent (15%), and its concentration in various organs and tissues is dependent on the relative blood flow (Koch-Weser and Klein, 1971; Koch-Weser, 1971; Giardina et al., 1974).

Independently from the administered dose, over a range of 0.5–1.5 g, the apparent volume of distribution of procainamide in normal subjects is about 2 L/kg, while in patients suffering from cardiac and renal diseases the apparent Vd may be reduced to 1.5 L/kg (Koch-Weser and Klein, 1971; Fremstad et al., 1973; Giardina et al., 1974).

The apparent plasma disappearance rate is fast, and the reported half-lives range from 2.2 to 3.5 h (Koch-Weser and Klein, 1971; Weily and Genton, 1972; Arstila et al., 1974; Giardina et al., 1974). In renal patients, the apparent plasma half-life may be prolonged up to 7–9 h, according to Gibson et al. (1975).

The major metabolite of procainamide identified in man is the N-acetyl derivative (Fig. 7). N-acetylprocainamide is usually present in urine for about 40 to 68% of the excreted material (Dreyfuss et al., 1972; Drayer et al., 1974; Karlsson et al., 1975). Plasma levels of the metabolite may be 2–3 times higher than those of procainamide, but its pharmacological potency is considerably less (Giardina et al., 1974; Karlsson et al., 1975). In a recent study, Reidenberg et al. (1975) described a ratio of NAPA to procainamide of 1.8 in fast and of 0.5 in slow acetylators, respectively.

The amount of drug excreted as such and as NAPA, in the first 6 h after administration, may range from 57–80% in normal subjects to 19–49% in renal and cardiac patients (Weily and Genton, 1972; Dreyfuss et al., 1972). Karlsson et al., more recently (1975), observed that in cardiac patients 60–90% of the dose is excreted in 24 h. Procainamide excretion appears to be directly related to creatinine clearance, according to Weily and Genton (1972). The total body clearance of procainamide may range from 316 to 680 ml/min. The renal clearance may vary from 179 to 309 ml/min, suggesting an active secretion at the tubular level.

A large variability in plasma levels, not related to the pro kilo dose, may be observed in the course of chronic treatment. Therapeutic plasma levels range from 4 to 8 μg/ml. For levels ranging from 8 to 16 μg/ml, about 30% of the subjects may present minor toxicity such as gastrointestinal disturbances, weakness and mild hypotension, while more serious cardiac toxic side effects (hypotension, cardiac conduction disturbances) are constantly associated with levels

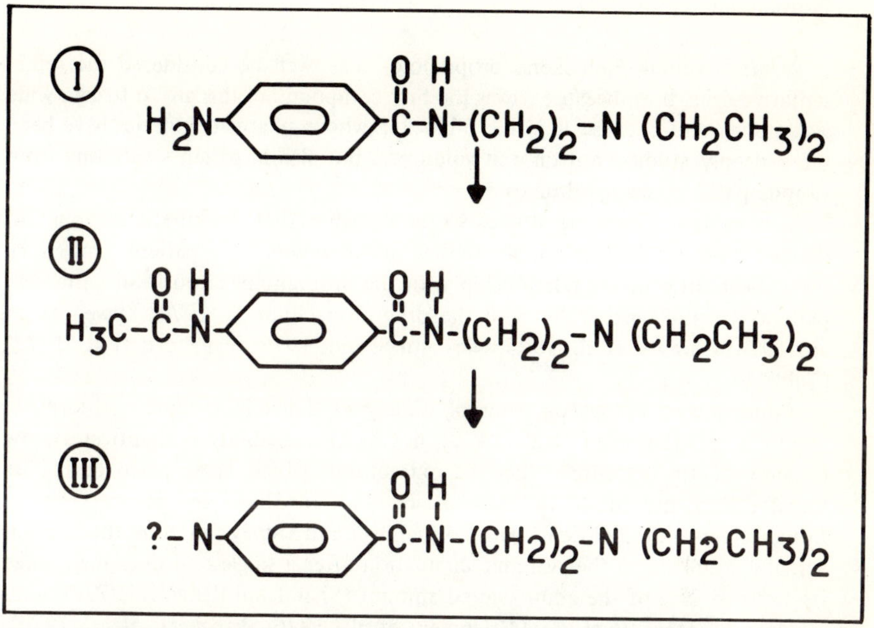

Fig. 7: Structural formula of procainamide and its main metabolites: I. Procainamide; II. N-acetylprocainamide; III. Metabolite not fully identified.

over 16 µg/ml (Koch-Weser and Klein, 1971; Collste and Karlsson, 1973; Karlsson et al., 1975; Shaw et al., 1974).

No data are available on procainamide disposition in infants and children.

BETA-ADRENERGIC RECEPTOR BLOCKING DRUGS

There is now a considerable number of therapeutic indications for the use of β-receptor blocking drugs both in adults and in children. These include angina pectoris, arrhythmias, hypertension, long Q-T syndrome, myocardial infarction, hypertrophic cardiomyopathy, palliation of tetralogy of Fallot, hyperthyroidism, migraine, and essential and drug-induced tremors. While a considerable body of information is available on their disposition in adults, the data on children and infants are practically nonexistent despite the increasing use of these compounds in pediatrics. In the following pages, a detailed description of the pharmacokinetics of propranolol will be given together with the few available data in children, while the other β-blockers will be treated very briefly together.

Propranolol

Adults. Among β-blockers, propranolol may well be considered the representative drug, both because it was the first compound of this group to gain wide acceptance and because it is the β-blocker whose pharmacokinetics have been more deeply studied not only in volunteers but also in patients suffering from various pathological syndromes.

It is evident, from the studies so far available, that the kinetic information derived from single-dose studies (either in volunteers or in patients) may very often bear little or no relationship with the propranolol disposition pattern in patients treated chronically with the drug (Morselli et al., 1974; Lowenthal et al., 1974; Chidsey et al., 1975; Nies and Shand, 1975; Bianchetti et al., 1976) (Table 1).

Administered orally, propranolol undergoes a nearly complete absorption from the gut (Paterson et al., 1970), but its bioavailability is significantly low because of the extensive "hepatic extraction" which takes place during its transfer from the gut to the systemic circulation (Shand and Rangno, 1972). In volunteers and in patients with normal liver and kidney function, the fraction actually available to the systemic circulation after a single oral dose may range from 10 to 25% of the administered amount (Shand and Rangno, 1972; Shand, 1974; Lowenthal et al., 1974; Gomeni et al., 1976; Bianchetti et al., 1976).

It has been reported several times that after a single oral dose of 30 mg the hepatic extraction is virtually complete and that for doses above 40 mg the avid extraction process becomes saturated, conditioning a disproportionate increase in plasma concentrations for higher dosages (Shand and Rangno, 1972; Evans and Shand, 1973; Shand, 1974; Nies and Shand, 1974; Sasyniuk and Ogilvie, 1975).

Recent observations of Gomeni et al. (1977) tend, however, to suggest that there is no evidence of a hepatic threshold nor of complete extraction even for oral doses as low as 10 mg. Taking advantage of a very specific and sensitive analytical method, these authors could in fact show that in healthy volunteers there is a simple and significant linear relationship between various administered doses and the area-under-the-plasma-concentration curves over a 24 h period. In this study, for doses ranging from 10 to 40 mg the fraction actually available to the systemic circulation was constant within each subject, with values ranging from 12 to 29%. Furthermore, as shown by Chidsey et al. (1975), in the course of chronic treatment, in patients suffering from mild hypertension, the fraction of propranolol actually available may range from 20 to 80% of the dose, independently from the administered amount. A bioavailability of 13 to 43% after a single oral dose of 80 mg has been described by Lowenthal et al. (1974) in chronic renal insufficiency, and, similarly, an increased bioavailability up to 68% has been observed by Bianchetti et al. (1976) in uremic patients not

Table 1. Propranolol
Pharmacokinetic Parameters in Various Physiopathological Conditions

Physiopathological Conditions	Dose (mg/kg)	Plasma Peak (ng/ml)	Apparent Kas (h^{-1})	Apparent Plasma T½ (h)	Apparent Vd (L/kg)	F (%)	Plasma Clearance (L/min)
Healthy volunteers	0.62 ±0.02	37 ±2	0.80 ±0.10	3.2 ±0.5	3.4 ±0.4	20 ±1	0.79 ±0.01
Hypertensive patients (single dose)	0.75	60 ±12	0.92 ±0.10	2.3 ±0.2	2.7 ±0.3	35 ±0.5	0.76 ±0.11
Hypertensive patients (chronic therapy)	0.73	80 ±20	0.55 ±0.12	5.6 ±0.2	4.1 ±0.8	46 ±10	0.60 ±0.07
Uremic patients not yet on R.D.T. (single dose)	0.75 ±0.02	176 ±50	1.07 ±0.05	3.9 ±0.8	2.4 ±0.3	51 ±6	0.44 ±0.08
R.D.T. patients (single dose)	0.67 ±0.05	47 ±9	1.27 ±0.08	2.8 ±0.2	3.1 ±0.3	25 ±3	0.77 ±0.04
R.D.T. patients (chronic therapy)	0.70 ±0.10	52 ±10	1.10 ±0.10	4.1 ±0.4	4.2 ±0.5	35 ±2	0.65 ±0.04
Cirrhotic patients (single dose)	0.65 ±0.04	51 ±4	0.50 ±0.20	15.3 ±1.1	7.8 ±0.8	64 ±6	0.35 ±0.6

Values refer to authors' published and unpublished observations.

yet on regular dialytic treatment (R.D.T.) after a single 40 mg dose. In agreement with previous data of Shand and Rangno (1972), an increased bioavailability (50–75%) has also recently been observed in cirrhotic patients with evidences of portocaval shunts and ascites (Sega et al., 1977).

Independently from the physiopathological status, peak levels are usually attained both in volunteers and in patients 60–120 min after the oral dose (Paterson et al., 1970; Shand et al., 1970; Shand and Rangno, 1972; George et al., 1972; Lowenthal et al., 1974; Bianchetti et al., 1975; Chidsey et al., 1975). Although there is a trend toward higher concentrations with higher dosages, absorption peak levels do not appear to be strictly dose-related and a 4- to 10-fold variation may be observed for each considered dosage (Fig. 8). Within the single patients, there is, however, a linear increase in plasma concentrations as the dose is increased (Chidsey et al., 1975). This fact suggests first that the effective absorption may be considered as the major determinant of the wide individual variability in propranolol plasma concentrations observed in patients in the course of chronic treatment, and second that no saturation of the hepatic extraction does occur, at least for doses up to 320 mg/day.

In volunteers, propranolol is bound to plasma proteins for about 90–96% (Evans and Shand, 1973), and no alteration of binding could be observed either in uremic terminal patients or in patients undergoing R.D.T. (Lowenthal et al., 1974; Bianchetti et al., 1975, 1976). An apparent volume of distribution of about 2–4 L/kg has been described for volunteers, hypertensive and chronic renal failure patients (Shand et al., 1970; Shand and Rangno, 1972; Evans and Shand, 1973; Morselli et al., 1974; Chidsey et al., 1975; Bianchetti et al., 1976). A remarkable increase of this parameter up to 6–8 L/kg was found in patients with portocaval shunts and ascites (Shand and Rangno, 1972; Sega et al., 1977).

Propranolol plasma concentrations decay biexponentially and, after a single administration (either by intravenous infusion or oral route), the apparent half-life of the terminal exponential phase may range from 2 to 3.5 h both in volunteers and in renal and hypertensive patients without liver function impairment (Paterson et al., 1970; Shand et al., 1970; George et al., 1972; Shand and Rangno, 1973; Lowenthal et al., 1974; Chidsey et al., 1975; Bianchetti et al., 1976; Gomeni et al., 1976). A very prolonged half-life (17–35 h) may, on the contrary, be observed in hepatopatic patients with evidence of portocaval shunts and ascites (Shand and Rangno, 1972; Sega et al., 1977). A prolonged plasma half-life has been recently reported also for elderly subjects (Castedlen et al., 1975).

At variance with the single-dose data, in the course of chronic treatment in patients with normal kidney and liver function, the apparent plasma half-life of propranolol usually ranges from 5 to 6 h independently from the route of administration (Morselli et al., 1974; Chidsey et al., 1975). The more rapid disappearance rate from plasma observed on single-dosing probably reflects the removal into a large volume of distribution and not the actual clearance

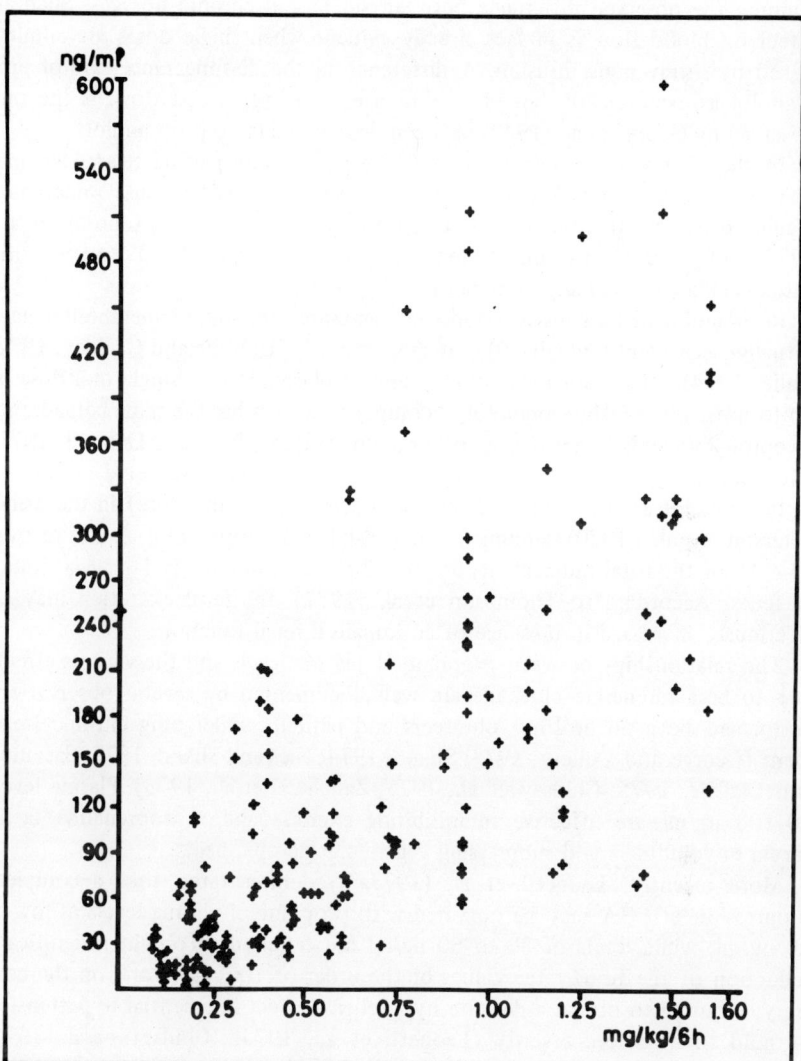

Fig. 8: Relationship between peak plasma levels of propranolol and the oral dose expressed as mg/kg/every 6 h. The wide individual variability is evident.

from the body by either excretion or metabolism (Chidsey et al., 1975). The propranolol effect on liver blood flow should not play a significant role in explaining the observed difference between single and chronic dosages. Such an effect on blood flow is in fact already evident when single doses are administered by intravenous infusion. A difference in the disappearance rate of propranolol isomers, clearly linked to this effect on liver blood flow, is the one observed by George et al. (1972) between dextro and laevo propranolol.

In the course of chronic treatment, the propranolol plasma clearances may vary from 0.5 to 0.9 L/min in hypertensive and renal patients undergoing regular dialytical treatment (R.D.T.) (Lowenthal et al., 1974; Chidsey et al., 1975) to 0.26–0.24 in terminal uremic patients not yet on R.D.T. and cirrhotic patients (Bianchetti et al., 1976; Sega et al., 1976).

Propranolol in humans is extensively metabolized, and 12 metabolites have actually been identified (Fig. 9) (Paterson et al., 1970; Walle and Gaffney, 1972; Walle, 1974). The main metabolite found in plasma after a single oral dose is, up to now, the 4-OH-propranolol, a compound which has the same betaadrenoreceptor antagonistic activity as propranolol (Fitzgerald and O'Donnell, 1971) but a shorter apparent half-life (Paterson et al., 1970; Thompson et al., 1972).

Propranolol as such is found only in traces (1% of the dose) in the urine. Paterson et al. (1970) administering C^{14}-labeled propranolol could recover 84–92% of the total radioactivity in the 48 h urine, while only 1–4% was found in feces. According to Thompson et al. (1972), the fecal excretion may be vicariously increased in presence of an impaired renal function.

The relationships between propranolol plasma levels and the various effects due to beta-adrenergic blockade are well documented by several observations performed both on healthy volunteers and patients undergoing chronic treatment (George and Dollery, 1973; Shand, 1974; Nies and Shand, 1975; Sasyniuk and Olgilvie, 1975; Chidsey et al., 1975; Zanchetti et al., 1975). Plasma levels 50–100 ng/ml are effective in inhibiting exercise and/or isoprenaline tachicardia in volunteers and suppressing ventricular ectopic beats.

More recently, Leonetti et al. (1975a,b) demonstrated that a complete suppression of PRA may be obtained with propranolol plasma levels as low as 20 ng/ml, while levels of 30 to 60 ng/ml are required to obtain a significant reduction of the heart rate. Values of the order of 100 ng/ml are, on the contrary, required to obtain a definite hypotensive effect in essential hypertension of mild to moderate severity (Leonetti et al., 1975b; Chidsey et al., 1975; Zanchetti et al., 1975). It must be noted that these observations suggest that the antihypertensive activity of propranolol does not appear to be mediated by means of reduction of cardiac output, or of renin secretion. Other mechanisms are probably involved in its antihypertensive effects.

At variance with previous reports, a sixfold variation both in the dose and plasma concentration of propranolol was recently observed in patients with angina when maximum benefit was obtained (Pine et al., 1975).

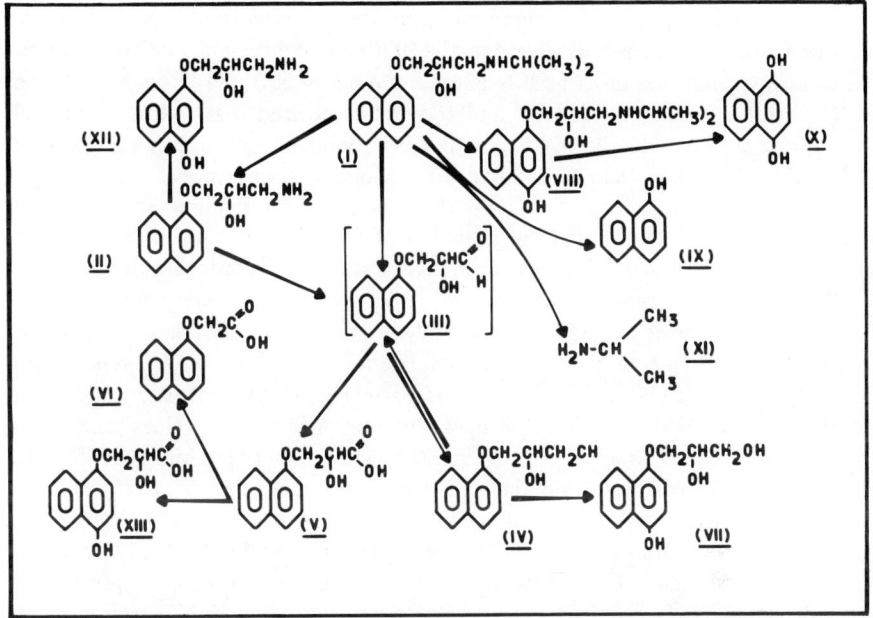

Fig. 9: Structural formula of propranolol and its metabolic pathway:
I. Propranolol; II. N-desisopropyl propranolol; III. Proposed aldehyde; IV. Propranolol glycol; V. Naphthoxyl acetic acid; VI. Naphthoxy hydroxy acetic acid; VII. 4-hydroxypropranolol glycol; VIII. 4-hydroxypropranolol; IX. alpha-naphthol; X. 1,4-dihydroxynaphthalene; XI. Isopropylamine; XII. 4-hydroxy-N-desisopropylpropranolol; XIII. 4-hydroxynaphthoxyl acetic acid.

Toxic effects of β-adrenergic blocking agents are mainly related to the blockade of adrenergic receptor per se. Serious cardiac depression, heart failure, cardiac conduction disturbances and broncoconstriction are infrequent but severe adverse effects, while more frequently occurring and less threatening undesirable effects are nausea, vomiting, diarrhea, insomnia and weakness. Toxic effects are said not to be related to plasma levels, but no controlled studies have been as yet performed with the specific objective of evaluating the possible toxic threshold.

Infants and children. In pediatrics, propranolol has been proven useful in palliation of tetralogy of Fallot, where it may relieve or prevent hypoxic spells, in hypertrophic cardiomyopathy, and in "long Q-T syndrome." It has also recently been recommended in prophylaxis of migraine in schoolchildren (Ludvigsson, 1974), while some doubts on its wide use in cardiac arrhythmias in pediatric patients have been put forward by Gelband and Rosen (1975). The available information on propranolol disposition in infants and children is limited to the two reports of Shand et al. (1970) and Ponce et al. (1973). In observations carried out on 2 infants (2 and 8 months old) and 2 young children (1.5 and 3 years old), Shand and co-workers noticed that following an oral dose of 0.57 mg/kg the mean plasma levels obtained over a 3 h period were considerably lower than those obtained in adults with an identical dose. According to the authors, these data support the need for the requirement of at least 1 mg/kg for effective long-term palliation of Fallot's tetralogy. In analogy with what is known for other drugs, an increased clearance is probably the reason of the lower levels observed in the two infants and two young children. More recently, Ponce et al. (1973), in a study conducted on 13 infants (< 2 years) and 9 children (2-11 years old), administering a dose of 1 mg/kg, reported in 11 infants peak plasma levels of 20-115 ng/ml (with 6 patients below 60 ng/ml) and peak levels of 25-80 ng/ml in 4 children. Again, these values tend to be lower than those obtained in adult patients with a similar pro kilo dose (Fig. 8). Extrapolation performed on the data reported by Ponce et al. (1973) suggests apparent plasma half-lives of about 1.5-4.0 h. In the same study, two infants with Down's syndrome had propranolol peak plasma levels of 211 and 467 ng/ml. Such high values, according to Ponce and co-workers, are suggestive of a defect in propranolol degradation associated with trisomy 21. However, another infant with Down's syndrome had low normal values. Complications and adverse toxic effects in children and infants are of the same magnitude and incidence as those observed in adults.

Other Beta-Blockers

Other compounds of the β-blockers group for which it is possible to describe the kinetic profile in humans are alprenolol, oxprenolol, tolamolol and pindolol (Reiss et al., 1970; Johansson et al., 1971a,b; Åblad et al., 1974; Gugler et al., 1974; von Bahr et al., 1974; Shand et al., 1974; Anavekar et al., 1975; Faulkner et al., 1975; Morselli and Bianchetti, 1975). They all are well absorbed by the gastrointestinal tract, and absorption peak levels are generally attained 60-180 min after an oral dose. The fraction actually available to the circulation after the "first pass extraction" may, however, vary considerably, and as reported in Table 2 it may range from 1-15% of the dose for alprenolol, and up to 80-90% of the dose for pindolol.

Remarkable differences are also present in regard to the plasma protein-binding, while the apparent volume of distribution is considerably large for all four compounds (Table 2).

Plasma levels decay biexponentially, and the terminal phases have an apparent plasma half-life which may range from 1.5 to 4 h. At variance with propranolol,

Table 2. Pharmacokinetic Profiles of Alprenolol, Oxprenolol, Tolamolol and Pindolol in Adults

	Alprenolol	Oxprenolol	Tolamolol	Pindolol
Absorption peak (min)	120-180	60-120	60-120	120-240
Protein-binding (% bound)	~30	90-95	90-92	50-60
Apparent Vd (L/kg)	3-6	2-3	2-5	~2
Fraction available (% of dose)	10-15	40-60	12-50	80-90
Apparent T½ (h)	2-3	2-3	2-5	2-4
Metabolism	Extensive (80%)	Extensive (80%)	Extensive (80%)	50%-60%
Total clearance (L/min)	~1	0.8-0.9	0.8-1.4	0.4-0.6
Effective plasma levels (ng/ml)	50-100	50-100	40-100	10-40

there are no data, up to now, suggesting a prolonged apparent half-life in the course of chronic treatment.

Metabolic degradation is extensive for alprenolol, oxprenolol and tolamolol, while it is considerably less for pindolol. Principal metabolites are the hydroxy derivatives which are further conjugated to inactive compounds. Pindolol may be found as such in the urine for about 40% of the administered dose, while the others are present as such only in traces. According to Ohnhaus (1973), a vicarious mechanism for the excretion of pindolol may take place in patients with renal insufficiency, since no differences in the apparent plasma disappearance rate could be observed between renal patients and control subjects. A prolonged apparent plasma half-life of oxprenolol (5-6 h) has recently been noted by Bianchetti and Sega (unpublished data) in patients suffering from chronic liver diseases.

On the basis of the available data, therapeutic plasma levels may range from 50 to 100 ng/ml for alprenolol, oxprenolol and tolamolol, while they may be lower for pindolol (10-50 ng/ml) (Johansson et al., 1971b; Gugler et al., 1974;

Shand, 1974; Anavekar et al., 1975; Morselli and Bianchetti, 1975).
It is evident that from a pharmacokinetic point of view the β-blockers cannot be considered a homogeneous group. Consequently, the various compounds cannot be considered as equivalent, and in programming therapeutic schedules the important pharmacokinetic differences (Table 2) must be taken into careful account.

It must further be remembered that most of the reported data have been obtained in volunteers. Whether the kinetic parameters are altered in the course of prolonged administration to patients is unknown. No data are available on the disposition of these drugs in pediatric patients.

CONCLUSIONS

It is clear that, with the exception of digoxin, our knowledge on the kinetic profile of cardiovascular drugs during development is practically inexistent. Their physicochemical properties suggest that important variations in the disposition rate in various age groups may be present. Their correct use may be critical in relation to the type of patient to whom they are administered and the very narrow therapeutic/toxic ratio. For these reasons, there is a great need for observations and studies which, through correct integrated monitoring of drug levels and effects, may help to achieve nor only more information but also safer use.

REFERENCES

Åblad, B., Borg, K.O., Johnson, G., Regårdh, C.-G and Sölvell, L. (1974): Combined pharmacokinetic and pharmacodynamic studies on alprenolol and 4-hydroxy-alprenolol in man. *Life Sciences, 14:* 693-704.

Abshagen, U., Remnekamp, H., Küchler, R. and Rietbrock, N. (1974): Formation and disposition of bis and monoglycosides after administration of ^{3}H04" '-methyldigoxin in man. *European Journal of Clinical Pharmacology, 7:* 177-181.

Adjepon-Yamoah, K.K. and Prescott, L.F. (1973): Lignocaine metabolism in man. *British Journal of Pharmacology, 47:* 672P-673P.

Anevekar, S.N., Louis, W.J., Morgan, T.O., Doyle, A.E. and Johnston, C.I. (1975): The relationship of plasma levels of pindolol in hypertensive patients to effects on blood pressure, plasma renin and plasma noradrenaline levels. *Clinical and Experimental Pharmacology and Physiology, 2:* 203-212.

Arstila, M., Katila, M., Sundquist, H., Anttila, M., Pere, A. and Tikkanen, R. (1974): Dosage, plasma concentration and antiarrhythmic effect of Procainamide in substained-release tablets. *Acta Medica Scandinavica, 195:* 217-222.

Assael, B.M., Mandelli, M., Visconti, V., Marini, A., Sereni, F. and Morselli, P.L. (1973): Farmacocientica della digossina nel neonato e nel lattante. In: *Atti del Convegno di Studio sulla Digitale,* Bergamo, 24-25 Nov.

Aviado, D.M. and Salem, H. (1975): Drug action, reaction, and interaction. I. Quinidine for

cardiac arrhythmias, *Journal of Clinical Pharmacology, 15:* 477-485.
Bahr, C., Von Alván, G., Lind, M., Mellström, B. and Sjoqvist, F. (1974): "First pass" effect and dose dependent availability as factors contributing to interindividual differences in equilibrium concentrations of alprenolol in man. *Acta Pharmaceutica Suecica, 11:* 649-650.
Beckett, A.H., Boyes, R.N. and Appleton, P.J. (1966): The metobolism and excretion of lingnocaine in man. *Journal of Pharmacy and Pharmacology, 18,* suppl.: 76S-81S.
Beller, G.A, Smith, T.W., Abelmann, W.H., Haber, E. and Hood, W.B., Jr. (1971): Digitalis intoxication. A prospective clinical study with serum level correlations. *New England Journal of Medicine, 284:* 989-997.
Bellet, S., Roman, L.R. and Boza, A. (1971): Relation between serum quinidine levels and renal function. *American Journal of Cardiology, 27:* 368-371.
Bertler, A., Gustafson, A. and Redfors, A. (1973): Massive digoxin intoxication. *Acta Medica Scandinavica, 194:* 245-249.
Bertler, A., Bergdahl, B. and Karlsson, E. (1974): Plasma-digoxin concentrations after an intravenous loading dose. *Lancet, 2:* 958,
Bertler, Å., Monti, M., Ohlin, P. and Redfors, A. (1975): Cardiac arrhythmias—electrolytes and digoxin concentration in plasma and urine in patients treated with digoxin. *Acta Medica Scandinavica, 197:* 391-401.
Bianchetti, G., Brancaccio, D., Leonetti, G., Graziani, G., Morganti, A. Ponticelli, C., Banfi, G., Terzoli, D. and Morselli, P.L. (1975): Pharmacokinetics of Propranolol in patients on regular dialytic treatment. (R.D.T.) In: *6th International Congress of Nephrology,* Firenze, 8-12 June, abstr. 450.
Bianchetti, G., Brancaccio, D., Graziani, D., Morganti, A., Leonetti, G., Manfrin, M., Ponticelli, C., Sega, R. and Morselli, P.L. (1976): Pharmacokinetics and effects of propranolol in terminal uraemic patients and in patients undergoing regular dialysis treatment. *Clinical Pharmacokinetics 1:* 373-386.
Binnion, P.F. (1974): The absorption of digoxin tablets. *Clinical Pharmacology and Therapeutics, 16:* 807-812.
Bissett, J.K., Doherty, S.E., Flanigan, W.J. and Dalrymple, G.V. (1973): Tritiated digoxin. XIX. Turnover studies in diabetes insipidus. *American Journal of Cardiology, 31:* 327-330.
Boyes, R.N., Scott, D.B., Jebson, P.J., Godman, M.J. and Julian, D.G. (1971): Pharmacokinetics of lidocaine in man. *Clinical Pharmacology and Therapeutics, 12:* 105-116.
Brown, D.D. and Abraham, G.N. (1973): Plasma digoxin levels in normal human volunteers following chronic oral and intramuscular administration. *Journal of Laboratory and Clinical Medicine, 82:* 201-207.
Butler, V.P., Jr. (1970): Digoxin: immunologic approaches to measurement and reversal of toxicity, *New England Journal of Medicine, 283:* 1150-1156.
Butler, V.P., Jr. and Lindenbaum, J. (1975): Serum digitalis measurement in the assessment of digitalis resistance and sensitivity. *American Journal of Medicine, 58:* 460-469.
Caldwell, J.H. and Greenberg, N.G. (1971): Interruption of enterophepatic circulation of digitoxin by cholestyramine. I. *Journal of Clinical Investigation, 50:* 2626-2637.
Carroll, F.I., Smith, D. and Wall, M.E. (1974): Carbon-13 magnetic resonance study. Structure of the metabolites of orally administered quinidine in humans. *Journal of Medicinal Chemistry, 17:* 985-987.
Castedlen, C.M., Kaye, C.M. and Parsons, R.L. (1975): The effect of age on plasma levels of propranolol and practolol in man. *British Journal of Clinical Pharmacology, 2:* 303-306.
Chidsey, C.A., Bianchetti, G., Morganti, A., Leonetti, G., Zanchetti, A. and Morselli, P.L. (1976): Pharmacokinetic and pharmacodynamic studies of propranolol in hypertension. Presented at the *International Symposium on Recent Advances in Clinical Pharmacology*

of Hypertension, Montecarlo, 25-26 April 1975.
Chidsey, C.A., Morselli, P.L., Bianchetti, G., Morganti, A., Leonetti, G. and Zanchetti, A. (1975): Studies of the absorption and removal of propranolol in hypertensive patients during therapy. *Circulation, 52:* 313-317.
Chien, Y.W., Lambert, H.J. and Karim, A. (1974): Comparative binding if disopyramide phosphate and quinidine sulfate to human plasma proteins. *Journal of Pharmaceutical Sciences, 63:* 1877-1879.
Chow, M.S.S. and Ronfeld, R.A., (1975): Pharmacokinetic data and drug monitoring. 1. Antibiotics and antiarrhythmics. *Journal of Clinical Pharmacology, 15:* 405-418.
Christiansen, N.J.B., Kølendorf, K., Siersbaek-Nielsen, K. and Mølholm Hansen, J. (1973): Serum digoxin values following a dosage regimen based on body weight, sex, age and renal function. *Acta Medica Scandinavica, 194:* 257-259.
Clark, D.R. and Kalman, S.M. (1974a): A reduction product of digoxin in man: dihydrodigoxin. *Clinical Pharmacology and Therapeutics, 15:* 202-203.
Clark, D.R. and Kalman, S.M. (1974b): Dihydrodigozin: a common metabolite of digoxin in man. *Drug Metabolism and Disposition, 2:* 148-150.
Cohen, L.S., Rosenthal, J.E., Horner, D.W., Atkins, J.M., Matthews, O.A. and Sarnoff, S.J. (1972); Plasma levels of lidocaine after intramuscular administration. *American Journal of Cardiology, 29:* 520-523.
Collste, P. and Karlsson, E. (1973): Arrhythmia prophylaxis with procaine amide: plasma concentrations in relation to dose. *Acta Medica Scandinavica, 194:* 405-411.
Coltart, D.J. Güllner, H.G., Billingham, M., Goldman, R.H., Stinson, E.B., Kalman, S.M. and Harrison, D.C. (1974): Physiological distribution of digoxin in human heart. *British Medical Journal, 4:* 733-736.
Cramer, G., Varnauskas, E. and Werkö, L. (1963): A new quinidine preparation with sustained release. *Acta Medica Scandinavica, 173:* 511-519.
Cree, J.E., Coltart, D.J. and Howard, M R. (1973): Plasma digoxin concentration in children with heart failure. *British Medical Journal, 1:* 443-444.
Crouthamel, W.G. (1973): Elimination of quinidine in congestive heart failure. *New England Journal of Medicine, 290:* 1379-1380.
Culhed, I., Hamfelt, A. and Malers, E. (1966): Serum quinidine concentration with two long-acting quinidine preparations. *Acta Medica Scandinavica, 179:* 401-405.
Dengler, H.J., Bodem, G. and Wirth, K. (1973): Pharmacokinetic and metabolic studies with lanatoside C,α-and β-acetyldigoxin and digoxin in man. In: *Pharmacology and the Future of man,* edited by G.T. Okita and G.H. Acheson, V.3, pp. 112-126, Karger, Basel.
Dettli, L., Ohnhaus, E.E. and Spring, P. (1972): Digoxin dosage in patients with impaired kidney function. *British Journal of Pharmacology, 44:* 373P-374P.
Doherty, J.E. (1973): Digitalis glycosides. Pharmacokinetics and their clinical implications. *Annals of Internal Medicine, 79:* 229-238.
Doherty, J.E., Ferrell, C.B. and Towbin, E.J. (1969): Localization of the renal excretion of the tritiated digoxin. *American Journal of Medical Sciences, 258:* 181-189.
Doherty, J.E., Flanigan, W.J., Perkins, W.H. and Ackerman, G.L. (1967a): Studies with tritiated digoxin in anephric human subjects. *Circulation 35:* 298-303.
Doherty, J.E., Perkins, W.H. and Flanigan, W.J. (1967b): The distribution and concentration of tritiated digoxin in human tissues. *Annals of Internal Medicine, 77:* 116-124.
Doherty, J.E., Flanigan, W.J., Murphy, M.L., Bulloch, R.T., Dalrymple, G.L., Beard, O W. and Perkins, W.H. (1970): Tritiated digoxin. XIV. Enterophepatic circulation, absorption and excretion studies in human volunteers. *Circulation, 42:* 867-873.
Doherty, J.E. and Kane, J.J. (1973): Clinical pharmacology and therapeutic use of digitalis

Glucosides. *Drugs, 6:* 167-221
Doherty, J.E. and Perkins, W.H. (1962): Studies with tritiated digoxin in human subjects after intravenous administration. *American Heart Journal, 63:* 528-536.
Doherty, J.E. and Perkins, W.H. (1965): Studies following intramuscular tritiated digoxin in human subjects. *American Journal of Cardiology, 15:* 170-174.
Drayer, D.E., Reidenberg, M.M. and Sevy, R.W. (1974): N-Acetylprocainamide: an active metabolite of procainamide. *Proceedings of the Society for Experimental Biology and Medicine, 146:* 358-363.
Dreyfuss, J., Bigger, J.T., Jr., Cohen, A.I. and Schreiber, E.C. (1972): Metabolism of procainamide in rhesus monkey and man. *Clinical Pharmacology and Therapeutics, 13:* 366-371.
Dungan, W.T., Doherty, J.E., Harvey, C., Char, F. and Dalrymple, G.V. (1972): Tritiated digoxin. XVIII. Studies in infants and children. *Circulation, 46:* 983-988.
Eisinger, A.J. and Hellier, M.D. (1969): Oral linocaine, *Lancet, 2:* 1303.
Evans, G.H. and Shand, D.G. (1973): Disposition of propranolol. VI. Independent variation in steady-state circulating drug concentrations and half-life as a result of plasma drug binding in man. *Clinical Pharmacology and Therapeutics, 14:* 494-500.
Falch, D. (1973): The influence of kidney function, body size and age on plasma concentration and urinary excretion of digoxin. *Acta Medica Scandinavica, 194:* 251-256.
Faulkner, J.K., Stopher, D.A., Walden, R., Singleton, W. and Taylor, S.H. (1975): Pharmacokinetic and pharmacological studies with Tolamolol in man. *British Journal of Clinical Pharmacology, 2:* 423-428.
Faulkner, S.L., Hopkins, J.T., Boerth, R.C., Young, J.L., Jr., Jellett, L.B., Nies, A.S., Bender, H.W. and Shand, D.G. (1973): Time required for complete recovery from chronic propranolol therapy. *New England Journal of Medicine, 289:* 607-609.
Finkelstein, F.O., Goffinet, J.A., Hendler, E.D. and Lindenbaum, J. (1975): Pharmacokinetics of digoxin and digitoxin in patients undergoing hemodialysis. *American Journal of Medicine, 58:* 525-531.
Fitzgerald, J.D. and O'Donnell, S.R. (1971): Pharmacology of 4-hydroxypropranolol, a metabolite of propranolol. *British Journal of pharmacology, 43:* 222-235.
Fleckenstein, L., Weintraub, M., Kroening, B. and Lasagna, L. (1974a): Assessment of the biologic availability of digoxin preparation in man. *Clinical Pharmacology and Therapeutics, 15:* 205.
Fleckenstein, L., Kroening, B. and Weintraub, M. (1974b): Assessment of the biologic availability of digoxin in man. *Clinical Pharmacology and Therapeutics, 16:* 435-443.
Fogelman, A.M., La Mont, J.T., Finkelstein, S., Rado, E. and Pearce, M.L. (1971): Fallibility of plasma digoxin in differentiating toxic from non-toxic patients. *Lancet, 2:* 727-729.
Fraser, E.J., Leach, R.H., Poston, J.W., Bold, A.M., Culank, L.S. and Lipede, A.B. (1973): Dissolution and bioavailability of digoxin tablets. *Journal of Pharmacy and Pharmacology, 25:* 968-973.
Fremstad, D., Dahl, S., Jacobsen, S., Lunde, P.K.M., Nödland, S. Aasness Marthinsen, A., Waaler, T. and Landmark, K.H. (1973): A new sustained-release tablet formulation of procainamide. *European Journal of Clinical Pharmacology, 6:* 251-255.
Gelband, H. and Rosen, M.R. (1975): Pharmacologic basis for the treatment of cardiac arrhythmias. *Pediatrics, 55:* 59-67.
George, C.F. and Dollery, C.T. (1973): Plasma concentrations and pharmacological effect of β-receptor blocking drugs. In: *Pharmacology and the Future of Man*, edited by Okita and G.H. Acheson, V. 3, pp. 86-97, Karger, Basel.
George, C.F., Fenyvesi, T., Conolly, M.E. and Dollery, C.T. (1972): Pharmacokinetics of

dextro-, laevo- and racemic propranolol in man. *European Journal of Clinical Pharmacology, 4:* 74-76.

Giardina, E.-G.V., Dreyfuss, J., Bigger, J.T., Jr. and Schreiber, E.C. (1974): N-Acetyl procaine amide after procaine amide-^{14}C treatment in man. *Ciculation, 49-50,* suppl. III: 227.

Gibson, T., Lowenthal, D., Nelson, H., Briggs, W. and Reed, W. (1975): Metabolism of procainamide in patients with reduced renal function. *Clinical Pharmacology and Therapeutics, 17:* 206.

Gomeini, R., Bianchetti, G., Sega, R. and Morselli, P.L. (1977: Pharmacokinetics of propranolol in normal health volunteers. *Journal of Biopharmaceutics and Pharmacokinetics.* In press.

Gorodischer, R.J., Jusko, W.J. and Yaffe, S.J. (1976a): Renal clearance of digoxin in young infants. In press.

Gorodischer, R., Jusko, W.J. and Yaffe, S.J. (1976b): Miocardium skeletal muscle and erythrocyte distribution of digoxin in infants. In press.

Gorodischer, R., Krasner, J. and Yaffe, S.J. (1974): Serum protein binding of digoxin in newborn infants. *Research Communications in Chemical Pathology and Pharmacology, 9:* 387-390.

Greenblatt, D.J., Duhme, D.W., Koch-Weser, J. and Smith, T.W. (1973): Evaluation of digoxin bioavailability in single-dose studies. *New England Journal of Medicine, 289:* 651-654.

Greenblatt, D.J., Duhme, D.W., Koch-Weser, J. and Smith, T.W (1974a): Bioavailability of digoxin tablets and elixir in the fasting and post prandial states. *Clinical Pharmacology and Therapeutics, 16:* 444-448.

Greenblatt, D.J., Duhme, D.W., Koch-Weser, J. and Smith, T.W. (1974b): Intra-venous digoxin as a bioavailability standard: slow infusion and rapid injection. *Clinical Pharmacology and Therapeutics, 15:* 510-513.

Greenblatt, D.J., Duhme, D.W., Koch-Weser, J. and Smith, T.W. (1974c): Comparison of one- and six-day urinary digoxin excretion in single-dose bioavailability studies. *Clinical Pharmacology and Therapeutics, 16:* 813-816.

Gugler, R., Herold, W. and Dengler, H.J. (1974): Pharmacokinetics of pindolol in man. *European Journal of Clinical Pharmacology, 7:* 17-24.

Güllner, M.-G., Stinson, E.B., Harrison, D.C. and Kalman, S.M. (1947): Correlation of serum concentrations with heart concentrations of digoxin in human subjects. *Circulation, 50:* 653-655.

Halkin, H., Meffin, P., Melmon, K.L. and Rowland, M. (1975a): Influence of congestive heart failure on blood levels of lidocaine and its active monodeethylated metabolite. *Clinical Pharmacology and Therapeutics, 17:* 669-676.

Halkin, H., Sheiner, L.B., Peck, C.C. and Melmon, K.L. (1975b): Determinants of the renal clearance of digoxin. *Clinical Pharmacology and Therapeutics, 17:* 385-394.

Hartel, G. and Korhonen, A. (1968): Thin-layer chromatography for the quantitative separation of quinidine and quinidine metabolites from biological fluids and tissues. *Journal of Chromatography, 37:* 70-75.

Hayes, C.J., Butler, V.P., Jr. and Gersony, W.M. (1973): Serum digoxin studies in infants and children. *Pediatrics, 52:* 561-568.

Hayes, C.J., Gersony, W.M., Smith, W.B. and Butler, V.P., Jr. (1971): Serum digoxin studies in infants and children. *Bulletin of the New York Academy of Medicine, 47:* 1226-1227.

Hernandez, A., Burton, R.M., Pagtakhan, R.D. and Goldring, D. (1969): Pharmacodynamics of ^{3}H-digoxin in infants. *Pediatrics, 44:* 418-428.

Hernandez, A., Jr., Kouchoukos, N., Burton, R.M. and Goldring, D. (1963): The effect of

extracorporeal circulation upon the tissue concentration of digoxin-H^3. *Pediatrics, 31:* 952-957.
Henning, R. and Nyberg, G. (1973): Serum quinidine levels after administration of three different quinidine preparations. *European Journal of Clinical Pharmacology, 6:* 239-244.
Hobson, J.D. and Zettner, A. (1973): Digoxin serum half-life following suicidal digoxin posioning. *Journal of the American Medical Association, 223:* 147-149.
Huffman, D.H. (1975): Relationship between digoxin concentrations in serum and saliva. *Clinical Pharmacology and Therapeutics, 17:* 310-312.
Huffman, D.H. and Azarnoff, D.L. (1972): Absorption of orally given digoxin preparations. *Journal of the American Medical Association, 222:* 957-960.
Huffman, D.H., Manion, C.V. and Azarnoff, D.L. (1975): Intersubject variation in absorption of digoxin in normal volunteers. *Journal of Pharmaceutical Sciences, 64:* 433-437.
Hutcheon, D.E. (1975): Cardiovascular drug interactions. *Journal of Clinical Pharmacology, 15:* 129-134.
Iisalo, E., Dahl, M. and Sundqvist, H. (1973): Serum digoxin in adults and children. *International Journal of Clinical pharmacology, 7:* 219-222.
Jelliffe, R.W., Buell, J., Kalaba, R., Sridhar, R. and Rockwell, R. (1970): A computer program for digitalis dosage regimens. *Mathematical Biosciences, 9:* 179-193.
Johanson, R., Regårdh, C.G. and Sjögren, J. (1971): Absorption of alprenolol in man from tablets with different rates of release. *Acta Pharmaceutica Suecica, 9:* 59-70.
Johnsson, G., Sjögren, J. and Sölvell, L. (1971): Beta-blocking effect and serum levels of alprenolol in man after administration of ordinary and substained release tablets. *European Journal of Clinical Pharmacology, 3:* 74-81.
Jounela, A.J., Pentikäinen, P.J. and Sothmann, A. (1975): Effect of particle size on the bioavailability of digoxin. *European Journal of Clinical Pharmacology, 8:* 365-370.
Jusko, W.J. (1974): Clinical pharmacokinetics of digoxin. In: *Clinical Pharmacokinetics,* edited by G. Levy, pp. 31-43, American Pharmaceutical Association, Washington.
Jusko, W.J., Szefler, S.J. and Goldfarb, A.L. (1974): Pharmacokinetic design of digoxin dosage regimens in relation to renal function. *Journal of Clinical Pharmacology, 14:* 525-535.
Jusko, W.J. and Weintraub, M. (1974): Myocardial distribution of digoxin and renal function. *Clinical Pharmacology and Therapeutics, 16:* 449-454.
Karjalainen, J., Ojala, K. and Reissell, P. (1974): Tissue concentrations of digoxin in an autopsy material. *Acta Phamacologica et Toxicoligica, 34:* 385-390.
Karlsson, E. (1973): Plasma levels of procaine amide after administration of conventional and substained release tablets. *European Journal of Clinical Pharmacology, 6:* 245-250.
Karlsson, E. Åberg, G., Collste, P., Molin, L., Norlander, B. and Sjöqvist, F. (1975): Acetylation of procaine amide in man. A preliminary communication. *European Journal of Clinical Pharmacology 8:* 79-81.
Keenaghan, J.B., and Boyes, R.N. (1972): The tissue distribution, metabolism and excretion of lidocaine in rats, guinea pigs, dogs and man. *Journal of Pharmacology and Experimental Therapeutics, 180:* 454-463.
Kessler, K.M., Lowenthal, D.T., Warner, H., Gibson, T., Briggs, W. and Reidenberg, M.M. (1974): Quinidine elimination in patients with congestive heart failure or poor renal function. *New England Journal of Medicine, 290:* 706-709.
Kim, P.W., Yanagi, R., Krasula, R.W., Soyka, L.F., Levitsky, S. and Hastreiter, A.R. (1974): Post-mortem digoxin concentrations in infants. In: *Proceedings, 47th Scientific Session, American Heart Association,* Nov. 18-21, Dallas, Texas.
Kirsten, E., Rodstein, M. and Iuster, Z. (1973): Digoxin in the aged. *Geriatrics, 28:* 95-101.

Koch-Weser, J. (1971): Pharmacokinetics of procainamide in man. *Annals of the New York Academy of Sciences, 179:* 370-382.
Koch-Weser, J. and Klein, S. W. (1971): Procainamide dosage schedules, plasma concentrations and clinical effects. *Journal of the American Medical Association, 215:* 1454-1460.
Kramer, P., Kethe, E., Saul, J. and Scheler, F. (1974): Uraemic and normal plasma protein binding of various cardiac glycosides under "in vivo" conditions. *European Journal of Clinical Investigation, 4:* 53-58.
Krasula, R.W., Pellegrino, P.A., Harstreiter, A.R. and Soyka, L.F. (1972): Serum levels of digoxin in infants and children. *Pediatrics, 81:* 566-569.
Krasula, R.W., Yanagi, R., Hastreiter, A.R., Levitsky, S. and Soyka, L.F. (1974): Digoxin intoxication in infants and children: correlation with serum levels. *Journal of Pediatrics, 84:* 265.
Larese, R.J. and Mirkin, B.L. (1974): Kinetics of digoxin absorption and relation of serum levels to cardiac arrhythmias in children. *Clinical Pharmacology and Therapeutics, 15:* 387-396.
Leonetti, G., Mayer, G., Morganti, A., Terzoli, L., Zanchetti, A., Morselli, P.L., Di Salle, E. and Chidsey, C.A. (1975a): Blood pressure decrease and responsiveness to renin-releasing stimuli under increasing doses of propranolol in patients with essential hypertension. *Clinical Sciences, Molecular Medicine, 48:* 77S-79S.
Leonetti, G., Mayer, G., Morganti, A., Terzoli, L., Zanchetti, A., Bianchetti, G., Di Salle, E., Morselli, P.L. and Chidsey, C.A. (1975b): Hypotensive and renin suppressing activities of propranolol in hypertensive patients. *Clinical Sciences, Molecular Medicine, 48:* 491-499.
Lindenbaum, J. (1973): Bioavailability of digoxin tablets. *Pharmacological Reviews, 25:* 229-237.
Lindenbaum, J. (1975): Bioavailability of different lots of digoxin tablets from the same manufacturer. *Clinical Pharmacology and Therapeutics, 17:* 296-301.
Lindseth Ditlefsen, E.M. and Löken, H.F. (1966): Quinidine concentrations in serum following two different types of delayed-absorption tablets. *Acta Medica Scandinavica, 179:* 333-336.
Lindseth Ditlefsen, E.M. and Bjerkelund, C. (1966): Quinidine concentration in serum. *Acta Medica Scandinavica, 180:* 537-542.
Lowenthal, D.T., Briggs, W.A., Gibson, T.P., Nelson, H. and Cirksena, W.J. (1974): Pharmacokinetics of oral propranolol in chronic renal disease. *Clinical Pharmacology and Therapeutics, 16:* 761-769.
Luchi, R.J. and Gruber, J.W. (1968): Unusually large digitalis requirements. A study of altered digoxin metabolism. *American Journal of Medicine, 45:* 322-328.
Ludvigsson, J. (1974): Propranolol used in prophylaxis of migraine in children. *Acta Neurologica Scandinavica, 50:* 109-115.
Lukas, D.S. (1971): Some aspects of the distribution and disposition of digitoxin in man. *Annals of the New York Academy of Sciences, 179:* 338-361.
Lukas, D.S. and De Martino, A.G. (1969): Binding of digitoxin and some related cardenolides to human plasma proteins. *Journal of Clinical Investigation, 48:* 1041-1053.
Manninen, V., Apajalahti, A., Melin, J. and Karesoja, M. (1973): Altered absorption of digoxin in patients given propantheline and metoclopramide. *Lancet, I:* 398-399.
Marcus, F.I. (1975): Digitalis pharmacokinetics and metabolism. *American Journal of Medicine, 58:* 452-459.
Marcus, F.I. and Kapadia, G.G. (1964): The metabolism of tritiated digoxin in cirrhotic patients. *Gastroenterology, 47:* 517-524.

Marcus F.I., Kapadia, G.J. and Kapadia, G.G. (1964): The metabolism of digoxin in normal subjects. *Journal of Pharmacology and Experimental Therapeutics, 145:* 203-209.
Marcus, F.I., Peterson, A., Salel, A., Scully, J. and Kapadia, G.G. (1966): The metabolism of tritiated digoxin in renal insufficiency in dogs and man. *Journal of Pharmacology and Experimental Therapeutics, 152:* 372-382.
Mason, D.T. and De Maria, A.N., Amsterdam, E.A., Zelis, R. and Massumi, R.A. (1973): Antiarrhythmic agents. I. Mechanisms of action and clinical pharmacology. *Drugs, 5:* 261-291.
Morselli, P.L. (1974): Drug disposition during development. *Acta Pharmaceutica Suecica. 11:* 647.
Morselli, P.L. (1975): Pediatric clinical pharmacology: routine monitoring or clinical trials? In: *Clinical Pharmacy and Clinical Pharmacology,* edited by Gouveia, Tognoni and Van der Klejin, pp. 279-289, Elsevier/North-Holland Biomedical Press.
Morselli, P.L., Assael, B.M., Gomeni, R., Mandelli, M., Marini, A., Reali, E., Visconti, U. and Sereni, F. (1975): Digoxin pharmacokinetics during human development. In: *Basic and Therapeutic Aspects of the Perinatal Pharmacology,* edited by P.L. Morselli, S. Garattini and F. Sereni, pp. 377-392, Raven Press, New York.
Morselli, P.L. and Bianchetti, G. (1975): Farmacocinetica dei β-bloccanti. In: *Temi di Terapia e Farmacologia Clinica,* Piccin, Padova, 15-25.
Morselli, P.L., Garattini, S. and Cohen, S.N. (eds.) (1974): *Drug Interactions,* Raven Press, New York.
Morselli, P.L., Morganti, A., Bianchetti, G., Di Salle, E., Leonetti, G., Chidsey, C.A. and Zanchetti, A. (1974): Plasma levels and pharmacokinetics studies of propranolol during chronic treatment in hypertensive patients. *European Journal of Clinical Investigation, 4:* 347.
Moss, A.J., Finkelstein, S., Crudup, C., Young, G.A., Dooley, R.R. and Osher, A.B. (1975): Absorption of digoxin in children with cystic fibrosis. *Journal of Pediatrics, 86:* 295-297.
Nies, A.S. and Shand, D.G. (1975): Clinical pharmacology of propranolol. *Circulation, 52:* 6-15.
Nyberg, L., Andersson, K.E. and Bertler, Å. (1974a): Bioavailability of digoxin from tablets. II. Radioimmunoassay and disposition pharmacokinetics of digoxin after intravenous administration. *Acta Pharmaceutica Suecica, 11:* 459-470.
Nyberg, L., Andersson, K.E. and Bertler, Å. (1974b): Bioavailability of digoxin from tablets. III. Availability of digoxin in man from preparations with different dissolutions rate. *Acta Pharmaceutica Suecica, 11:* 471-492.
Ohnhaus, E.E. (1973): The pharmacokinetics of unchanged pindolol in patients with impaired renal function. *British Journal of Pharmacology, 47:* 620P-621P.
Ohnhaus, E.E., Spring, P. and Dettli, L. (1972): Protein binding of digoxin in human serum. *European Journal of Clinical Pharmacology, 5:* 34-36.
Ohnhaus, E.E., Spring, P. and Dettli, L. (1974): Eliminationskinetik und Dosierung von Digoxin bei Patienten mit Niereninsuffizienz. *Deutsche Medizinische Wochenschrift, 99:* 1797-1803.
Okita, G.T., Plotz, E.J. and Davis, M.E. (1956): Placental transfer of radioactive digitoxin in pregnant women and its fetal distribution. *Cardiovascular Research, IV:* 376-380.
Okita, G.T., Talso, P.J., Curry, J.H., Jr., Smith, F.D., Jr. and Geiling, E.M.K. (1955): Metabolic fate of radioactive digitoxin in human subjects. *Journal of Pharmacology and Experimental Therapeutics, 115:* 371-379.
O'Malley, K., Coleman, E.N., Doig, W.B. and Stevenson, I.H. (1973): Plasma digoxin levels in infants. *Archives of Disease in Childhood, 48:* 55-57.

Palmer, K.H., Martin, B., Baggett, B. and Wall, M.E. (1969): The metabolic fate of orally administered quinidine gluconate in humans. *Biochemical Pharmacology, 18:* 1845-1860.
Paterson, J.W., Conolly, M.E., Dollery, C.T., Hayes, A. and Cooper, R.G. (1970): The pharmacodynamics and metabolism of propranolol in man. *Pharmacologia Clinica, 2:* 127-133.
Peck, C.C., Sheiner, L.B., Martin, C.M., Combs, D.T. and Melmon, K.L. (1973): Computer-assisted digoxin therapy. *New England Journal of Medicine, 289:* 441-446.
Perkins, W.H. and Doherty, J.E. (1967): Serum protein binding of tritiated digoxin. *Clinical Research, 15:* 58.
Peters, U., Hausamen, T.U., Grosse-Brockhoff, F. (1974): Therapie mit digitoxin unter kontrolle des serum-digitoxinspiegels. *Deutsche Medizinische Wochenschrift, 99:* 1701-1707.
Pine, M., Favrot, L., Smith, S., McDonald, K. and Chidsey, C.A. (1975): Correlation of plasma propranolol with therapeutic response in patients with angina pectoris. *Circulation,* in press.
Ponce, F.E., Williams, L.C., Webb, H.M., Riopel, D.A. and Hohn, A.R. (1973): Propranolol palliation of tetralogy of Fallot: experience with long-term drug treatment in pediatric patients. *Pediatrics, 52:* 100-116.
Rasmussen, K., Jervell, J., Storstein, L. and Gjerdrum, K. (1972): Digitoxin kinetics in patients with impaired renal function. *Clinical Pharmacology and Therapeutics, 13:* 6-14.
Reidenberg, M.M. and Affrime, M. (1974): Influence of disease on binding of drugs to plasma proteins. *Annals of the New York Academy of Sciences, 226:* 115-126.
Reidenberg, M.M., Drayer, D.E., Levy, M. and Warner, H. (1975): Polymorphic acetylation of procainamide in man. *Clinical Pharmacology and Therapeutics, 17:* 722-730.
Reuning, R.H., Sams, R.A. and Notari, R.E. (1973): Role of pharmacokinetics in drug dossage adjustment. I. Pharmacologic effect kinetics and apparent volume of distribution of digoxin. *Journal of Clinical Pharmacology, 13:* 127-141.
Riess, W., Rajagopalan, T.G., Imhof, P., Schmid, K. and Keberle, H. (1970): Metabolic studies on oxprenolol in animals and man by means of radio-tracer techniques and GLC-analysis. *Postgraduate Medical Journal,* suppl. Nov.: 32-43.
Ritzmann, L.V., Bangs, C.C., Coiner, D., Custis, J.M. and Walsh, J.R. (1973): Serum glycoside levels by rubidium assay. *Archives of Internal Medicine, 132:* 823-830.
Rogers, M.K., Willerson, J.T., Goldblatt, A. and Smith, T.W. (1972): Serum digoxin concentrations in the human fetus, neonate and infant. *New England Journal of Medicine, 267:* 1010-1013.
Ronfeld, R.A. and Chow, M.S.S. (1975): Volume of distribution of quinidine. *New England Journal of Medicine, 292:* 981.
Rowland, M. (1974): Clinical Pharmacokinetics of lidocaine: general approach to drug administration and individualized therapy. In: *Clinical Pharmacokinetics,* edited by G. Levy, pp. 53-66, American Pharmaceutical Association, Washington.
Rowland, M., Thomson, P.D., Guichard, A. and Melmon, K.L. (1971): Disposition kinetics of lidocaine in normal subjects. *Annals of the New York Academy of Sciences, 179:* 383-398.
Sanchez, N., Sheiner, L.B., Halkin, H. and Melmon, K.L. (1973): Pharmacokinetics of digoxin: interpreting bioavailability. *British Medical Journal, 4:* 132-134.
Sasyniuk, B.I. and Ogilvie, R.I. (1975): Antiarrhythmic drugs: electrophysiological and pharmacokinetic considerations. *Annual Review of Pharmacology, 15:* 131-155.
Scott, D.B., Jebson, P.J., Vellani, C.W. and Giulian, D.J. (1968): Plasma-levels of linocaine after intramuscular injection, *Lancet, II:* 1209-1210.

Sega, R., Bianchetti, G. and Morselli, P.L. (1977): Propranolol in cirrhosis. In preparation.
Shand, D.G. (1974): Pharmacokinetics properties of the β-adrenergic receptor blocking drugs. *Drugs, 7:* 39-47.
Shand, D.G., Nuckolls, E.M. and Oates, J.A. (1970): Plasma propranolol levels in adults. With observations in four children. *Clinical Pharmacology and Therapeutics, 11:* 112-120.
Shand, D.G. and Rangno, R.E. (1972): The disposition of propranolol. I. Elimination during oral absorption in man. *Pharmacology, 7:* 159-168.
Shaw, T.R.D. and Carless, J.E. (1974): The effect of particle size on the absorption of digoxin. *European Journal of Clinical Pharmacology, 7:* 269-273.
Shaw, T.R.D., Howard, M.R. and Hamer, J. (1972): Variation in the biological availability of digoxin. *Lancet, 2:* 303-307.
Shaw, T.R.D., Kumana, C.R., Royds, R.B., Padgham, C.M. and Hamer, J. (1974): Use of plasma levels in evaluation of procainamide dosage. *British Heart Journal, 36:* 265-270.
Sheiner, L.B., Rosenberg, B., Marathe, V.V. and Peck, C. (1974): Differences in serum digoxin concentrations between outpatients and inpatients. An effect of compliance? *Clinical Pharmacology and Therapeutics, 15:* 239-246.
Smith, T.W. (1975): Digitalis toxicity: epidemiology and clinical use of serum concentration measurements. *American Journal of Medicine, 58:* 470-476.
Smith, T.W. and Haber, E. (1970): Digoxin intoxication: the relationship of clinical presentation to serum digoxin concentration. *Journal of Clinical Investigation, 49:* 2377-2386.
Smith, T.W. and Haber, E. (1973): Digitalis. *New England Journal of Medicine, 289:* 945-952, 1010-1015, 1063-1072, 1125-1129.
Smith, T.W. and Willerson, J.T. (1971): Suicidal and accidental digoxin ingestion. Report of five cases with serum digoxin level correlations. *Circulation, XLIV:* 29-36.
Smith, E., Barkan, S., Ross, B., Maienthal, M. and Levine, J. (1973): Examination of quinidine and quinine and their pharmaceutical preparations. *Journal of Pharmaceutical Sciences, 62:* 1151-1155.
Solomon, H.M. and Abrams, W.B. (1972): Interactions between digitoxin and other drugs in man. *American Heart Journal, 83:* 277-280.
Soyka, L.F. (1972): Clinical pharmacology of digoxin. *Pediatric Clinics of North America, 19:* 241-256.
Soyka, L.F., Krausula, R.W., Yanagi, R., Hastreiter, A.R. and Levitsky, S. (1975): Changes in serum, tissue and urinary excretion of digoxin in children undergoing cardiopulmonary by pass. In: *Basic and Therapeutic Aspects of Perinatal Pharmacology,* edited by P.L. Morselli, S. Garattini and F. Sereni, pp. 367-375, Raven Press, New York.
Steiness, E. (1974): Renal tubular secretion of digoxin. *Circulation, 50:* 103-107.
Steiness, E., Christensen, V. and Johansen, H. (1973): Bioavailability of digoxin tablets. *Clinical Pharmacology and Therapeutics, 14:* 949-954.
Steiness, E., Svendsen, O. and Rasmussen, F. (1974): Plasma digoxin after parenteral administration. Local reaction after intramuscular injection. *Clinical Pharmacology and Therapeutics, 16:* 430-434.
Stenson, R.E., Constantino, R.T. and Harrison, D.C. (1971): Interrelationships of hepatic blood flow, cardiac output and blood levels of lidocaine in man. *Circulation, 43:* 205-211.
Storstein, L. (1974a): Studies on digitalis. 1. Renal excretion of digitoxin and its cardioactive metabolites. *Clinical Pharmacology and Therapeutics, 16:* 14-24.

Storstein, L. (1974b): Studies on digitalis. II. The influence of impaired renal function on the renal excretion of digitoxin and its cardioactive metabolites. *Clinical Pharmacology and Therapeutics, 16:* 25-34.
Storstein, L. (1975): Studies on digitalis. III. Biliary excretion and enterohepatic circulation of digitoxin and its cardioactive metabolites. *Clinical Pharmacology and Therapeutics, 17:* 313-320.
Strong, J.M. and Atkinson, A.G., Jr. (1972): Simultaneous measurement of plasma concentrations of lidocaine and its desethylated metabolite by mass fragmentography. *Analytical Chemistry, 44:* 2287-2290.
Thompson, F.D., Joekes, A.M. and Foulkes, D.M. (1972): Pharmacodynamics of propranolol in renal failure. *British Medical Journal, 2:* 434-436.
Thomson, P., Cohn, K., Steinbrunn, W., Rowland, M. and Melmon, K.L. (1969): The influence of heart failure (HF) and liver disease (LD) on plasma concentration and clearance of lidocaine (L) in man. *Circulation, 39,* suppl. III: 203.
Thomson, P.D., Rowland, M. and Melmon, K.L. (1971): The influence of heart failure, liver disease, and renal failure on the disposition of lidocaine in man. *American Heart Journal, 82:* 417-421.
Thomson, P.D., Melmon, K.L., Richardson, J.A., Cohn, K., Steinbrunn, W., Cudihee, R. and Rowland, M. (1973): Lidocaine pharmacokinetics in advanced heart failure, liver disease, and renal failure in humans. *Annals of Internal Medicine, 78:* 499-508.
Vöhringer, H.F. and Rietbrock, N. (1974): Metabolism and excretion of digitoxin in man. *Clinical Pharmacology and Therapeutics, 16:* 796-806.
Wagner, J.G. (1974a): Loading and maintenance doses of digoxin in patients with normal renal function and those with severely impaired renal function. *Journal of Clinical Pharmacology, 14:* 329-338.
Wagner, J.G. (1974b): Appraisal of digoxin bioavailability and pharmacokinetics in relation to cardiac therapy. *American Heart Journal, 88:* 133-138.
Wagner, J.G., Yates, J.D., Willis, P.W., III, Sakmar, E. and Stoll, R.G. (1974): Correlation of plasma levels of digoxin in cardiac patients with dose and measures of renal function. *Clinical Pharmacology and Therapeutics, 15:* 291-301.
Wallace, S. and Whiting, B. (1974): Some clinical implications of the protein binding of digoxin. *British Journal of Clinical Pharmacology, 1:* 325-328.
Walle, T. (1974): GLC determination of propranolol, other blocking drugs, and metabolites in biological fluids and tissues. *Journal of Pharmaceutical Sciences, 63:* 1885-1891.
Walle, T. and Gaffney, T.E. (1972): Propranolol metabolism in man and dog: mass spectrometric identification of six new metabolites. *Journal of Pharmacology and Experimental Therapeutics, 182:* 83-92.
Watson, E., Clark, D.R. and Kalman, S.M. (1973): Identification by gas-chromatography-mass spectroscopy of dihydrodigoxin. A metabolite of digoxin in man. *Journal of Pharmacology and Experimental Therapeutics, 184:* 424-431.
Weily, H.S. and Genton, E. (1972): Pharmacokinetics of procainamide. *Archives of Internal Medicine, 130:* 366-369.
Weliky, I. and Neiss, E.S. (1975): Absorption of procainamide from the human intestine. *Clinical Pharmacology and Therapeutics, 17:* 248.
Wettrell, G., Andersson, K.-E., Bertler, A. and Lundstrom, N.R. (1974): Concentrations of digoxin in plasma, urine and tissues in infants and children with heart disease. *Acta Paediatrica Scandinavica, 63:* 480-481.
White, R.J., Chamberlain, D.H., Howard, M. and Smith, T.W. (1971): Plasma concentrations of digoxin after oral administration in the fasting and postprandial state. *British Medical Journal, 1:* 380-381.
Yanagi, R., Woong Kim, P., Krasula, R.W., Soyka, L.F. and Hastreiter, A.R. (1975): Urinary

excretion of digoxin in infants and children. In: *Proc., 47th Scientific Session,* American Heart Assoc., Nov. 18-21, 1974, Dallas, Texas, in press.

Zanchetti, A., Leonetti, G., Morganti, A., Terzoli, L., Chidsey, C.A., Bianchetti, G. and Morselli, P.L. (1975): Correlation between renin-suppressive and hemodynamic effects of beta-adrenoceptor blocking agents. In: *Regulation of Blood Pressure by Central Nervous System,* Grune & Stratton, New York, in press.

Zilly, W., Richter, E. and Rietbrock, N. (1975): Pharmacokinetics and metabolism of digoxin and β-methyl-digoxin-12 α-^{3}H in patients with acute hepatitis. *Clinical Pharmacology and Therapeutics, 17:* 302-309.

Zito, R. and Reid, P. (1975): Lidocaine kinetics in man. *Clinical Pharmacology and Therapeutics, 17:* 248.

14

Psychotropic Drugs

PAOLO LUCIO MORSELLI

The term "psychotropic drugs" is inclusive of a variety of compounds which may go from those used in the clinical treatment of mental disturbances, to others which, as amphetamines and psychotomimetics compounds, find very little use at a clinical level. In this chapter, we have restricted our comments to neuroleptics, tricyclic antidepressants and benzodiazepines, taken as representative of 3 classes of drugs widely used in clinics. The information today available on the above-mentioned compounds permits a definite evaluation of the effects of age on drug disposition, and hence a correct usage only for the benzodiazepines. Scanty data may be found on the pharmacokinetics of tricyclic antidepressants in infants and children, while no data exist for the antipsychotic group. Their use in pediatrics, however, does not reflect the available body of kinetic knowledge, and, even if blindly, major tranquilizers and tricyclic antidepressants are widely administered, often without real or correct motivation, to "nervous" infants and children. For these reasons, we report here at least the data available in adults, as a basis for a further work and/or a revision of our therapeutic approach in children.

ANTIPSYCHOTIC DRUGS

The therapeutic response to antipsychotic drugs is dependent upon several factors not always strictly correlated with the pharmacodynamics of the administered drug. On the other hand, correct use of this class of compounds is of extreme importance, considering the category of patients who are treated with antipsychotic drugs. Today, there are still no means of establishing the right dose or the right dosage schedule, and therapy is largely depending on "impressions" and "trial and error" approach.

As described in the following pages, the kinetic information on antipsychotic drugs is still very scarce, fragmentary and not always reliable for the technical problems related to the chemical lability of several of these agents. Despite the lack of established evidence, there are few reports which clearly suggest that antipsychotic therapy may be considerably improved by the monitoring of plasma levels. Furthermore, even if the risk of acute toxicity with these agents is low, the risk of severe delayed complications and side effects in the course of prolonged overdosage is not a remote one.

Drugs described in this section include chlorpromazine, thioridazine, thioxanthenes and butyrophenones.

Chlorpromazine

Chlorpromazine (CPZ) administered by the oral route is incompletely absorbed from the gastrointestinal tract, with peak plasma levels attained between 2 and 4 h after dosing (Curry et al., 1969, 1970a; Curry and Marshall, 1968; Curry, 1971; Sakalis et al., 1972; March et al., 1972). As shown by Curry et al. (1971) in the rat, in all likelihood in man chlorpromazine is degraded in the gut, even before entering the portal circulation (Curry, 1971). Furthermore, differences in formulation, the presence of food, as well as concomitant treatment with other drugs such as antacids and/or anti-parkinson drugs, are all factors which may significantly modify the drug's absorption pattern (Curry et al., 1970a; Forrest et al., 1970; Rivera-Calimlin et al., 1973). Following intramuscular administration, absorption of chlorpromazine is much more efficient, leading to plasma levels which may be 4-10 fold higher than those obtained with a similar oral dose. With intramuscular administration, peak plasma levels are usually reached in 2-3 h; the absorption, however, does not follow a first-order process, since wide fluctuations and secondary peaks can frequently be observed during the absorptive phase (Curry et al., 1969, 1970a). Precipitation of chlorpromazine at the injection site, and the influence of the drug itself on the autonomic regulation of the vascular bed, might be two possible explanations for this phenomenon. Once absorbed, the drug diffuses widely to all tissues and body organs, with an apparent volume of distribution of about 7 L/kg (Curry et al., 1970a). In animals, brain concentrations parallel those in the plasma but are about 4-5 times greater (Curry, 1971). Under normal conditions, chlorpromazine, in adult volunteers and in patients, is 90-95% bound to plasma proteins, mainly to the albumin fraction, with an affinity constant of 1.9×10^5 M^{-1} (Curry et al., 1970a).

After a single intravenous or intramuscular administration, chlorpromazine plasma concentrations follow a biesponential decay, with an apparent plasma half-life of about 1 h for the alpha-phase and 4-5 h for the β-phase (Curry et al., 1970a). In patients who are dosed chronically with chlorpromazine in association with other drug therapy, the apparent plasma half-life of the terminal exponential phase may vary from 3 to 30 h. Steady-state plasma levels of the drug ranging from 10 to 1,300 ng/ml have been reported in psychotic patients (Huang and Ruskin, 1964; Curry et al., 1970b; March et al., 1972; Rivera-Calimlin et al., 1973). Differences in absorption and metabolic degradation, as well as drug-interaction phenomena and poor compliance, most likely contribute to such wide interindividual variability.

Chlorpromazine is extensively degraded in the body. Over the last 20 years, more than 40 derivatives have either been identified or described as possible metabolites in man by several authors (Salzman and Brodie, 1956; Lin et al., 1959; Fishman and Goldenberg, 1960, 1963, 1965; Goldenberg and Fishman, 1961; Fishman et al., 1962; Emmerson and Miya, 1963; Beckett et al., 1963; Posner, 1963; Huang et al., 1963; Huang and Riskin, 1964; Williams and Parke, 1964; Johnson et al., 1965; Gillette and Kamm, 1966; Bolt et al., 1966; Rodriguez and Johnson, 1966; Wechsler et al., 1967; Huang, 1967; Coccia and Westerfeld, 1967; Curry and Marshall, 1968; Curry et al., 1969; Hammar and Holmstedt, 1968; Usdin, 1970, 1971; Turano et al., 1972, 1974; Chan et al., 1974; Craig et al., 1974). The major metabolic steps involved in the degradation of chlorpromazine are demethylation, hydroxylation, sulfoxidation, O-methylation, side-chain dealkylation and N-oxidation. In general, the phenolic metabolites are further conjugated to glucuronide derivatives (Fishman and Goldenberg, 1963; Posner et al., 1963; Huang and Ruskin, 1964; Bolt et al., 1966; Lin et al., 1969; Curry, 1971; March et al., 1972), but there is also the possibility of sulfate conjugate formation (Beckett et al., 1963). Despite the large number of papers that document the existence of this plethora of derivatives in experimental animals and in man, critical investigation initiated during the last 3-4 years tends to suggest that only 10-12 compounds are of true metabolic origin in man (Turano et al., 1972, 1973, 1974; Kaul et al., 1974); these include didemethyl compounds, 7- and 8-hydroxy derivatives, methoxy derivatives and 2-chlorophenothiazine (Fig. 1). Other compounds such as the monodemethyl derivatives, the N-oxide and the sulfoxide might be of metabolic origin but also might be formed during the extraction procedure, in either the aqueous or the solvent phase. As reported recently by Turano et al. (1974), the formation of such derivatives can occur even in the dark at room temperature. Furthermore, some of these derivatives may be formed in the intestinal lumen or in the gut wall (Curry et al., 1971). At present, it is very difficult to determine how many (and how much) of the compounds described in Fig. 1 are formed by enzymatic action or nonenzymatic processes and to ascertain how many are artefact due to the chemical lability of the molecule.

434 DRUG DISPOSITION DURING DEVELOPMENT

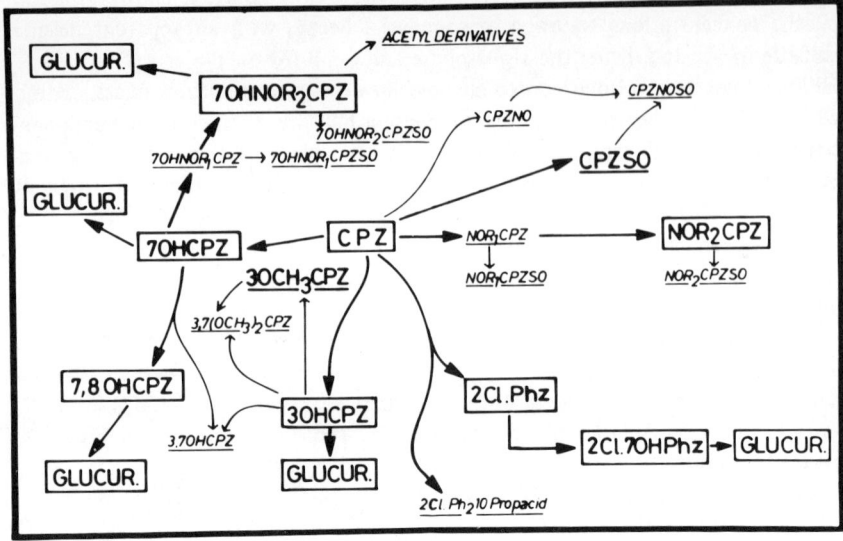

Fig. 1: Metabolism of chlorpromazine in man. Compounds included in the rectangles are today considered to be of true metabolic origin. The other compounds may be of metabolic origin or may be partial artifacts as well. CPZ = chlorpromazine; CPZSO = chlorpromazine sulfoxide; CPZNO = chlorpromazine N-oxide; NOR_1 CPZ = desmethyl chlorpromazine; NOR_2 CPZ = didesmethyl chlorpromazine; 2 ClPhz = 2-chlorphenothiazine; 7OH CPZ = 7-hydroxy chlorpromazine; $3OCH_3$ CPZ = 3-methoxy chlorpromazine; $7OHNOR_2$ CPZ = 7-hydroxydidesmethyl chlorpromazine; 2 Cl Phz 10 propacid = 2-chlorphenothiazine-10-propacid.

Unchanged chlorpromazine has been found present only in traces in human urine and feces (Goldenberg and Fishman, 1961; Bolt et al., 1966; Curry et al., 1969, 1970a). Phenolic compounds, mostly free and conjugated 7-hydroxy derivatives, and didemethyl chlorpromazine account for the majority of chlorpromazine derivatives found in human urine (Bolt et al., 1966; Forrest et al., 1970; Chan et al., 1974). Phenolic glucuronides can account for 60-70% of the urinary-excreted, solvent-extractable material, while nonphenolic compounds represent 20-30% of the total (Chan et al., 1974). In a recent study run on 3 animal species with tritiated chlorpromazine, Forrest et al. (1974) showed that measuring with chemical methods yielded only about 30% of the amount of compounds indicated by radioactive measurements. These data suggest that additional unidentified derivatives may be present in the excreta. With phenobarbital included in the therapeutic regimen, the metabolic breakdown of chlorpromazine may be increased significantly, as is documented by the augmented urinary excretion of hydroxy derivatives, mostly glucuronide conjugates (Forrest et al., 1970). Several of these metabolites have been shown to possess pharmacological activity in the experimental animal. However, as yet no data indicate any possible antipsychotic effects of these compounds in man (Davison et al., 1957; Usdin, 1970). The possible existence of metabolites with central action has recently been hypothesized by Sakalis et al. (1972) to explain the apparent lack of correlation between chlorpromazine plasma levels and some of the drug's central effects.

After a single dose, a clear relationship has been observed in the individual patient between peak plasma levels and effects, such as sedation and orthostatic hypotension, but the threshold for response may vary significantly from patient to patient (Curry et al., 1970b). A definite tolerance toward the sedative hypotensive action of the drug usually develops in 6-7 days of constant treatment, while the antipsychotic effect becomes manifest (Curry et al., 1970b). A progressive decline in the chlorpromazine plasma level after 2-3 weeks of treatment has been reported (Sakalis et al., 1972; March et al., 1972). Possible explanations of this phenomenon are that chlorpromazine impairs its own absorption through its recognized slowing effect on gastrointestinal motility or that chlorpromazine accelerates its own metabolism through enzyme induction. As far as the plasma levels of the metabolites are concerned, levels ranging from 100 to 900 ng/ml, have been found for phenolic derivatives (Huang and Ruskin, 1964; Curry and Marshall, 1968; Curry et al., 1970a; March et al., 1972; Chan et al., 1974). Perry et al. (1964) have hypothesized that 7-hydroxychlorpromazine may be involved in the hyperpigmentation and corneal opacities seen in chronically treated patients. Steady-state plasma levels, between 100 and 300 ng/ml, have been found to be associated with good clinical response, whereas poor responders had plasma levels below 30-50 ng/ml (Curry et al., 1970b; Rivera-Calimlin et al., 1973). Patients with severe side effects, such as dystonia, tremor and convulsions, had steady-state plasma levels higher than 600 ng/ml, as did those individuals in whom there was a clear worsening of the psychic symptomatology (Curry et al., 1970b; Rivera-Calimlin et al., 1973). In all instances, a reduction in dosage, followed by a prompt drop in chlorpromazine plasma levels, resulted in an amelioration of the clinical picture. The most common side effects of chlorpromazine, not always linked to overdosage, are the following: excessive sedation, orthostatic hypotension with reflex tachycardia, tremor, dystonia, extrapyramidal syndrome, skin rashes, dry mouth, blurred vision and photosensitivity. In addition, cholestatic jaundice may occur, and, rarely, blood dyscrasias have been observed.

There are no kinetic data on chlorpromazine in newborns, infants and children. The drug and its metabolies, easily cross the placenta (O'Donoghue, 1971); therefore, the possibility of central and peripheral effects on newborns, as well as photosensitive reactions, must be kept in mind. Data on the human fetus (Pelkonen et al., 1972) indicate a very slow metabolic degradation of chlorpromazine. This would suggest that, in analogy with what is known for other drugs, there is a reduced capability to dispose of the drug in the newborn. Chlorpromazine and a substantial number of derivatives were found in urine of neonates whose mothers received chlorpromazine before delivery (O'Donoghue, 1971). According to the same author, the same metabolites may be found in the 72 h urine of neonates of non-treated mothers, who received immediately after birth 1 mg of chlorpromazine. The possibility of induction due to exposure to other chemical in utero was not taken into consideration. In view of what is actually known on the analytical technical problems related to chlorpromazine and its derivatives, the possibility of artefacts must also be considered. No data on the analytical methods used are in fact available.

Thioridazine

When given by the oral route at doses of 100 mg, thioridazine reaches peak plasma levels of 130-150 ng/ml within 1-4 h (Martenson and Roos, 1973). During chronic treatment, plasma levels ranging from 100 to 1,800 ng/ml have been described by the same authors, who also reported a positive correlation between the daily dose and the morning blood levels. These plasma concentrations are considerably lower than those previously reported by other authors (Mellinger et al., 1965; Pacha, 1969; Berling et al., 1975). The difference is probably due to the use of a more specific method of analysis; in fact, the specificity of the fluorimetric method on samples from chronically treated patients is questionable. According to Martenson and Roos (1973), the absorption of thioridazine may be impaired for dosages over 5 mg/kg; this may be due to the strong anticholinergic effect of the drug, which might influence gastric emptying and, hence, its own absorption. The apparent plasma half-life of thioridazine is about 10 h (Pacha, 1969; Martenson and Roos, 1973). A clear effect of age on the level/dose ratio has been reported by Martenson and Roos, but no data are available for patients below 17 years of age, despite the wide use of thioridazine in the pediatric age group (at least in Europe).

As with chlorpromazine, thioridazine is extensively degrated in the body, and only trace amounts of the unchanged drug may be found in the urine. The metabolites which have been identified mostly from animal studies include the 5-sulfoxide, the 3-sulfoxide, the disulfoxide and the sulfone, and demethylated derivatives. Demethylation appears to occur at a very high rate (Zehnder et al., 1962). Eiduson and Geller (1963), after a single dose of radioactive thioridazine was given to psychiatric patients, found 30% of the administered radioactivity in the feces. Surprisingly, very little conjugated material was found in the urine. No relationship between the plasma levels and the clinical effects of the drug could be established by Berling et al. (1975) in their investigations.

Other Phenothiazines

Among the other phenothiazines, only limited data are available on the disposition and metabolism of *levopromazine* (Allgen et al., 1960), *perphenazine* (Huang and Kurland, 1964; Larsen and Naestoft, 1975) and *trifluperazine* (Sprites, 1974). These compounds have a kinetic and metabolic pattern which is very similar to that of chlorpromazine, since they all undergo demethylation, sulfoxidation, N-oxidation and hydroxylation, with subsequent conjugation. On the other hand, *butaperazine,* at variance with chlorpromazine, seems to be absorbed more efficiently by the oral than by the intramuscular route (Simpson et al., 1973). This drug has an apparent plasma half-life, after both acute and chronic administration, that varies from 5 to 30 h (Davis et al., 1974). Steady-state plasma levels may range from 50 to 300 ng/ml on a daily intake of 20-40 mg and from 800 to 1,100 ng on daily doses of 80 mg (Simpson et al., 1973; Davis et al., 1974).

Thioxanthenes

The thioxanthene nucleus is a 6,6,6 tricyclic system, closely related to the phenothiazine nucleus. The double bond in 10 position appears to be necessary for its CNS action (Petersen and Nielsen, 1964). It is worthwhile to remember that, in contrast with what is reported by Ban (1972), the "cis," and not the "trans," isomers are the pharmacologically active compounds (Dunitz, 1964; Schaefer, 1967; Weissman, 1968, 1974). The psychopharmacological activities of thioxanthenes generally parallel those of analogous phenothiazines but are usually less potent in producing extrapyramidal symptoms. Kinetic data are available on chlorprothixene and thiothixene.

Chlorprothixene is promptly absorbed from the gastrointestinal tract and within 15-30 min after administration is present in all organs, both as chlorprothixene and chlorprothixene sulfoxide (Petersen and Nielsen, 1964; Bann, 1972; Raaflaub, 1967). The compound appears to have a greater stability than CPZ in solution and a lesser sensitivity to light. The metabolic fate of chlorprothixene (CPTX) has been studied extensively in animals and man. In animals (rats and dogs), Huus and Khan (1967) detected the presence of sulfoxide, norsulfoxide, norchlorprothixene and chlorprothixene N-oxide. Phenolic derivatives were observed in dog urine but not in that of the rat. In human urine, Allgen et al. (1960) found chlorprothixene sulfoxide as the major metabolite, but, according to Wallace (1967), only 7% of the administered dose may be recovered as such and as heptane-extractable metabolites within 72 h.

The kinetics of *thiothixene* have been studied more extensively in chronically treated schizophrenic patients. This drug is rapidly absorbed, with peak plasma levels (10-22 ng/ml) attained 1-3 h after dosing. The absorption rate appears to be quite rapid, with an apparent absorption half-life of 0.5 h (Hobbs et al., 1973). The plasma levels reported by Hobbs are considerably lower than those described by Mjorndal and Oreland (1971) (45 ng/ml), and, once more, this may be due to analytical problems since a fluorimetric method was used by the latter authors and N-demethylthiothixene was probably also measured. The drug disappears from circulation following a biexponential decay, the alpha-phase half-life being 3.5 h and the β-phase apparent plasma half-life 34 h. In animal studies using S^{35}-labeled thiothixene, Hobbs (1968) observed that the compound was rapidly absorbed from the g.i. tract. Following a single dose, the radioactivity was primarily excreted in the feces 48 h later, as the results of extensive biliary excretion. Recently, Hobbs et al. (1974) found evidence of an enterohepatic circulation of the drug in man. Thiothixene and metabolites appear to be widely distributed in all body tissues, but only thiothixene seems to be present in the brain. According to Hobbs et al. (1971), effective plasma levels in the course of chronic treatment range between 10-20 ng/ml at peak time, with pre-dose levels varying between 2.7 and 6.4 ng/ml. More recently, Berling et al. (1975), using a modified version of the fluorimetric method of Mjorndal and Oreland (1971), described plasma levels of 10-150 ng/ml during chronic treatment. These same authors reported a drop in plasma levels after 6-8 weeks of treatment; this suggests both the possibility of induction and the formation of an active metabolite, since no changes in the pharmacological effects were noticed concomitantly with the fall in plasma levels. No relationships between the dose administered and plasma levels, nor between clinical symptoms, rating scores and plasma levels could be demonstrated. The adverse effects usually observed with thioxanthenes are similar to those induced by phenothiazines.

Butyrophenones

The butyrophenones, although structurally different from phenothizines, share many of their pharmacological and therapeutic activities. The prototype of this class is *haloperidol,* introduced in Europe in 1958 and in the United States in 1967. The drug is rapidly absorbed both after oral and intramuscular administration. After an i.m. dose of 2 mg, peak levels of 2-10 ng/ml were observed within 10 min by Cressman et al. (1974), while levels of 260 ng/ml were reported by Marcucci et al. (1971) 60 min after a 4 mg dose. No data are available on plasma protein-binding. Steady-state plasma levels of 55-188 ng/ml were found in four patients receiving a chronic oral dose of 9 mg. Similarly, in two other patients in whom the plasma levels were followed during a gradual increasing of the dose from 3 to 12 mg/day, relatively constant plasma levels of about 120-150 ng/ml were observed after 4-5 days of constant treatment (Marcucci et al., 1971). Haloperidol plasma levels decay according to a multicompartment model. The apparent plasma half-life of the terminal elimination phase may range from 12.8 to 35.5 h (Cressman, et al., 1974).

Penfluridol, a more potent analog not yet marketed in the United States, has a different pharmacokinetic profile. Administered once a week, at doses of 20-120 mg, it usually provides adequate effect for 6-7 days. Peak concentrations occur between 8 and 12 h after the oral intake, and after a dose of 120 mg they may range from 20 to 40 ng/ml (Cooper et al., 1975). The plasma concentrations decline rapidly for about 20 h, when the decline becomes much slower and plasma levels of 4-5 ng/ml are still measurable after 6-7 days. The calculated apparent plasma half-life of the terminal exponential phase is about 72-92 h (Cooper et al., 1975a). In the course of chronic treatment, "steady-state" plasma concentrations appear to be linearly related to the dose expressed as mg/kg. At dosages of 60-120 mg, steady-state plasma levels may range from 6 to 25 ng/ml, according to Cooper et al. (1975b).

There are no data yet available on the possible relationships between effects and plasma concentrations, nor on the possible toxic thresholds of these compounds. Such data may be very important for the elevated incidence of extrapyramidal reactions, considerably higher in children and adolescents. On the contrary, side effects linked to an autonomic unbalance are considerably less frequent and of minor intensity.

ANTIDEPRESSANT DRUGS

The introduction of tricyclic antidepressants drugs (TCA) in the medical armamentarium has represented a considerable step forward in the treatment of depressive illness. Today, this class of compounds is also used in behavioral disturbances in children. The pharmacokinetics of tricyclic antidepressant drugs has been extensively studied in man, and a consistent body of data is available relative to the adult patient. Such information points out the fact that monitoring of plasma concentrations of tricyclic antidepressants may be of real value for an individualized approach to the therapy of depressive states (Garattini and Morselli, 1975). The data available on pediatric patients are, on the contrary, very few despite the wide use of these drugs in preschool and school age, and despite the fact that very severe side effects may be induced by inappropriate dosages. The drugs discussed in this section include imipramine, desipramine, amitriptyline and nortiptyline, taken as examples of the overall class. No data are reported on MAO inhibitors because of their limited use and the limited data available on their kinetics in humans.

Imipramine and Desmethylimipramine

Imipramine (IMI) and desmethylimipramine (DMI) are completely absorbed from the gastrointestinal tract (Herman, 1963; Bickel et al., 1967; Christiansen et al., 1967; Gram and Christiansen, 1975). Peak plasma levels of 10-25 ng/ml may be obtained 4-8 h after a single oral administration of 50-75 mg of commercially available preparations of both compounds (Rizzo et al., 1973; Garattini and Morselli, 1975; Belvedere et al., 1975). Earlier (2-4 h) and higher (30-100 ng/ml) peak plasma levels have been reported for both desmethylimipramine and imipramine, administered either in capsule form (1 mg/kg) or in aqueous solution (35-50 mg) (Alexanderson, 1972b; Gram and Christiansen, 1975). Occasionally, in the course of chronic treatment using the commercially available preparations, peak plasma levels may be attained as late as 12-14 h. This delay is most likely due to the anticholinergic effect of the drug itself on gastric emptying, as shown to occur in animals and men by Consolo et al. (1970). Concomitant administration of antacids does not seem to modify desmethylimipramine absorption substantially; however, significant differences in bioavailability may be observed for different preparations (Garattini and Morselli, 1975). Following imipramine administration, desmethylimipramine reaches measurable concentrations in plasma within 2-3 h and may attain levels higher than the parent compound 10-12 h after dosing (Belvedere et al., 1975; Gram and Christiansen, 1975). According to these authors, the systemic availability of imipramine among different individuals may vary from 29 to 77% of the dose. This factor may partially account for the very large apparent volume of distribution observed on certain occasions with this class of compounds. Alexanderson (1972b) has reported that the apparent volume of distribution for DMI may vary from 22 to 59 L/kg with a mean value of 41 ± 12 L/kg.

Imipramine and desmethylimipramine are bound to plasma proteins to a considerable extent. Binding values, ranging from 75 to 90% for imipramine and from 70 to 92% for desmethylimipramine, has been reported by various authors (Borga et al., 1968, 1969; Campbell and Todrick, 1970; Pruitt and Dayton, 1971; Glassman et al., 1974; Sharpless, 1975). Sharpless has reported a K for albumin of 0.239×10^5 liter mol^{-1} for IMI and of 0.702×10^5 liters mol^{-1} for DMI. However, as seen by Pruitt and Dayton (1971), globulin also may be involved in the plasma protein-binding of these compounds. Other drugs, such as diphenylhydantoin, phenylbutazone, aspirin, aminopyrine, scopolamine, phenothiazines, and other tricyclic antidepressants, may significantly increase the free fraction of imipramine and desmethylimipramine by displacing them from binding sites (Sharpless, 1975; Borga et al., 1969). The large apparent volume of distribution of both IMI and DMI is indicative of an extensive high tissue-binding for both drugs.

Animal observations performed under steady-state conditions indicate a brain/plasma ratio of about 20 and an atria/plasma ratio of 30 (Franco and Morselli, unpublished data). Moreover, similar ratios may be obtained by extrapolating from reports on post-mortem observations in suicide cases (Herrmann and Pulver, 1960; Bickel et al., 1967). Tissue concentration found after suicide attempts with doses varying from 2,500 to 4,500 mg ranged from 136 to 300 μg/g in brain, 150-230 μg/g in liver and 50-27 μg/g in the heart. Maximum concentrations in the brain were found in the amygdala and in the basal nuclei, and the lowest were in cortical white matter, cerebellum and the pons. The relative ratio between IMI and DMI in the available reports varies considerably, according to the time elapsed between ingestion and death (Herrmann and Pulver, 1960; Herrmann, 1963; Bickel et al., 1967; Siridopoulos and Bickel, 1971; Christiansen and Gram, 1973). Following oral or intravenous administration, plasma levels of IMI and/or DMI decay biexponentially, with a distribution phase (alpha) which may last as long as 8-12 h. Apparent plasma half-lives of the β terminal phase may range from 10 to 16 h for imipramine (Gram and Christiansen, 1975) and from 12 to 77 h for desmethylimipramine (Alexanderson, 1972b; Rizzo et al., 1973). According to the same authors, plasma clearance rates of both drugs range between 0.76 and 2.8 L/h/kg.

Imipramine and its main active metabolite, desmethylimipramine, are extensively degraded in the body. The major common metabolic pathway to the formation of inactive compounds is via the aromatic hydroxylation in position 2, which yields 2-hydroxyimipramine and 2-hydroxydesmethylimipramine. These compounds are then either excreted as such or further conjugated to glucuronide derivatives (Herrmann and Pulver, 1960; Fishman and Goldenberg, 1962; Crammer and Scott, 1966; Christiansen et al., 1967; Bickel and Weder, 1968; Gram, 1974). Other minor metabolic pathways include the N-oxidation of imipramine (Fishman and Goldenberg, 1962; Herrmann, 1963), dealkylation of the whole side chain, resulting in the formation of the iminodibenzyl (Imobersteg and Baumler, 1962; Crammer et al., 1969), and demethylation of DMI to yield didesmethylimipramine (Herrmann and Pulver, 1960; Christiansen et al., 1967). The concomitant administration of neuroleptic drugs may significantly inhibit imipramine and desipramine metabolism (Gram and Fredricson-Overö, 1972; Rizzo et al., 1973). According to Minder et al. (1971), the possibility of a limited imipramine demethylation by human gastrointestinal contents cannot be excluded.

Radioactive studies performed with C^{14} imipramine have shown that 70-85% of the administered dose is recovered in the urine within 6-8 days (Christiansen et al., 1967; Crammer et al., 1968). The amount excreted during the first 24 h may vary from 15 to 68% of the dose. The maximal rate of urinary excretion is reached 3 to 6 h after administration. Imipramine and desmethylimipramine, as such, represent only 1-3% of the excreted material, while the major part consists of the glucuronides of the hydroxy derivatives (35-40%) free hydroxy compounds account for about 15%. About 23% of the excreted radioactivity is represented by nonextractable, polar compounds, not as yet unidentified. Ten to 20% of the administered radioactivity may be found in the feces, suggesting either incomplete absorption or extensive enterohepatic recycling. From the data of Crammer et al. (1968), the second possibility seems the more likely.

Both imipramine and desmethylimipramine are filtered at the glomerular level and are then subject to passive reabsorption in the distal tubule. Gram et al. (1971) have shown that acidification of the urine may lead to an increase in the

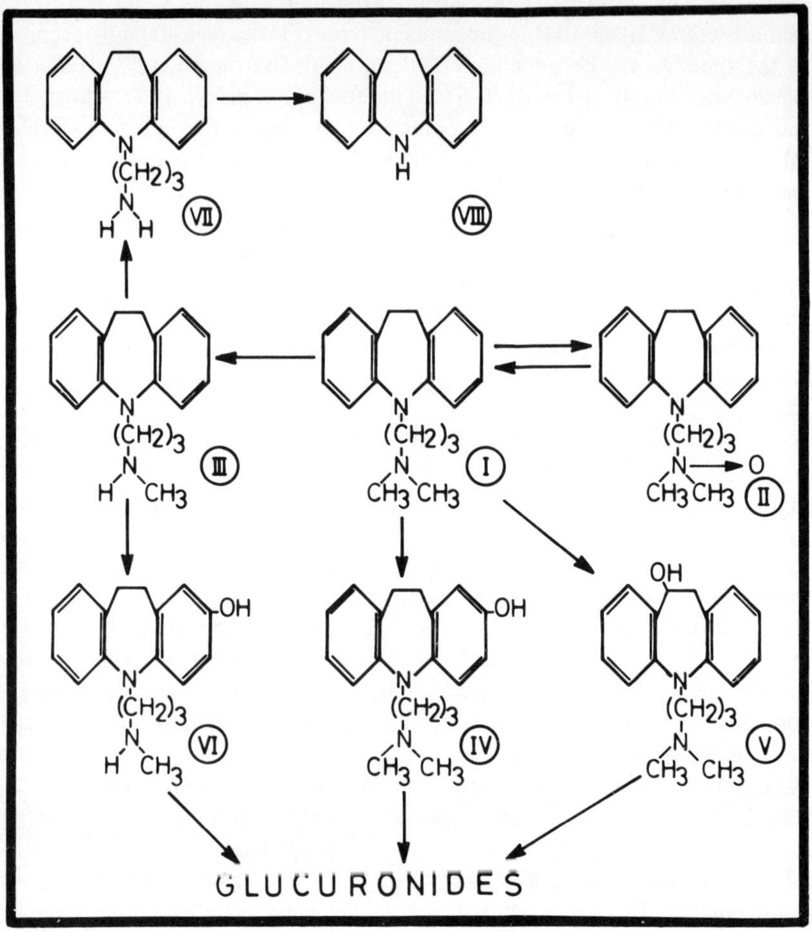

Fig. 2: Metabolism of imipramine in man. I = imipramine (IMI); II = imipramine-N-oxide; III = desmethyl imipramine (DMI); IV = 2-hydroxy imipramine; V = 10-hydroxy imipramine; VI = 2-hydroxydesmethyl imipramine; VII = didesmethyl imipramine; VIII = iminodibenzyl.

total drug excretion of about 10-40%. This increase is due to a 50-100 fold increase in the amount of unconjugated derivatives, mainly imipramine and desmethylimipramine.

During chronic treatment, great variability in the steady-state plasma levels of imipramine and desmethylimipramine has been reported by several authors. For oral doses of from 75 to 150 mg/day, plasma levels may vary from 10 to 300 ng/ml for imipramine and from 5 to 350 ng/ml for desmethylimipramine (Sjoqvist et al., 1968; Alexanderson, 1972a; Tuck et al., 1972; Frigerio et al., 1972; Rizzo et al., 1973; Belvedere et al., 1975; Garattini and Morselli, 1975; Olivier-Martin et al., 1975). In patients receiving imipramine, the ratio between desmethylimipramine and the parent compound may vary considerably from subject to subject and appears to be linked both to genetic differences in drug metabolism and to first-pass effect (Moody et al., 1967; Gram and Christiansen, 1975; Belvedere et al., 1975).

Amitriptyline and Nortriptyline

Amitriptyline (AMI) and its demethylated, pharmacologically active metabolite, nortriptyline (NT), are also completely absorbed by the gastrointestinal tract. Following doses of 25-50 mg, peak plasma levels of 20-100 ng/ml are usually attained within 4-8 h, while higher and earlier peak levels are obtained by intramuscular route (Eschenhof and Rieder, 1969; Alexanderson, 1972a,b; Alexanderson and Sjöqvist, 1973; Alexanderson et al., 1973). The systemic availability of NT has been shown to be 56 to 70% of the administered dose; a first-pass effect very likely occurs for both the compounds (Alexanderson et al., 1973). Amitriptyline and nortriptyline are about 90-95% bound to plasma proteins, and several drugs can displace them from their binding sites (Borgå et al., 1969). The apparent volume of distribution of nortriptyline, after correction for systemic availability, may vary from 11 to 23 L/kg, suggesting, again, extensive tissue binding of the drug (Alexanderson et al., 1973). Amitriptyline and nortriptyline plasma concentrations decay biexponentially, with an apparent plasma half-life of the terminal phase of about 40-75 h for amitriptyline and 12-35 h for nortriptyline (Eschenhof and Rieder, 1969; Braithwaite and Widdop, 1971; Alexanderson, 1972a,b, 1973). Reported plasma clearances for NT range from 0.4 to 1.4 L/kg (Alexanderson, 1972a,b).

According to Braithwaite and Widdop (1971), the demethylation of amitriptyline is a slower process than that of imipramine. Amitriptyline metabolites include, in addition to nortriptyline (Hucker, 1962), desmethylnortriptyline (Eschenhof and Rieder, 1969) and the hydroxy derivatives of the 3 above-mentioned compounds. At variance with imipramine, the hydroxylation of amitriptyline, nortriptyline and desmethylnortriptyline is an aliphatic process, taking place in the 10-11 position. The hydroxylation is stereospecific and gives rise to cis- and trans-isomers in a constant ratio; the hydroxy derivatives are then further conjugated with glucuronic acid (Hammer et al., 1971; de Leenheer and Heyndrick, 1971; Bertilsson and Alexanderson, 1972; Knappe et al., 1972; Alexanderson and Borgå, 1973).

The metabolic breakdown of nortriptyline may be reduced significantly by the concomitant administration of neuroleptics (Gram and Fredricson-Overö, 1972; Garattini and Morselli, 1975) and enhanced by phenobarbital (Sjöqvist et

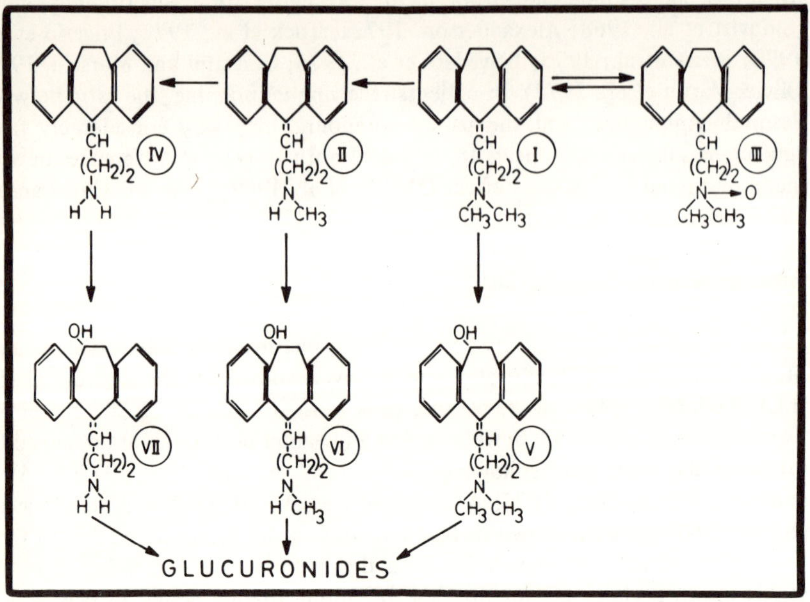

444 DRUG DISPOSITION DURING DEVELOPMENT

Fig. 3: Metabolism of amitriptyline in man. I = amitriptyline (AMI); II = nortriptyline (NT); III = amitriptyline-N-oxide; IV = desmethyl nortriptyline; V = 10-hydroxy amitriptyline; VI = 10-hydroxy nortriptyline; VII = 10-hydroxydesmethyl nortriptyline.

al., 1969). Oral contraceptives may significantly impair the metabolic breakdown of amitriptyline (Rizzo et al., 1973; Garattini and Morselli, 1975).

About 60 to 80% of the nortriptyline administered orally can be recovered as metabolites in the urine. Nortriptyline and amitriptyline, as such, are present only in negligible amounts (2-5% of the dose). About 80% of the excreted material (50% of the dose) is represented by conjugated and unconjugated 10-hydroxynortriptyline (Eschenhof and Rieder, 1969, Alexanderson, 1972a; Borga and Garle, 1972; Alexanderson and Borgå, 1973). Steady-state plasma levels observed in the course of chronic treatment do not bear many relationship to the administered doses, and may range, according to the various reports, from 50 to 380 ng/ml for nortriptyline, and from 20 to 250 ng/ml for amitriptyline (Sjoqvist et al. 1969; Asberg et al., 1971; Braithwaite and Widdop, 1971; Alexanderson and Sjoqvist, 1971; Burrows et al., 1972; Braithwaite et al., 1972; Rizzo et al., 1973; Kragh-Sørensen et al., 1973a,b, 1974; Lyle et al., 1974). Blood levels as high as 18 µg/ml for amitriptyline, and 5 µg/ml for nortriptyline, have been observed in cases of suicide attempts (Munksgaard, 1969).

Other Tricyclic Antidepressants

The limited information available on other tricyclic antidepressants such as *chloroimipramine, butriptyline, protriptyline, maprotyline, trimepromine* and *doxepine* suggest that all behave very similarly from a pharmacokinetic point of view (Charalampous and Johnson, 1967; Hobbs, 1969; Sisenwine et al., 1970; Faigle and Dieterle, 1973; Reiss et al., 1972; Cameron et al., 1974). With regard to protiptyline, it is interesting to note that its metabolic breakdown may lead to the formation of a stable epoxide, as recently shown by Hucker et al. (1975) in the rat.

Plasma Levels and Effects

Clinical observations have shown that there is no direct relationship between the administered daily dose of tricyclic antidepressants and their therapeutic outcome. This lack of correlation is probably sustained by the wide individual variability in steady-state plasma levels usually observed in the course of chronic treatment (Hammer et al., 1967; Hammer and Sjöqvist, 1967; Sjöqvist et al., 1968; Alexanderson and Sjöqvist, 1973). Genetic factors contribute significantly to this variability, but other factors, such as previous or concomitant exposure to chemicals and to other drugs, plus first-pass effect, may also play an important role (Alexanderson et al., 1969; Asberg et al., 1971b; Alexanderson and Sjöqvist, 1971; Gram, 1974; Garattini and Morselli, 1975). There is no general agreement on the existence of a therapeutic range for tricyclic antidepressant plasma levels. A consistent body of data indicates a good relationship between plasma levels and therapeutic effects, maximal benefit being achieved for concentrations ranging from 60 to 200 ng/ml (Asberg et al., 1971a; Braithwaite et al., 1972; Alexanderson and Sjöqvist, 1973; Rizzo et al., 1973; Krag-Sørensen et al., 1973a,b, 1974; Garattini and Morselli, 1975; Olivier-Martin et al., 1975). Other authors, however, were unable to find any relationship between plasma levels and clinical effects (Burrows et al., 1972, 1974; Lyle et al., 1974). According to two recent critical reviews on this topic, some of the quoted studies (on both sides) were deficient in several respects, therefore, it is felt that further data are needed to clarify this point (Glassman and Perel., 1974; Lader, 1974). Two of the main reasons for the apparent discrepancies are, on the one hand, the heterogenicity of the disease and its phasic behavior and, on the other, the fact that the diagnostic criteria were not always the same nor as strict as they should have been in the different studies.

A wide variety of side effects may occur during chronic treatment with tricyclic antidepressants. The most commonly reported symptoms include dry mouth, blurred vision, fatigue, sweating, tremor, headache, dizziness, paresthesias, difficulty in micturition, constipation and orthostatic hypotension with tachycardia (Cole and Davis, 1967). In general, if patients are carefully followed, the reported side effects are not so disturbing and tend to diminish within 7-10 days. However, in the case of inappropriate dosage, seen mainly in elderly people, paralytic ileus and cardiovascular complications are not rare events. No difference in the incidence of side effects between responders and nonresponders were found in the study by Watt et al. (1968), and no relationship between plasma levels and side effects could be demonstrated by Braithwaite et al. (1972) or Burrows et al. (1972). On the contrary, Asberg et al. (1970), Asberg and Germanis (1972) and Asberg (1974) reported a significant correlation.

It is a common observation that many of the above-mentioned symptoms may occur at varying plasma concentrations and may be related to different effects of tricyclic antidepressants. However, very severe adverse reactions are usually associated with high plasma levels, and a reduction of the plasma concentration is followed by a reduction in the adverse effects (Rizzo et al., 1973; Olivier-Martin, 1975). This is particularly true for the cardiovascular toxicity, which in some cases may be very severe and may even result in death. Evidence of minor electrocardiographic changes, such as depression of ST segment, T wave flattening or inversion, can be observed in about one-fifth to one-third of patients on chronic therapy with tricyclic antidepressants (Kristiansen, 1961; Rasmussen and Kristiansen, 1963). More serious changes, including bundle branch block, profound bradycardia, infarction and/or cardiac arrest, may occasionally be observed in patients on therapeutic dosages (Sloman, 1960; Smith and Rusbatch, 1967; Freyschuss et al., 1970; Williams and Sherter, 1971; Singh, 1972; Moccetti et al., 1972).

The presence of predisposing factors, such as age, hypertension and cardiac insufficiency, may be very important in determining the severity of the cardiotoxicity which, as mentioned, may even result in death (Muller et al., 1961; Coull et al., 1970; Moir et al., 1972, 1973; Brackenridge, 1972). Up to now there has been no specific or definite proof that cardiotoxicity is related to high plasma concentrations; however, in our experience, in depressed patients with normal heart, modifications of the ECG become manifest when plasma levels are over 250-300 ng/ml. Recent observations on animal levels, run under steady-state conditions, confirm that alteration of the ECT pattern becomes evident for S.S. plasma levels of 300-600 ng/ml which correspond to atria concentrations of 6,000-12,000 ng/g (Franco and Morselli, unpublished data). The possibility of cardiac complications should be borne in mind every time one treats a depressed patient with tricyclic antidepressant drugs.

In the case of acute voluntary overdosage, the toxic effects of tricyclic antidepressants may appear within 20-30 min. After a short period of restlessness, the picture is that of profound CNS depression, with hypothermia, depressed respiration, changes in deep tendon reflexes and coma with mydriasis, followed in many instances by seizures. If treated symptomatically, this picture does not last more than 30-77 h and is not life-threatening as long as vital functions are supported. The period of awakening is followed by CNS excitement, with agitation, incoherent speech, disorientation and, in some cases, hallucinations. Much more important, and potentially fatal, are the effects on the heart: after an initial moderate tachycardia, the picture may evolve versus supraventricular tachycardia, atrioventricular block, ventricular tachycardia and cardiac arrest. Severe hypotension is usually present (Rasmussen, 1965; Brackenridge et al., 1968; Barnes et al., 1968; Freeman et al., 1969; Williams, 1971; Thompson, 1973; Vohra and Burrows, 1974). Post-mortem data have revealed heart concentrations 10-30 times higher than those in the serum (Curry, 1964; Rasmussen, 1965). Propranolol and diphenylhydantoin may be useful in such cases (Marshall and Green, 1968; Freeman and Loughhead, 1973; Vohra and Burrows, 1974). In a recent study on moderately or severely poisoned patients, during the comatose phase of the intoxication, Thorstrand (1974) observed a lowered arteriovenous pressure difference and a high cardiac putput, while the stroke volume appeared unchanged. This suggests a clinical picture of hyperkinetic circulation, which could partially explain the efficacy of β-blockers, despite the marked prolongation of time QRS (>0.12 min).

Newborns, Infants and Children

Tricyclic antidepressants are used in children for a variety of clinical conditions, such as enuresis, hyperactive aggressive behavior, school phobias and autism (Agarwala and Heycock, 1968; Schaffer et al., 1968; Liederman et al., 1969; Rabiner and Klein, 1969; Campbell et al., 1971; Saraf et al., 1974). The information available up to now on dosages, safety margins and incidence of toxic reactions is quite fragmentary. The same holds true for pharmacokinetic data.

It is known that this class of compounds can readily cross the placenta, and when there is administration of any of these drugs in the days preceding the delivery, concentrations similar to those present in the mother's plasma may be found in the cord or newborn plasma (Douglas and Hume, 1967; Pruitt and Dayton, 1971; Sjoqvist et al., 1972; Van Petten, 1975). The unbound fraction of imipramine in human cord plasma may be 2 times higher (26%) than that found in the plasma of adults (13%), according to Pruitt and Dayton (1971). Similar results have been reported by Rane et al. (1971) for desmethylimipramine in pooled cord plasma at drug concentrations ranging from 160 to 1,450 ng/ml. Taking these data into account and considering the very high liped/water partition coefficient of these agents, the possibility of attaining toxic concentrations in the brain and other tissues is very likely in newborns exposed in utero to tricyclic antidepressants. Marked EKG abnormalities were present at birth, with plasma concentrations of nortriptyline of about 200 ng/ml, in a newborn whose mother took an overdose of the drug 20 h before delivery. The EKG tracing finally appeared normal 5 days later, when the baby's plasma levels fell below 100 ng/ml (Sjoqvist et al., 1972). The apparent plasma half-life of nortriptyline was 56 h in the newborn and 17 h in the mother, suggesting a limited metabolic capacity for this drug in the neonate. Considerable amounts of conjugated and unconjugated 10-hydroxynortriptyline were recovered in the newborn's urine 24 and 96 h after birth. It was not established, however, whether the metabolites were of maternal or neonatal origin. The first possibility seems the more likely, considering several reports on other drugs which suggest limited hydroxylating and conjugating capabilities in the newborn. No kinetic data are available for infants.

In older children, Winsberg et al., (1974) observed that following an oral dose of 50 mg of imipramine, absorption can be very rapid, with peak levels of 150 ng/ml reached within 30-60 min after drug intake. According to the same authors, the binding of imipramine to plasma proteins in children of 7 to 10 years is less (81% ± 1.6) than that observed in adults, and only in children over 13 years of age are adult-like binding values obtained. In the same study, the apparent plasma half-life of imipramine was very variable (from 25 to 40 h); however, the reported ratio (>2) between desmethylimipramine and imipramine plasma levels suggests a very rapid turnover of the latter.

In observations made on children from 5 to 12 years of age who were receiving nortriptyline at dosages ranging from 0.4 to 1.0 mg/kg, we also observed rapid drug absorption, with peak levels of 20-25 ng/ml occurring at about 3-4 h in 70% of the cases. Nortriptyline steady-state plasma levels of 30 to 90 ng/ml were reached within 4-5 days. Mean apparent half-life was 18 ± 3 h, with about 50% of the cases showing values below 14 h (Garattini and Morselli, 1975). As suggested by Winsberg et al. (1974), the rapidity of absorption in children, the greater amount of free drug and the greater proportion of lean body mass (for the smaller adipose tissue compartment) could cause higher drug concentrations in the CNS and could partially account for the relative immediacy of clinical response in children. For the same reason, the usage of a single, large dose at bedtime should be discouraged, in order to avoid the possible occurrence of toxic peak tissue concentrations. On the other hand, an increased catabolism is suggested by the shorter apparent plasma half-life and by the high ratio between DMI and IMI, and this could partially explain the fact that children do require, in many instances, daily dosages which on a per kilo basis are considerably greater (5-7 mg/kg) than those usually administered to adults.

The use of tricyclic antidepressants in childhood does, however, require careful monitoring, as dosages over 5 mg/kg may lead to very troublesome and dangerous side effects. According to Di Mascio and Solty (1970), the incidence of side effects in children is similar to that reported in adults. The most commonly encountered symptoms include dizziness, gastric distress, anorexia, constipation, drowsiness, lethargy and tremors, while blurred vision, increased sweating and skin rashes are less frequently seen (Saraf et al., 1974). The more severe reactions, such as the cardiovascular problems, occur more rarely, but they may be life-threatening. A case of sudden death is reported by Saraf et al. (1974) in a

6-year old girl after 3 days of therapy with IMI at a dosage of 14.7 mg/kg; her plasma levels were 1,800 ng/ml. Evidence of pulmonary edema, pericardial hemorrhage and congestion of the leptomeningeal vessels was found on autopsy. Several authors have reported that acute overdosage of tricyclic antidepressants (10-190 mg/kg) in children is followed by severe CNS depression, seizures and severe electrocardiographic alterations which become evident shortly after drug intake (Arneson, 1961; Alajem-Albagli, 1962; Sunshine and Yaffe, 1963; McGiles, 1963; Steel et al., 1967; Sacks et al., 1968; Freeman et al., 1969; Falletta et al., 1970; Brown et al., 1972; Roberts et al., 1973). Serum concentrations of 100 to 7,000 ng/ml have been reported by Steel et al. (1967) in 3 cases that eventually had positive outcomes. Brain concentrations of 43,000 ng/g for IMI and 35,000 ng/g for DMI are reported by Dingell et al. (1963) in a 2½-year old boy who ingested a lethal dose of IMI 3 days previously. Plasma levels in this child were 1,000 ng/ml for IMI and 3,500 ng/ml for DMI. Sunshine and Yaffe also reported on a case of lethal poisoning with 1,000 mg amitriptyline in a 15-month old boy, a serum level of 2,500 ng/ml, with a heart concentration of 26,000 ng/g. As stressed by Steel et al. (1967) and by Schrober and Mantel (1970), the concomitant use of this drug with digoxin may lead to immediate death. Symptomatic treatment, such as purging and administration of charcoal, is very important for this class of drug, since, due to their anticholinergic activity, peristaltic activity is reduced, thus contributing to prolonged drug absorption. Intravenous administration of a large volume of fluids has no effect on the TCA excretion and, furthermore, may be harmful if the myocardium is severely depressed. Forced acidification of urine may also be dangerous in children. Peritoneal and extracorporeal dialysis are totally ineffective (Sunshine and Yaffe, 1963). As reported by Ramsay (1967) for a 14-year-old girl who ingested 2,500 mg of imipramine, the use of propranolol may be very effective. The successful use of β-blockers in a 2½-year-old boy and in a 26-month-old girl, after massive accidental ingestion of tricyclic antidepressants, has been also reported by both Brown et al. (1972) and Roberts et al. (1973).

BENZODIAZEPINES

Benzodiazepines today are the most widely used minor tranquilizers. There is no branch of medicine in which their use has not been either recommended or proposed. Among the various compounds belonging to this group there are no real differences as far as either the mechanism of action of the type of drug effects is concerned. However, because of the different pharmacokinetic profiles (mainly due to the number of halogens and to the presence or absence of methyl or other groups on the nitrogen in position 1 and/or of an hydroxy group in position 3), the dosages employed and the duration and intensity of the effects may vary substantially from one benzodiazepine to another. This implies that the various benzodiazepines, although very similar in their effects, cannot be considered as equivalent from a practical point of view. The choice of one or the other of these drugs, in other words, should be dictated by the clinical situation and by a precise knowledge of their pharmacokinetic profile.

The metabolic breakdown is very similar for the various benzodiazepines. With the exception of those possessing a NO_2 group, all the compounds sooner or later undergo dealkylation at the nitrogen in position 1 and hydroxylation in position 3. These two derivatives are, in fact, the main metabolites for a variety of compounds, and are subsequently conjugated to glucuronide derivatives, which are promptly excreted in the urine. On the basis of the available data, the formation of parahydroxyphenyl derivatives has not appeared to be an important metabolic pathway in man. In this section, we will take into consideration diazepam and N-desmethyldiazepam as representative compounds of this class. The body of knowledge available for these two drugs does permit an evaluation of the effect of age on drug disposition. For other compounds, such as chlordiazepoxide, oxazepam, temazepam, lorazepam, prazepam, medazepam, ketazolam, bromazepam, oxazolam, etc., we refer the reader to the recent monograph of Greenblatt and Shader (1974).

Diazepam

In adults, diazepam administered by the oral route is readily absorbed, with maximal plasma concentrations attained within 30-90 min. According to the various reports, dosages of 10-20 mg, given as a single dose, lead to peak plasma levels of 100-500 ng/ml, and concentrations of 70-100 ng/ml may be present as early as 15 min after drug intake (De Silva et al., 1964, 1966; Schwartz et al., 1965, 1966; Garattini, 1969, Marcucci et al., 1970; Baird and Hailey, 1972; Garattini et al., 1973; Kaplan et al., 1973; Bliding et al., 1974; Hillestadt et al., 1974a; Arnold, 1975). During chronic treatment, and especially when associated with tricyclic antidepressant medication, peak plasma levels may be attained as late as 4 to 8 h after oral dosing (Garattini and Morselli, 1974). When administered intramuscularly, diazepam is also efficiently absorbed, peak plasma levels comparable to the oral ones being attained within 1 to 3 h (Hillestadt et al., 1974; Kanto et al., 1975; Morselli, unpublished results). On the contrary, reduced and erratic diazepam absorption has been described following administration via rectal suppository, with peak plasma concentrations at 2-5 h after dosing and reaching levels of about one-third of those after oral ingestion (Schwartz et al., 1966; Arnold, 1975).

Differences in bioavailability among the various preparations have been reported (Schwartz et al., 1966; Berlin et al., 1972; Arnold, 1975), and for the commercially available tablets a bioavailability of about 75% has been recently estimated by Klotz et al. (1975). According to Sellman et al. (1975), a reduced absorption of diazepam following oral administration is a constant finding in alcoholics. In the study reported, the possible influence of concomitant drugs that might be capable of significantly modifying g.i. motility was not taken into consideration; thus further data are needed to confirm this alteration in absorption. A secondary peak may frequently be seen in plasma levels 6-12 h after a single morning drug intake and has been considered as being suggestive of an enterohepatic cycle (Baird and Hailey, 1972). A recent hypothesis, however, tends to attribute this secondary peak to an increase in postprandial plasma lipoprotein-binding (Klotz et al., 1975b; Korttila et al., 1975).

Diazepam is highly bound to plasma proteins, the free fraction ranging from 3 to 10%, according to various authors (van der Kleijn, 1969a; van der Kleijn et al., 1971; Muller and Wallert, 1973; Klotz et al., 1975; Kanto et al., 1975). The apparent volume of distribution may vary from 1.6 to 2.3 L/kg, according to Kaplan et al. (1973) and to Morselli (1977), while lower values have been reported by van der Kleijn et al. (1971) and Klotz et al. (1975). Diazepam is distributed in all body tissues, but higher amounts are usually found in adipose tissue and brain, where the drug is found present at maximal concentrations in only a few minutes after an i.v. injection (Marcucci et al., 1968; Garattini et al., 1973a; Morselli et al., 1973a; Placidi et al., 1976). Animal experiments indicate that diazepam accumulates quite differently in various parts of the brain, maximal concentrations being attained in the white matter structures in 1-3 h after drug intake (Morselli et al., 1973a; Placidi et al., 1976). The high accumulation of diazepam in adipose tissue might be an important factor in programming dosage schedules for obese patients (Garattini et al., 1973a).

The apparent plasma half-life of the terminal exponential phase may range from 15 to 60 h (mean: about 24 h) in normal, healthy volunteers, whereas it may be prolonged up to 100 h or more in elderly people and in patients with liver disease (Schwartz et al., 1965; De Silva et al., 1966; van der Kleijn et al., 1969b, 1971; Berlin et al., 1972; Garattini et al., 1973; Kaplan et al., 1973; Hillestadt et al., 1974b; Arnold, 1975; Morselli, 1977). Diazepam is extensively metabolized in the body, mainly through demethylation and hydroxylation. The major degradation products that have been so far identified are N-desmethyldiazepam, methyloxazepam (or temazepam) and oxazepam, all of which are then conjugated with glucuronic acid and excreted in the urine, mainly as glucuronide derivatives. The desmethylated metabolite (which will be discussed more extensively later), is detectable in plasma as early as 15 min after diazepam administration, and tends to accumulate in the course of repeated treatment because of its longer plasma half-life (Schwartz et al., 1965; De Silva et al., 1966; Garattini, 1969; Marcucci et al., 1969; Berlin, 1972; Hendel, 1975; Arnold, 1975). According to Kaplan et al. (1973), in humans the overall elimination of diazepam occurs via the desmethyldiazepam pathway. However, the significant amount of methyloxazepam recoverable in the urine in several cases tends to suggest that this metabolic pathway, too, may be of similar importance in man. Increased formation and elimination of methyloxazepam may frequently be ob-

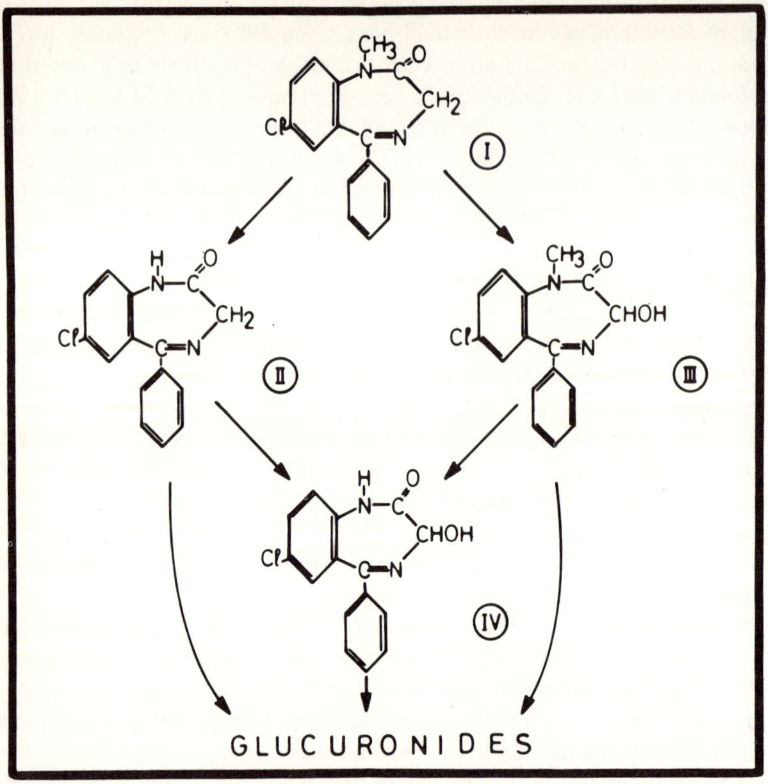

Fig. 4: Metabolism of diazepam in man. I = diazepam; II = N-desmethyl diazepam; III = N-methyloxazepam; IV = oxazepam

served in cases where concomitant administration of known metabolic inducers has occurred.

Diazepam as such is excreted in the urine only in negligible amounts (<0.5% of the dose), while 6-80% of the dose is excreted as conjugated derivatives and 10% can be recovered in feces; about 20% of the compounds present in the urine have not yet been identified (Schwartz et al., 1965). Over a period of 72-120 h, N-desmethyldiazepam found in the urine may account for 3.6-5% of the dose, methyloxazepam for 6-8% and oxazepam for 8-17% (Schwartz et al., 1965; Kaplan et al., 1973; Morselli, unpublished results). Kaplan et al. (1973) reported that following an intravenous injection of diazepam, N-desmethyldiazepam is excreted in higher amounts than after oral intake. This data is suggestive of a first-pass effect and is in apparent agreement with the more recent data of Klotz et al. (1975) indicating a bioavailability of 75%.

The possibility that diazepam may induce its own metabolism as well as that of other drugs has been postulated on several occasions (Heubel and Frank, 1970; Kanto et al., 1974). Up to now, however, no direct evidence has been presented to support such a hypothesis. The data reported by Kanto et al. (1974) as evidence of autoinduction may be open to criticism; in fact, it is very difficult to understand both how, with an augmentation in the drug's catabolism, there is an increased level of nonterminal metabolites and why the hydroxy derivatives, which are usually quickly conjugated and excreted in the urine, were found present as free compounds in the plasma. In our experience, the increased catabolism of diazepam is accompanied by a faster disappearance rate of the metabolites and, also, by the increased formation and excretion of glucuronide derivatives. An explanation of the data reported by Kanto et al. (1974) might be given on taking into consideration previous or concomitant treatments and/or direct effects of diazepam on the gastrointestinal motility. Reduced absorption, as well as a reduction in the metabolic degradation of N-desmethyldiazepam, could also explain the lower diazepam levels and the higher metabolite concentrations. The only possible direct evidence of autoinduction, i.e., the shortening of the apparent plasma half-life without modification in the apparent Vd, was not given. At variance with such data, controlled studies tend to indicate that diazepam as an inducer in man is very unlikely at the usual dosages (Breckenridge and Orme, 1973).

Diazepam steady-state plasma levels are generally achieved within 7-10 days of treatment. For dosages of 10-20 mg/day, plasma concentrations may range from 200 to 1200 ng/ml (Marcucci et al., 1970; Van der Kleijn et al., 1971; Berlin et al., 1972; Garattini et al., 1973; Dasberg et al., 1974; Hillestadt et al., 1974b; Kanto et al., 1974; Bliding, 1974; Dasberg, 1975). In all of these reports, the presence of N-desmethyldiazepam at concentrations higher than those of the parent compound has been described. From the available data on volunteers, it appears that subjective and objective effects of diazepam are evident at plasma concentrations between 80-150 ng/ml, while drowsiness, sedation and impairment of performance may be present for plasma levels over 300 ng/ml (Marcucci et al., 1970; Baird and Hailey, 1972; Bliding, 1975). Although the therapeutic threshold has not yet been clearly defined, preliminary data tend to indicate that the minimal effective concentrations in the treatment of neurotic patients in steady-state conditions are around 400-500 ng/ml (Dasberg et al., 1974; Hillestadt et al., 1975a,b). In our experience, the appearance of disturbing side effects, such as marked drowsiness, vertigo, ataxia, impairment of performance and impairment of memory, is usually associated with plasma concentrations of over 900-1000 ng/ml.

N-desmethyldiazepam

N-desmethyldiazepam is a metabolic product common to several benzodiazepines (Greenblatt and Shader, 1974). It is usually present in the plasma at concentrations higher than those of the parent compound after repeated administration of chlordiazepoxide, chlorazepate, diazepam, medazepam, prazepam and pinazepam. Animal studies have shown that N-desmethyldiazepam is the compound which is present in higher concentrations in the brain in the course of repeated administration (Placidi et al., 1976). As shown by several reports, N-desmethyldiazepam itself possesses all the properties of the compounds from which it is derived and may be considered as a key product for the hypnotic and antianxiety effects (Curry, 1970; Biscaldi et al., 1971; Tosi et al., 1973; Tansella et al., 1974, 1975; Tognoni et al., 1975; Dasberg, 1975).

Preliminary data on its kinetics in volunteers and patients were reported by Marcucci et al. (1970), van der Kleijn (1969b) and van der Kleijn et al. (1971). Following a single oral administration of 10-20 mg, the compound is readily absorbed, with peak plasma levels of 200-800 ng/ml attained 1-4 h after dosing. During the course of repeated treatment, a delay in the absorption peak of up to 8-12 h may be observed, especially after bedtime administration. *In vitro* studies indicate that the drug is about 94-97% bound to plasma protein (Van der Kleijn, 1971; Klotz et al., 1975), but a recent report from Hendel (1975) suggests that with chronic treatment the *in vivo* free fraction may be as high as 10-30%. The apparent volume of distribution at steady-state, assuming complete bioavailability, may range from 0.8 to 2.54 L/kg, according to Tognoni et al. (1975). The apparent plasma half-life of N-desmethyldiazepam is considerably longer than that of diazepam and of the other benzodiazepines from which it is derived—a fact which explains its accumulation in the course of repeated treatment. The T½ values reported may range from 30 to 90 h following single or multiple administration (van der Kleijn, 1971; Tognoni et al., 1975). A biexponential decay after discontinuation of repeated treatment, suggesting the possibility of a saturation kinetics for this class of drugs, has been recently observed by Tognoni et al. (1975).

The drug is mainly degraded via both hydroxylation to oxazepam and conjugation with glucuronic acid. Only 1-2% of the administered dose is found in the urine as free N-desmethyldiazepam. In the urine, the main fraction is represented by oxazepam glucuronide (about 50-60%). While Tognoni et al. (1975) found no clear relationship between the hypnosedative effect and the N-desmethyldiazepam steady-state plasma levels, according to Curry (1970) and Dasberg (1975) a relationship may be observed between rating of anxiety and performance tests and the plasma levels of the drug. More recently, a clear relationship between N-desmethyldiazepam plasma levels and objective measures of "hangover" was reported by Tansella et al. (1975), who noticed that higher levels were associated with a lower increment of performance.

The side effects of N-desmethyldiazepam are similar to those encountered with other benzodiazepines: somnolence, vertigo, slurring of speech, blurred vision, incoordination of motor performance, impairment of memory, ataxia, weakness and muscular hypotonia. As in the case of diazepam, the abrupt discontinuation of prolonged treatment with the drug may provoke withdrawal symptoms in some individuals. For a more complete review of the undesirable reactions to benzodiazepines, the reader should refer to the excellent monograph recently published by Greenblatt and Shader (1974).

Newborns, Infants and Children

Diazepam and other benzodiazepines are widely used during pregnancy and labor, either to induce sedation and muscular relaxation or for the treatment of eclampsia and severe pre-eclampsia (Bepko et al., 1965; Toulouse and Maffei, 1965; Berger, 1966; Flowers et al., 1969; Friedman et al., 1969; Joyce and Kenyon, 1972; Lean et al., 1972; Shannon et al., 1972; Eliot et al., 1975). While their use has been considered completely safe for years, recent reports have pointed out that the administration of large doses of diazepam to the mother in the days preceding the delivery may lead to undesirable effects in the newborn such as low Apgar scores, hypotonia, hypothermia, impaired response to cold stress and respiratory and neurological depression (Flowers et al., 1969; Shannon et al., 1972; Owen et al., 1972; Scher et al., 1972; André et al., 1972; Cree et al., 1973; McCarthy et al., 1973; Thearle et al., 1973). As documented by several reports, diazepam and its metabolites can readily and promptly cross the placenta and may also be administered to the newborn through breast-feeding (Cavanagh and Condo, 1964; De Silva et al., 1964; Idanpaan-Heikkila et al., 1971; Shannon et al., 1972; Erkkola and Kanto, 1972; Patrick et al., 1972; Sereni et al., 1973a, Erkkola et al., 1973; Thearle et al., 1973; Kanto et al., 1973, 1974; Mandelli et al., 1975; Eliot et al., 1975).

Concentrations similar to those present in maternal plasma, for both diazepam and N-desmethyldiazepam, may be observed as early as 20-40 min after a single administration of 10 mg by either intravenous or intramuscular route (Mandelli et al., 1975). An equilibrium between maternal and fetal concentrations is usually achieved within 3-4 h. Following repeated treatment to the mother, the concentrations of both diazepam and N-desmethyldiazepam tend to be higher in the cord than in the mother.

Mandelli et al. (1975) have recently reported *in vivo* evidence for the presence of enzymatic N-demethylating activity in the fetus. On the contrary, hydroxylated metabolites, present in cord blood in a few cases, were of maternal origin. The concentrations usually found in the cord plasma at birth, after 10 or 20 mg of diazepam have been administered to the mother a few hours before the delivery, may range from 20 to 300 ng/ml for both diazepam and N-desmethyldiazepam; however, during the course of repeated treatment, concentrations as high as 1800 ng/ml have been observed (Owen et al., 1972; Kanto et al., 1973, 1974; Cree et al., 1973; Mandelli et al., 1975; Eliot et al., 1975). Concentrations of over 300-400 ng/ml are usually associated with the undesirable effects described above.

Table 1. Effect of Age and/or Exposure to Inducing Agents on Diazepam Disposition

Age Group	Type of Treatment	Apparent Half Life (h)	Apparent Vd (L/kg)	Metabolites Present in 24 h Urine*		
				NDZ	MOX	OX
Premature newborns	a	75 ± 35	1.8 ± 0.3	90-95	<1	<1
	b	11	n.d.	n.d.	n.d.	n.d.
Full-Term newborns	a	31 ± 2	n.d.	66-90	0.2-12	0-13
	b	18 ± 1	n.d.	18-21	23-41	37-58
	c	29 ± 1	n.d.	34-35	48-63	2-14
Infants	a	10 ± 2	1.3 ± 0.2	25-35	30-40	30-34
Children	a	17 ± 3	2.6 ± 0.5	26-40	18-52	18-53

[a]Single dose of diazepam either directly to the child or to the mother, no exposure to barbiturates.
[b]Previous exposure to barbiturates either during intrauterine life or during first days of extrauterine life.
[c]Repeated administration to the mother without concomitant treatment with barbiturates.
*Data are expressed as relative percentage of the excreted material.
n.d.: No data available.
Figures are derived from personal data and from data available in the literature reported in the text.

Given either orally or intramuscularly, diazepam is readily and efficiently absorbed in *newborns*, with peak plasma levels attained within 30–60 min after oral intake and 1 to 4 h after intramuscular administration. Although Krasner and Yaffe (1975) did not observe any difference for diazepam in the binding properties between cord and adult serum, this does not exclude differences in binding due to the variation in protein concentrations. In fact, Kanto et al. (1974) reported a binding of 86% for diazepam in cord serum, against a corresponding protein-binding of 96% in the mothers. The apparent volume of distribution in premature newborns is lower than the range observed in adults, and the computed mean values may vary from 1.1 to 1.8 L/kg (Morselli et al., 1973; Morselli, 1977).

The apparent plasma disappearance rate of diazepam, either administered directly to the newborn in the first few days of life or transferred transplacentally, is extremely slow. The rate of disappearance appears to be related to the degree of maturation. An apparent plasma half-life of 40 to 100 h (mean: 75 h) has been reported for premature newborns (Morselli et al., 1972, 1973; Morselli, 1974, 1977), whereas in full-term newborns the apparent plasma half-life may range from 20 to 45 h (mean: 31 h) (Sereni et al., 1973b; Morselli, 1974; Morselli et al., 1974a; Mandelli et al., 1975). Similar data for full-term newborns (T½ = 40–50 h) can be obtained by computing the mean data from other authors (Cree et al., 1973; Eliot, 1975). The slower disposition rate of diazepam in newborns is due to the reduced metabolic degradation of the compound, which is documented both by a slower formation rate of N-desmethyldiazepam (K = 0.097 in newborns against a K of 0.179 in children) and by a limited hydroxylation of both diazepam and N-desmethyldiazepam (Morselli et al., 1973; Cree et al., 1973; Sereni et al., 1973; Morselli, 1974, 1976; Kanto et al., 1974; Eliot, 1975).

In fact, very limited amounts of hydroxylated metabolites, if any, can be found in the 24–48 h urine of premature or full-term newborns who have received the drug, either directly or through the mother a few hours before delivery. In these cases, 70–80% of the benzodiazepines present in the urine are in the form of conjugated N-desmethyldiazepam, while methyloxazepam and oxazepam represent only 10–20% (Morselli et al., 1972, 1973; Sereni et al., 1973b; Mandelli et al., 1975). Our data have been recently confirmed by Eliot et al. (1975), who observed that during the first 24 hours of life N-desmethyldiazepam accounted for 66% for urinary metabolites while methyloxazepam and oxazepam represented only 13% and 12%, respectively. A consistent amount of hydroxy derivatives can be found in the urine of newborns whose mothers have received repeated diazepam administration (Kanto et al., 1974; Morselli et al., 1974a; Mandelli, 1975). Most of these hydroxylated derivatives, free and conjugated, are of maternal origin, as was well-documented by Mandelli et al. (1975), and are not due to the newborns' metabolism.

On the contrary, after diazepam administration, an increased output of hydroxylated benzodiazepine derivatives, due to an increased metabolic degradation of diazepam by the newborn, may be observed in those cases with previous exposure to inducing agents (such as phenobarbital) either during intrauterine life or immediately after birth (Sereni et al., 1973; Morselli et al., 1974a, 1977). In such cases, a consistent drop in the apparent plasma half-life (10–12 h), together with marked excretion of methyloxazepam and oxazepam (80–90% of urinary metabolites), may be observed (Morselli, 1974a, 1976) (Table 1). These data emphasize the need to be more cautious in evaluating newborn metabolizing activities solely from urinary data; this fact is especially relevant in those cases in which the mothers have received repeated and multiple drug treatment.

In *infants,* diazepam administered by the oral route, as a syrup, is readily absorbed, and peak plasma levels of 300–600 ng/ml are achieved 15–30 min after a dose of 0.3 mg/kg. In a recent report, Agurell et al. (1975) described peak plasma levels of 380 and 420 ng/ml within 30 min in two infants given 0.4 and 0.8 ng/kg by intramuscular injection. The same authors reported that, following administration by the rectal route through "rectiols," the absorption appeared to be considerably faster, with peak levels of 435–1135 ng/ml achieved after doses of 0.23 and 0.45 mg/kg, respectively. As in adults, the use of suppositories is not advisable because of inefficient and erratic absorption.

The apparent volume of distribution in infants may range from 1.3 to 1.5 L/kg (Morselli, 1975); unfortunately, no data on plasma protein-binding are available. As observed for other drugs, the apparent plasma half-life of diazepam in infants is remarkably faster than in neonates and in children, the values ranging from 8 to 14 h (Morselli and Tognoni, 1974; Morselli, 1974, 1975). The increase in the apparent disposition rate is accompanied by enhanced formation of hydroxylated metabolites which are mainly excreted as the glucuronide derivatives. Hydroxy derivatives, in the 48 h urine following a single administration, may account for 60–70% of the urinary metabolites (Morselli, 1975). It may be of interest to note that no impairment of diazepam absorption has been observed in the course of malabsorption syndromes (Mandelli and Sereni, unpublished results).

In children, as in infants, oral absorption of diazepam is more rapid than in adults. Peak plasma levels of 400–500 ng/ml are achieved within 15–30 min after an oral dose of about 0.25 mg/kg (Marcucci et al., 1970; Garattini et al., 1973). According to our experience, following intramuscular administration, peak levels are usually attained within 1 to 4 h; however, more recently, Agurell et al. (1975) reported a much faster absorption, with peak levels 20–30 min after an intramuscular injection of 0.23–0.36 mg/kg. Differences in the injection site (see Chapter 2) could possibly explain the discrepancy. In children as in infants, the administration by "rectiols" give a very fast and reliable absorption, with peak plasma levels achieved within 10–30 min, and plasma concentrations ranging from 200 to 1200 ng/ml are attained at doses of 0.23–0.39 mg/kg (Agurell et al., 1975). There are no data on the plasma protein-binding of diazepam in children, and the computed apparent volume of distribution may range from 2.2 to 3.0 L/kg (Morselli, 1975).

According to the available data, the apparent plasma half-life of diazepam in children may range from 15 to 21 h, the mean value being 18 h (Morselli and Tognoni, 1974; Morselli, 1974, 1977). About 59–93% of the metabolites found in the 24 h urine collection are represented by conjugated hydroxy derivatives, while N-desmethyldiazepam, present mostly as the glucuronide, may account for 26 to 40% of the excreted material (Morselli et al., 1973; Morselli, 1977).

From the data reported, it appears that diazepam disposition may vary significantly with development (Table 1). Premature and full-term newborns dispose of diazepam and its metabolites at a much lower rate than do infants and children. The latter two groups, on the other hand, metabolize the drug faster than adults and elderly people. The reduced disposition in newborns is apparently due to a slow rate of demethylation and hydroxylation, which leads to elevated, prolonged plasma levels of diazepam. The persistence of high concentrations of diazepam and of its metabolites, together with the reduced serum protein-binding reported by Kanto et al. (1973), would seem to indicate that special care may be necessary for neonates whose mothers have received large doses of diazepam during labor. It is also important to note that an increase in plasma levels at 5–7 days of age, probably due to release of the drug from tissue stores, has been reported in some cases by various authors (Cree et al., 1973; Kanto et al., 1974; Eliot, 1975).

The situation may, however, be completely different if the premature and full-term newborns were exposed to phenobarbital. In such cases, the metabolic degradation of diazepam may proceed at a rate that is higher than that observed in infants and children. On the other hand, infants and children absorb diazepam faster and more efficiently than do adults and, also, dispose of it at a higher rate.

CONCLUSIONS

Our knowledge on the pharmacokinetics of psychotropic drugs in pediatric age is very poor. The need for more detailed information not only on drug kinetics but also on therapeutic and toxic levels is so evident that further stress is unnecessary in the light of the wide use of these agents both in preschool and in school-age children. On the basis of the limited information available, there are few considerations which can be made. It appears that newborns dispose of lipophilic drugs (which most of the psychoactive drugs are) at an extremely low rate, mainly for a relative deficiency of hydroxylative pathways. Hydroxylation is a common metabolic route for most of the compounds in this class.

Many of the psychotropic agents considered produce their effects through a modification of biogenic amine neurotransmitters. The possibility that active concentrations of the above mentioned compounds may be present in the brain of newborns who received them transplacentally must be borne in mind. Since nothing is practically known on the acute or long-term effects of a prolonged exposure to these agents in the first days of life, it would probably be safer to consider newborns exposed to psychotropic drugs as "at risk." On the other hand, the data available on infants and children suggest that they absorb and dispose of many of these agents at a rate considerably higher than do adults.

These observations should challenge the increasing usage of a single high dose at night, considering on the one hand the possibility of severe side effects (such as cardiac effects) during the absorption peak, and on the other the wide fluctuations in plasma levels due to the higher disposition rate. It appears that at least up to 7–10 years, 2–3 divided doses during the day would provide a safer and more rational dosage schedule.

Finally, on the basis of what has been observed with benzodiazepines, the possibility of a completely different kinetic situation due to exposure to agents capable of drug interaction at various levels must always be considered, especially when treating newborns and infants.

REFERENCES

Agarwala, S. and Heycock, J.B. (1968): A controlled trial of imipramine in the treatment of childhood enuresis. *British Journal of Clinical Practice, 22:* 296-298.

Agurell, S., Berlin, A., Ferngren, H. and Hellström, B. (1975): Plasma levels of diazepam after parenteral and rectal administration in children. *Epilepsia, 16:* 277-283.

Alajem, M. and Albagli, C. (1962): Severe imipramine poisoning in an infant. *American Journal of Diseases of Children, 103:* 702-705.

Alderton, H.R. (1970): Imipramine in childhood enuresis: further studies on the relationship of time and administration to effect. *Canadian Medical Association Journal, 102:* 1179-1180.

Alexanderson, B. (1972): Pharmacokinetics of nortriptyline in man after single and multiple oral doses: the prectability of steady-state plasma concentrations from single dose plasma level data. *European Journal of Clinical Pharmacology, 4:* 82-91.

Alexanderson, B. (1973): Prediction of steady-state plasma levels of nortriptyline from single oral dose kinetics: a study in twins. *European Journal of Clinical Pharmacology, 6:* 44-53.

Alexanderson, B., Åsberg, M. and Tuck, D. (1973a): Relationships between the steady-state plasma concentration of nortriptyline and some of its pharmacological effects. In: *Biological Effects of Drugs in Relation to their Plasma Concentrations,* edited by D.S. Davies and B.N.C. Prichard, pp. 191-199, Macmillan, London.

Alexanderson, B. and Borgå, O. (1972): Interindividual differences in plasma protein binding of nortriptyline in man. A twin study. *European Journal of Clinical Pharmacology, 4:* 196-200.

Alexanderson, B. and Borgå, O. (1973): Urinary excretion of nortriptyline and five of its metabolites in man after single and multiple oral doses. *European Journal of Clinical Pharmacology, 5:* 174-180.

Alexanderson, B., Borgå, O. and Alván, G. (1973b): The availability of orally administered nortriptyline. *European Journal of Clinical Pharmacology, 5:* 181-185.

Alexanderson, B., Evans, P.D.A. and Sjöqvist, F. (1969): Steady-state plasma levels of nortriptyline in twins: influence of genetic factors and drug therapy. *British Medical Journal, 4:* 764-768.

Alexanderson, B. and Sjöqvist, F. (1971): Individual differences in the pharmacokinetics of monomethylated tricyclic antidepressants role of genetic and environmental factors and clinical importance. *Annals of the New York Academy of Sciences, 171:* 739-751.

Alexanderson, B. and Sjöqvist, F. (1973): Pharmacokinetic and genetic studies of nortriptyline and desmethylimipramine in man. In: *Pharmacology and the Future of Man,* edited by G.T. Okita and G.H. Acheson, V. 3, pp. 150-162, Karger, Basel.

Allgen, L.G., Jönsson, B., Nauckhoff, B., Andersen, M.L. Huus, I. and Møller Nielsen, I. (1960): On the elimination of chlorprotixene in rat and man. *Experientia, 16:* 325.

Allgen, L.G., Hellström, L. and Sant'Orp, C.J. (1963): On the metabolism and elimination of the psychotropic phenothiazine drug levomepromazine (Norzinan R) in man. *Acta Psychiatrica Scandinavica, 39,* suppl. 169: 366-381.

André, M., Sibout, M., Petry, J.-M. and Vert, P. (1973): Depression respiratoire et neurologique chez le prematuré nouveau-né de mère traitée par Diazepam. *Journal of Gynecologie, Obsterique et Biologie de la Reproduction, 2:* 375-366.

Arneson, G.A. (1961): A near fatal case of imipramine overdosage. *American Journal of Psychiatry, 117:* 934-936.

Arnold, E. (1975): A simple method for determining diazepam and its major metabolites in biological fluids: applications in bioavailability studies. *Acta Pharmacologica et Toxicologica, 36:* 335-350.

Åsberg, M. (1974): Plasma nortriptyline levels—relationship to clinical effects. *Clinical Pharmacology and Therapeutics, 16:* 215-229.

Åsberg, M., Cronholm, B., Sjöqvist, F. and Tuck, D. (1970): Correlation of subjective side effects with plasma concentrations of nortriptyline. *British Medical Journal, 4:* 18-21.

Åsberg, M., Cronholm, B., Sjöqvist, F. and Tuck, D. (1971a): Relationship between plasma level and therapeutic effect or nortriptyline. *British Medical Journal, 3:* 331-334.

Åsberg, M., Evans, D.A.P. and Sjöqvist, F. (1971b): Genetic control of nortriptyline kinetics in man: a study of relatives of propositi with high plasma concentrations. *Journal of Medical Genetics, 8:* 129-135.

Åsberg, M. and Germanis, M. (1972): Ophthalmological effects of nortriptyline-relationship to plasma level. *Pharmacology, 7:* 349-356.

Baird, E.S. and Hailey, D.M. (1972): Delayed recovery from a sedative: correlation of the plasma levels of diazepam with clinical effects after oral and intravenous administration. *British Journal of Anaesthesiology, 44:* 803-803.

Ban, T. (1969): The thioxanthenes. In: *Psychopharmacology,* edited by T. Ban, p. 258, Williams & Wilkins, Baltimore.

Barnes, R.J., Kong, S.M. and Wu, R.W. (1968): Electrocardiographic changes in amitriptyline poisoning. *British Medical Journal, 3:* 222.

Beckett, A.H., Beaven, M.A. and Robinson, A.E. (1963): Metabolism of chlorpromazine in humans. *Biochemical Pharmacology, 12:* 779-794.

Beckett, A.H. and Al Sarraj, S. (1973): Metabolism of amitriptyline, nortriptyline, imipramine and desipramine to yield hydroxylamines. *Journal of Pharmacy and Pharmacology, 25:* 335-336.

Belvedere, G., Burti, L., Frigerio, A. and Pantarotto, C. (1975): Gas chromatographic-mass fragmentographic determination of "steady-state" plasma levels of imipramine and desipramine in chronically treated patients. *Journal of Chromatography, 111:* 313-321.

Bepko, F., Lowe, E. and Waxman, b. (1965): Relief of the emotional factor in labor with parenterally administered isazepam. *Obstetrics and Gynecology, 26:* 852-857.

Berger, M. (1966): Die anwendung von 7-Chlor-1,3-dihydro-1-methyl-5-phenyl-2H1,4-benzodiazepin-2-on (Diazepam) bei 3000 Gebärenden. *Arzneimittel Forschung, 16:* 1110-1113.

Berling, A., Siwers, B., Agurell, S., Hiort, A., Sjöqvist, F. and Ström, S. (1972): Determination of bioavailability of diazepam in various formulations from steady state plasma concentration data. *Clinical Pharmacology and Therapeutics, 13:* 733-744.

Berling, R., Mjorndal, J., Oreland, L., Rapp, W. and Wold, S. (1975): Plasma levels and clinical effects of thioridazine and thiothixene. *Journal of Clinical Pharmacology, 15:* 178-186.

Bertilsson, L. and Alexanderson, B. (1972): Stereospecific hydroxylation of nortriptyline in man in relation to interindividual differences in its steady-state plasma level. *European Journal of Clinical Pharmacology, 4:* 201-205.

Bickel, M.H. (1969): Pharmacokinetic studies in animals as a model system for human therapy. In: *The present status of psychotropic drugs.* Proc. VI Int. Congr. Collegium Internationale Neuropsychopharmacologicum, Tarragona, 1968, Excerpta Medica, Amsterdam.

Bickel, M.H., Brochon, R., Friolet, B., Hermann, B. and Stofer, A.R. (1967): Clinical and biochemical results of a fatal case of desipramine intoxication. *Psychopharmacologia, 10:* 431-436.

Bickel, M.H. and Weder, H.J. (1969): Buccal absorption and other properties of pharmacokinetic importance of imipramine and its metabolites. *Journal of Pharmacy and Pharmacology, 21:* 160-168.

Biscaldi, G.P., Hattab, J., Montanaro, N. and Scoz, R. (1971): Quantitative polygraphic evaluation of emotional tension in the study of a new benzodiazepine. *Current Therapeutic Research, 13:* 606-615.

Bliding, Å. (1974): Effects of different rates of absorption of two benzodiazepines on subjective and objective parameters. *European Journal of Clinical Pharmacology, 7:* 201-211.

Bolt, A.G., Forrest, I.S. and Serra, M.T. (1966): Quantitative studies of urinary excretion of chlorpromazine metabolites in chronically-dosed psychiatric patients. *Journal of Pharmaceutical Sciences, 55:* 1205-1208.

Borgå, O., Azarnoff, D.L. and Sjöqvist, F. (1968): Species differences in the plasma protein binding of desipramine. *Journal of Pharmacy and Pharmacology, 20:* 571.

Borgå, O., Azarnoff, D.L., Forshell, G.P. and Sjöqvist, F. (1969): Plasma protein binding of tricyclic antidepressants in man. *Biochemical Pharmacology, 18:* 2135-2143.

Borgå, O. and Garle, M. (1972): A gas chromatographic method for the quantitative determination of nortriptyline and some of its metabolites in human plasma and urine. *Journal of Chromatography, 68:* 77-88.

Brackenridge, R.G. (1972): Cardiotoxicity of amitriptyline. *Lancet, II:* 929-930.

Brackenridge, R.G., Peters, T.J. and Watson, J.M. (1968): Myocardial damage in amitriptyline and nortriptyline poisoning. *Scottish Medical Journal, 13:* 208-210.

Braithwaite, R.A. and Widdop, B. (1971): A specific gas-chromatographic method for the measurements of "steady-state" plasma levels of amitriptyline and nortriptyline in patients. *Clinica Chimica Acta, 35:* 461-472.

Braithwaite, R.A., Goulding, R., Theano, G., Bailey, J. and Coppen, A. (1972): Plasma concentration of amitriptyline and clinical response. *Lancet, I:* 1297-1300.

Breckenridge, A. and Orme, M. (1973): Interaction of benzodiazepines with oral anticoagulants. In: *The Benzodiazepines,* edited by S. Garattini, E. Mussini and O. Randall, pp. 647-654, Raven Press, New York.

Brown, K.G.E., McMichen, H.U.S. and Briggs, D.S. (1972): Tachyarrhythmia in severe imipramine overdose controlled by practolol. *Archives of Diseases in Childhood, 47:* 104-106.

Burrows, G.D., Davies, B. and Scoggins, B.A. (1972): Plasma concentration of nortriptyline and clinical response in depressive illness. *Lancet, II:* 629-623.

Burrows, G., Scoggins, B.A., Turecek, L.R. and Davies, B. (1974): Plasma nortriptyline and clinical response. *Clinical Pharmacology and Therapeutics, 16:* 639-644.

Cameron, B.D., Chasseaud, L.F., Lewis, J.D. and Taylor, T. (1974): The disposition of butriptyline in rats, dogs and man. *Arzneimittel-Forschung, 24:* 93-96.

Campbell, I.C. and Todrick, A. (1970): Plasma protein binding of tricyclic antidepressive drugs. *Journal of Pharmacy and Pharmacology, 22:* 226.

Campbell, M., Fish, B. and Shapiro, T. (1971): Imipramine in preschool autistic and schizophrenic children. *Journal of Autism and Childhood Schizophrenia, 1:* 267-282.

Cavanagh, D. and Condo, C.S. (1964): Diazepam—a pilot study of drug concentrations in maternal blood, amniotic fluid and cord blood. *Current Therapeutic Research, 6:* 122-126.

Chan, T.L., Sakalis, G. and Gershon, S. (1974): Quantitation of chlorpromazine and its metabolites in human plasma and urine by direct spectrodensitometry of thin-layer chromatograms. In: *The Phenothiazines and Structurally Related Drugs,* edited by I.S. Forrest, C.J. Carr and E. Usdin, pp. 323-333, Raven Press, New York.

Charalampous, K.D. and Johnson, P.C. (1967): Studies of C^{14}-protriptyline in man: plasma levels and excretion. *Journal of Clinical Pharmacology, 7:* 93-96.

Christiansen, J., Gram, L.F., Kofod, B. and Rafaelsen, O.J. (1967): Imipramine metabolism in man. *Psychopharmacologia, 11:* 255-264.
Christiansen, J. and Gram, L.F. (1973): Imipramine and its metabolites in human brain. *Journal of Pharmacy and Pharmacology, 25:* 604-608.
Coccia, P.F. and Westerfeld, W.W. (1967): The metabolism of chlorpromazine by liver microsomal enzyme systems. *Journal of Pharmacology and Experimental Therapeutics, 157:* 466-458.
Cole, J.O. and Davis, J.M. (1967): Antidepressant drugs. In: *Comprehensive Textbook of Psychiatry*, edited by A.M. Freedman and H.I. Kaplan, pp. 1263-1275, Williams & Wilkins, Baltimore.
Consolo, S., Morselli, P.L., Zaccala, M. and Garattini, S. (1970): Delayed absorption of phenylbutazone caused by desmethylimipramine in humans. *European Journal of Pharmacology, 10:* 239-242.
Cooper, S.F., Albert, J.M. and Dugal, R. (1975a): Gas-liquid chromatographic determination of penfluridol in plasma. *International Pharmacopsychiatry, 10:* 78-88.
Cooper, S.F., Dugal, R. Albert, J.M. and Bertrand, M. (1975b): Penfluridol steady-state pharmacokinetics in psychiatric patients. *Journal of Clinical Pharmacology*, in press.
Coull, D.C., Crooks, J., Dingwall-Fordyce, I., Scott, A.M. and Weir, R.D. (1970): A method of monitoring drugs for adverse reactions. II. Amitryptiline and cardiac disease. *European Journal of Clinical Pharmacology, 3:* 51-55.
Craig, J.C., Garland, W.A., Gruenke, L.D., Kray, L.R. and Walker, K.A.M. (1974): The use of combined gas chromatography-mass spectrometry techniques for the identification of hydroxylated and dihydroxylated metabolites of phenothiazines drug. In: *The Phenothiazines and Structurally Related Drugs*, edited by I.S. Forrest, C.J. Carr and E. Usdin, p. 405, Raven Press, New York.
Crammer, J.L. and Scott, B. (1966): New metabolites of imipramine. *Psychopharmacologia* (Berlin), *8:* 461-468.
Crammer, J.L., Scott, B., Woods, H. and Rolfe, B. (1968): Metabolism of ^{14}C-imipramine. Excretion in the rat and in man. *Psychopharmacologia* (Berlin), *12:* 263-277.
Crammer, J.L., Scott, B. and Rolfe, B. (1969): Metabolism of [^{14}C]-imipramine. II. Urinary metabolites in man. *Psychopharmacologia* (Berlin), *15:* 207-225.
Cree, J.E., Meyer, J. and Hailey, D.M. (1973): Diazepam in labour: its metabolism and effect on the clinical condition and thermogenesis of the newborn. *British Medical Journal, 4:* 251-255.
Cressman, W.A., Bianchine, J.R., Slotnick, V.B., Johnson, P.C. and Plostnieks, J. (1974): Plasma level profile of haloperidol in man following intramuscular administration. *European Journal of Clinical Pharmacology, 7:* 99-103.
Curry, A.S. (1964): Seven fatal cases involving imipramine in man. *Journal of Pharmacy and Pharmacology, 16:* 265-267.
Curry, S.H. (1971): Chlorpromazine: concentrations in plasma, excretion in urine and duration of effect. *Proceedings of The Royal Society of Medicine, 64:* 285-289.
Curry, S.H. (1974): Concentration-effect relationship with major and minor tranquilizers. *Clinical Pharmacology and Therapeutics, 16:* 192-197.
Curry, S.H., Davis, J.M., Janowsky, D.S. and Marshall, J.H.L. (1969): Interpatient variation in physiological availability of chlorpromazine as a complicating factor in correlation studies of drug metabolism and clinical effect. In: *The Present Status of Psychotropic Drugs*, edited by A. Cerletti and F.J. Bovè, pp. 72-76. Excerpta Medica, Amsterdam.
Curry, S.H., Davis, J.M., Janowsky, D.S. and Marshall, J.H.L. (1970a): Factors affecting chlorpromazine plasma levels in psychiatric patients. *Archives of General Psychiatry, 22:* 209-215.
Curry, S.H., O'Millo, A. and Mould, G.P. (1971): Destruction of chlorpromazine during

absorption in the rat in vivo and in vitro. *British Journal of Pharmacology, 42:* 403-411.
Curry, S.H. and Marshall, J.H.L. (1968): Plasma levels of chlorpromazine and some of its relatively non-polar metabolites in psychiatric patients. *Life Sciences, 7:* 9-17.
Curry, S.H., Marshall, J.H.L., Davis, J.M. and Janowsky, D.S. (1970b): Chlorpromazine plasma levels and effects. *Archives of General Psychiatry, 22:* 289-296.
Daly, J.W. and Manian, A.A. (1969): The action of catechol-o-methyltransferase on 7,8-dihydroxychlorpromazine formation of 7-hydroxy-8-methoxychlorpromazine and 8-hydroxy-7-methoxychlorpromazine. *Biochemical Pharmacology, 18:* 1235-1238.
Dasberg, H.H. (1975): Effects and plasma levels of N-desmethyldiazepam after oral administration in normal volunteers. *Psychopharmacologia* (Berlin), *43:* 191-198.
Dasberg, H.H. van der Kleijn, E., Guelen, P.J.R. and Van Praag, H.M. (1974): Plasma concentrations of diazepam and its metabolite N-desmethyldiazepam in relation to anxiolytic effect. *Clinical Pharmacology and Therapeutics, 15:* 473-483.
Davidson, J.D., Terry, I.L. and Sjoerdsma, A. (1957): Action and metabolism of chlorpromazine sulfoxide in man. *Journal of Pharmacology and Experimental Therapeutics, 125:* 8-12.
Davis, J.M., Janowsky, D.S., Sekerke, H.J., Manier, H. and Khaled El-yousef, M. (1974): The pharmacokinetics of butaperazine in serum. In: *The Phenothiazines and Structurally Related Drugs,* edited by I.S. Forrest, C.J. Carr and E. Usdin, pp. 433-443, Raven Press, New York.
De Silva, J.A.F., Schwartz, M.A., Stefanovic, V., Kaplan, J. and D'Arconte, L. (1964a): Determination of diazepam (Valium) in blood, by gas liquid chromatography. *Analytical Chemistry, 36:* 2099-2105.
De Silva, J.A.F., D'Arconte, L. and Kaplan, J. (1964b): The determination of blood levels and the placental transfer of diazepam in humans. *Current Therapeutic Research, 6:* 115-121.
De Silva, J.A.F., Koechlin, B.A. and Bader, G. (1966): Blood level distribution patterns of diazepam and its major metabolite in man. *Journal of Pharmaceutical Sciences, 55:* 692-702.
Di Mascio, A. and Solty, J.J. (1970): Psychotropic drug side effects in children. In: *Psychotropic Drug Side Effects. Clinical and Theoretical Perspective,* edited by A. Di Mascio and R.I. Shader, pp. 235-260, Williams & Wilkins, Baltimore.
Dingell, J.V., Sulser, F. and Gillette, J.R. (1964): Species differences in the metabolism of imipramine and desmethylimipramine (DMI). *Journal of Pharmacology and Experimental Therapeutics, 143:* 14-22.
Douglas, B.H. and Hume, A.S. (1967): Placental transfer of imipramine, a basic lipid-soluble drug. *American Journal of Obstetrics and Gynecology, 99:* 573-575.
Drew, L.R.H. (1966): Control of enuresis by imipramine. *Medical Journal of Australia, 2:* 1225-1227.
Dunitz, J.D., Eser, H. and Strickler, P. (1964): Die konfiguration des physiologisch wirksamen 2-Chlor-9-(w-dimethylaminopropyliden)-thioxanthens. *Helvetica Chimica Acta, 47:* 1897-1902.
Eiduson, S. and Geller, E. (1963): The excretion and metabolism of ^{35}S-labeled thioridazine in urine, blood, bile and feces. *Biochemical Pharmacology, 12:* 1529-1435.
Eliot, B.W., Hill, J.G., Cope, A.P. and Hailey, D.M. (1975): Continuous pethidine/diazepam infusion during labour and its effects on the newborn. *British Journal of Obstetrics and Gynecology, 82:* 126-131.
Emmerson, J.L. and Miya, T.S. (1963): Metabolism of phenothiazine drugs. *Journal of Pharmaceutical Sciences, 52:* 411-419.
Erkkola, R. and Kanto, J. (1972): Diazepam and breast-feeding. *Lancet, I:* 1235.
Erkkola, R., Kangas, L. and Pekkarinen, A. (1973): The transfer of diazepam across the placenta during labour. *Acta Obstetrica Gynecologica Scandinavica, 52:* 167-170.

Eschenhof, E. and Rieder, J. (1969): Untersuchungen über das Schicksal des Antidepressivums Amitriptylin im Organismus der Ratte und des Menschen. *Arzneimittel Forschung, 19:* 957-966.
Faigle, J.W. and Dieterle, W. (1973): The metabolism and pharmacokinetic of clomipramine (Anafranil). *Journal of Internal Medical Research, 1:* 281-290.
Falletta, J.M., Stansey, C.R. and Mintz, A.A. (1970): Amitriptyline poisoning treated with physostigmine. *Southern Medical Journal, 63:* 1492-1493.
Fishman, V. and Goldenberg, H. (1960): Metabolism of chlorpromazine: organic extractable fraction from human urine. *Proceedings of the Society for Experimental Biology and Medicine, 104:* 99-103.
Fishman, V. and Goldenberg, H. (1962): Identification of a new metabolite of imipramine. *Proceedings of the Society for Experimental Biology and Medicine, 110:* 187-190.
Fishman, V. and Goldenberg, H. (1963): Metabolism of chlorpromazine. IV. Identification of 7-hydroxychlorpromazine and its sulfoxide and desmethyl derivatives. *Proceedings of the Society for Experimental Biology and Medicine, 112:* 501-506.
Fishman, V. and Goldenberg, H. (1965): Side-chain degradation and ring hydroxylation of phenothiazine tranquilizers. *Journal of Pharmacology and Experimental Therapeutics, 150:* 122-127.
Fishman, V., Heaton, A. and Goldenberg, H. (1962): Metabolism of chlorpromazine-N-oxide. *Proceedings of the Society for Experimental Biology and Medicine, 109:* 548-552.
Flowers, C.E., Rudolph, A.J. and Desmond, M.M. (1969): Diazepam (Valium) as an adjunct in obstetric analgesia. *Obstetrics and Gynecology, 34:* 68-81.
Forrest, F.M., Forrest, I.S. and Serra, M.T. (1970): Modification of chlorpromazine metabolism by some other drugs frequently administered to psychiatric patients. *Biological Psychiatry, 2:* 53-58.
Forrest, I.S., Fox, J., Green, D.E., Melkian, A.P. and Serra, M.T. (1974): Total excretion of 3H-chlorpromazine and 3H-prochlorperazine in chronically dosed animals: balance sheet. In: *Phenothiazines and Structurally Related Drugs,* edited by I.S. Forrest, C.J. Carr and E. Usdin, pp. 347-356, Raven Press, New York.
Freeman, J.W., Mundy, G.R., Beattie, R.R. and Ryan, C. (1969): Cardiac abnormalities in poisoning with tricyclic antidepressants. *British Medical Journal, 2:* 610-611.
Freeman, J.W. and Loughhead, M.G. (1973): Beta blockade in the treatment of tricyclic antidepressant overdosage. *Medical Journal of Australia, 1:* 233-238.
Freyschuss, U., Sjöqvist, F., Tuck, D. and Åsberg, M. (1970): Circulatory effects in man of nortriptyline, a tricyclic antidepressant drug. *Pharmacologia Clinica, 2:* 68-71.
Friedman, E.A., Niswander, K.R. and Sachtleben, M.R. (1969): Effect of diazepam on labor. *Obstetrics and Gynecology, 34:* 82-86.
Frigerio, A., Belvedere, G., De Nadai, F., Fanelli, R., Pantarotto, C., Riva, E. and Morselli, P.L. (1972): A method for the determination of imipramine in human plasma by gas-liquid chromatography-mass fragmentography. *Journal of Chromatography, 74:* 201-208.
Fruthaler, G.J. and Snyder, C.H. (1962): Poisoning in childhood. *Pediatrics Clinics of North America, 9:* 41-62.
Garattini, S. (1969): Metabolism of diazepam in animals and man. In: *The Present Status of Psychotropic Drugs,* edited by A. Cerletti and F.J. Bovè, pp. 84-89, Excerpta Medica, Amsterdam.
Garattini, S., Marcucci, F., Morselli, P.L. and Mussini, E. (1973): The significance of measuring blood levels of benzodiazepines. In: *Biological Effects of Drugs in Relation to Their Plasma Concentrations,* edited by D.S. Davies and B.N.C. Prichard, pp. 211-225, Macmillan, London.
Garattini, S. and Morselli, P.L. (1974): *Interazioni tra Farmaci,* Ferro Edizioni, Milano.

Garattini, S. and Morselli, P.L. (1975): Monitoring plasma levels of tricyclic antidepressant agents: an individualized approach to depression therapy. In: *Physician's Guide to Depression,* edited by R.R. Fieve, pp. 101-131, P.W. Communic, Inc., New York.

Garrison, H.F., Jr., Moffitt, E.M. and Jackson, O. (1962): Imipramine hydrochloride intoxication. *Journal of the American Medical Association, 179:* 156-158.

Gillette, J.R. and Kamm, J.T. (1966): The enzymatic formation of sulphoxides: the oxidation of chlorpromazine and 4,4'-diamino-diphenyl-sulphide by guinea pig liver microsomes. *Journal of Pharmacology and Experimental Therapeutics, 130:* 262-267.

Glassman, A.H., Hurwic, M.J., Kanzler, M., Shostak, M. and Perel, J.M. (1974): Imipramine steady-state studies and plasma binding. In: *The Phenothiazines and Structurally Related Drugs,* edited by I.S. Forrest, C.J. Carr and E. Usdin, pp. 457-461, Raven Press, New York.

Glassman, A.H. and Perel, J.M. (1974): Plasma levels and tricyclic antidepressants. *Clinical Pharmacology and Therapeutics, 16:* 198-200.

Goldenberg, H. and Fishman, V. (1961): Species dependence of chlorpromazine metabolism. *Proceedings of the Society for Experimental Biology and Medicine, 108:* 178-182.

Gram, L.F. (1974): Metabolism of tricyclic antidepressants. *Danish Medical Bulletin, 21:* 218-231.

Gram, L.F. and Christiansen, J. (1975): First-pass metabolism of imipramine in man. *Clinical Pharmacology and Therapeutics, 17:* 555-563.

Gram, L.F., Christiansen, J. and Fredicson Överö, K. (1973): Pharmacokinetic interaction between tricyclic antidepressants and other psychopharmaca. *Acta Psychiatrica Scandinavica,* suppl. *243:* 52-53.

Gram, L.F., Christiansen, J. and Fredicson Överö, K. (1974): Interaction between neuroleptics and tricyclic antidepressants. In: *Drug Interactions,* edited by P.L. Morselli, S. Garattini and S.N. Cohen, pp. 271-276, Raven Press, New York.

Gram, L.F. and Fredricson Överö, K. (1972): Drug interaction: inhibitory effect of neuroleptics on metabolism of tricyclic antidepressants in man. *British Medical Journal, 1:* 463-465.

Gram, L.F., Kofod, B., Christiansen, J. and Rafaelsen, O.J. (1971): Imipramine metabolism: pH-dependent distribution and urinary excretion. *Clinical Pharmacology and Therapeutics, 12:* 239-244.

Greenblatt, D.J. and Shader, R.I. (1974): *Benzodiazepines in Clinical Practice,* p 17, Raven Press, New York

Hammar, C.-G., Alexanderson, B., Holmstedt, B. and Sjöqvist, F. (1971): Gas chromatography-mass spectrometry of nortriptyline in body fluids of man. *Clinical Pharmacology and Therapeutics, 12:* 496-505.

Hammar, C.G. and Holmstedt, B. (1968): Utilisation de la chromatographie en phase gaseuse en combination avec la spectrometrie de masse pour l'identification de la chlorpromazine et ses metabolites. *Aggressologie, 9:* 109-110.

Hammer, W. and Sjöqvist, F. (1967): Plasma levels of monomethylated tricyclic antidepressants during treatment with imipramine like compounds. *Life Sciences, 6:* 1895-1903.

Hammer, W., Ideström, C.M. and Sjöqvist, F. (1967): Chemical control of antidepressant drug therapy. In: *Antidepressant Drugs,* edited by S. Garattini and M.N.G. Dukes, pp. 301-310, Excerpta Medica, Amsterdam.

Hendel, J. (1975): Cumulation in cerebrospinal fluid of the N-desmethyl-metabolite after long-term treatment with diazepam in man. *Acta Pharmacologica et Toxicologica, 37:* 17-22.

Herrmann, B. (1963): Quantitative methoden zur Untersuchungen des Stoffwechsels von Tofranil. *Helvetica Physiologica Acta, 21:* 402-408.

Herrmann, B. (1967): Aspects of the metabolism of imipramine. In: *Proc. V. Interna-*

tional Congress Collegium—Internationale Neuro-Psychopharmacologicum, pp. 347-351, Excerpta Medica, Amsterdam.
Herrmann, B. and Pulver, R. (1960): Der Stoffwechsel des Psychopharmakons Tofranil. *Archives Internationales de Pharmacodynamie, 126:* 454-469.
Heubel, F. and Frank, R. (1970): Zur induktiven Wirkung von Diazepam. *Arzneimittel-Forsch Ung, 20:* 1706-1708.
Hillestad, L., Hansen, T., Melsom, H. and Drivenes, A. (1974a): Diazepam metabolism in normal man. I. Serum concentrations and clinical effects after intravenous, intramuscular and oral administration. *Clinical Pharmacology and Therapeutics, 16:* 479-484.
Hillestad, L., Hansen, T. and Melsom, H. (1974b): Diazepam metabolism in normal man. II. Serum concentration and clinical effect after oral administration and cumulation. *Clinical Pharmacology Therapeutics, 16:* 485-489.
Hobbs, D.C. (1969): Distribution and metabolism of doxepin. *Biochemical Pharmacology, 18:* 1941-1954.
Hobbs, D.C., Welch, W.M., Short, M.J., Moody, W.A. and Van der Velde, C.D. (1974): Pharmacokinetics of thiothixene in man. *Clinical Pharmacology and Therapeutics, 16:* 473-478.
Huang, C.L. (1967): Isolation and identification of urinary chlorpromazine metabolites in man. *International Journal of Neuropharmacology, 6:* 1-13.
Huang, C.L. and Kurland, A.A. (1964): Perphenazine (Trelafon) metabolism in psychotic patients. *Archives of General Psychiatry, 10:* 639-646.
Huang, C.L. and Ruskin, B.H. (1964): Determination of serum chlorpromazine metabolites in psychotic patients. *Journal of Nervous and Mental Diseases, 139:* 381-386.
Huang, C.L., Sands, F.L. and Kurland, A.A. (1963): Urinary thorazine metabolites in psychotic patients. *Archives of General Psychiatry, 8:* 301-307.
Hucker, H.B. (1962): Metabolism of amitriptyline. *Pharmacologist, 4:* 171.
Hucker, H.B., Balletto, A.J., Demetriades, J., Arison, B.H. and Zacchei, A.G. (1975): Epoxide metabolites of protriptyline in rat urine. *Drug Metabolism and Disposition, 3:* 80-83.
Huus, I. and Khan, A.R. (1967): Studies on the metabolism of chlorprothixene in rats and dogs. *Acta Pharmacologica Toxicologica, 25:* 397-404.
Idänpään-Heikkilä, J.E., Jouppila, P.I., Puolakka, J.O. and Vorne, M.S. (1971): Placental transfer and fetal metabolism of diazepam in early human pregnancy. *American Journal of Obstetrics and Gynecology, 109:* 1011-1016.
Im Obersteg, J. and Bäumler, J. (1962): Suicid mit dem psychopharmakon Tofranil. *Archiv für Toxikologie, 19:* 339-344.
Johnson, D.E., Rodriguez, C.F. and Burchfield, H.P. (1965): Determination by microcolorimetric gas chromatography of chlorpromazine metabolites in human urine. *Biochemical Pharmacology, 14:* 1453-1469.
Joyce, D.N. and Kenyon, V.G. (1972): The use of diazepam and hydralazine in the treatment of severe pre-eclampsia. *Journal of Obstetrics and Gynaecology of the British Commonwealth, 79:* 250-254.
Kanto, J., Kangas, L. and Sürtola, T. (1975): Cerebrospinal fluid concentrations of diazepam and its metabolites in man. *Acta Pharmacologica et Toxicologica, 36:* 328-334.
Kanto, J., Erkkola, R. and Sellman, R. (1973): Accumulation of diazepam and N-demethyldiazepam in the fetal blood during labor. *Annals of Clinical Research, 5:* 375-379.
Kanto, J., Iisalo, E., Lehtinen, V. and Salminen, J. (1974a): Concentrations of diazepam and its metabolites in plasma after an acute and chronic administration. *Psychopharmacologica, 36:* 123-131.
Kanto, J., Erkkola, R. and Sellman, R. (1974b): Perinatal metabolism of diazepam. *British Medical Journal, 1:* 641-642.

Kaplan, S.A., Jack, M.L., Alexander, K. and Weinfeld, R.E. (1973): Pharmacokinetic profile of diazepam in man following single intravenous and oral and chronic oral administration. *Journal of Pharmaceutical Sciences, 62:* 1789-1796.

Kaul, P.K., Conway, M.W. and Clark, M.L. (1974): Pharmacokinetics of chlorpromazine metabolites. A colossal problem. In: *The Phenothiazines and Structurally Related Drugs,* edited by I.S. Forrest, C.J. Carr and E. Usdin, p. 391, Raven Press, New York.

Klotz, U., Antonin, K.H., Müller, W.A. and Bieck, P. (1975): Influence of dosing and liver disease on the pharmacokinetics of diazepam in man. *Sixth Int. Congress of Pharmacology,* Helsinki, July 20-25, Abst. 120.

Klotz, U., Avant, G.R., Hohyumpa, A., Schenker, S. and Wilkinson, G.R. (1975): The effect of age and liver disease on the disposition and elimination of diazepam in man. *Journal of Clinical Investigation, 55:* 347-359.

Knapp, D.R., Gaffney, T.E., McMahon, R.E. and Kiplinger, G. (1972): Studies of human urinary and biliary metabolites of nortriptyline with stable isotope labelling. *Journal of Pharmacology and Experimental Therapeutics, 180:* 784-790.

Korein, J., Fish, B., Shapiro, T., Gerner, E.W. and Levidow, L. (1971): EEG and behavioral effects of drug therapy in children. *Archives of General Psychiatry, 24:* 552-563.

Korttila, K., Mattila, M.J. and Linnoila, M. (1975): Factors modifying the pharmacokinetics of diazepam. *Sixth Int. Congress of Pharmacology,* Helsinki, Finland, July 20-25, Abst. 120.

Kragh-Sørensen, P., Asberg, M. and Eggert-Hansen, C. (1973a): Plasma-nortriptyline levels in endogenous depression. *Lancet, I:* 113-115.

Kragh-Sørensen, P., Hansen, C.E. and Asberg, M. (1973b): Plasma levels of nortriptyline in the treatment of endogenous depression. *Acta Psychiatrica Scandinavica, 49:* 444-456.

Kragh-Sørensen, P., Eggert-Hansen, C., Larsen, N.-E., Naestoft, J. and Hvidberg, E.F. (1974): Long-term treatment of endogenous depression with nortriptyline with control of plasma levels. *Psychological Medicine, 4:* 174-180.

Krasner, J. and Yaffe, S.J. (1975): Drug protein binding in the neonate. In: *Basic and Therapeutic Aspects of Perinatal Pharmacology,* edited by P.L. Morselli, S. Garattini and F. Sereni, pp. 357-366, Raven Press, New York.

Kristiansen, E.S. (1961): Cardiac complications during treatment with imipramine. *Acta Psychiatrica et Neurologica Scandinavica, 36:* 427-442.

Kuhn, R. (1965): Untersuchungen über mogliche Zusammenhänge swischen Metabolitenausscheidung und Krankheitsverlauf depressiver Zustande Unter Imipramin-Medikation. *Psychopharmacologia, 8:* 201-222.

Lader, M. (1974): Plasma concentrations of tricyclic antidepressive drugs. *British Journal of Clinical Pharmacology, 1:* 281-283.

Larsen, N.E. and Naestoft, J. (1970): Determination of perphenazine and its sulphoxide metabolite in human plasma after therapeutic doses by gaschromatography. *Journal of Chromatography, 109:* 259-264.

Lean, T.H., Ratnam, S.S. and Sivasamboo, R. (1968): Use of benzodiazepines in the management of eclampsia. *Journal of Obstetrics and Gynaecology of the British Commonwealth, 75:* 856-862.

Leenheer, A. de and Heyndrick, A. (1971): Identification of a major metabolite of nortriptyline in human urine. *Journal of Pharmaceutical Sciences, 60:* 1403-1405.

Liederman, P.C., Wasserman, D.H. and Liederman, V.R. (1969): Desipramine in the treatment of enuresis. *Journal of Urology, 101:* 314-316.

Lin, J.H., Reynolds, L.W., Rondish, I.M. and Van Loon, E.J. (1959): Isolation and characterization of glucuronic acid conjugates of chlorpromazine in human urine. *Proceedings of the Society for Experimental Biology and Medicine, 102:* 602-605.

Lyle, W.H., Braithwaite, R.A., Brooks, P.W., Cuthill, J.M., Early, D.F., Goulding, R., Leggett, W.P., Pearson, I.B., Silverman, G., Snaith, R.P. and Strang, G.E. (1974): Plasma concentration of nortriptyline as a guide to treatment. *Postgraduate Medical Journal, 50:* 282-287.
Mandelli, M., Morselli, P.L., Nordio, S., Pardi, G., Principi, N., Sereni, F. and Tognoni, G. (1975): Placental transfer of diazepam and its disposition in the newborn. *Clinical Pharmacology and Therapeutics, 17:* 564-572.
Manian, A.A., Efron, D.H. and Goldberg, M.E. (1965): A comparative pharmacological study of a series of monohydroxylated and methoxylated chlorpromazine derivatives. *Life Sciences, 4:* 2425-2438.
Manian, A.A., Watzman, N., Steenberg, M.L. and Buckley, J.P. (1968): A pharmacologic study of two bis-alkoxy-chlorpromazine derivatives. *Life Sciences, 7:* 731-740.
March, J.E., Donato, D., Turano, P. and Turner, W.J. (1972): Interpatient variation and significance of plasma levels of chlorpromazine in psychotic patients. *Journal of Medicine, 3:* 146-162.
Marcucci, F., Fanelli, R., Frova, M. and Morselli, P.L. (1968): Levels of diazepam in adipose tissue of rats, mice and man. *European Journal of Pharmacology, 4:* 464-466.
Marcucci, F., Mussini, E.E., Morselli, P.L., Garattini, S., Libretti, A. and Zaccala, M. (1970): Osservazioni sul metabolismo delle benzodiazepine nell'uomo. In: *Atti II ruinione Nazionale Societa Italiana di Neuropsicofarmacologia*, Tirrenia (Pisa), 14-16 June, 1969, 63-70, Arti Grafiche Pacini Mariotti, Pisa.
Marcucci, F., Mussini, E., Airoldi, L., Fanelli, A., Frigerio, A., De Nadai, F., Bizzi, A., Rizzo, M., Morselli, P.L. and Garattini, S. (1971): Analytical and pharmacokinetic studies on butyrophenones. *Clinica Chimica Acta, 34:* 321-332.
Marshall, L.J. and Green, V.A. (1968): Propranolol and diazepam for imipramine poisoning. *Lancet, 2:* 1249.
Martensson, E. and Roos, B.-E. (1973): Serum levels of thioridazine in psychiatric patients and healthy volunteers. *European Journal of Clinical Pharmacology, 6:* 181-186.
McCarthy, G.T., O'Connell, B. and Robinson, A.E. (1973): Blood levels of diazepam in infants of two mothers given large doses of diazepam during labour. *Journal of Obstetrics and Gynaecology of the British Commonwealth, 80:* 349-352.
McGiles, H. (1963): Imipramine poisoning in childhood. *British Medical Journal, 2:* 844-846.
Mellinger, T.J., Mellinger, E.M. and Smith, W.T. (1965): Thioridazine blood levels in patients receiving different oral forms. *Clinical Pharmacology and Therapeutics, 6:* 486-491.
Minder, R., Schnetzer, F. and Bickel, M.H. (1971): Hepatic and extrahepatic metabolism of the psychotropic drugs, chlorpromazine, imipramine and imipramine-N-oxide. *Naunyn-Schmiedebergs Archiv für Pharmakologie und Experimentelle Pathologie, 268:* 334-347.
Mjorndal, T. and Oreland, L. (1971): Determination of thioxanthens in plasma at therapeutic concentrations. *Acta Pharmacologica et Toxicologica, 29:* 295-302.
Moccetti, T., Lichtlen, P., Casaccia, M., Halter, J. and Mohr, P. (1972): Tossicita cardiaca negli antidepressivi triciclici. *Giornale Italiano di Cardiologia, 2:* 442-451.
Moir, D.C. (1973): Tricyclic antidepressants and cardiac disease. *American Heart Journal, 86:* 841-842.
Moir, D.C., Crooks, J., Cornwell, W.B., O'Malley, K., Dingwall-Fordyce, I., Turnbull, M.J. and Weir, R.D. (1972): Cardiotoxicity of amitriptyline. *Lancet, II:* 561-564.
Moir, D.C., Dingwall-Fordyce, I. and Weir, R.D. (1973): Medicines evaluations and monitoring group. A follow-up study of cardiac patients receiving amitriptyline. *European Journal of Clinical Pharmacology, 6:* 98-101.

Moody, J.P., Tait, A.C. and Todrick, A. (1967): Plasma levels of imipramine and desmethylimipramine during therapy. *British Journal of Psychiatry, 113:* 183-193.
Morselli, P.L. (1974): Drug disposition during development. *Acta Pharmaceutica Suecica, 11:* 645-652.
Morselli, P.L. (1975): Problemas de terapia en la edad pediatrica. In: *Advances in Therapeutica,* edited by J. La Porte and J.A. Salva, Salvat, Barcelona, in press.
Morselli, P.L. (1976): Pediatric clinical pharmacology–routine monitoring for clinical trials? In: *Clinical Pharmacy and Clinical Pharmacology,* edited by Gouveia, Tognoni and van der Kleijn, pp. 279-289, Elsevier/North-Holland Biomedical Press.
Morselli, P.L., Mandelli, M., Pardi, G., Principi, N., Tognoni, G. and Sereni, F. (1974b): Diazepam placental transfer in humans and its metabolism in the premature and full term newborns. In: *Proceedings XIV International Congress of Pediatrics,* Editorial Medica Panamericana, Buenos Aires, pp. 35-41.
Morselli, P.L., Mandelli, M., Tognoni, G., Principi, N., Pardi, G. and Sereni, F. (1974a): *Drug Interactions,* edited by P.L. Morselli, S. Garattini and S.N. Cohen, pp. 259-270, Raven Press, New York.
Morselli, P.L., Principi, N., Tognoni, G. and Sereni, F. (1972): Diazepam metabolism in premature infants. *Pediatric Research, 6:* 53.
Morselli, P.L., Principi, N., Tognoni, G., Reali, E., Belvedere, G., Standen, S.M. and Sereni, F. (1973): Diazepam elimination in premature and full term infants and children. *Journal of Perinatal Medicine, 1:* 133-141.
Morselli, P.L. and Tognoni, G. (1974): Il servizio di farmacologia clinica in pediatria. *Prospettive in Pediatria, 14:* 167-174.
Muller, O.F., Goodman, N. and Bellet, S. (1961): The hypotensive effect of imipramine hydrochloride in patients with cardiovascular disease. *Clinical Pharmacology and Therapeutics, 2:* 300-307.
Müller, W. and Wollert, U. (1973): Characterization of the binding of benzodiazepines to human serum albumin. *Naunyn-Schmiedeberg's Archives of Pharmacology, 280:* 229-237.
Munksgaard, E.C. (1969): Concentrations of amitriptyline and its metabolites in urine, blood and tissue in fatal amitriptyline poisoning. *Acta Pharmacologica et Toxicologica, 27:* 129-134.
O'Donoghue, S.E.F. (1971): Distribution of pethidine and chlorpromazine in maternal, foetal and neonatal biological fluids. *Nature (London), 229:* 124-125.
Oliver-Martin, R., Marzin, D., Buschenschutz, E., Pichot, P. and Boissier, J. (1975): Concentrations plasmatiques de l'imipramine et de la desmethylimipramine et effet antidepresseur au cours d'un traitment controlé. *Psychopharmacologia, 41:* 187-195.
Owen, J.R., Irani, S.F. and Blair, A.W. (1972): Effect of diazepam administered to mothers during labour on temperature regulation of neonate. *Archives of Disease in Childhood, 47:* 107-110.
Pacha, W.L. (1969): A method for the fluorimetric determination of thioridazine (Mellaril R) or Mesoridazine (Lidanil R) in plasma. *Experientia, 25:* 103-104.
Patrick, M.J., Tilstone, W.J. and Reavey, P (1972). Diazepam and breast-feeding. *Lancet, 1:* 542-543.
Pelkonen, O., Vorne, M., Jouppila, P. and Kärki, N.T. (1971): Metabolism of chlorpromazine and p-nitrobenzoic acid in the liver, intestine, and kidney of the human foetus. *Acta Pharmacologica et Toxicologica, 29:* 284-294.
Perry, T.L., Culling, C.F.A., Berry, K. and Hansen, S. (1964): 7-hydroxychlorpromazine: potential toxic drug metabolite in psychiatric patients. *Science, 146:* 81-82.
Petersen, P.V. and Nielsen, M.I. (1964): Thioxanthene derivatives. In: *Psychopharmacological Agents,* edited by M. Gordon, pp. 301-325, Academic Press, New York.

Placidi, G.F., Tognoni, G., Pacifici, G.M., Cassano, G.B. and Morselli, P.L. (1976): Regional distribution of diazepam and its metabolites in the brain of cat after chronic treatment. *Psychopharmacologia, 48:* 133-137.

Posner, H.S., Culpan, R. and Levine, J. (1963): Quantification and probable structure in human urine, of the nonphenolic and phenolic metabolites of chlorpromazine. *Journal of Pharmacology and Experimental Therapeutics, 150:* 377-391.

Posner, H.S. and Hearst, E. (1964): Pharmacological activity of 1-,2-, and 3-hydroxypromazine and 7-methoxychlorpromazine. *International Journal of Neuropharmacology, 3:* 635-641.

Posner, H.S., Hearst, E., Taylor, W.L. and Cosmides, G.J. (1962): Model metabolites of chlorpromazine and promazine: relative activities in some pharmacological and behavioral tests. *Journal of Pharmacology and Experimental Therapeutics, 137:* 84-90.

Pruitt, A.W. and Dayton, P.G. (1971): A comparison of the binding of drugs to adult and cord plasma. *European Journal of Clinical Pharmacology, 4:* 59-62.

Raablaub, J. (1967): Zum metabolismus des chlorprothixen. *Arzneitittel-Forschung, 17:* 1393-1395.

Rabiner, C.J. and Klein, D.F. (1969): Imipramine treatment of school phobia. *Comprehensive Psychiatry, 10:* 387-390.

Ramsay, I.D. (1967): Survival after imipramine poisoning. *Lancet, II:* 1308-1309.

Rane, A., Lunde, P.K.M., Jalling, B., Yaffe, S.J. and Sjöqvist, F. (1971): Plasma protein binding of diphenylhydantoin in normal and hyperbilirubinemic infants. *Journal of Pediatrics, 78:* 877-882.

Rasmussen, E.B. (1965): Amitriptyline and imipramine poisoning. *Lancet, II:* 850.

Rasmussen, E.B. and Kristijansen, P. (1963): ECG changes during amitriptyline treatment. *American Journal of Psychiatry, 119:* 781-790.

Riess, W., Rajagopalan, T.G., Schmid, K. and Keberle, H. (1972): Pharmacokinetics studies on maproptyline (Ludiomil R). In: *Depressive Illness,* edited by P. Kielholz, pp. 140-148, Huber Publ., Bern.

Riess, W., Rajagopalan, T.G., Schmid, K. and Keberle, H. (1973): Studi farmacocinetici con maprotilina (Ludiomil R). *Bollettino Chimico Farmaceutico, 112:* 677-683.

Rivera-Calimlin, L. and Lasagna, L. (1973): Effects of mode of management on plasma chlorpromazine in psychiatric patients. *Clinical Pharmacology and Therapeutics, 14:* 978-986.

Rizzo, M., Giannelli, A., Jogan, E., Standen, S.M. and Morselli, P.L. (1973): Alcune osservazioni sulle correlazioni tra livelli plasmatici degli antidepressivi triciclici monometilati ed effetti terapeutici. *Rivista Sperimentale di Freniatria, 47:* 3-27.

Roberts, R.J., Mueller, S. and Lauer, R.M. (1973): Propranol in the treatment of cardiac arrhythmias associated with amitriptyline intoxication. *Journal of Pediatrics, 82:* 65-67.

Rodriguez, C.F. and Johnson, D.E. (1966): A new metabolite of chlorpromazine in human urine. *Life Sciences, 5:* 1283-1290.

Sacks, M.H., Bonforte, R.J., Lasser, R.P. and Dimich, I. (1968): Cardiovascular complications of imipramine intoxication. *Journal of the American Medical Association, 205:* 588-590.

Sakalis, G., Curry, S.H., Mould, G.P. and Lader, M.H. (1972): Physiologic and clinical effects of chlorpromazine and their relationship to plasma level. *Clinical Pharmacology and Therapeutics, 13:* 931-946.

Salzman, N.P. and Brodie, B.B. (1956): Physiological disposition and fate of chlorpromazine and a method for its estimation in biological material. *Journal of Pharmacology and Experimental Therapeutics, 118:* 46-54.

Saraf, K.R., Klein, D.F., Gittelman-Klein, R. and Groff, S. (1974): Imipramine side effects in children. *Psychopharmacologia, 37:* 265-274.

Schaefer, J.P. (1967): The structure of thiothixene. *Chemical Communications, 15:* 743-744.
Schaffer, D., Costello, A.J. and Hill, D. (1968): Control of enuresis with imipramine. *Archives of Disease in Childhood, 43:* 665-671.
Scher, J., Hailey, D.M. and Beard, R.M. (1972): The effects of diazepam on the fetus. *Journal of Obstetrics and Gynaecology of the British Commonwealth, 79:* 635-638.
Schober, J.C. and Mantel, K. (1970): Letale vergiftungen-mit thymoleptica im Kleinkindesalter. *Monatschrift fur Kinderheilkunde, 6:* 340-341.
Schwartz, M.A., Koechlin, B.A., Postma, E., Palmer, S. and Krol, G. (1965): Metabolism of diazepam in rat, dog and man. *Journal of Pharmacology and Experimental Therapeutics, 149:* 423-435.
Schwartz, D.E., Vecchi, M., Ronco, A. and Kaiser, K. (1966): Blood levels after administration of 7-chloro-1,3-dihydro-1-methyl-5-phenyl-2H-1,4-benzodiazepine-2-one (diazepam) in various forms. *Arzneimittel-Forschung, 16:* 1109-1110.
Sellman, R., Pekkarinen, A., Kangas, L. and Raijola, E. (1975): Reduced concentrations of plasma diazepam in chronic alcoholic patients following an oral administration of diazepam. *Acta Pharmacologica et Toxicologica, 36:* 25-32.
Sereni, F., Morselli, P.L. and Pardi, G. (1973a): Postnatal development of drug metabolism in human infants. In: *Perinatal Medicine,* edited by H. Bossart, J.M. Cruz, A. Huber, L.S. Prod'Hom and J. Sistek, pp. 63-77, Huber Publ., Bern.
Sereni, F., Mandelli, M., Principi, N., Tognoni, G., Pardi, G. and Morselli, P.L. (1973b): Induction of drug metabolizing enzyme activities in the human fetus and in the newborn infant. *Enzyme, 15:* 318-329.
Shannon, R.W., Fraser, G.P., Aitken, R.G. and Harper, J.R. (1972): Diazepam in preclamptic toxaemia with special reference to its effect on the newborn infant. *British Journal of Clinical Practice, 26:* 271-275.
Sharples, D. (1975): Competition for plasma protein binding sites between phenothiazine tranquilizers and iminodibenzyl antidepressants. *Journal of Pharmacy and Pharmacology, 27:* 379-381.
Sidiropoulos, D. and Bickel, M.H. (1971): Eine tödliche Vergiftung mit Imipramin in kleiner Dosis bei einem Kleinkind. *Schweizerische Medizinische Wochenschrift, 101:* 851-854.
Simpson, G., Lament, R., Cooper, B.T., Lee, J.H. and Bruce, R.B. (1973): The relationship between blood levels of different forms of butaperazine and clinical response. *Journal of Clinical Pharmacology, 13:* 288-297.
Singh, G. (1972): Cardiac arrest with clomipramine. *British Medical Journal, 3:* 698.
Sjöqvist, F., Bergfors, P.G., Borga, O., Lind, M. and Ygge, H. (1972): Plasma disappearance of nortriptyline in a newborn infant following placental transfer from an intoxicated mother: evidence for drug metabolism. *Journal of Pediatrics, 80:* 496-500.
Sjöqvist, F., Hammer, W., Ideström, C.M., Lind, M., Tuck, D. and Asberg, M. (1968): Plasma level of monomethylated tricyclic antidepressant and side-effects in man. In: *Toxicity and Side Effects of Psychotropic Drugs,* Proc. European Society Study of Drug Toxicity, V. 9, pp. 246-257, Excerpta Medica, Amsterdam.
Sjöqvist, F., Hammer, W., Borga, O. and Azarnoff, D.L. (1969): Pharmacological significance of the plasma level of monomethylated tricyclic antidepressants. In: *The Present Status of Psychotropic Drugs,* edited by A. Cerletti and F.J. Bové, pp. 128-136, Excerpta Medica, Amsterdam.
Sloman, L. (1960): Myocardial infarction during imipramine treatment of depression. *Canadian Medical Association Journal, 82:* 20-22.
Smith, R.B. and Rusbatch, B.J. (1967): Amitriptyline and heart block. *British Medical Journal, 3:* 311.

Spirtes, M.A. (1974): Two types of metabolically produced trifluoroperazine N-oxides. In: *Phenothiazines and Structurally Related Drugs*, edited by I.S. Forrest, Carr and E. Usdin, pp. 399-404, Raven Press, New York.
Steel, C.M., O'Duffy, J. and Brown, S.S. (1967): Clinical effects and treatment of imipramine and amitriptyline poisoning in children. *British Medical Journal, 3:* 663-667.
Sunshine, P. and Yaffe, S.J. (1963): Amitriptyline poisoning: clinical and pathological findings in a fatal case. *American Journal of Diseases of Children, 106:* 501-506.
Tansella, M., Zimmermann-Tansella, C. and Lader, M. (1974): The residual effects of N-desmethyldiazepam in patients. *Psychopharmacologia, 38:* 81-90.
Tansella, M., Burti, L., Siciliani, O., Zimmermann, C., Schiavon, M., Gerna, M., Tognoni, G. and Morselli, P.L. (1975): N-desmethyldiazepam and amylobarbitone sodium as hypnotics in anxious patients: correlations between plasma levels and behavioral tests. *Psychopharmacologia, 41:* 81-85.
Thearle, M.J., Dunn, P.M. and Hailey, D.M. (1973): Exchange transfusion for diazepam intoxication at birth followed by jejunal stenosis. *Proceedings of the Royal Society of Medicine, 66:* 349-350.
Thompson, G.A. (1973): Amitriptyline overdose. *Drug Intelligence and Clinical Pharmacy, 7:* 451-458.
Thorstrand, C. (1974): Cardiovascular effects of poisoning with tricyclic antidepressants. *Acta Medical Scandinavica, 195:* 505-514.
Tognoni, G., Gomeni, R., De Maio, D., Alberti, G.G., Franciosi, P. and Scieghi, G. (1975): Pharmacokinetics of N-demethyldiazepam in patients suffering from insomnia and treated with nortriptyline. *British Journal of Clinical Pharmacology, 2:* 227-232.
Toulouse, R. and Maffei, J.L. (1965): Utilisation du Valium en obstétrique. *Revue Franaise de Gynecologie et d'Obstetrique, 60:* 263-270.
Tosi, G.C., Tosi, E.C. and Hattab, J.R. (1974): The use of N-demethyldiazepam in outpatients suffering from insomnia. *Current Therapeutic Research, 15:* 460-464.
Tuck, R.J., Kahan, E. and Siwers, B. (1973): Biological and pharmacokinetic evidence for generic preparations: comparison with a new imipramine analogue. *Acta Pharmacologica et Toxicologica, 32:* 304-313.
Turano, P., March, J.E., Turner, W.J. and Merlis, S. (1972): Qualitative and quantitative report on chlorpromazine and metabolites in plasma, erythrocytes and erythrocyte washings from chronically medicated schizophrenic patients. *Journal of Medicine, 3:* 109-120.
Turano, P., Turner, W.J. and Manian, A.A. (1973): Thin-layer chromatography of chlorpromazine metabolites. Attempts to identify each of the metabolites appearing in blood, urine and feces of chronically medicated schizophrenics. *Journal of Chromatography, 75:* 277-293.
Turano, P., Turner, W.J. and Donato, D. (1974): Further studies of chlorpromazine metabolism in schizophrenic men. In: *The Phenothiazines and Structurally Related Drugs*, edited by I.S. Forrest, C.J. Carr and E. Usdin, pp. 315-322, Raven Press, New York.
Usdin, E. (1970): Absorption, distribution and metabolic fate of psychotropic drugs. *Psychopharmacology Bulletin, 6:* 4-25.
Usdin, E. (1971): The assay of chlorpromazine and metabolites in blood urine and other tissues. *CRC Critical Reviews in Clinical Laboratory Sciences, 2:* 347-391.
van der Kleijn, E. (1969a): Protein binding and lipophilic nature of atarectics of the meprobamate- and diazepine-group. *Archives Internationales de Pharmacodynamie, 179:* 225-250.
van der Kleijn, E. (1969b): Kinetics of distribution and metabolism of diazepam in animals and humans. *Archives Internationales de Pharmacodynamie, 182:* 433-436.
van der Kleijn, E., van Rossum, J.M., Muskens, E.T.J.M. and Rijntjes, N.V.M. (1971):

Pharmacokinetics of diazepam in dogs, mice and humans. *Acta Pharmacologica et Toxicologica, 29,* suppl. 3, 109-127.

Van Petten, G.R. (1975): Fetal cardiovascular effects of maternally administered tricyclic antidepressants. In: *Basic and Therapeutic Aspects of Perinatal Pharmacology,* edited by P.L. Morselli, S. Garattini and F. Sereni, pp. 83-88, Raven Press, New York.

Vohra, J. and Burrows, G.D. (1974): Cardiovascular complications of tricyclic antidepressant overdosage. *Drugs, 8:* 432-437.

Wallace, J.E. (1967): Ultraviolet spectrophotometric determination of chlorprothixene in biologic specimens. *Journal of Pharmaceutical Sciences, 56:* 1437-1441.

Watt, D.C., Crammer, J.L. and Elkes, A. (1969): The relation of side effects to therapeutic outcome of imipramine in depressive illness. In: *The Present Status of Psychotropic Drugs,* edited by A. Cerletti and F.J. Bové, pp. 553-555, Excerpta Medica, Amsterdam.

Wechsler, M.B., Wharton, R.N., Tanaka, E. and Malitz, S. (1967): Chlorpromazine metabolite pattern in psychotic patients. *Journal of Psychiatric Research, 5:* 327-333.

Weissman, A. (1968): Psychopharmacological effects of thiothixene and related compounds. *Psychopharmacologia, 12:* 142-157.

Weissman, A. (1974): Chemical, pharmacological and metabolic considerations on thiothixene. In: *The Phenothiazines and Structurally Related Drugs,* edited by I.S. Forrest, C.J. Carr and E. Usdin, pp. 471-480, Raven Press, New York.

Williams, R.T. and Parke, D.V. (1964): The metabolic fate of drugs. *Annual Reviews of Pharmacology, 4:* 85-114.

Williams, R.B. and Sherter, C. (1971): Cardiac complications of tricyclic antidepressant therapy. *Annals of Internal Medicine, 74:* 395-398.

Winsberg, B.G., Perel, J.M., Hurwic, M.J. and Klutch, A. (1974): Imipramine protein binding and pharmacokinetics in children. In: *The Phenothiazines and Structurally Related Drugs,* edited by I.S. Forrest, C.J. Carr and E. Usdin, pp. 425-431, Raven Press, New York.

Zehnder, K., Kalberer, F., Kreis, W. and Rutschmann, J. (1962): The metabolism of thioridazine (Mellaril R) and one of its pyrrolidine analogues in the rat. *Biochemical Pharmacology, 11:* 535-550.

15

Conclusion

PAOLO LUCIO MORSELLI

The material reported in this volume may appear rather fragmentary and incomplete; moreover, a correct comparison between infants or children and adults has always not been possible because of the lack of available data. Differences in the analytical techniques used, in the goals of the various studies, in the "kinetic criteria" followed by the authors further complicate the problem. Very probably, many of the data already acquired should be reevaluated with more specific techniques and/or reconsidered in the light of more recent kinetic information.

Despite these drawbacks, it clearly emerges that, for several classes of drugs, very important differences in the pharmacokinetic parameters may be present during development. These differences may be magnified or reduced by concomitant administration of several drugs or by the severity of the diseases. In all instances, however, they may be very important from a practical, clinical point of view, since they can lead to either a positive or negative outcome of the therapeutic intervention.

Summarizing we can say that in the newborn there is a modified absorption, a reduced plasma protein-binding, a modified volume of distribution and a markedly reduced ability to metabolize and excrete drugs. The neonatal period is followed by 2-3 years in which the absorption and elimination rate constants appear to be considerably faster than in adults, while differences in apparent volume of distribution are related both to the physicochemical properties of the compounds and to the maturational stage. After the first 3 years of life, there is a progressive leveling toward adult values, with the possibility of sudden variations in concomitancy with the sexual maturation.

As already said, this general picture, linked to the development of various physiological variables, may be at any juncture modified by previous or concomitant exposition to other therapeutic agents or by the severity of the pathological syndromes.

For all these reasons, we must be very cautious in administering drugs to children. To improve our knowledge, we must monitor the plasma levels of the drugs we are administering. To monitor drug plasma levels should not and must not be considered experimentation; on the contrary, it means performing the therapeutic act in a more conscientious and informed manner. Monitoring of drug levels in children should be performed in every situation "at risk," where risk means not only possibility of adverse reactions but also lack of therapeutic efficacy. It should be performed on a wider scale, as a routine service that every hospital should be able to offer.

Due to the continuous changing and maturation of various physiological variables, it is in fact practically impossible to make any prediction on drug kinetic patterns in infancy and childhood and hence to perform a rational dosage assignation in a single case. As a consequence, it appears that the only way to provide children, as in the case of adults, with a safer and better therapy is to monitor drug levels during their "naturalistic" usage.

The effort and the price to be paid for a drug assay service are no larger than those needed for a drug research lab. However, the differences in the outcome are substantial, since by routine monitoring we may benefit the individual patient, understand him better and, in the meantime, gain valuable information on drug disposition in various developmental stages and physiopathological conditions. By routine monitoring of drug plasma levels, we can understand more about toxic reactions and lack of responses, and we can establish therapeutic and toxic thresholds. In other words, we can, by integrating pharmacokinetics and physiopathology, achieve a more rational individualized therapy. For such an effort, we need more trained personnel in universities, hospitals and industries, new analytical techniques and new methods for evaluating both adverse reactions and therapeutic efficacy, but, more important, we need a closer cooperation and a steady flow of information among the various people interested in this fascinating but neglected area.

This volume, as we said in the preface, had the ambitious aim to cooperate in such a mutual effort. We hope now it can contribute, at least partially, to improving awareness of how much is still needed to be done in this branch of medicine.

Index

Absorption, 51
   Age variations of A, 52, 53, 54, 55, 56, 475
   Cutaneous, 54
   Factors influencing A, 52
   Intramuscular, 53, 54, 55
   Oral, 52, 55
Accumulation Ratio, 416
Acenocoumarol, 262
   Absorption, 262
   Plasma levels in chronic treatment, 262
   Plasma protein binding, 262, 263
   Plasma half-life, 262
   Urinary excretion, 264
Acetaminophen, 293
   Absorption
      Adults, 293
      Newborns, 296
   Interactions with other drugs, 294
   Metabolism
      Adults, 294
      Newborns, 296
   Plasma protein binding, 294
   Plasma half-life
      Adults, 294
      Newborns, 296
   Toxic effects, 294
      Adults, 295
      Children, 295
   Toxic plasma levels, 295
   Urinary excretion
      Adults, 294
      Newborns, 296
Acetanilid, 292
   Absorption, 292
   Plasma protein binding, 292
   Plasma half-life, 292
Actinomycin-D, 114
   Absorption, 114
   Biliary excretion, 114
   Mechanism of action, 114
   Tissues concentrations, 114
   Toxic effects
      Adults, 114, 115
      Children, 114, 115
      Infants, 114, 115
   Urinary excretion, 114
Adriamycin, 115
   Biliary excretion, 116
   CSF Concentrations, 116
   Metabolism, 115
   Plasma half life, 116

INDEX

Tissues concentrations, 116
Toxic effects
  Adults, 117
  Children, 117
  Infants, 117
Urinary excretion, 116
Alprenolol, 416
  Absorption, 416-417
  Plasma levels in chronic treatment, 417
  Plasma protein binding, 417
  Plasma half-life, 417
  Total body clearance, 417
  Volume of distribution, 417
Aminoglycosides, 115
  Absorption, 159, 160, 161
    Adults, 160
    Newborns, 164
  Biliary excretion, 157, 162
  CSF Concentrations, 159, 162
    Infants, 159
    Newborns, 165
  Individual Agents
    Amikacin, 172
    Gentamycin, 159-170
    Kanamycin, 156-159
    Tobramycin, 170-172
  Interactions with other drugs, 163
  Metabolism 163
  Plasma levels in chronic treatment
    Adults, 156
    Children, 168
    Infants, 168, 171
    Newborns, 158, 166
  Plasma protein binding
    Adults, 162
    Newborns, 164
  Plasma half-life
    Adults, 156, 160
    Children, 168
    Infants, 168, 171
    Newborns, 158, 165, 166, 172
  Renal clearance, 157, 160
  Therapeutic plasma levels, 162, 169
  Tissues concentrations, 163, 165
  Total body clearance, 157, 160, 171
  Toxic effects, 155, 170
  Toxic plasma levels, 169, 170
  Urinary excretion
    Adults, 157, 164
    Infants, 171
    Newborns, 158, 165, 168, 172

Volume of distribution, 157, 160
  Adults, 157, 160
  Children, 168
  Infants, 168
Amitriptyline, 443
  Absorption, 443
  Interactions with other drugs, 443-444
  Metabolism, 443-444
  Overdosage
    Adults, 446-447
    Children, 449
  Plasma levels in chronic treatment, 444
  Plasma protein binding, 443
  Plasma half-life, 443
  Therapeutic plasma levels, 445
  Tissues concentrations, 449
  Total body clearance, 443
  Toxic effects
    Adults, 445-446
    Children, 449
  Urinary excretion, 444
  Volume of distribution, 443
Amobarbital, 371
  Absorption, 371
  Metabolism, 371-372
  Plasma protein binding, 371
  Plasma half-life
    Adults, 371
    Newborn, 378
  Therapeutic plasma levels, 373
  Urinary excretion, 371
  Volume of distribution, 371
Aminopyrine, 289
  Absorption, 289
  Interactions with other drugs, 289
  Metabolism, 289
  Plasma protein binding, 289
  Plasma half-life
    Adults, 289
    Newborns, 290
  Urinary excretion, 289
Antiarrhythmic Agents, 404
Antibiotics, 123
  Significance plasma levels of, 124
Anticoagulants, 251
  Oral A, 254
Antidepressant Drugs, 439
Antiepileptics, 311
Antiinflammatory Drugs, 271
Antineoplastic Agents, 101
Antipsychotic Drugs, 431

INDEX **479**

Antipyrine, 290
    Absorption, 290
    Interactions with other drugs, 290
    Metabolism, 291
    Plasma half-life
        Adults, 290
        Children, 291
    Urinary excretion, 291
    Volume of distribution, 290
Antitubercular Agents, 177
    Absorption
        Adults, 177, 178, 179, 180
        Children, 182
        Infants, 177, 182
        Newborns, 177, 182, 183
    Biliary excretion, 182
    CSF concentrations, 178
        Newborns, 183
    Enterohepatic circle, 181
    Individual Agents
        Isoniazid, 178-179
        Rifampicin, 179-183
        Streptomycin, 177-178
    Interaction with other drugs, 179, 180, 181, 182
    Metabolism, 178
    Plasma protein binding
        Adults, 180
        Newborns, 183
    Plasma half-life
        Adults, 177, 181
        Newborns, 178
    Therapeutic plasma levels
        Adults, 177, 178, 180
        Children, 182
        Infants, 182
        Newborns, 182
    Tissues concentrations, 180, 181
    Urinary excretion
        Adults, 178, 182
        Infants, 178
        Newborns, 183
    Volume of distribution
        Adults, 182
        Children, 182
        Infants, 182
        Newborns, 182
Apparent Volume of Distribution
    Definition of, 2

Area Under the Concentration Curve, 2
Benzodiazepines, 449
Bioavailability, 7
Bishydroxycoumarin, 261
    Absorption, 261
    Interaction with other drugs, 261, 262
    Metabolism, 262
    Plasma protein binding, 261
    Plasma half-life, 261
    Volume of distribution, 261
Butaperazine, 437
    Absorption, 437
    Plasma levels in chronic treatment, 437
    Plasma half-life, 437
Butyrophenones, 438

Capacity Limited Processes, 12, 16
Carbamazepine, 336
    Absorption, 336-337
    CSF concentrations, 337
    Interaction with other drugs, 338
    Metabolism, 338-339
    Plasma levels in chronic treatment, 338-339
    Plasma protein binding
        Adults, 337-339
    Plasma half-life
        Adults, 338
        Newborns, 340
    Therapeutic plasma levels, 339
    Total body clearance
        Adults, 340
        Children, 340
    Toxic effects, 340
    Toxic plasma levels, 339
    Urinary excretion, 339
    Volume of distribution, 337
Cephalosporins, 146
    Absorption
        Adults, 147, 149, 153, 155
        Children, 152, 153, 155
        Infants, 152, 153
        Newborns, 152, 153
    Biliary excretion, 151
    Individual Agents
        Cephadrine, 155
        Cephalexin, 153-154
        Cephaloridine, 152-153
        Cephalotin, 152
        Cephazoline, 153

Interaction with other drugs, 150-151
Metabolism, 150
Plasma levels in chronic treatment
  Adults, 148, 153
  Children, 153, 154
  Infants, 153, 154
  Newborns, 153, 154
Plasma protein binding, 148, 150, 152
Plasma half-life
  Adults, 148, 152
  Children, 152, 153
  Infants, 152, 153
  Newborns, 153
Tissues concentrations, 151, 152
Total body clearance, 148
Urinary excretion
  Adults, 148-150
  Children, 153, 154
  Infants, 153, 154
  Newborns, 153, 154
Volume of distribution, 148, 150
Chloral Hydrate, 362
  Absorption, 363
  Interaction with other drugs, 363
  Metabolism, 362-363
  Plasma protein binding, 363
  Plasma half-life
    Adults, 362
    Children, 364
  Toxic effects, 364
Chloramphenicol, 183
  Absorption, 184
  CSF concentrations, 184
  Interaction with other drugs, 184
  Metabolism, 184
  Plasma protein binding, 184
  Plasma half-life
    Adults, 184
    Children, 184
    Infants, 184
    Newborns, 184
  Tissues concentrations, 184
  Urinary excretion, 184
Chlorpromazine, 432
  Absorption, 432
  Interaction with other drugs, 432-435
  Metabolism, 433-434
  Plasma levels in chronic treatment, 433
  Plasma protein binding, 432
  Plasma half-life, 433
  Therapeutic plasma levels, 435
  Toxic effects, 435
  Toxic plasma levels, 435
  Urinary excretion
    Adults, 434, 435
    Newborns, 436
  Volume of distribution, 432
Chlorprothixene, 437
  Absorption, 437
  Metabolism, 437
  Urinary excretion, 437
Clindamycin, 187
  Absorption
    Adults, 187, 188
    Children, 187, 189
  Biliary excretion, 190
  Metabolism, 187, 190
  Plasma protein binding, 190
  Plasma half-life
    Adults, 187, 188
    Children, 189
  Tissues concentrations, 190
  Urinary excretion
    Adults, 188, 190
    Children, 189, 190
    Infants, 190
    Newborns, 190
  Volume of distribution
    Adults, 188
    Children, 189
Clonazepam, 340
  Absorption, 341
  Metabolism, 342-343
  Plasma level in chronic treatment, 343
  Plasma half-life, 341
  Therapeutic plasma levels, 343
  Toxic plasma levels, 343
  Urinary excretion, 341-343
  Volume of distribution, 341
Compartment Models, 9
Cotrimoxazole, 231
  Absorption
    Adults, 233
    Children, 236
    Infants, 236
  Biliary excretion, 234
  Metabolism, 233, 235
  Plasma levels in chronic treatment
    Adults, 233, 235
    Children, 236
    Infants, 236
  Plasma protein binding, 233

INDEX **481**

Plasma half-life
  Adults, 233
  Children, 236
  Infants, 236
  Newborns, 236
Tissues concentrations, 234, 235
Toxic effects, 235
Urinary excretion, 233
Curve Fitting, 43, 45, 46
Cyclophosphamide, 102
  Absorption, 103
  Interaction with other drugs, 104, 105
  Mechanism of action, 103
  Metabolism, 103
  Plasma protein binding, 104
  Plasma half-life, 104
  Renal clearance, 104
  Tissues concentrations, 104
  Toxic effects, 105, 106
  Urinary excretion, 104
Cytosine-Arabinoside, 109
  Absorption, 109
  Mechanism of action, 109
  Metabolism, 110
  Plasma half-life
    Adults, 110
    Children, 110
  Renal clearance, 110
  Toxic effects
    Adults, 110
    Children, 110
    Newborns, 110
  Urinary excretion
    Adults, 110
    Children, 110

Daunomycin, 115
  Biliary excretion, 116
  SCF Concentrations, 116
  Metabolism, 115
  Plasma half-life
  Tissues concentrations, 116
  Toxic effects
    Adults, 117
    Children, 117
    Infants, 117
  Urinary excretion, 116
Desmethylimipramine, 439
  Absorption, 439-440
  Interaction with other drugs, 440-441
  Metabolism, 441-442

Overdosage
  Adults, 440, 446-447
  Children, 449
Plasma levels in chronic treatment, 442
Plasma protein binding
  Adults, 440
  Newborns, 447
Plasma half-life, 441
Therapeutic plasma levels, 445
Tissues concentrations, 440, 449
Total body clearance, 441
Toxic effects
  Adults, 445-446
  Children, 448
Toxic plasma levels
  Adults, 448
  Children, 449
Urinary excretion, 441
Volume of distribution, 440
Diazepam, 450
  Absorption
    Adults, 450-451
    Children, 458
    Infants, 457-458
    Newborns, 456
  Enterohepatic circle, 451
  Interactions with other drugs, 453-457
  Metabolism
    Adults, 451
    Newborns, 457
  Plasma level in chronic treatment
    Adults, 453
    Newborns, 455
  Plasma protein binding
    Adults, 451
    Newborns, 456
  Plasma half-life
    Adults, 451
    Children, 458
    Infants, 458
    Newborns, 456
  Therapeutic plasma levels, 453
  Toxic effects
    Adults, 453
    Newborns, 455
  Toxic plasma levels, 453
  Urinary excretion
    Adults, 452
    Children, 458
    Infants, 458
    Newborns, 457

Volume of distribution
    Adults, 451
    Children, 458
    Infants, 458
    Newborns, 456
Digitalis Glycosides, 393
Digitoxin, 401
    Absorption, 401
    Enterohepatic circle, 402
    Metabolism, 402-403
    Plasma protein binding, 401
    Plasma half-life, 402
    Renal clearance
    Toxic effects, 403
    Toxic plasma levels, 403
    Urinary excretion, 403
    Volume of distribution, 402
Digoxin, 394
    Absorption
        Adults, 394-395
        Infants, 399
        Newborns, 398
    Metabolism
        Adults, 396-397
        Children, 400
        Infants, 400
    Plasma levels in chronic treatment
        Adults, 396-392
        Children, 400
        Newborns, 399
    Plasma protein binding
        Adults, 392-396
        Newborns, 398
    Plasma half-life
        Adults, 395-396
        Infants, 399-400
        Newborns, 399
    Renal clearance, 396-397, 400
    Tissues concentrations, 399
    Toxic effects, 398
    Toxic plasma levels
        Adults, 398
        Children, 400
        Infants, 400
    Urinary excretion, 396
    Volume of distribution
        Adults, 396
        Children, 400
        Infants, 399
        Newborns, 398-399

Di-l-Propylacetate, 344
    Absorption, 344
    Interactions with other drugs, 345
    Plasma protein binding, 344
    Plasma half-life
        Adults, 344
        Children, 344
    Toxic effects, 344
    Urinary excretion, 344
    Volume of distribution, 344
Diphenylhydantoin, 312
    Absorption, 312-313
        Adults, 312-313
        Children, 319-320
        Infants, 319
        Newborns, 317
    CSF concentrations
        Adults, 313
        Children, 320
    Enterohepatic circle, 313
    Interactions with other drugs, 313-315
    Metabolism
        Adults, 313-314
        Children, 321
        Newborns, 318
    Plasma levels in chronic treatment, 315
        Adults, 315
        Children, 319
    Plasma protein binding
        Adults, 313-317
        Children, 319
    Plasma half-life, 314-315
        Adults, 314-315
        Children, 320
        Newborns, 318
    Renal clearance, 315
    Therapeutic plasma levels
        Adults, 315
        Children, 321
    Tissues concentrations, 313
    Toxic effects
        Adults, 315-317
        Children, 322
    Toxic plasma levels
        Adults, 315
        Children, 322-323
    Urinary excretion
        Adults, 315
        Children, 320-321

INDEX **483**

Volume of distribution
  Adults, 313
  Newborns, 318
Dose Interval, 36, 37

Erytromycin, 185
  Biliary excretion, 186
  CSF concentrations, 186
  Interactions with other drugs, 186
  Plasma levels in chronic treatment
    Adults, 186
    Newborns, 186
  Plasma protein binding
    Adults, 186
    Newborns, 186
  Plasma half-life
    Adults, 186
    Newborns, 186
  Urinary excretion
    Adults, 186
    Newborns, 186
Ethylbiscoumacetate, 263
  Absorption, 263
  Plasma protein binding, 263
  Total body clearance, 263
  Urinary excretion, 263
  Volume of distribution, 263
Ethosuximide, 333
  Absorption, 333
    Adults, 333
    Children, 335
  CSF concentration, 333
  Metabolism
    Adults, 334
    Newborns, 335
  Plasma half-life
    Adults, 334
    Children, 336
  Renal clearance, 335
  Therapeutic plasma levels
    Adults, 335
    Children, 336
  Toxic effects, 335
  Urinary excretion
    Adults, 334
    Newborns, 335
  Volume of distribution
    Adults, 334
    Children, 335

Feathering, 43
First Order Processes, 10, 14, 21, 27, 30
First Pass Effect, 8
Fluorophenindione, 263
  Absorption, 264
  Interaction with other drugs, 264
  Plasma protein binding, 264
  Plasma half-life, 264
  Urinary excretion, 264
Flurazepam, 378
  Absorption, 379
  Metabolism, 379-380
  Plasma protein binding, 380
  Plasma half-life, 379
  Urinary excretion, 379

Glutethimide, 365
  Absorption, 365
  Biliary excretion, 366
  CSF concentrations, 367
  Enterohepatic circle, 366
  Metabolism, 365-366
  Overdosage, 367
  Plasma protein binding, 365
  Plasma half-life, 365
  Toxic effects, 367
  Toxic plasma levels, 367
  Urinary excretion, 365-366

Half Life
  Definition of, 2
Haloperidol, 438
  Absorption, 438
  Metabolism, 438
  Plasma level in chronic treatment, 438
  Plasma protein binding, 438
  Plasma half-life, 438
  Urinary excretion, 438
  Volume of distribution, 438
Heparin, 251
  Absorption, 253
  Mechanism of action, 252, 253
  Plasma protein binding, 253
  Plasma half-life, 253
Hexobarbital, 375
  Absorption, 375
  Metabolism, 376
  Plasma protein binding, 375
  Plasma half-life, 375-376
  Urinary excretion, 376
  Volume of distribution, 375
Hypnotics, 361

484 INDEX

Imipramine, 439
  Absorption
    Adults, 440
    Children, 448
  Interactions with other drugs, 440-441
  Metabolism, 441-442
  Overdosage
    Adults, 446-447
    Children, 449
  Plasma levels in chronic treatment, 442
  Plasma protein binding
    Adults, 440
    Children, 448
    Newborns, 447
  Plasma half-life
    Adults, 441
    Children, 448
  Therapeutic plasma levels, 445
  Tissues concentrations, 440, 449
  Total body clearance, 441
  Toxic effects
    Adults, 445-446
    Children, 448
  Toxic plasma levels
    Adults, 445
    Children, 449
  Urinary excretion, 441
  Volume of distribution, 440
Indomethacin, 285
  Absorption, 285
  Biliary excretion, 286
  CSF concentrations, 286
  Enterohepatic circle, 286
  Interactions with other drugs, 286
  Metabolism, 287
  Plasma protein binding, 285-286
  Plasma half-life
    Adults, 286
    Newborns, 288
Intravenous Infusion, 24

l-Asparaginase, 110
  Absorption, 111
  Biliary excretion, 111
  Mechanism of action, 111
  Plasma protein binding, 111
  Plasma half-life, 111
  Toxic effects
    Adults, 112
    Children, 112
  Urinary excretion, 111

Lidocaine, 406
  Absorption, 406
  Metabolism, 406-407
  Plasma protein binding, 406
  Plasma half-life, 406
  Therapeutic plasma levels, 407
  Toxic effects, 407
  Toxic plasma levels, 407
  Volume of distribution, 406

Mathematical Models, 38
6-Mercaptopurine, 107
  Absorption, 108
  CSF concentration, 108
  Interactions with other drugs, 108
  Mechanism of action, 108
  Metabolism
    Adults, 108
    Children, 109
  Plasma protein binding, 108
  Plasma half-life
    Adults, 108
    Children, 108
  Urinary excretion, 109
  Volume of distribution, 108
Metabolism (liver), 71-87
  Conjugation, 80, 81
  Cyt P-450, 73, 74, 76
  Development phase I reactions, 75, 76, 77, 78, 79
  Development phase II reactions, 80, 81, 82
  Endogenous substrate competition, 76
  Endoplastic reticulum, 72, 73
  Liver development, 74, 75
  Liver blood supply, 74
  Microsomal phospholipids, 74
  Microsomes, 72, 73
  Mixed function oxidase, 73, 74, 75
  NADP - NAD - NADPH2, 73, 74, 77, 78, 79
Methaqualone, 368
  Absorption, 368
  Biliary excretion, 369
  Enterohepatic circle, 369
  Interactions with other drugs, 369
  Metabolism, 369-370
  Plasma levels in chronic treatment, 369
  Plasma protein binding, 368-369
  Plasma half-life, 369
  Therapeutic plasma levels, 369

INDEX **485**

Toxic effects, 369-370
Toxic plasma levels, 369
Urinary excretion, 369
Volume of distribution, 368
Methotrexate, 106
   Absorption, 106
   Enterohepatic circle, 107
   Interactions with other drugs, 107
   Mechanism of action, 106
   Plasma protein binding, 106
   Plasma half-life
      Adults, 107
      Children, 107
      Infants, 107
      Newborns, 107
   Urinary excretion, 107

Nalidixic Acid, 239
   Absorption
      Adults, 239, 240
      Children, 242, 243
      Infants, 242, 243
      Newborns, 242, 243
   Interactions with other drugs, 242
   Metabolism
      Adults, 240, 241
      Children, 243
   Overdosage
      Adults, 243
      Infants, 243
   Plasma levels in chronic treatment, 242
   Plasma protein binding, 240
   Plasma half-life
      Adults, 240
      Children, 242, 243
      Infants, 242, 243
      Newborns, 242, 243
   Therapeutic plasma levels, 242
   Toxic effects
      Adults, 243
      Infants, 243
   Urinary excretion, 242
   Volume of distribution
      Adults, 240
      Children, 243
      Infants, 243
      Newborns, 243
N-Desmethyldiazepam, 453
   Absorption, 454
   Plasma protein binding, 454
   Plasma half-life, 454

   Toxic effects, 454
   Urinary excretion
      Adults, 454
      Children, 458
      Newborns, 457
   Volume of distribution, 454
Nitrazepam, 381
   Absorption, 381
   Metabolism, 381
   Plasma protein binding, 381
   Plasma half-life, 381
   Toxic effects, 382
   Urinary excretion, 382
Nitrofurantoin, 236
   Absorption, 237
   Interactions with other drugs, 238
   Metabolism, 238
   Plasma levels in chronic treatment, 237
   Plasma half-life, 238
   Therapeutic plasma levels, 237
   Toxic effects
      Adults, 237
      Newborns, 238
   Urinary excretion, 238
Nortriptyline, 443
   Absorption, 443
   Interactions with other drugs, 443-444
   Metabolism, 443-444
   Overdosage
      Adults, 446-447
      Children, 445
   Plasma levels in chronic treatment
      Adults, 444
      Children, 448
   Plasma protein binding, 443
   Plasma half-life
      Adults, 444
      Children, 448
      Newborn, 447
   Therapeutic plasma levels, 445
   Toxic effects
      Adults, 445-446
      Children, 448
      Newborns, 447
   Toxic plasma levels
      Adults, 444
      Children, 449
   Urinary excretion
      Adults, 444
      Newborns, 448
   Volume of distribution, 443

One Compartment Open Model, 14, 16, 24, 27, 29
Oxprenolol, 417
  Absorption, 417
  Metabolism, 417
  Plasma protein binding, 417
  Therapeutic plasma levels, 417
  Total body clearance, 417
  Volume of distribution, 417

Peeling Method, 23, 43
Penfluridol, 439
  Absorption, 439
  Plasma levels in chronic treatment, 439
    Adults, 439
    Children, 439
    Infants, 439
    Newborns, 439
  Plasma half-life, 439
Penicillins, 126
  Absorption
    Adults, 130-141
    Children, 142
    Infants, 142
    Newborns, 141
  Biliary excretion, 132
  CSF concentrations
    Adults, 131, 140
    Children, 140
    Infants, 140
  Individual Agents
    Amoxicilline, 140-142
    Ampicillin, 140-142
    Benzathine Penicillin, 134-138
    Carbenicillin, 142-146
    Metcillin, 142
    Penicillin G, 134-138
    Procaine Penicillin, 134-138
  Interaction with other drugs, 134, 142, 145
  Metabolism, 132
  Plasma levels in chronic treatment
    Adults, 136
    Children, 136
    Infants, 136
    Newborns, 136, 137, 138, 139, 140, 143, 144
  Plasma protein binding, 127, 128, 129, 132, 135, 140
  Plasma half-life
    Adults, 127, 128, 129, 134, 141, 145
    Children, 134, 141, 145
    Infants, 134, 142, 145
    Newborns, 135, 137, 139, 140, 143, 144, 145
  Renal clearance, 127, 128, 129
  Therapeutic plasma levels, 132, 135, 138
  Tissues concentrations, 131
  Total body clearance, 127, 128, 129
  Urinary excretion
    Adults, 127, 128, 129, 133, 135
    Children, 135
    Newborns, 135, 137, 138, 139, 140, 143, 145
  Volume of distribution
    Adults, 127, 128
    Newborns, 143, 145
Pentobarbital, 373
  Absorption, 373
  Metabolism, 374
  Plasma protein binding, 373
  Plasma half-life, 373
  Urinary excretion, 374-375
  Volume of distribution, 373-374
Pharmacokinetic Models
  Comparison of, 46
Phenacetin, 292
  Absorption, 292
  Metabolism, 292-293
  Plasma half-life, 292
  Toxic effects, 293-294
Phenylbutazone, 281
  Absorption
    Adults, 281
    Children, 284
    Infants, 284
    Newborns, 284
  Biliary excretion, 282
  Enterohepatic circle, 282
  Interactions with other drugs, 282
  Metabolism, 283
  Plasma levels in chronic treatment
    Adults, 284
    Children, 284
  Plasma protein binding
    Adults, 282
    Children, 284
    Infants, 284
    Newborns, 284
  Plasma half-life
    Adults, 282
    Children, 284-285
    Infants, 284-285

INDEX **487**

Newborns, 284-285
Therapeutic plasma levels, 284
Tissues concentrations, 282-284
Toxic effects, 284
Toxic plasma levels, 284
Urinary excretion, 283
Volume of distribution
   Adults, 282
   Children, 284-285
   Infants, 284-285
   Newborns, 284-285
Phenobarbital, 323
  Absorption
   Adults, 323
   Children, 329
   Infants, 327
   Newborns, 325
  CSF concentrations
   Infants, 327
   Newborns, 326
  Interactions with other drugs, 327-331
  Metabolism
   Adults, 324
   Children, 330
   Newborns, 327
  Plasma levels in chronic treatment, 325
  Plasma protein binding
   Adults, 324
   Children, 329
   Newborns, 326
  Plasma half life
   Adults, 324-328
   Children, 328-329
   Infants, 328-329
   Newborns, 326-328
  Therapeutic plasma levels
   Adults, 325
   Children, 331
   Infants, 329
   Newborns, 327
  Toxic effects
   Adults, 325
   Children, 331
   Infants, 329
  Toxic plasma levels
   Adults, 325
   Children, 331
   Infants, 329
   Newborns, 327
  Urinary excretion, 325

Volume of distribution
   Adults, 324-328
   Children, 328
   Infants, 327-328
   Newborns, 326-327
Pindolol, 417
  Absorption, 417
  Metabolism, 417
  Plasma protein binding, 417
  Plasma half-life, 417
  Therapeutic plasma levels, 417
  Total body clearance, 417
  Volume of distribution, 417
Plasma Protein Binding, 61
  Age variations of, 63, 64, 65, 61
  Children, 65
  Displacement, 63, 64, 475
  Infants, 65
  Newborns, 63
Primidone, 331
  Absorption, 331-332
  CSF concentrations, 332
  Metabolism, 332
  Plasma half-life, 332
  Therapeutic plasma levels, 333
  Toxic effects, 333
Procainamide, 407
  Absorption, 407
  Metabolism, 408
  Plasma protein binding, 408
  Plasma half-life, 408
  Therapeutic plasma levels, 408
  Total body clearance, 408
  Toxic effects, 409
  Toxic plasma levels, 408
  Urinary excretion, 408
  Volume of distribution, 408
Propranolol, 410
  Absorption, 410-411-412
  Metabolism, 414-415
  Plasma levels in chronic treatment
   Adults, 414
   Children, 416
   Infants, 416
  Plasma protein binding, 412
  Plasma half-life
   Adults, 411-412
   Children, 416
   Infants, 416
  Therapeutic plasma levels, 414

488 INDEX

Total body clearance, 411-414
Toxic effects, 415
Urinary excretion, 414
Volume of distribution, 411-412
Psychotropic Drugs, 431

Quinidine, 404
    Absorption, 404
    Metabolism, 405
    Plasma protein binding, 404
    Plasma half-life, 404
    Therapeutic plasma levels, 405
    Tissues concentrations, 404
    Toxic effects, 405
    Toxic plasma levels, 405
    Urinary excretion, 405
    Volume of distribution, 404

Rate Method, 34
Rate Processes, 9
Renal Function, 89
    Age dependent effectiveness of diuretic, 96
    Age dependnt electrolite excretion, 96
    Age dependent toxicity, 96
    Development of, 91, 92, 93, 94
    Diurnal rhythm of, 89
    Glomerular filtration, 90, 91, 92
    Induction of, 95
    Tubular resorption, 94
    Tubular secretion, 92, 93, 94
Routine Monitoring, 476

Salicylates, 271
    Absorption
        Adults, 271-272
        Children, 280
        Infants, 280
        Newborns, 277
    CSF concentrations, 280
    Interactions with other drugs, 273-278-279
    Metabolism
        Adults, 274-275
        Newborns, 278-279
    Plasma levels in chronic treatment, 276
    Plasma protein binding
        Adults, 272-273
        Children, 280
        Infants, 280
        Newborns, 277

    Plasma half-life
        Adults, 274
        Children, 280
        Infants, 280
        Newborns, 278
    Renal clearance, 275
    Tissues concentrations, 273-274
    Toxic effects
        Adults, 276
        Children, 281
        Infants, 281
        Newborns, 279
    Toxic plasma levels, 276
    Urinary excretion
        Adults, 275
        Newborns, 279
    Volume of distribution
        Adults, 273
        Children, 280
        Infants, 280
        Newborns, 278
Secobarbital, 377
    Absorption, 377
    Metabolism, 377
    Plasma half-life, 377
    Toxic effects, 377
    Urinary excretion, 377
Sigma Minus Method, 34
Steady State Concentrations, 36
Sulfadiazine, 223
    Absorption, 223
    Metabolism, 224
    Plasma protein binding, 223
    Plasma half-life, 224
    Renal clearance, 224
    Therapeutic plasma levels, 224
    Toxic effects, 224
    Urinary excretion, 224
    Volume of distribution, 223
Sulfamethopyrazine, 225
    Absorption, 225
    Metabolism, 226
    Plasma protein binding
        Adults, 226
        Children, 226, 227
        Infants, 226, 227
        Newborns, 226, 227
    Plasma half-life
        Adults, 225
        Children, 226
        Infants, 226

INDEX **489**

Newborns, 226
Volume of distribution
  Adults, 225
  Children, 226
  Infants, 226
  Newborns, 226
Sulfamethoxypyridazine, 224
  Absorption, 224
  CSF concentrations, 225
  Plasma levels in chronic treatment
    Adults, 224
    Newborns, 225
  Plasma protein binding, 224
  Plasma half-life, 225
  Tissues concentrations, 225
  Urinary excretion, 225
  Volume of distribution, 224
Sulfasalazine, 227
  Absorption, 228
  Biliary excretion, 228
  Interactions with other drugs, 228
  Metabolism, 228, 229, 231
  Plasma levels in chronic treatment, 230, 231
  Plasma half-life, 230
  Renal clearance, 230
  Toxic effects, 231
  Toxic plasma levels, 231
  Urinary excretion, 228, 230
Sulfisoxazole, 220
  Absorption
    Adults, 220
    Infants, 222
  CSF concentrations, 221
  Metabolism, 221, 222
  Plasma protein binding, 220
  Plasma half-life
    Adults, 221, 223
    Children, 222, 223
    Infants, 222, 223
    Newborns, 222, 223
  Urinary excretion
    Adults, 221, 222
    Children, 223
    Infants, 223
    Newborns, 223
  Volume of distribution
    Adults, 221, 223
    Children, 222, 223
    Infants, 222, 223
    Newborns, 222, 223
Sulfonamides, 219

Tetracyclines, 172
  Absorption, 174, 175
  Biliary excretion, 176
  CSF Concentrations, 177
  Enterohepatic circle, 175, 176
  Interactions with other drugs, 174
  Metabolism, 176
  Plasma half-life, 175
  Renal clearance, 175, 176
  Tissues concentrations, 177
  Urinary excretion, 174, 176, 177
  Volume of distribution, 177
Thiamphenicol, 183
  Absorption, 184
  Plasma protein binding, 184
  Plasma half-life, 184
  Renal clearance, 185
  Total body clearance, 185
  Urinary escretion
    Adults, 185
    Children, 185
    Newborns, 185
  Volume of distribution, 185
Thioridazine, 436
  Absorption, 436
  Interaction with other drugs, 436
  Metabolism, 436
  Plasma half-life, 436
  Urinary excretion, 436
Thiothixene, 437
  Absorption, 437
  Biliary excretion, 438
  Metabolism, 438
  Plasma half-life, 438
  Therapeutic plasma levels, 438
Tolamolol, 417
  Absorption, 417
  Metabolism, 417
  Plasma protein binding, 417
  Plasma half-life, 417
  Therapeutic plasma levels, 417
  Volume of distribution, 417
Total Body Clearance
  Definition of, 6, 7
Two-Compartment Open Model, 21, 26, 30

Urinary Antiseptics, 236
Urinary Excretion
  Renal clearance, definition of, 33
  Rate of elimination, defintion of, 33

Vincristine, 112
　Absorption, 113
　Biliary excretion, 113
　Mechanism of action, 112
　Metabolism, 113
　Plasma protein binding, 113
　Plasma half-life
　　Adults, 113
　　Children, 113
　Toxic effects
　　Adults, 113
　　Children, 113
　Urinary excretion, 113
　Volume of distribution, 113

Warfarin, 257
　Absorption, 257
　Interactions with other drugs, 258, 260
　Metabolism, 259
　Plasma protein binding, 258
　Plasma half-life, 258
　Toxic effects, 255, 257
　Urinary excretion, 260
　Volume of distribution, 258, 260

Zero Order Processes, 12, 24, 26